ENDURANCE IN SPORT

VOLUME II OF THE ENCYCLOPAEDIA OF SPORTS MEDICINE

AN IOC MEDICAL COMMISSION PUBLICATION

IN COLLABORATION WITH THE

INTERNATIONAL FEDERATION OF SPORTS MEDICINE

EDITED BY

R.J. SHEPHARD & P.-O. ÅSTRAND

OXFORD

BLACKWELL SCIENTIFIC PUBLICATIONS

LONDON EDINBURGH BOSTON

MELBOURNE PARIS BERLIN VIENNA

© 1992 International Olympic Committee

Published by
Blackwell Scientific Publications
Editorial Offices:
Osney Mead, Oxford OX2 0EL
25 John Street, London WC1N 2BL
23 Ainslie Place, Edinburgh EH3 6AJ
238 Main Street, Cambridge
  Massachusetts 02142, USA
54 University Street, Carlton
  Victoria 3053, Australia

Other Editorial Offices:
Librairie Arnette SA
2, rue Casimir-Delavigne
75006 Paris
France

Blackwell Wissenschafts-Verlag
Meinekestrasse 4
D-1000 Berlin 15
Germany

Blackwell MZV
Feldgasse 13
A-1238 Wien
Austria

First published 1992
Reprinted 1993

Set by Setrite Typesetters, Hong Kong
Printed and bound in Great Britain by
Butler & Tanner Ltd, Frome and London

Part title illustrations by Grahame Baker

DISTRIBUTORS

Marston Book Services Ltd
PO Box 87
Oxford OX2 0DT
(*Orders*: Tel: 0865 791155
       Fax: 0865 791927
       Telex: 837515)

USA
  Human Kinetics Books
  Human Kinetics Publishers, Inc.
  Box 5076, Champaign
  Illinois 61825–5076
  (*Orders*: Tel: 1 800–747–4457)

Canada
  Human Kinetics Publishers, Inc.
  Box 2503, Windsor
  Ontario N8Y 4S2
  (*Orders*: Tel: 1 800–465–7301)

Australia
  Blackwell Scientific Publications Pty Ltd
  54 University Street
  Carlton, Victoria 3053
  (*Orders*: Tel: 03 347–5552)

British Library
Cataloguing in Publication Data

Endurance in sport.
  1. Sports. Physical fitness
  I. Shephard, R.J.   II. Åstrand, P.-O.   III. Series
  613.711

Library of Congress
Cataloging-in-Publication Data

Endurance in sport/edited by R.J. Shephard and
P.-O. Åstrand.
        p.   cm. — (The Encyclopaedia of sports
  medicine)
  Includes index.
  1. Endurance sports.   2. Exercise — Physiological
  aspects.
  3. Physical fitness.   I. Shephard, Roy J.   II. Åstrand,
  Per-Olof.   III. Series.
  RC1220. E53E53   1992
613.7'1 — dc20

Contents

v

List of Contributors

PER-OLOF ÅSTRAND, MD PhD, *Department of Physiology III, Karolinska Institutet, Stockholm, Sweden*

ULF BERGH, PhD, *National Defence Research Establishment, Sundyberg, Sweden*

EVA BLOMSTRAND, PhD, *Pripps Bryggerier, Research Laboratory, Bromma, Sweden*

CLAUDE BOUCHARD, PhD, *Laboratoire des sciences de l'activitié physique, Université Laval, Quebec, Canada*

STEVEN R. BUSSOLARI, PhD, *Department of Aeronautics & Astronautics, Massachusetts Institute of Technology, Cambridge, Massachusetts, USA*

ENZO CAFARELLI, PhD FACSM, *Department of Physical Education, York University, Toronto, Ontario, Canada*

JOAN F. CARROLL, MA, *Department of Exercise & Sport Sciences, University of Florida, Gainsville, Florida, USA*

ROBERTO COLLI, Trainer, *Department of Physiology & Biomechanics, Istituto Scienza dello Sport-CONI-Roma, Rome, Italy*

ANTONIO DAL MONTE, MD, *Department of Physiology & Biomechanics, Istituto Scienza dello Sport-CONI-Roma, Rome, Italy*

JACK T. DANIELS, PhD, *Department of Physical Education, State University of New York, Cortland, New York, USA*

JEROME A. DEMPSEY, PhD, *Department of Preventive Medicine, University of Winsconsin-Madison, Madison, Wisconsin, USA*

PIETRO E. DI PRAMPERO, MD *Istituto di Biologia, Facolta di Medicina, Udine, Italy*

RICHARD H.T. EDWARDS, PhD FRCP, *Department of Medicine, University of Liverpool, Liverpool, UK*

KRISTINE E. ENSRUD, MD, *Division of Epidemiology, School of Public Health, University of Minnesota, Minneapolis, Minnesota, USA*

PIERO FACCINI, MD, *Department of Physiology & Biomechanics, Istituto Scienza dello Sport-CONI-Roma, Rome, Italy*

MARCELLO FAINA, MD, *Department of Physiology & Biomechanic, Istituto Scienza dello Sport-CONI-Roma, Rome, Italy*

LAWRENCE J. FOLINSBEE, PhD, *C-E Environmental Inc., Chapel Hill, North Carolina, USA*

AARON R. FOLSOM, MD MPH, *Division of Epidemiology, School of Public Health, University of Minnesota, Minneapolis, Minnesota, USA*

ARTUR FORSBERG, Phys Ed, *Department of Physiology III, Karolinska Institutet, Stockholm, Sweden*

EDWARD C. FREDERICK, PhD, *Exeter Research Inc., Brentwood, New Hampshire, USA*

HENRIK GALBO, MD DMSc, *Department of Medical Physiology B, The Panum Institute, University of Copenhagen, Copenhagen, Denmark*

HENRY GIBSON, PhD, *Department of Medicine, University of Liverpool, Liverpool, UK*

NORMAN GLEDHILL, PhD, *Department of Physical Education, York University, Toronto, Ontario, Canada*

JAMES E. GRAVES, PhD, *Departments of Medicine, Physiology and Exercise & Sport Sciences, University of Florida, Gainsville, Florida, USA*

PAUL L. GREENHAFF, PhD, *Department of Clinical Chemistry II, Karolinska Institutet, Huddinge University Hospital, Huddinge, Sweden*

LENNART GULLSTRAND, D. Phys Ed, *Bosön Institute of Sport, Lidingö, Sweden*

L. HOWARD HARTLEY, MD, *Division of Cardiology, Brigham & Women's Hospital, Boston, Massachusetts, USA*

JAN HENRIKSSON, MD PhD, *Department of Physiology III, Karolinska Institutet, Stockholm, Sweden*

WILDOR HOLLMAN, MD, *Institute for Cardiology & Sports Medicine, German Sports University, Cologne, Germany*

THOMAS F. HORNBEIN, MD, *Department of Anesthesiology, University of Washington, Washington, USA*

RICHARD L. HUGHSON, PhD, *Department of Kinesiology, University of Waterloo, Waterloo, Ontario, Canada*

ERIC HULTMAN, MD PhD, *Department of Clinical Chemistry II, Karolinska Institutet, Huddinge University Hospital, Huddinge, Sweden*

PEKKA KANNUS, MD PhD, *Tampere Research Station of Sports Medicine, Tampere, Finland*

LARRY M. LEITH, PhD, *School of Physical & Health Education, University of Toronto, Toronto, Ontario, Canada*

DAVID T. LOWENTHAL, MD PhD, *Departments of Medicine, Pharmacology and Exercise & Sport Sciences, University of Florida, and Gregg V.A. Medical Center, Gainsville, Florida, USA*

NEIL McANDREW, MA, *Department of Biochemistry, University of Oxford, Oxford, UK*

DONALD C. McKENZIE, PhD, *Departments of Sport Science and Family Practice, University of British Columbia, Vancouver, British Columbia, Canada*

MURLI MANOHAR, DVM PhD, *Department of Veterinary Biosciences, University of Illinois at Urbana-Champaign, Champaign, Illinois, USA*

CLAUDIO MENCHINELLI, MD, *Department of Physiology & Biomechanic, Istituto Scienza dello Sport-CONI-Roma, Rome, Italy*

ETHAN R. NADEL, PhD, *The John B. Pierce Laboratory and Yale University School of Medicine, New Haven, Connecticut, USA*

SANDRA L. NEHLSEN-CANNARELLA, PhD, *Departments of Surgery, Pathology and Microbiology, Loma Linda University, Loma Linda, California, USA*

GEORG NEUMANN, MD, *Research Institute for Physical Culture & Sports, Leipzig, Germany*

ERIC A. NEWSHOLME, MA PhD DSc, *Department of Biochemistry, University of Oxford, Oxford, UK*

BODIL NIELSEN, PhD, *August Krogh Institute, Copenhagen University, Copenhagen, Denmark*

DAVID C. NIEMAN, DHSc MPH FACSM, *Department of Health, Leisure & Exercise Science, Appalachian State University, Boone, North Carolina, USA*

HUGH O'BRODOVICH, MD, *Hospital for Sick Children Research Institute, University of Toronto, Toronto, Ontario, Canada*

PATRICK J. O'CONNOR, PhD, *Exercise & Sport Research Institute-PEBE 210, Arizona State University, Tempe, Arizona, USA*

KENT B. PANDOLF, PhD, *US Army Research Institute of Environmental Medicine, Natick, Massachusetts, USA*

MARK PARRY-BILLINGS, BSc DPhil, *Department of Biochemistry, University of Oxford, Oxford, UK*

MICHAEL J. PLYLEY, MD PhD DPE, *School of Physical & Health Education, University of Toronto, Toronto, Ontario, Canada*

MICHAEL L. POLLOCK, PhD, *Departments of Medicine, Physiology and Exercise & Sport Sciences, University of Florida, Gainsville, Florida, USA*

JERILYNN C. PRIOR, MD FRCP, *Department of Medicine, University of British Columbia, Vancouver, British Columbia, Canada*

PER RENSTRÖM, MD PhD, *McClure Musculoskeletal Research Center, Department of Orthopedics & Rehabilitation, University of Vermont, Burlington, Vermont, USA*

RICHARD ROST, PhD, *Institute for Cardiology & Sports Medicine, German Sports University, Cologne, Germany*

THOMAS W. ROWLAND, MD, *Department of Pediatrics, Baystate Medical Center, Springfield, Massachusetts, USA*

ROBERT B. SCHOENE, MD, *Pulmonary Function & Exercise Laboratory, University of Washington, Washington, USA*

NIELS H. SECHER, MD PhD, *Department of Anaesthesia, Rigshospitalet, University of Copenhagen, Copenhagen, Denmark*

ROY J. SHEPHARD, MD PhD DPE, *School of Physical & Health Education, University of Toronto, Toronto, Ontario, Canada*

JAN SVEDENHAG, MD PhD, *Department of Clinical Physiology, Karolinska Institutet, Huddinge University, Huddinge, Sweden*

KURT TITTEL, MD, *Department of Functional Anatomy, German University for Physical Culture, Leipzig, Germany*

LARS-ERIC UNESTÅHL, PhD, *Department of Psychology, Scandinavian International University, Örebro, Sweden*

R. PETER WELSH, MB ChB FRCSC FACS, *Orthopaedic & Arthritic Hospital, Toronto, Ontario, Canada*

JACK H. WILMORE, PhD, *Department of Kinesiology & Health Education, University of Texas at Austin, Austin, Texas, USA*

LINDA J. WOODHOUSE, BA BSc MA, *Orthopaedic & Arthritic Hospital, Toronto, Ontario, Canada*

HEINZ WUTSCHERK, PhD, *Department of Sports Anthropology, German University for Physical Culture, Leipzig, Germany*

ANDREW J. YOUNG, PhD, *US Army Research Institute of Environmental Medicine, Natick, Massachusetts, USA*

Foreword

The idea behind the launching of the series of publications entitled *Encyclopaedia of Sports Medicine* was to present state-of-the-art information about current topics of clinical and scientific importance for competitive sport to professional personnel working with athletes and sports teams. While the information to be presented is intended to be of interest to individuals and groups representing a wide range of disciplines, the primary groups for whom the series is intended are sports scientists, sports medicine doctors, medical doctors in family practice, physical therapists and athletic trainers, and graduate students in the sports sciences and other health-related professions.

The collaboration of the Medical Commission of the International Olympic Committee and the Scientific Commission of the International Federation of Sports Medicine resulted in the publication of the series' initial volume, *The Olympic Book of Sports Medicine* in 1989. The success of this publication resulted in the establishment of the IOC Publications Advisory Committee which was formed for the purpose of planning and producing succeeding volumes of the *Encyclopaedia of Sports Medicine*.

For the ensuing publications, it was decided that each volume should address a specific issue or problem area central to sports performance, sports conditioning, or clinical sports medicine. The initial three such areas that were selected were: endurance in sport, strength and power in sport, and the prevention of injury in sport.

For this volume on *Endurance in Sport*, the Publications Advisory Committee selected for its editorial leadership two distinguished scientists, each of whom possesses a wealth of experience in scientific publications: Professor Roy Shephard of the University of Toronto (Canada) and Professor Per-Olof Åstrand of the Karolinska Institute in Stockholm (Sweden). In turn, the coeditors successfully recruited a team of contributing authors made up of prominent scientists and clinicians, all of whom have established themselves as world leaders in their particular areas of interest and scientific investigation.

The product of the efforts of this eminent group does, indeed, represent the leading edge of knowledge regarding endurance performance. The combination of basic information about the biological mechanisms of endurance, measurement techniques, conditioning programmes for sports participation, and clinical considerations regarding endurance performance provides a wealth of information for persons involved with endurance sports.

The Publications Advisory Committee of the International Olympic Committee is extremely pleased to present *Endurance in Sport* as the second volume published in the *Encyclopaedia of Sports Medicine* series. The scientific and clinical information contained in this volume constitutes a major contribution to the body of literature in sports medicine and sports science.

Prince Alexandre de Merode (Chairman)
IOC Medical Commission

Howard G. Knuttgen (Chairman)
Francesco Conconi
Per Renström
Richard H. Strauss
Kurt Tittel
IOC Medical Commission
Publications Advisory Sub-committee

Preface

Relatively brief physical activities such as a 1500-m race have sometimes been characterized as 'endurance sport'. However, in this book we have deliberately focussed our attention upon events where the competition itself and/or the required training lasts for 1 hour or longer. There were several reasons for this decision. Certainly, we were instructed to do this by the series editors, since they are currently planning other volumes that will cover shorter periods of activity. However, we are not exactly famous for following arbitrary directives from editors, and our eventual compliance with the 1-hour criterion was assured by more persuasive arguments.

Firstly, we both view international competition as the ultimate challenge to the various regulatory systems of the body, physiological, biochemical, biomechanical and psychological. If the body finds difficulty in regulating the constancy of the *milieu intérieur* over a 4-min mile, how much greater is the challenge to accommodate the metabolic, thermal and other demands of a marathon race run in the heat of summer, or the Vasa Loppet in the depths of winter, and how much more exciting it is to unravel details of the adaptive mechanisms that allow such feats to be accomplished!

We recognize that there have been a number of previous monographs looking at various physiological aspects of prolonged exercise, but much of the work described in such texts has been conducted in the laboratory. There remains a dearth of scientific information on the stresses encountered and the adaptive responses demanded by actual participation in the various potential forms of prolonged athletic competition. The present volume was thus conceived to fill this void in a comprehensive fashion.

In completing such a major undertaking, we have been fortunate to draw upon more than 60 of the world's authorities in all areas of the sport sciences. The volume thus offers a broad international perspective upon the challenge of human participation in endurance events. The material is divided into seven sections: (1) a brief definition of fundamental terms and concepts, (2) a full review of basic scientific considerations that ranges over anatomy, biomechanics, physiology, biochemistry, nutrition, humoral and immune function, psychological factors, genetics and environmental constraints, (3) methods of measuring the various determinants of endurance performance in the field and in the laboratory, (4) optimal principles of preparation for various types of endurance competition, (5) endurance training in special population groups, (6) prevention of medical and surgical problems during endurance training and competition, with a discussion of the potential health benefits of such activities, and (7) an exploration of issues specific to individual types of endurance performance ranging from cross-country skiing to human-powered flight.

The material is presented in a format that will be accessible to all with some background in the sport sciences. It is anticipated that the volume will appeal particularly to sport scientists and physicians involved in the preparation of endurance competitors, but the broad picture of human regulatory mechanisms during extended exercise will also attract the interest of a much wider audience in physiology, biochemistry and psychology, and this volume will undoubtedly become required reading for many graduate programmes in medicine and the science of sport.

Roy J. Shephard, *Toronto*
Per-Olof Åstrand, *Stockholm*
1991

PART 1

DEFINITIONS

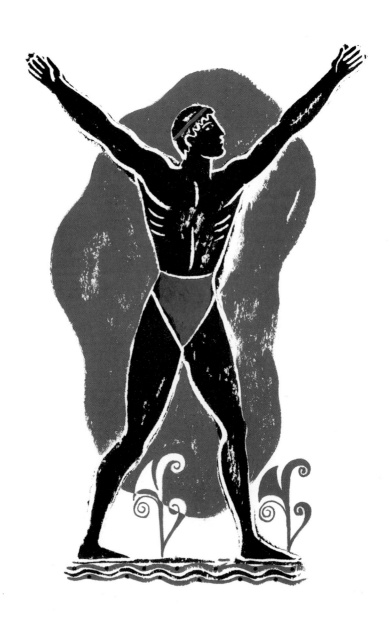

Chapter 1

Semantic and Physiological Definitions

ROY J. SHEPHARD

Physical activity, exercise and physical fitness

The distinction between such terms as physical activity, exercise and physical fitness has been sharpened through the contributions of Caspersen *et al.* (1985), and is discussed below.

Physical activity: This may be considered as any form of body movement that makes a significant metabolic demand. Thus defined, physical activity encompasses not only preparation for, and participation in, a wide range of competitive sports, but also other aspects of an athlete's life, such as the pursuit of many strenuous physical occupations, the undertaking of household chores (including the production of food in some countries), transportation (walking, cycling, the operation of hand-propelled watercraft) and engagement in voluntary leisure activity unrelated to the primary athletic interests.

Exercise: Physical exercise may be considered as the voluntary component of the overall physical activity inventory. It is occasionally spontaneous and playful, but more usually it is performed with a specific objective in view (such as preparation for a competition or the maintenance of personal fitness). Some forms of play and recreational exercise may contribute to the primary performance of a major athlete, either by the development of biological function (for example, the introduction of land exer-

cises when a rower cannot exercise on water) or by offering relaxation and psychological *détente* between competitive seasons. However, other physically active pursuits can be disadvantageous to the performance of an athlete, encouraging an inappropriate development of physique, occupying time that should have been allocated to more specific forms of training and (through a process of 'negative transfer') degrading established psychomotor skills.

Physical fitness: The concept of physical fitness has been discussed in detail elsewhere (Shephard, 1977). The definition remains controversial, but in our context of high-performance sport, it implies an optimal combination of those physical, physiological, biochemical, biomechanical and psychological characteristics that contribute to competitive success. The physical fitness of an athlete is highly specific to a given class of competition, but given the multiplicity of biological determinants of fitness, there is not necessarily a single optimal solution for a given event; for example, psychological hardiness has sometimes allowed very successful competitive performance by a person with a body form that is very unfavourable from a biomechanical standpoint.

Physical activity, in the form of rigorous training, normally enhances the fitness of an individual, but this is not inevitably the case. An

3

inappropriate form of training may lead to disadvantageous changes — for example, an overemphasis upon strength training could lead to a substantial handicap due to excessive body mass in a distance runner. Moreover, if the product of intensity and duration of training is carried to excess, a combination of physiological and psychological reactions leads to a deterioration of fitness (the situation of 'overtraining' or 'staleness').

Argument continues as to how far physical fitness is inherited, and how far it can be acquired through an appropriate programme of preparation (Bouchard & Malina, 1983). Plainly, body build makes a major contribution to success in many events, and the shape of the adult body is largely immutable. With respect to physiological characteristics such as the peak oxygen transport, an attempt can be made to divide the observed interindividual differences into components of variance attributable to constitution, domestic environment (for example, birth into a family where high-level competition is the expected norm), a constitutional susceptibility to training, and a cumulative response to training that could have been elicited through adequate motivation of any growing child or young adult. Clarification of the relative contributions of genes and en-

vironment is important for the coach, who must decide whether to allocate resources to talent scouting or to an improvement of training methods (Fig. 1.1). Unfortunately, the answers obtained to date have proved rather unstable. Some authors have suggested that physical fitness has a very large genetic component, but others have found a negligible influence of constitution. Given such major uncertainty in the interpretation of easily quantitated physiological data, it is hardly surprising that little is known about the contribution of inheritance to other aspects of fitness.

Force, work and power

The terms force, work and power have a long-standing mechanical significance, and have been defined in a biological context by Knuttgen (1984).

Force: Early reports on muscle strength measured peak forces in pounds weight or kilogram force. Force is more properly expressed in newtons, the SI units of force (Ellis, 1971; Table 1.1). for example, a mass of 1 kg exerts a force of 9.81 N in unit gravitational field. Small variations of gravitational acceleration (and thus the weight of objects) occur with changes of

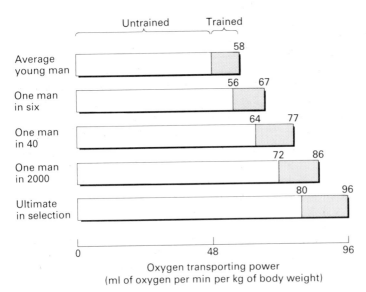

Fig. 1.1 Diagram illustrating the relative importance of athletic selection and rigorous training to the development of a competitor with a large maximal oxygen intake. The assumption is made that the peak effect of training is a 20% increase of oxygen transport. From Shephard (1978), with permission.

Table 1.1 Recommended standard international (SI) units of force, work and power (based on recommendations of Ellis, 1971).

Force	= newton (N) (1 kg·m·s^{-2}; a mass of 1 kg exerts a force of 9.81 N in a standard gravitational field)
Distance	= metre (m)
Time	= second (s)
Work	= force × distance = N·m = joule (J)
Power	= work/time = J·s^{-1} = watt (W)
Pressure	= force/area = N·m^{-2} = pascal (Pa)

latitude or altitude, both reflecting differences in the distance separating the object from the centre of the earth.

Work: Work is the product of force and distance. If a force of 1 N is sustained over a distance of 1 m, 1 J of work is performed. Older texts of nutrition refer to calories; under standard conditions, 1 calorie is equal to 4.186 J.

The body must perform physical work whenever activity is undertaken. Stores of potential energy are modified, viscous work is performed against internal or external resistance, and the kinetic energy of the body and associated equipment is altered. Body stores of chemical energy are used to effect these changes, and reserves are later replenished through the consumption of food.

The athlete may increase *potential energy* stores by performing sustained work against gravity, for example when propelling a bicycle up a steep incline. The energy cost is given by the product of the vertical ascent (in metres) and the mass of the rider plus machine (in newtons). Segmental potential energy may also change during the course of exercise (for instance, when an arm and racket are raised in a tennis serve).

A good example of external *viscous work* is encountered when cross-country skis glide over a snow-covered surface. The viscous work performed by the competitor may be calculated as the distance travelled times the resisting force (the product of gravitational acceleration, the mass of competitor plus skis, and the coef-ficient of sliding friction for a given wax, temperature and snow condition).

The body accumulates *kinetic energy* when a sprinter accelerates from the blocks. A single limb and associated equipment may also gain kinetic energy (for example, as the arm accelerates during a tennis serve). The developed force is proportional to the product of mass and acceleration, and the work performed is again the product of this force and the distance over which it has operated. Work may be performed not only in accelerating the body or its parts, but also in deceleration (for instance, the eccentric contractions that control the descent of the body when running downhill).

Power: The quantity of work performed in unit time has the dimensions of power, and is best expressed in watts (1 W = 1 N·m·s^{-1}, or 1 J·s^{-1}). A distinction must again be drawn between the external power output, readily measured on a device such as a cycle ergometer, and the internal energy consumption (usually at least four times as great, reflecting not only the energy consumed by the muscles engaged in performing a particular task, but also the resting energy consumption and unavoidable ancillary costs of the activity, such as increases of energy expenditure in the heart and the respiratory muscles).

Mechanical efficiency

Like most machines designed by humans, the body is an imperfect device for converting stored energy into external work. Mechanical efficiency expresses the ratio of the external work performed to the food energy that is consumed; commonly, the resting energy consumption is deducted from the energy cost to yield a *net efficiency* value. The net efficiency varies from around 25%* when operating an efficient machine such as a bicycle (Fig. 1.2) to a

* The mechanical efficiency can sometimes rise above the theoretical maximum value of 25% if energy is stored by the stretching of tendons (for example, the rebound of a runner).

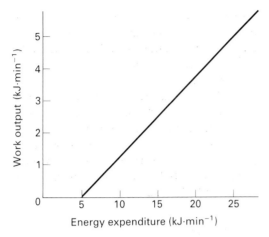

Fig. 1.2 Relationship of energy expended to output of useful athletic work. The intercept on the abscissa reflects the resting energy expenditure, and the slope of the line indicates net efficiency (25% in the example illustrated). From Shephard (1982), with permission.

figure as low as 1% in a novice swimmer. In highly skilled activities such as swimming, the difference in mechanical efficiency (and thus the energy cost of a given performance) be-

tween a novice and an international competitor is at least fourfold, and very substantial gains of performance can result from an upgrading of technique.

The difference between the external work performed and the food energy that is consumed normally appears as heat. In many circumstances, the endurance athlete has problems in dissipating this waste heat, although in some types of event (such as distance swimming in very cold water), the heat production helps to conserve a minimum body core temperature.

Strength and endurance

Sports may be broadly classified into events that demand great strength (well typified by competitive weight-lifting) and events that demand tremendous endurance (for example, participation in an ultramarathon run). The first type of competition requires an unusual development of the skeletal muscles (particularly fast-twitch, type II muscle fibres), but the second category is favoured by the pre-

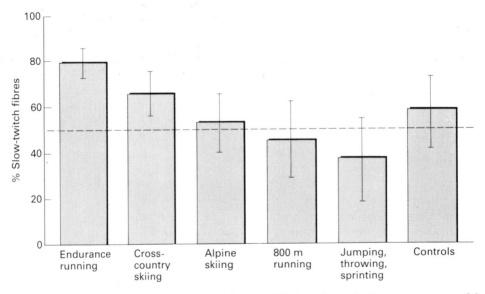

Fig. 1.3 Bar chart illustrating the preponderance of slow-twitch (type I) muscle fibres among successful endurance competitors. From Dirix *et al.* (1988), with permission.

dominance of slow-twitch, type I fibres (Fig. 1.3); endurance performance depends on an ability to supply the active muscle cells with adequate amounts of oxygen and essential nutrients, while eliminating heat, carbon dioxide and other waste-products and sustaining homoeostasis in other parts of the body.

Strength events will be examined in a separate volume of this series, and the present volume is thus limited to endurance events, which we are arbitrarily assuming to involve an hour or more of sustained physical activity.

In many forms of prolonged competition central factors (particularly the pumping ability of the heart) appear important to success, but in some events (for example, the dinghy sailor who must make repeated 'hiking' movements to counterbalance a small boat) the ability to make sustained load-bearing muscle contractions (isometric muscle endurance) is a critical factor. In other instances (such as a prolonged tennis tournament) repeated powerful arm movements (isotonic muscular endurance) are needed.

The distance runner requires, above all, cardiovascular endurance — the ability to sustain a large blood flow to the working muscles — as preloading of the heart is reduced by sweating and an extravasation of fluid into the active tissues, and peripheral resistance is lowered by a rising core temperature.

In ultra-long distance events, performance is threatened by other events — a depletion of intramuscular and hepatic glycogen reserves, a dispersal of the calcium ion reserves needed to initiate muscle contraction, and an escape of intracellular potassium ions that threatens the normal electrical function of the muscle membranes.

Finally, irrespective of the type of event, there is a need for psychological toughness — a motivation to endure and to excel in the face of pain and discouragement. Individual competitors may have an advantage in any of these domains that offers them an unusual endurance relative to their rivals.

References

Bouchard, C. & Malina, R. (1983) Genetics of physiological fitness and motor performance. *Exerc. Sport Sci. Rev.* **11**, 306–339.

Caspersen, C.J., Powell, K.E. & Christenson, G.M. (1985) Physical activity, exercise and physical fitness: definitions and distinctions for health related research. *Public Health Rep.* **100**, 126–131.

Dirix, A., Knuttgen, H.G. & Tittel, K. (eds) (1988) *The Olympic Book of Sports Medicine.* Blackwell Scientific Publications, Oxford.

Ellis, G. (1971) *Units, Symbols and Abbreviations. A Guide for Biological and Medical Editors and Authors.* Royal Society of Medicine, London.

Knuttgen, H.G. (1984) Instructions to authors. *Med. Sci. Sports Exerc.* **16**, xviii–xix.

Shephard, R.J. (1977) *Endurance Fitness,* 2nd edn. University of Toronto Press, Toronto.

Shephard, R.J. (1978) *The Fit Athlete.* Oxford University Press, Oxford.

Shephard, R.J. (1982) *Physiology and Biochemistry of Exercise.* Praeger Publishers, New York.

Chapter 2

Endurance Sports

PER-OLOF ÅSTRAND

Introduction

Which sport events call for endurance? Certainly running a marathon, bicycling 180 km and, still more so, partaking in the triathlon. What about running 10 000 m? Rather arbitrarily, physical activity that lasted for 1 h or longer was taken as a guidance in this volume. However, each training session for a 10 000-m race usually lasts for many hours. A tennis match can last for 4 h or more. Team sports are activities with intermittent exercises: the effective time in team handball is two periods of 30 min, in basketball it is 2 × 20 min, American football is 4 × 15 min, Australian football is 4 × 25 min, volleyball consists of three sets and the time for a set is from 15 to 30 min, field hockey is 2 × 35 min, waterpolo is 4 × 5 min and netball is 4 × 15 min; in ice hockey, where the effective time is 3 × 20 min the individual player participates for only part of this time (except for the goalkeeper).

The total time taken for a game is often much longer than the 'effective time'. In the recent world cup soccer championship held in Italy, many matches were not settled after two 45-min periods, so two 15-min periods were added with short breaks in between.

The physiological response to exercise can be very different in continuous exercise compared with intermittent exercise, i.e. short bursts of intensive exercise. This chapter describes the physiology of intermittent exercise (time of less than 1 min), interval exercise (2–6 min bouts) and continuous exercise (over longer periods of time).

Intermittent exercise

A man was able to exercise at a high work rate, 412 W, but after 3 min of continuous cycling he was exhausted. When exercising intermittently for 1 min and resting for 2 min, etc., he was able to continue for 24 min before being totally exhausted, with a blood lactate concentration of 15.7 mM. On another day, the periods of exercise were reduced to 10 s and the rest periods to 20 s. He could then complete the intended production of 247 kJ within 30 min with no severe feeling of strain. His blood lactate concentration did not exceed 2 mM, indicating an almost balanced oxygen supply to his heavily stressed muscles (Fig. 2.1a.) With periods of exercise and rest of 30 s and 60 s respectively, intermediate results were obtained. With 10-s exercise bouts interrupted by 20-s rest periods the engaged muscles and their metabolic processes could be subjected to great demands without undue fatigue. How can we explain that power which actually demands an oxygen consumption exceeding the subject's maximal oxygen intake, measured at the 'lung level', can be performed without noticeable support from anaerobic processes? Figure 2.1b attempts to give an answer.

When a person exercises intermittently in 10-s periods there is vasodilatation of the vessels supplying more active muscles, which

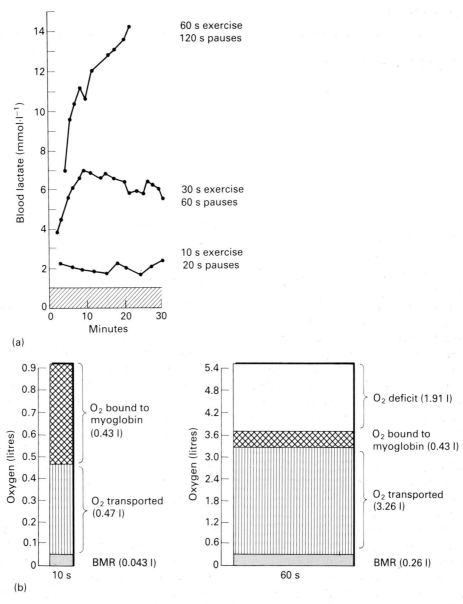

Fig. 2.1 (a) Blood lactate concentration in a total work production of 247 kJ (25 200 kpm) in 30 min. The exercise was accomplished with a power of 412 W (2520 kpm·min⁻¹), the exercise periods being 10, 30 and 60 s, and the rest periods 20, 60 and 120 s, respectively. The lower shaded area shows lactate concentration at rest. (b) Oxygen requirement for 10 s and 60 s power of 412 W. The schematic drawing indicates the basal metabolic rate (BMR), the calculated fractions of oxygen bound to myoglobin and transported by the blood, and the oxygen deficit. From Åstrand *et al.* (1960).

will secure a good blood supply, and therefore a good oxygen supply, during exercise as well as at rest periods. In addition there is an oxygen store in the myoglobin which can be consumed during the bout of exercise. During the following period of rest, this depot is quickly refilled with oxygen. The calculated oxygen store in this experiment was approximately 0.4 litres. With the period of exercise prolonged to 60 s it was calculated that 1.9 litres of oxygen was missing (Fig. 2.1b) and therefore anaerobic processes must be contributing.

In another experiment, with running for 10 s and resting for 5 s, a subject was able to prolong the total exercise plus rest period to 30 min at a speed that normally exhausted him after about 4 min of continuous running. During exercise there is a reduction of adenosine triphosphate (ATP) and phosphocreatine concentrations which, however, can be restored during the period of rest, evidently by aerobic processes. In intermittent exercise at the same work rate as in continuous exercise, less glycogen is utilized and the lactate concentration in the muscles is much lower. It should be emphasized that 13 times more ATP can be replenished when glycogen is metabolized aerobically compared with the efficiency of anaerobic breakdown of glycogen to lactate (for references to

these studies see Åstrand & Rodahl, 1986, pp. 304–307).

With maximal effort extended to 1 min followed by rest for 4 min, repeating the sequence four or five times, very high lactate concentrations can be attained in the active muscles (>25 mM·kg^{-1} wet muscle) and in the blood (>20 mM·l^{-1}), and the pH in arterial blood can drop to 7.0. To train using this protocol is very fatiguing, and such a regimen is usually not introduced until a month or two before the competitive season.

Interval exercise

Figure 2.2 illustrates interval exercise performed with the purpose of bringing oxygen intake and heart rate (and cardiac output) up to maximal values. After warming up, maximal rates can actually be reached within 1 min. When running, maximal oxygen intake can, in well trained and highly motivated athletes, be

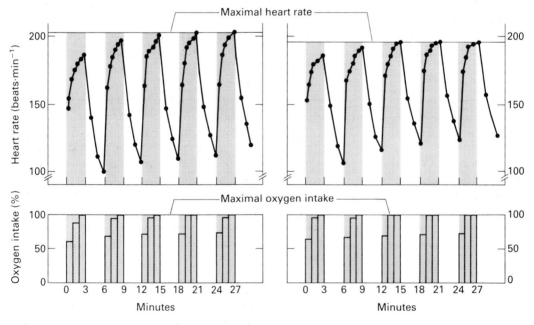

Fig. 2.2 Heart rate and oxygen uptake recorded in two subjects during training with alternating 3-minute periods of running (■) and rest (□). The efforts were not maximal, but the oxygen uptake reached maximal values, as did the heart rate. From Saltin *et al.* (1968).

maintained for some 20 min but a more 'normal' time is well below 10 min. It should be emphasized that '100% maximal oxygen intake' can be attained even if speed and perceived exertion are submaximal. If oxygen demand exceeds the individual's maximal oxygen intake the deficit must be covered by anaerobic processes, with the consequence that muscle and blood proton (and lactate) concentrations increase. We cannot explain the mechanisms but marked proton accumulations interfere negatively with performance and are correlated with fatigue. Training at maximal oxygen intake is an effective way of improving this maximal aerobic power (see Wenger & Bell, 1986). The balancing act is to find a work rate just high enough to tax this maximum without too much anaerobic support. On a cycle ergometer 300 W may cause exhaustion after 5 min but 250 W is enough to engage the oxygen transport system at maximal power (Åstrand & Rodahl, 1986, p. 300). When running on a treadmill at a speed of 13 $km \cdot h^{-1}$, maximal time was 4 min. The speed could be reduced by several $km \cdot h^{-1}$ without reducing maximal oxygen intake (see Åstrand & Rodahl, 1986, p. 443). These examples illustrate how maximal aerobic power can be attained at submaximal work rates.

There are no studies indicating that an aerobic training is more effective if combined with hypoxia and anaerobic conditions. There is an ongoing discussion about training at high altitude. In endurance events at high altitude a period of acclimatization is an essential part of the preparation for competition, at 2000 m or higher for several weeks (see Jackson & Sharkey, 1988). It is unfortunate that organizers of world cups, world championships and the Olympic games give in to pressure groups for economic reasons and select places for competition at high altitudes. Data indicate that athletes with a very high oxygen intake per kilogram of body weight are particularly handicapped at high altitudes due to limitations in the peak oxygen diffusing capacity of the lungs (see Shephard *et al.*, 1988). In addition,

countries with no good sports facilities at high altitudes within their borders have an economic handicap.

Performance at sea level is, as far as we know, not enhanced by a period of acclimatization at high altitude. It should be noted that in 1968, following the Olympic games in Mexico City (altitude 2300 m), no world records were broken in middle and long distance running events when world-class runners returned to sea level conditions after weeks at high altitude.

As discussed in Chapter 7, there is convincing evidence that the central circulation limits the maximal oxygen uptake. It therefore makes sense that stress on this system should elicit a positive adaptation. It should, however, be emphasized that training at a percentage of maximal oxygen intake lower than 100% will improve maximal oxygen intake (see Chapter 29). Peak blood pressures, heart rate and cardiac output are attained at approximately the same work rate as when oxygen intake reaches its maximum. However, stroke volume is already at a maximum when oxygen intake is 40−50% of maximum (Fig. 2.3).

Cross-country running or skiing is 'natural' interval training, with peak efforts uphill and moderate demands when running on the horizontal or downhill.

During the periods between bouts of vigorous exercise, walking or jogging at a rate of up to about 50% of maximal oxygen intake ($\dot{V}O_{2\,max}$) will speed up the rate of removal of lactate, which is a substrate in aerobic metabolism. Lactate is definitely not a waste-product! From a theoretical point of view in 'anaerobic training' that includes intermittent exercise, the periods between bursts of activity should be for rest because then the removal rate of lactate is slow.

Continuous exercise

Endurance time in exercises demanding maximal oxygen intake is limited. Therefore, continuous exercise for 10−20 min and longer, as in running, bicycling, skiing, swimming or

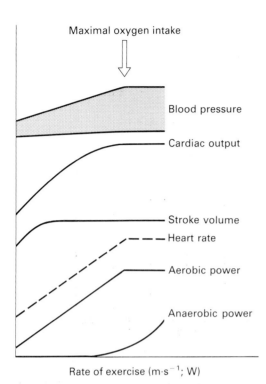

Maximal oxygen intake

Blood pressure

Cardiac output

Stroke volume

Heart rate

Aerobic power

Anaerobic power

Rate of exercise (m·s^{-1}; W)

Fig. 2.3 Schematic diagram showing some of the major cardiovascular responses to exercise of increasing intensity up to a maximum. From Åstrand & Rodahl (1986).

canoeing, must be at submaximal oxygen intake. The skeletal muscle cells of endurance-trained individuals are characterized by a high density of mitochondria and therefore a high concentration of the enzymes involved in aerobic metabolism. Actually, fast-twitch (type II) and slow-twitch (type I) muscle fibres have similar metabolic profiles in those subjects. Capillary density is also high and, at any given time, more blood is available for exchange of gases, nutrients and waste-products with the tissue. Promotion of oxidation of free fatty acids has a glycogen-saving effect (see Chapter 12). It was mentioned above that the central circulation seems to be the limiting factor for maximal aerobic power. In endurance events peripheral factors are quite decisive. An élite marathon runner has a high maximal oxygen uptake per kilogram of body mass, a good

running economy, and she or he can run at a high percentage of maximal aerobic power without accumulation of protons and lactate (see Sjödin & Svedenhag, 1985; Pate *et al.*, 1987). As indicated in Fig. 2.4 marathon runners are not necessarily champions in maximal oxygen uptake. Other qualities, just mentioned, are very important for success. Élite marathon runners and cross-country skiers have a high percentage of slow-twitch fibres, about 80% compared with about 50% in unselected groups. It is still an open question whether the high percentage of those fibres is a consequence of adaptation to endurance training or is an innate characteristic (see Chapter 5). In a recent study Coggan *et al.* (1990) found that master athletes in endurance events, with a mean age of 63 years, had a similar distribution of fibre types to younger runners with a mean age of 26 years (60% type I and very few type IIb fibres in the gastrocnemius muscle). One interpretation of their finding could be that years of endurance training do not modify fibre distribution (from type II to I).

The literature related to exercise physiology reveals a great interest in the anaerobic threshold concept, i.e. the work rate or percentage of maximal oxygen intake that can be attained at a given concentration of blood lactate. Alternative methods to establish the threshold are non-invasive. With increasing work rate, pulmonary ventilation increases linearly with oxygen intake to a point where ventilation increases non-linearly (the ventilation per litre of oxygen intake increases). There are data indicating that this 'ventilatory threshold' occurs at the work rate that causes an increase in blood lactate concentration. However, there are also reports that do not support this idea of similar thresholds. There are also large individual variations in the responses (for discussion see Åstrand & Rodahl, 1986, pp. 327–330; Orok *et al.*, 1989; Chapter 22). Droghetti *et al.* (1985) found a linear relationship between power and heart rate up to a submaximal rate beyond which the increase in heart rate slowed down. This deflection point

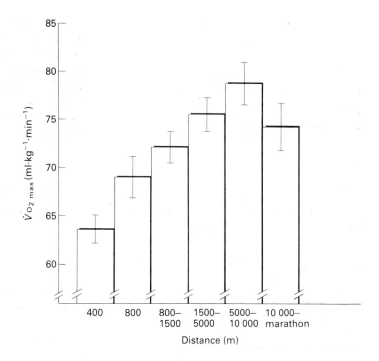

Fig. 2.4 Maximal oxygen intake in track athletes who represented the Swedish national team. From Svedenhag & Sjödin (1984).

of non-linearity in the heart rate response was found to correlate significantly to the anaerobic threshold ('Conconi test'). Other researchers have not been able to confirm this finding (see Francis *et al.*, 1989).

For a physiologist, the anaerobic threshold concept is not simple to interpret: should one consider a threshold for a single muscle fibre, a muscle group, regulatory systems (e.g. the centres generating impulses that activate the respiratory muscles), the behaviour of blood lactate concentration (which does not necessarily mirror events within a muscle), or some other lactate and pH-dependent functions? How important is the establishment of a threshold as a guide in coaching? Can data obtained in the laboratory be applied to field situations? When running outdoors, physiological responses at a given speed are modified by track conditions, terrain and wind. If heart rate is taken as a guide to demands on the oxygen transport system one must keep in mind that a hot environment and dehydration can dramatically increase the heart rate at a given oxygen intake. After all, the experienced endurance athlete knows quite well the speed that can be tolerated without undue fatigue caused by proton and lactate accumulation. However, training becomes much more sophisticated when the coach can give instructions based on blood lactate data.

Recommendations about endurance training intensity are often based on a percentage of maximal oxygen intake or heart rate. Perceived exertion is also used as a guide (see Purvis & Cureton, 1981).

From a practical viewpoint, few coaches have access to laboratories that can measure pulmonary ventilation, oxygen intake and lactate concentration, particularly in developing countries. Therefore heart rate recordings or, if equipment is not available, just recording the time taken for a fixed number of heart beats, are often the only objective measurements available. Taking group mean values at 50% of $\dot{V}_{O_2 \, max}$ gives a heart rate which is about 65% of maximal heart rate; 80% of $\dot{V}_{O_2 \, max}$ corresponds to 87% of maximal heart rate. However, if heart rate is calculated as a percentage of 'heart rate reserve' the value comes, on average, very close to the corresponding percentage of $\dot{V}o_{2\,max}$. One can generalize and take 60 beats·min^{-1} as resting heart rate. If maximal heart rate is 190 beats·min^{-1}, the 'reserve' is $190 - 60 = 130$ beats·min^{-1}. If the purpose is to train at 80% of 'heart rate reserve', it is 104 beats·min^{-1}. Then we again add 60 and end up with a heart rate of $104 + 60 = 164$ beats·min^{-1}. In the example given above, 80% of $\dot{V}o_{2\,max}$ should correspond to 87% of the maximal heart rate: 87% of $190 = 165$ beats·min^{-1}. If the maximal heart rate is not known, a mean value for the individual's age group is often used. However, because this mean value has a standard deviation of ± 10 beats·min^{-1} it is quite useless as a guide. In healthy, trained people, like athletes, the individual's maximal heart rate can easily be established with a stopwatch. After warming up, the subject runs at a speed close to maximum for a couple of minutes and then makes a 1-minute spurt, at the end preferably uphill. Immediately afterwards the subject sits down and a stopwatch is used to record the time taken for exactly 10 beats, with palpation over the carotid artery, radial artery or on the chest over the heart. Because the heart rate drops rapidly it is important that counting of the heart rate should start immediately after exercise (make a countdown of $5-4-3-2-1-0$ and on '0', start the stopwatch). A table can be constructed to convert the 10-beat time to heart rate in beats·min^{-1}.

A similar protocol can be applied when the exercise is skiing, cycling, swimming or rowing; the peak heart rate in these activities is similar to that of running. Again it should be emphasized that exercise in a hot environment and dehydration will gradually increase the heart rate at a given oxygen intake.

Conclusion

This volume concentrates on scientific analysis of endurance sports, particularly on events with continuous activation of large muscle groups for 1 h or more. However, it is important to include a basic discussion of training for many sports events of short duration because they may demand hours of daily exercise. In this chapter the physiological responses involved in three different training principles have been discussed: (i) intermittent exercise with repeated bursts of vigorous activity of short duration (less than 1 min followed by rest). Intermittent exercise in periods of 10 s or less can be performed almost exclusively aerobically thanks to unloading and recharging of myoglobin oxygen stores ; (ii) interval exercise with repeated 3–6-minute periods of vigorous activity with periods of walking or jogging in between can effectively load the oxygen transport system up to maximum. A balancing act is to find a power level high enough to tax this maximum but with only a modest contribution from the anaerobic breakdown of glycogen; (iii) continuous exercise at submaximal oxygen intake of relatively long duration. This type of training seems to be effective as a stimulus to increase the mass and density of mitochondria in skeletal muscle. The oxidation of free fatty acids will be enhanced, which has a glycogen-saving effect.

A simple method of establishing an individual's maximal heart rate is described, and a formula is given by which the percentage of maximal oxygen intake can be converted to the percentage of maximal heart rate.

Other chapters give more detailed discussion of muscular endurance, including the 'anaerobic threshold' (Chapter 22), endurance conditioning (Chapter 29) and training for specific sport events (Chapters 48–57).

References

Åstrand, I., Åstrand, P.-O., Christensen, E.H. & Hedman, R. (1960) Myoglobin as an oxygen-store in man. *Acta Physiol. Scand.* **48**, 454–460.

Åstrand, P.-O. & Rodahl, K. (1986) *Textbook of Work Physiology*. McGraw-Hill, New York.

Coggan, A.R., Spina, R.J., Rogers, M.A. *et al.* (1990) Histochemical and enzymatic characteristics of skeletal muscle in master athletes. *J. Appl. Physiol.* **68**, 1896–1901.

Droghetti, P., Borsetto, C., Casoni, I., Cellini, M., Ferrari, M., Paolini, A.R. & Conconi, F. (1985)

Noninvasive determination of the anaerobic threshold in canoeing, cross-country skiing, rolling, and ice skating, rowing and walking. *Eur. J. Appl. Physiol.* **53**, 299–303.

Francis, K.T., McClatchey, P.R., Sumsion, J.R. & Hansen, D.E. (1989) The relationship between anaerobic threshold and heart rate linearity during cycling ergometry. *Eur. J. Appl. Physiol.* **59**, 273–277.

Jackson, C.G.R. & Sharkey, B.J. (1988) Altitude, training and human performance. *Sports Med.* **6**, 279–284.

Orok, C.J., Hughson, R.L., Green, H.J. & Thomson, J.A. (1989) Blood lactate responses in incremental exercise as predictors of constant load performance. *Eur. J. Appl. Physiol.* **59**, 262–267.

Pate, R.R., Sparling, P.B., Wilson, G.E., Cureton, K.J. & Miller, B.J. (1987) Cardiorespiratory and metabolic responses to submaximal and maximal exercise in elite women distance runners. *Int. J. Sports Med.* **8**, 91–95.

Purvis, J.W., & Cureton, K.J. (1981) Ratings of perceived exertion at the anaerobic threshold. *Ergonomics* **16**, 595–600.

Saltin, B., Blomqvist, G., Mitchell, J.H., Johnson, R.L. Jr, Wildenthal, K. & Chapman, C.B. (1968) Response to submaximal and maximal exercise after bed rest and training. *Circulation* **38**, (Suppl. 7), 1–78.

Shephard, R.F., Bouhlel, E., Vanderwalle, H. & Monod, H. (1988) Peak oxygen intake and hypoxia: influence of physical fitness. *Int. J. Sports Med.* **9**, 279–283.

Sjödin, B. & Svedenhag, J. (1985) Applied physiology of marathon running. *Sports Med.* **2**, 83–99.

Svedenhag, J. & Sjödin, B. (1984) Maximal and submaximal oxygen uptakes and blood lactate levels in elite male middle- and long-distance runners. *Int. J. Sports Med.* **5**, 255–261.

Wenger, H.A. & Bell, G.J. (1986) The interactions of intensity, frequency and duration of exercise training in altering cardiorespiratory fitness. *Sports Med.* **3**, 346–356.

PART 2

BASIC SCIENTIFIC CONSIDERATIONS

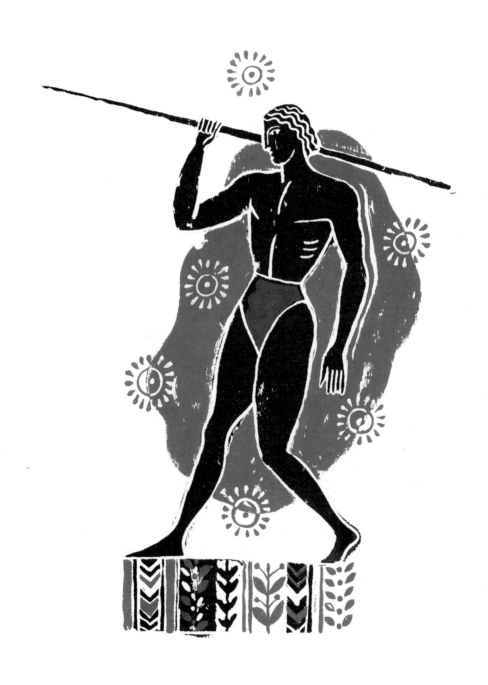

Part 2a

Biological Bases of Endurance Performance
and the Associated Functional Capacities

Chapter 3

General Considerations

ROY J. SHEPHARD

This section of the monograph examines the basic determinants of endurance performance — biological, psychological, genetic and physical. In essence, competitive success depends on the individual's ability to maximize biological function and psychological preparedness, thus optimizing the ability to perform athletically useful work against the inevitable constraints imposed by body form and environment.

Because the human body obeys the basic laws of thermodynamics, the energy needed to perform external work must be derived from body stores. Discounting the special case of the athlete who is reducing reserves of potential energy by descending a hill, the primary resource available to the active muscle fibres is a small local reserve of high energy phosphate compounds (adenosine triphosphate (ATP) and creatine phosphate). During a bout of physical activity, ATP is degraded to adenosine diphosphate (ADP) or, occasionally, to adenosine monophosphate (AMP), while creatine phosphate (CP) is converted to creatine. Each gram molecule of phosphate that is liberated yields a 'free' energy of about 46 $kJ \cdot mol^{-1}$ that can be applied to the actin/myosin interaction needed for muscle contraction. Unfortunately, the total usable muscle store of high energy phosphates is only about 30 $mmol \cdot kg^{-1}$ muscle (wet weight), a reserve that can be exhausted by 2 s or less of all-out effort. The endurance competitor must thus repeatedly resynthesize ATP and creatine phosphate, using energy

derived from the metabolic breakdown of other food reserves (Newsholme, 1983; Shephard, 1984).

Individuals differ greatly in their mechanical efficiency when converting chemical energy into athletically useful work. This reflects differences of body build, differing levels of technical skill, and differing tactical decisions in such matters as choice of pace (for example, anaerobic effort is more costly than aerobic effort). One of the important goals of prolonged, sport-specific training is the realization of the individual's potential in terms of technical skill and choice of tactics.

Prolonged athletic performance depends not only upon the extent of food reserves (both locally, within the active muscles, and elsewhere in the body), but also upon the ability to mobilize such reserves and transport them to the working tissues, together with the ability to supply the oxygen needed for their metabolic breakdown and to remove the waste-products of metabolism (carbon dioxide, heat and such substances as lactate). Moreover, function must be sustained in regions of the body other than muscle while the exercise is proceeding. For instance, an inadequate blood flow to the brain may lead to a poor competitive performance from mental confusion or impaired muscular coordination, while in sports that demand teamwork or forward planning, an excessive rise of core temperature or a drop of blood sugar concentration may lead to irritability and impaired thinking.

The psychological make-up of the individual determines the willingness to sustain rigorous training over many months, as well as the hardiness that may allow a continuation of all-out competitive effort in the face of physical pain and psychological discouragement. Genetic factors influence initial physical and physiological status, as well as the individual's responsiveness to training (in terms of conditioning both whole organs and specific enzyme systems). Finally, the physical circumstances of the competitive environment (for example, a change in the type of equipment that is permitted, or the choice of high altitude as the site of competition) can substantially influence the performance that is achieved for a given expenditure of metabolic energy.

Conductance theory

The physiological and biochemical systems involved in metabolism are arranged as a tightly interlinked gas-transporting sequence that extends from the chest bellows to the enzymes of the mitochondrial cristae within the active cells (Shephard, 1977). One purpose of conductance analysis is thus to identify potential bottlenecks in the transport process, subsequently bettering performance as these bottlenecks are eliminated through an appropriate combination of initial selection and extensive conditioning of the competitor. We shall look first at the conductance chain for the transport of oxygen, and will then examine more briefly analogous systems for the transport of carbon dioxide, lactate, heat and metabolic fuels (Shephard, 1976; 1982).

Oxygen conductance

A conductance (g) is the reciprocal of the corresponding resistance (r): $\dot{g} = 1/r$, or $r = 1/\dot{g}$. Thus, it is conventional to think of the bellows function of the chest as the respiratory minute volume that can be sustained during vigorous exercise (a maximum of perhaps $100 \, l \cdot min^{-1}$). It is immediately possible to think in terms of an electrical or a mechanical analogue for any conductance. The electrical analogue is governed by Ohm's law, with the electrical driving pressure or voltage (e) across an individual link in the system being proportional to the product of flux (I) and resistance ($e = Ir$, or $e = I/g$). The overall resistance of the system is given by the reciprocal sum of the individual conductances: $R = 1/G = 1/g_1 + 1/g_2 + 1/g_3 \ldots$. Notice that when analysing conductances in the human model, the driving pressure must be expressed in appropriate (dimensionless) units. For example, air normally contains 20.9% oxygen, so that the total driving pressure from ambient air to the muscle mitochondria is $209 \, ml \cdot l^{-1}$ (0.209). To take a practical example, if the maximal oxygen flux of an endurance competitor is $6 \, l \cdot min^{-1}$, then the overall conductance for oxygen ($G = I/E$) = 6/0.209, or $28.7 \, l \cdot min^{-1}$. If the driving pressure from the atmosphere to alveolar gas is 0.06, and the maximal exercise ventilation is $100 \, l \cdot min^{-1}$, then the overall oxygen flux can be derived from the product of the regional pressure and the corresponding conductance ($I = e\dot{g}$, 100×0.06, or again $6 \, l \cdot min^{-1}$).

It becomes more difficult to analyse data for the transfer of oxygen from the lungs to the pulmonary capillaries, and from the muscle capillaries to the muscle itself, because the driving pressures change continually on moving along the capillaries; both in the lungs and the muscles, there is almost complete equilibration at the venous end of the capillaries. Because equilibration is almost complete in both of these locations, to a first approximation the overall conductance process from air to muscle can be simplified to respiratory and cardiovascular conductances, arranged in series (Fig. 3.1).

There is a change of phase on passing from alveolar gas into the blood stream, and it is thus necessary to introduce a solubility factor in order to describe the cardiovascular conductance. In precise terms, this corresponds to the average slope of the oxygen dissociation curve between arterial and muscle venous blood;

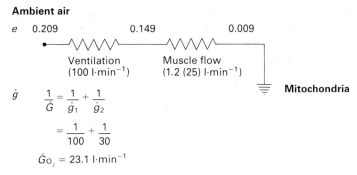

$$\frac{1}{\dot{G}} = \frac{1}{\dot{g}_1} + \frac{1}{\dot{g}_2}$$

$$= \frac{1}{100} + \frac{1}{30}$$

$$\dot{G}_{O_2} = 23.1 \ l \cdot min^{-1}$$

Fig. 3.1 Diagram illustrating the main conductances for the transport of oxygen from ambient air to the working muscles. The total pressure gradient (E) from ambient air to mitochondria (0.209 atm) is distributed between ventilation ($e = 0.06$), muscle blood flow ($e = 0.14$) and residual ($e = 0.009$) according to the reciprocal of the individual conductances (for ventilation, $\dot{g}_1 = 100 \ l \cdot min^{-1}$, and for muscle blood flow, $\dot{g}_2 = 30 \ l \cdot min^{-1}$ after allowing for a solubility coefficient of 1.2, see Fig. 3.2).

during endurance exercise, a linear average value of 1.2 may be assumed (Fig. 3.2). A peak muscle blood flow of 25 $l \cdot min^{-1}$ thus yields a blood stream oxygen conductance of 30 $l \cdot min^{-1}$. Plainly, when considering oxygen transport,

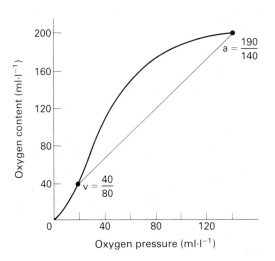

Fig. 3.2 Graph illustrating the calculation of an average blood solubility factor for oxygen from the oxygen dissociation curve of blood. At the arterial point, an oxygen content of 190 ml·l^{-1} is associated with an oxygen pressure of 140 ml·l^{-1}, while at the venous point the corresponding figures are 40 and 18 ml·l^{-1}. The slope between arterial and venous points thus averages 150/122, or 1.2.

the cardiovascular conductance is smaller (and thus the cardiovascular resistance is higher) than the corresponding values for the ventilatory term, a point that is confirmed by looking at the corresponding driving pressures (0.06 for the respiratory part of the circuit, and 0.14 for the circulation). It may finally be noted that because the driving pressure at the venous end of the muscle capillaries is close to zero, it is unlikely that peripheral factors such as enzyme activities have a major influence upon the peak rate of energy release during endurance effort.

The overall oxygen conductance is calculated by reciprocal summation of the respiratory and cardiovascular components. In our example, it amounts to 23.1 $l \cdot min^{-1}$ (see Fig. 3.1).

Carbon dioxide conductance

Similar general principles apply to the conductance of carbon dioxide from the working muscles to ambient air (Fig. 3.3). However, the gradient of driving pressure is in the opposite direction, and in a normal, well-ventilated environment, the pressure of carbon dioxide in ambient air remains close to zero. A ceiling of perhaps 100 ml·l^{-1} (0.10) is set to driving pressure at the muscular end of the system by local toxic effects of carbon dioxide (specifically, a rising hydrogen ion concentration in the

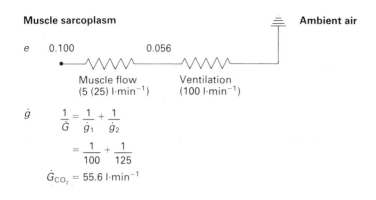

Muscle sarcoplasm   **Ambient air**

e 0.100   0.056

Muscle flow   Ventilation
(5 (25) l·min^{-1})   (100 l·min^{-1})

$\dot{g}$ $\dfrac{1}{\dot{G}} = \dfrac{1}{\dot{g_1}} + \dfrac{1}{\dot{g_2}}$

$\phantom{\dot{g}}$ $= \dfrac{1}{100} + \dfrac{1}{125}$

$\dot{G}_{CO_2} = 55.6\ \text{l·min}^{-1}$

Fig. 3.3 Diagram illustrating the conductance of carbon dioxide from the working muscles to the atmosphere. The total pressure gradient from the working muscles to ambient air (E, 0.100 atm) is distributed between ventilation ($e = 0.056$) and muscle blood flow ($e = 0.044$) according to the reciprocal of the individual conductances (for ventilation, $\dot{g_1} = 100$ l·min^{-1}, and for muscle blood flow, $\dot{g_2} = 125$ l·min^{-1} after allowing for a solubility coefficient of 5.0).

working muscles, with inhibition of key enzymes of glycogen metabolism such as phosphorylase and phosphofructokinase). Very high concentrations of carbon dioxide may also have adverse effects on cerebral function. The peak flux of carbon dioxide through the system is usually a little less than for oxygen. At the beginning of an endurance event, the respiratory quotient (the ratio of carbon dioxide output to oxygen intake) is likely to exceed 0.9, signifying that carbohydrate metabolism is providing most of the required food energy. Thus, in our example, the total flux of carbon dioxide would be 5.4 l·min^{-1}. However, as an event continues, the reserves of glycogen become exhausted and the quotient may drop to 0.8 or lower, corresponding to a carbon dioxide flux of 4.8 l·min^{-1}.

The blood solubility factor is higher for carbon dioxide than for oxygen; we are in essence dealing with the carbon dioxide dissociation curve, and over the normal operating range from muscle veins to arterialized blood, this curve may be approximated by a linear solubility coefficient of 5.0. Thus, in our hypothetical example, the overall conductance for carbon dioxide is $1/100 + 1/5(25)$, or 55.5 l·min^{-1}. Given also the smaller peak flux of carbon dioxide, it is unlikely that carbon dioxide transport will be severely taxed by most types of competition, despite the fact that the limiting overall pressure gradient is smaller for carbon dioxide than for oxygen.

Lactate conductance

Lactic acid accumulates in muscle whenever the local oxygen supply is inadequate to support aerobic metabolism (Shephard, 1982). Transport of lactate proceeds from the working muscles to the blood stream (Fig. 3.4), and thence to the liver (where glycogen is synthesized from the lactate residues) or to inactive tissues (where it is converted to pyruvate and then metabolized to carbon dioxide and water through Krebs' cycle (Gladden, 1989). The driving pressure is the local lactate concentration; the maximum intramuscular value of $30-40$ mmol·l^{-1} is set by the rising local hydrogen ion concentration and the resultant inhibition of glycolytic enzymes (Shephard, 1984). The peak arterial concentration is normally about 10 mmol·l^{-1}, although a figure of some 30 mmol·l^{-1} can be reached if several brief bouts of exhausting large muscle work are repeated over the space of 20 min. The flux of lactate from muscle to blood stream during maximal effort typically occurs at a rate of 10 mmol·min^{-1}, although some authors have suggested ceiling values as low as 2 mmol·min^{-1} (Shephard, 1976). Taking the 10 mmol·min^{-1} figure and assuming a muscle blood flow of 20 l·min^{-1}, the arteriovenous concentration gradient would reach the typical experimental value of 0.5 mmol·l^{-1}, about one sixtieth of the muscle/capillary gradient of 30 mmol·l^{-1}.

Fig. 3.4 Diagram illustrating pathways for the conductance of lactate from the working muscles. The pressure gradient E is a lactate concentration of 40 mmol·l^{-1}, extending from the muscle sarcoplasm to the sites of lactate metabolism in resting muscle and liver. The main gradient (and thus the smallest conductance) is from the muscle sarcoplasm into the blood stream.

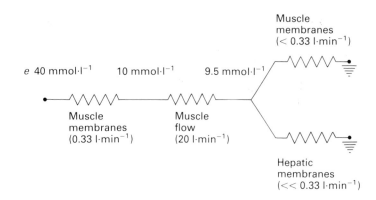

We may conclude that the outward conductance of lactate from muscle to blood is only about one sixtieth of the blood stream transport, being equivalent to a local blood flow of only 0.33 l·min^{-1}. The figure still remains relatively imprecise, and there have been suggestions that lactate conductance can be increased substantially by the administration of bicarbonate solutions, giving rise to a temptation of 'bicarbonate doping' (Gledhill, 1984). The reverse lactate conductance, from the blood stream into resting or moderately active muscle, also proceeds more rapidly, probably reaching a rate of about 40 mmol·min^{-1}.

Heat conductance

Heat follows a pathway from muscle to skin (Fig. 3.5), where it is normally dissipated by a combination of sweating and convection (Nadel, 1977; 1987). The driving pressure is a temperature difference, measured between the active deep tissues and either the skin surface (in a partial analysis) or the ambient air (in a total analysis).

There is some competition between muscle and skin blood flow in a hot environment, but the latter usually peaks at about 5 l·min^{-1}. When analysing thermal conductances, it is again necessary to apply a 'solubility factor'; for the blood, this is its specific heat (about 3.4 kJ·l^{-1} per degree centigrade). The total heat conductance is then approximated by reciprocal summation as $(1/20 + 1/5)\ 1/3.4$, or 14 kJ·l^{-1}·min^{-1}. The total flux is the energy equivalent of at least 75% of the maximal oxygen intake, 0.75 (6.0) 21 kJ·min^{-1}, or (since an oxygen consumption of 1 l·min^{-1} is equivalent to about 21 kJ·min^{-1}), about 95 kJ·min^{-1} in

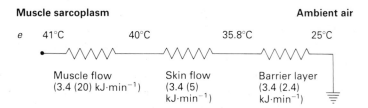

Fig. 3.5 Diagram illustrating pathways for the conductance of heat from the working muscles. The total pressure gradient (measured in degrees centigrade) depends on the ambient air temperature (25°C in the example). The blood stream conductance of heat is given by the product of flow and a 'heat solubility factor' of 3.4 kJ·l^{-1}·°C^{-1}. If transfer of heat across the barrier layer of still air around the body is expressed in the same terms, it can be seen that this is the smallest of the three conductances, and thus has the largest influence upon heat loss from the body.

our example. Given also the conductance of $14 \text{ kJ}^{-1} \cdot \text{min}^{-1}$, a thermal gradient of about $7°C$ becomes necessary to transfer all of the heat that is produced from the working muscles to the skin surface. A core temperature in excess of $41°C$ is regarded as a dangerous level of hyperthermia; the implication is that a skin temperature of $34°C$ is needed for thermal equilibrium during prolonged physical activity. A peak oxygen intake of $4 \text{ l} \cdot \text{min}^{-1}$ is more usual than $6 \text{ l} \cdot \text{min}^{-1}$ during endurance events, so that the total heat flux drops to about $65 \text{ kJ} \cdot \text{min}^{-1}$; moreover, some heat is conducted directly from muscle through the overlying tissues. The required skin temperature for thermal equilibrium can thus rise to at least $35.8°C$ rather than $34°C$. Nevertheless, it is difficult to hold readings even to the higher limit under hot and humid conditions, so that a rising core temperature is commonly a factor limiting sustained physical activity.

It is finally worth noting that under temperate environmental conditions, a major portion of the overall thermal gradient is from the skin to the ambient air. A thin film of stationary air (the 'boundary layer') offers a major barrier to heat dissipation. Assuming an air temperature of $25°C$, the thermal gradient from skin to air ($10.8°C$ in our example) is more than twice that from core to skin ($5.2°C$), implying that the air barrier to heat exchange is at least twice as important as that offered by maximal skin blood flow.

Rapid body movement displaces the boundary layer of still air, so that it is a much less important barrier to heat exchange for a cyclist than for a runner. The conductance of heat across the barrier layer is also influenced by the density and the chemical composition of the environment. Conductance is decreased at high altitudes, but is greatly increased in the diver who is using a breathing system containing helium (a gas with a high thermal conductivity). In water, boundary layer effects are much less important than in air, so that the outward heat flux is much greater than when on land. As a consequence, the distance swimmer may encounter problems due to a falling core temperature and hypothermia.

Conductance of metabolites

Depending somewhat upon the state of training of the individual, carbohydrate initially provides about three quarters of the metabolic fuel needed by the endurance performer. Intramuscular reserves of glycogen are used at a rate of about $2{-}4 \text{ g} \cdot \text{min}^{-1}$ (about $16 \text{ mmol} \cdot \text{min}^{-1}$ of the equivalent glucosyl units), while a further $1 \text{ g} \cdot \text{min}^{-1}$ ($5.3 \text{ mmol} \cdot \text{min}^{-1}$ of glucosyl units) is transported from the liver to the active tissues. There is no evidence that the transport of these substances limits endurance performance, at least until the local reserves of glycogen have dropped to quite low levels (Hultman, 1978; Karlsson, 1979; Conlee, 1986). At this stage, the speeds of the distance competitor begin to show an appreciable decline.

The rate of glycogen depletion depends on the tactics adopted by the competitor. Fat metabolism is oxygen dependent, so that the choice of an over-rapid pace increases the likelihood of local oxygen lack, boosting the proportion of carbohydrate that is metabolized in the early part of a race. The ideal plan for the competitor is to operate just below his or her anaerobic threshold, and the experienced participant in endurance events normally adopts this pattern of exercise, reserving a burst of anaerobic activity for the final sprint to the finishing line.

On occasion, an attempt is made to boost the carbohydrate reserves of the athlete by the drinking of glucose or glucose/polymer solutions during competition (Murray, 1987; Shephard & Leatt, 1987). The maximum rate of ingestion of sweetened fluid during endurance effort is achieved when drinking a 5% solution of glucose. The peak intake is then about $600 \text{ ml} \cdot \text{h}^{-1}$, $0.5 \text{ g} \cdot \text{min}^{-1}$ glucosyl equivalents ($2.6 \text{ mmol} \cdot \text{min}^{-1}$). This represents a relatively small fraction of the total carbohydrate metabolism, at least until muscle glycogen reserves have been depleted.

In very prolonged endurance effort, performance may be limited by the ability to mobilize fat from the adipose tissue and/or the ability to transport it to the working muscles (Bülow, 1987). In view of the limited blood supply of adipose tissue and the variations in the rates of triglyceride metabolism with changes in the blood levels of fatty acids, one might suspect the problem is of limited vascular conductance. On the other hand, training increases the peripheral mobilization of triglyceride metabolites, and also increases the activity of fat-metabolizing enzymes within the working muscle, presumably as a mechanism of glycogen-sparing in the earlier stages of a competition.

Nature and location of fatigue

Acute and chronic forms of fatigue (Simonson, 1971; Green, 1987; MacLaren et al., 1989) are common complaints of the endurance competitor. The problem may be physiological, psychological, or occasionally medical in nature, and can be local (confined to a particular group of muscles) or general (affecting the body as a whole).

Physiological fatigue

Physiological fatigue is seen as a deterioration of performance, either during a specific type of competition or as a task is repeated from one day to another. For example, the pace of a runner may slow or the force of repeated maximal isotonic muscular contractions may diminish. There are associated signs of failing homoeostasis, for example a rising heart rate, respiratory rate, minute volume or respiratory gas exchange ratio for a given intensity of effort. However, there remain substantial interindividual differences in the limiting values for variables such as intravascular or intramuscular lactate concentration, and often there is only a limited relationship between subjective reports of tiredness and objective data, indicating a substantial gap between the physiologically possible and the psychologically acceptable.

The proximate cause of fatigue may be a lack of appropriate signals to the active muscle fibres, a failure of mechanisms for replenishing the high energy phosphate molecules needed to power muscle contractions, or more general problems of homoeostasis.

Failure of drive mechanisms: Muscle contractions are normally initiated by a coordinated volley of impulses originating in the motor cortex and/or the cerebellum. The signal passes through synapses in the brain and spinal cord, traverses the neuromuscular junction and penetrates the transverse tubules of the active muscle fibre, finally liberating calcium ions from the sarcoplasmic reticulum. The calcium ions are a key component of the trigger mechanism that initiates the formation of cross-bridges between actin and myosin molecules, using energy stored in ATP. In theory, fatigue could originate at any point in the chain of command, and some evidence for a neural component to fatigue can be seen in an altered pattern of movement as a person becomes tired (Green, 1987; Bigland-Ritchie, 1990; Figs 3.6 & 3.7). Specifically, recordings of action potentials from the working muscles show that the slow frequency component of the electromyogram is increased. This could represent an attempt to recruit (from an alternative muscle group) fibres that are not yet fatigued. Suggested mechanisms for the slower average rate of firing include an alteration in the synchronization of individual motor units, the recruitment of slowly firing, high threshold motor fibres, or alterations in the electrophysiological characteristics of the conducting membranes.

The brain is able to metabolize only carbohydrate, so that the development of a decreasing blood sugar level after several hours of large muscle activity may lead to errors of judgment, loss of teamwork, and a failure of coordination. In some instances (for example, soccer matches), team performance has improved and individual motor reactions have increased when players have been given small

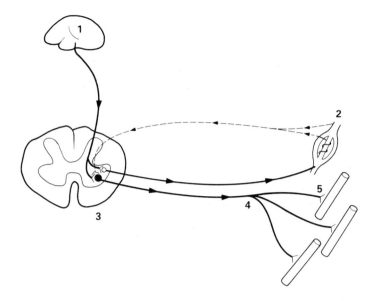

Fig. 3.6 Potential sites of central fatigue: 1, supraspinal failure; 2, segmental afferent inhibition; 3, depression of motoneuron excitability; 4, loss of excitation at branch points; 5, presynaptic failure. From Green (1987), with permission.

doses of glucose or sugar at half-time (Shephard & Leatt, 1987). A poor coordination of movement is another expression of cerebral fatigue, although this may indicate either a poor circulation to the brain or a low blood sugar level. Clumsiness is exacerbated by changes in the sensitivity of the spindle organs that detect muscle tension, and by attempts to sustain performance using muscle groups other than those trained to undertake a given task.

There is little evidence that the carriage of impulses along the nerve fibres is affected by the fatigue of endurance competition, but in some instances there has been evidence of a slowing of the calcium pumping needed during recovery intervals, both at the neuromuscular junction and also at the level of the sarcoplasmic reticulum within the active muscle fibres. Fatiguing exercise, both local and general, further leads to a substantial leakage of potassium ions from the active muscle fibres (Sjögaard *et al.*, 1985), with adverse effects upon the electrical charge on the membrane and the conduction of the signal along the transverse tubules of the muscle fibres to the site of calcium release.

Failure of power supply: We have noted that the supply of energy needed for the resynthesis of ATP can be threatened by an inadequate supply of oxygen, an accumulation of carbon dioxide or lactic acid which inhibits the enzymes involved in glycogen breakdown, and a lack of food reserves locally within the active muscle fibres.

While a competitor can use 100% of maximal oxygen transport for a few minutes of large muscle effort, during an extended competition such as a marathon run, fatigue develops if the intensity of effort reaches more than about 75% of maximal oxygen intake (Costill, 1972). The probable explanation of the latter finding is that the blood supply to the muscle fibres is non-uniform; thus, if the intensity of effort exceeds 75% of the overall oxygen transporting capacity, the capillary supply is insufficient to avert anaerobic metabolism in some muscle fibres. One factor that influences the local blood supply in both rhythmic and heavy isotonic activity is the development of a high intramuscular pressure as the muscles contract; thus, factors that reduce intramuscular pressure (use of a lower gear ratio on a bicycle, or the strengthening of the active muscles by appropriate isotonic training) may enable a well prepared distance competitor to exercise for long periods at more than 75% of maximal oxygen

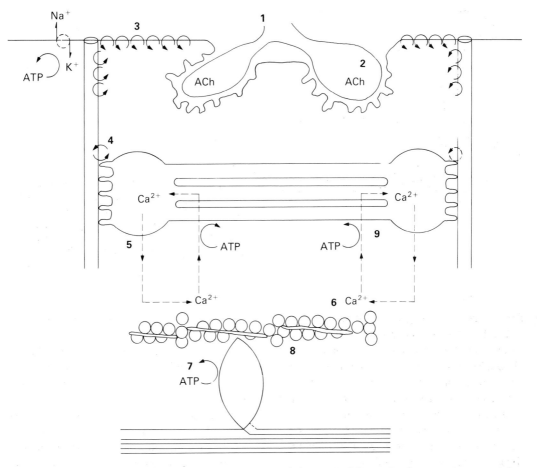

Fig. 3.7 Potential peripheral sites of fatigue: 1, presynaptic failure; 2, inability to develop an action potential at motor endplate (ACh, acetyl choline); 3, failure of sarcolemma to sustain an action potential; 4, loss of coupling of excitation between t-tubule and sarcoplasmic reticulum; 5, depressed release of calcium ions from the sarcoplasmic reticulum; 6, reduced binding affinity of the receptor protein troponin on the actin molecule; 7, a failure in the actin/myosin cross-bridge cycle; 8, delayed cross-bridge dissociation; 9, depressed reaccumulation of calcium ions by sarcoplasmic reticulum. From Green (1987), with permission.

intake without experiencing fatigue. Likewise, in a sport that requires repeated vigorous isotonic efforts, the decrease of force over 50 repetitions of a maximal contraction will be much less than before training.

Carbon dioxide accumulation does not contribute significantly to either local or general fatigue except in special circumstances such as prolonged underwater exploration, where the ventilatory conductance (more important for

the elimination of carbon dioxide than for the intake of oxygen) is limited by the added deadspace and external resistance of breathing equipment.

Glycogen reserves are almost completely depleted by about 100 min of endurance work (Hultman, 1971; Conlee, 1986), and they can equally be exhausted by 10 or a dozen nearmaximal contractions of a muscle group, if each individual effort has been sustained to the point of fatigue. Subsequently, transport of triglycerides from fat depots to the working muscles can sustain an intensity of aerobic activity equivalent to about 50% of maximal oxygen intake, but it cannot provide fuel for anaerobic activity. The potential to produce glucose in the liver (the process of hepatic gluconeogenesis (Wahren & Björkman, 1981; Winder, 1985), drawing upon such resources as hepatic glycogen, amino acids, glycerol and lactate) is extremely limited, so that blood sugar concentration drops, sometimes as low as 3 mmol·l^{-1}. A sensation of intense weakness and fatigue then develops whenever postural, isometric, or heavy isotonic muscle activity is required.

Failure of homoeostasis: With very prolonged activity, a general failure of homoeostasis may develop, involving the circulation, the kidneys or the endocrine glands, and sometimes accompanied by an excessive rise or fall of body temperature. A local failure of homoeostasis is also possible when a specific group of muscles is engaged in repeated isotonic or isometric effort.

General circulatory problems arise from a decrease in the amount of blood in the central part of the circulation (Saltin, 1964; Senay & Pivarnik, 1985; Convertino, 1987). Factors contributing to this challenge include a dilatation of the peripheral capacitance vessels (the major veins), sweating (which may cause a fluid loss of as much as 2 l·h^{-1}), exudation of fluid into the active tissues (a potential loss of about 20% of the total blood volume over the course of 30 min of physical activity), and possible exhaustion of the neural and hormonal regulatory systems. Dominant features are a decline of the cardiac stroke volume and an increase of heart rate for any given intensity of effort.

Local circulatory problems arise when blood flow is restricted by a forceful muscle contraction. Blood flow is impeded when the force of contraction exceeds 15% of the maximal voluntary force for a given muscle group, and occlusion of the blood vessels becomes complete

at 70% of maximal voluntary force (Shephard, 1982). The situation is worsened if the arm is held above the head (as in a tennis serve), since the perfusion pressure is then decreased by the need to pump the blood to a greater height, but the force of the muscle contraction and thus the vascular compression is unchanged.

If subjects compete repeatedly in a very hot environment, there may be a progressive failure of circulatory homoeostasis over a period of weeks (Wyndham & Strydom, 1972). Here, the problem is a chronic depletion of minerals such as sodium ions, with an associated loss of water and thus blood volume.

There have been occasional reports of renal failure following prolonged events such as marathon and ultramarathon races. Generally, there has been evidence of an associated hyperthermia, and the basis of the problem has been a restriction of visceral blood flow in an attempt to maintain blood flow to other more vital areas of the circulation.

Restriction of visceral flow may also cause a failure of the adrenal cortex (the final stage of Selye's stress reaction); this causes an inadequate production of the hormones regulating potassium and sodium ions (aldosterone) and water and carbohydrate stores (cortisol). If competition is perceived as unusually stressful from a psychological perspective, this can interact with physiological stress to exacerbate hormonal fatigue. There may be an associated deterioration of immune function (Keast *et al.*, 1988), leaving the athlete more vulnerable to minor infections, and this can further exacerbate both physical and psychological fatigue.

A failure of circulatory homoeostasis may be linked with an excessive rise of core temperature (Nadel, 1987). Because the rising core temperature diverts blood flow from the brain and the working muscles to the skin, it can exacerbate feelings of fatigue and precipitate a loss of circulatory homoeostasis (Rowell, 1983). Repeated bouts of prolonged exercise in hot environments can also produce the chronic fatigue associated with mineral and water depletion.

Too low a core temperature can be equally

fatiguing, since the local muscle blood flow is reduced, an increase of muscle viscosity augments the internal work that must be performed during physical activity, and a cooling of peripheral neural receptors leads to a more clumsy performance of many tasks.

Psychological fatigue

Although psychological fatigue is hard to pinpoint, it is a very real phenomenon in many athletes who have pursued heavy training schedules to the point of 'staleness'.

While the tiredness can arise acutely, the onset is more often gradual and chronic. Typically, it has a situational or even an emotional rather than a firm physiological basis. Factor analyses of the subjective reports from athletes (Kinsman et al., 1973) have distinguished three elements: projected fatigue (noted in such sensations as leg weakness, shaking or aching muscles, a pounding heart, shortness of breath and a dry mouth — many of the somatic manifestations of an anxiety state); task aversion (perceived as sweating, discomfort and a wish to do something other than train or compete); and poor motivation, encompassing feelings of reduced drive, lack of vigour and a want of determination.

The athlete becomes bored with seemingly endless and unchanging training sessions, there is an aversive reaction to the restrictions imposed by the coach and the associated loss of social life, and discouragement develops as the rewards of improving performance disappear despite the ever-increasing demands of the training programme. The affected individual is typically underaroused, and fails to achieve his or her physiological potential. An associated loss of vigilance may increase the risk of accidents. In contrast with physical exhaustion, the psychologically fatigued athlete demands a change rather than a rest. An unpleasant or unfamiliar environment (for example, competing in a foreign city, sleeping in an uncomfortable hotel room at an unaccustomed altitude or temperature, conflict with the coach, or a

series of defeats) can all exacerbate the problem, not by any direct physiological mechanism, but rather by increasing task aversion.

Highly trained athletes undoubtedly habituate themselves to situations that lesser competitors would find psychologically fatiguing. However, short-term training programmes apparently do little to change the perception of effort (Pandolf, 1983).

Medical aspects of fatigue

Fatiguing effort may induce tissue injuries that are only slowly reversed. These range from a slight muscular stiffness reported for a day or two following intensive competition to chronic tendon injuries, fatigue fractures of bones, and disturbances of immune function that can affect the susceptibility of a competitor to intercurrent infections.

The minor lesions are subcellular in type. Evidence of altered membrane permeability can be found in modifications of ionic balance (a shift of potassium ions from the active muscles into the plasma and inactive tissues), the escape of various intracellular enzymes such as lactate dehydrogenase and creatine kinase into the blood stream, and the appearance of low molecular weight proteins in the urine (Poortmans, 1985; Rogers et al., 1985; Armstrong, 1986). Ultrastructural changes are also visible in muscle, heart and nerve at electron microscopy (Banister, 1971; Oscai & Palmer, 1988). It has been suggested that such subcellular changes are a necessary concomitant of an adaptive response to heavy training. However, the dividing line that separates such phenomena from irreversible tissue injury is fine, and it seems very likely that ultrastructural changes often contribute to chronic fatigue — particularly in terms of feelings such as stiffness and muscle pain.

In some instances, reports of fatigue may be an indication that an athlete is developing an anxiety state, possibly as a reaction to the stresses of competition, or possibly as a reaction to other personal circumstances.

Central versus peripheral limitations of endurance effort

There has been much debate as to whether a typical endurance performance such as distance running is limited by central or peripheral mechanisms (Shephard, 1982). The issue is important for those who seek to augment human performance, since it indicates whether the sports scientist should focus his or her endeavours upon an improvement of cardiorespiratory function, or whether greater attention should be directed to changing cellular and subcellular events.

In forms of exercise that involve activation of a large proportion of the total musculature, the conductance theory offers persuasive arguments for a central limitation of effort, as discussed above. Other arguments for a peripheral limitation of effort have been considered and rejected (Shephard, 1982). Given 20 kg of active muscle, and a peak muscle blood flow of 25 l·min^{-1}, the regional blood flow averages about 80 ml·min^{-1}·100 ml^{-1} tissue. There are good reasons to believe that the blood vessels in a large muscle could accept three to four times this blood flow if the heart were able to sustain a greater rate of tissue perfusion (Savard et al., 1987).

However, the arguments favouring a central limitation of endurance performance become less clear as the determinants of cardiac output are examined. These determinants include the preloading of the ventricles, myocardial contractility, the chronotropic response of the heart, and the after-loading of the ventricles. Preloading reflects the rate of venous return to the heart. Thus, in wheelchair athletes with muscular paralysis, a peripheral loss of the muscle pump may cause blood to accumulate in the paralysed limbs, reducing preloading and restricting cardiac output (Shephard, 1990). The sympathetically controlled increase of myocardial contractility quickly augments the stroke volume during exercise, and the chronotropic increase of heart rate is also mediated largely via sympathetic β-receptors. However,

some authors have argued that local, limb-specific peripheral responses to training modify the extent of these responses; perhaps there is less peripheral stimulation of ergo-receptors as the active muscles become stronger, or perhaps there is a reduction of central command to the working muscles and thus a lesser irradiation of impulses to the cardiovascular control centres in the brain. Finally, the extent of after-loading, the force opposing ventricular emptying, is strongly influenced by the exercise-induced rise of systemic blood pressure; this depends in turn upon the fraction of maximal voluntary force exerted by the working muscles, and thus local muscular strength (Shephard, 1982). From many points of view, the distinction between central and peripheral limitation is thus somewhat arbitrary, and tends to be a matter of semantics.

In forms of exercise where the volume of active muscle is limited, the likelihood of a peripheral limitation of effort is correspondingly increased. During cycling, a surprisingly large proportion of the total effort is sustained by the quadriceps muscle, and poorly trained individuals tend to complain that their maximal effort is limited by muscular fatigue rather than by indications of impending cardiovascular failure such as incoordination, mental confusion, and loss of consciousness (Shephard, 1977). Because of local hypertrophy of the limb muscles, there is a lesser likelihood that muscle fatigue will limit effort in those who are well trained. Wheelchair athletes, for example, can develop as large a maximal oxygen intake as an average person while using only the greatly hypertrophied muscles of the arms and shoulder girdle.

During many forms of heavy dynamic work, the volume of active muscle is further restricted, and the intensity of effort that is demanded often approaches the maximum voluntary force. Local blood flow is now entirely occluded, and a peripheral limitation of exercise becomes the norm.

References

Armstrong, R.B. (1986) Muscle damage and endurance events. *Sports Med.* **3**, 370–381.

Banister, E. (1971) Energetics of muscular contraction. In R.J. Shephard (ed.) *Frontiers of Fitness*, pp. 5–36. C.C. Thomas, Springfield, Illinois.

Bigland-Ritchie, B. (1990) Discussion: nervous system and sensory adaptation. In: C. Bouchard & R.J. Shephard (eds) *Exercise, Fitness and Health*, pp. 377–384. Human Kinetics, Champaign, Illinois.

Bülow, J. (1987) Regulation of lipid mobilization in exercise. *Can. J. Sport Sci.* **12** (Suppl. 1), 117S–119S.

Conlee, R.K. (1986) Muscle glycogen and exercise endurance. *Exerc. Sport Sci. Rev.* **15**, 1–28.

Convertino, V.A. (1987) Fluid shifts and hydration state: effects of long-term exercise. *Can. J. Sport Sci.* **12** (Suppl. 1), 136S–139S.

Costill, D.L. (1972) Physiology of marathon running. *J. Am. Med. Assoc.* **221**, 1024–1029.

Gladden, L.B. (1989) Lactate uptake by skeletal muscle. *Exerc. Sport Sci. Rev.* **17**, 115–156.

Gledhill, N. (1984) Bicarbonate ingestion and anaerobic performance. *Sports Med.* **1**, 177–180.

Green, H.J. (1987) Neuromuscular aspects of fatigue. *Can. J. Sport Sci.* **12** (Suppl. 1), 7S–19S.

Hultman, E. (1971) Muscle glycogen stores and prolonged exercise. In: R.J. Shephard (ed.) *Frontiers of Fitness*. C.C. Thomas, Springfield, Illinois.

Hultman, E. (1978) Regulation of carbohydrate metabolism in the liver during rest and exercise, with special reference to diet. In: F. Landry & W.A.R. Orban (eds) *Third International Symposium on the Biochemistry of Exercise*, pp. 99–126. Symposia Specialists, Miami, Florida.

Karlsson, J. (1979) Localized muscular fatigue: role of muscle metabolism and substrate depletion. *Exerc. Sport Sci. Rev.* **7**, 1–42.

Keast, D., Cameron, K. & Morton, A.R. (1988) Exercise and the immune response. *Sports Med.* **5**, 248–267.

Kinsman, R.A., Weiser, P.C. & Stamper, D.A. (1973) Multidimensional analysis of subjective symptomatology during prolonged strenuous exercise. *Ergonomics* **16**, 211–226.

MacLaren, D.P., Gibson, H., Parry-Billings, M. & Edwards, R.H.T. (1989) A review of metabolic and physiological factors in fatigue. *Exerc. Sport Sci. Rev.* **17**, 29–66.

Murray, R. (1987) The effects of consuming carbohydrate–electrolyte beverages on gastric emptying and fluid absorption during and following exercise. *Sports Med.* **4**, 322–351.

Nadel, E.R. (1977) *Problems with Temperature Regulation During Exercise*. Academic Press, New York.

Nadel, E.J. (1987) Prolonged exercise at high and low ambient temperatures. *Can. J. Sport Sci.* **12** (Suppl. 1), 140S–142S.

Newsholme, E.A. (1983) Control of metabolism and the integration of fuel supply for the marathon runner. In: H.G. Knuttgen, J.A. Vogel & J. Poortmans (eds) *Biochemistry of Exercise*, pp. 144–150. Human Kinetics, Champaign, Illinois.

Oscai, L.B. & Palmer, W.K. (1988) Muscle lipolysis during exercise: an up-date. *Sports Med.* **6**, 23–28.

Pandolf, K.B. (1983) Advances in the study and application of perceived exertion. *Exerc. Sport Sci. Rev.* **11**, 118–158.

Poortmans, J.R. (1985) Effects of long-lasting physical exercise and training on protein metabolism. In: H. Howald & J.R. Poortmans (eds) *Metabolic Adaptation to Prolonged Physical Exercise*, pp. 212–228. Birkhauser Verlag, Basel.

Rogers, M.A., Stull, G.A. & Apple, F.S. (1985) Creatine kinase isoenzyme activities in men and women following a marathon race. *Med. Sci. Sports Exerc.* **17**, 679–682.

Rowell, L.B. (1983) Cardiovascular adjustment to thermal stress. In: J.T. Shepherd & F.M. Abbound (eds) *Handbook of Physiology, 2. The Cardiovascular System*, Vol. III, pp. 967–1023. American Physiological Society, Bethesda, Maryland.

Saltin, B. (1964) Aerobic work capacity and circulation at exercise in man. *Acta Physiol. Scand.* **62** (Suppl.), 230.

Savard, G., Kiens, B. & Saltin, B. (1987) Limb blood flow in prolonged exercise: magnitude and implication for cardiovascular control during muscle work in man. *Can. J. Sport Sci.* **12**, (Suppl. 1), 89S–101S.

Senay, L.C. & Pivarnik, J.M. (1985) Fluid shifts during exercise. *Exerc. Sport Sci. Rev.* **13**, 335–387.

Shephard, R.J. (1976) A new look at aerobic power. In: E. Jokl, R.L. Anand & H. Stoboy (eds) *Medicine and Sport*, Vol. 9, pp. 61–84. Karger Publishing, Basel.

Shephard, R.J. (1977) *Endurance Fitness*, 2nd edn. University of Toronto Press, Toronto.

Shephard, R.J. (1982) *Physiology and Biochemistry of Exercise*. Praeger Publishing, New York.

Shephard, R.J. (1984) *Biochemistry of Exercise*. C.C. Thomas, Springfield, Illinois.

Shephard, R.J. (1990) *Fitness in Special Populations*. Human Kinetics, Champaign, Illinois.

Shephard, R.J. & Leatt, P. (1987) Carbohydrate and fluid needs of the soccer player. *Sports Med.* **4**, 164–176.

Simonson, E. (1971) *Physiology of Work Capacity and Fatigue*. C.C. Thomas, Springfield, Illinois.

Sjögaard, G., Adams, R.B. & Saltin, B. (1985) Water and ion shifts in skeletal muscle of humans with intense dynamic knee extension. *Am. J. Physiol.* **248**, R190–R196.

Wahren, J. & Björkman, O. (1981) Hormones, exercise

and regulation of splanchnic glucose output in normal man. In: J. Poortmans & G. Nisset (eds) *Biochemistry of Exercise*, IVa. University Park Press, Baltimore.

Winder, W. (1985) Regulation of hepatic glucose production during exercise. *Exerc. Sport Sci. Rev.* **13**, 1–32.

Wyndham, C. & Strydom, N.B. (1972) Körperliche Arbeit bei höher Temperatur. In: W. Hollmann (ed.) *Zentrale Themen der Sport Medizin*, pp. 131–149. Springer Verlag, Berlin.

Chapter 4

Anatomical and Anthropometric Fundamentals of Endurance

KURT TITTEL AND HEINZ WUTSCHERK

Introduction

A large number of recent publications seeking to identify the effects of somatotypical variability on athletic capacity have either described the athlete's constitution or given measurements of body dimensions. Statistical values are presented as means, standard deviations and percentiles. The standard deviations show that individual values diverge widely from the reported mean values for a given type of sport. The resultant difficulties increase as a larger number of individual body measurements is assessed. Kunze et al. (1976) have claimed that 'exact anthropometrical studies enable us to deduce ideal values for athletes in different sports'; they qualify their claim, however, noting that 'deviations from the sport-type do not necessarily mean bad results in competitions'. The contradiction evident in this statement is caused by a focus on description of the phenotype, which lacks an immediate relationship to the variability of athletic performance. Investigators have looked mainly for differences of characteristics, relative to other populations. The method of comparison has typically been between:

1 athletes and non-athletes;

2 athletes participating in a given sport and those from other disciplines (Tittel & Wutscherk, 1972; DeGaray et al., 1974);

3 individual values and averaged data registered for a particular sport discipline;

4 individual values and group values using hypothetical reference values such as the unisex model (Ross & Wilson, 1974; Ross, 1978) or a determination of somatotype (Tittel & Wutscherk, 1972; Carter et al., 1978, 1982; Stepnicka, 1981) relative to a distributive spectrum representing the total population.

The results of such investigations represent the characteristic differences mathematically and/or visually, but cannot indicate their effects upon athletic abilities (Tittel & Wutscherk, 1972; DeGaray et al., 1974). These authors do not exclude the possibility of obvious differences in mean somatotypic characteristics for specific athletic requirements (for example, extremes of strength or endurance), a point first made by Kohlrausch as early as 1927, and which gives some competitors a predisposition towards certain sports (Grimm, 1966). The state of knowledge has not changed decisively with more sophisticated analytical procedures based upon correlational statistics, including factorial analysis. Knowledge of the mechanisms that determine endurance capacity is fundamental to athletic preparation. Such study calls for a causal—analytic procedure, as published some time ago (Wutscherk, 1981; Wutscherk & Tittel, 1982), but reflected only insignificantly in other authors' more recent publications.

Terminology and methodological aspects

'Endurance' here refers to the ability to maintain an actual, quantified, muscular performance for a period characteristic of the event concerned. Endurance depends on the intensity and duration of the exerted force. If $F_{max} \rightarrow t_{min}$ expresses the maximum force to be exerted, its reciprocal $F_{min} \rightarrow t_{max}$ is the counterpole, or endurance. A causal analysis of the functional−anatomical and anthropometric fundamentals of endurance should begin, therefore, with the question as to what measurable parameters correlate closely with muscular force and determine its variability.

The force of every single muscle can be estimated anthropometrically only by measuring the circumferences of the extremities concerned. Such an approach is vague, because agonistic and antagonistic muscles, subcutaneous fat and bones are all included in the circumference. The same is true if extremity volumes are assessed by the displacement procedure (Davies, 1978), or if the masses of the extremities are determined by processing anthropometric data in regression equations (Martirosov, 1982). Body masses correlate most strongly with the total strength of the skeletal musculature (absolute force). Anthropometric procedures allow the estimation of muscle mass, fat mass, fat-free or lean body mass, bone mass and total body mass. Good correlations could probably be found between the absolute force and the summed circumferences of the extremities. Factor analyses have confirmed correlations of these body characteristics with dynamometrically registered values by showing high rankings of both − somatotypical characteristics and dynamometric values − in the same factors (Wutscherk, 1981).

Muscle mass is the fundamental structural element that determines muscle strength. It can be estimated from a series of anthropometric measurements (four circumferences of the extremities, corrected by the appropriate skinfold values (Matiegka, 1921)) or it can be quantified by determinations of the total potassiums (^{40}K). The correlations between the other body masses and muscular strength support the assumption that body mass and lean or fat-free mass change in parallel with muscular mass, in a stochastic manner.

The variability in endurance capacity is due in part to differences in these body masses, but the importance of total body mass to specific ability is less clear. In answering this question, note that body dimensions affect endurance capacity in at least two ways (Fig. 4.1).

1 Muscular strength is correlated with muscle mass.

2 Total body mass (BM) is subject to the force of gravity (F_{grav}), although the impact on a particular endurance sport is not always given by the relationship BM/F_{grav}. This ratio is appropriate in track events, but the relationship is more complex in rowing, canoeing, swimming and cycling (where the gravitational effect of body mass is partly or almost completely offset by buoyancy, water displacement and/or the mass of auxillary equipment), and air or water resistance becomes the dominant influence (Fig. 4.2).

Terms stressing just one aspect, such as 'strength-endurance' or 'short, medium and long-term endurance' have become established in training circles (Thiess & Schnabel, 1985). The profile of sport-specific endurance which conditions the dominance of certain phenotypes in different types of endurance event is, however, determined by the relationship between the relative strength needed for a given sport and its duration (as stipulated by the rules and regulations of competition).

Anthropometric fundamentals

Effect of total body mass on endurance capacity

Differences of mean body mass (Table 4.1) reflect the differing profiles appropriate to various types of endurance sport (see Fig. 4.2). The lowest mean values are seen in sports where the body mass acts unrestrictedly against gravity. The average values are considerably higher in events requiring strength-endurance. Competitive duration also influences optimal body mass. The highest values are seen in sports of relatively short competitive duration (rowing, 6−7 min; swimming, 4−16 min), and

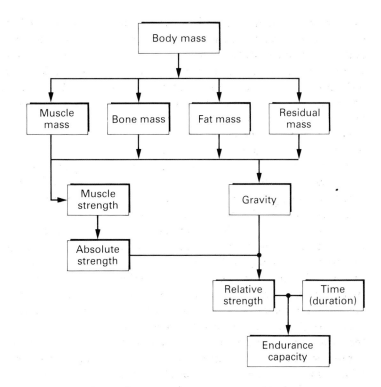

Fig. 4.1 Diagram showing the functional relationship between body mass and endurance.

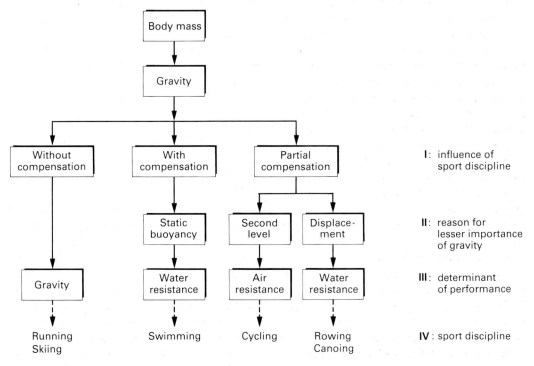

Fig. 4.2 Diagram illustrating the varying effects of gravity in different endurance disciplines.

Table 4.1 Typical body measurements in male endurance athletes.

Measurement	Running (m)					Walking (km)		Swimming (m)		Rowing
	1500	5000	10 000	Marathon	3000[‡]	20	50	400	1500	
Body height (cm)	178.6	176.6	174.7	171.8	173.7	177.4	178.4	179.5	179.4	189.5
Body mass (kg)	66.5	63.5	60.7	60.1	63.3	66.0	64.3	76.3	75.3	86.7
Sitting height (cm)	91.4	90.9	95.6	88.9	90.6	93.2	93.0	94.5	93.0	98.5
Arm length (cm)	76.9	77.1	76.6	74.9	76.1	78.2	78.3	79.1	81.3	82.9
Leg length* (cm)	88.0	87.4	85.4	83.6	84.3	84.8	85.9	86.6	88.2	92.6
Sitting height (%)[†]	51.2	51.5	54.7	51.7	52.2	52.5	52.1	52.6	51.8	52.0
Arm length (%)[†]	43.1	43.7	43.8	43.6	43.8	44.1	44.0	44.1	45.3	43.7
Leg length* (%)[†]	49.3	49.5	48.9	48.7	48.5	47.8	48.2	48.2	49.2	48.9

* Leg length = length of thigh + lower leg; [†] percentage of body height; [‡] steeplechase.

lower values are seen as the distance increases.

Relative strength can be optimized by increasing muscularity or by reducing body mass (thereby reducing the influence of gravity). A large body mass is advantageous in sports where the influence of gravity is partly or fully compensated. The ranking of mean body mass in various sports remains unchanged in spite of balancing differences of mean body height in the various types of endurance sport (Table 4.2).

The mean values of body mass also show sexual–morphological differences. In endurance-dominated sports (among others, increasing distances of track and field) the relative body mass values for women* show much larger reductions than those for men as the competitive distance is increased. In sports where strength-endurance is required (for example in rowing) women's relative values are again higher. Women achieve a higher relative strength in long-distance events by reducing their gravitational load (Tittel & Wutscherk, 1972), but they also need absolute strength: women must therefore accept greater amounts of bulk tissue (fat mass). This disadvantage

* The 'relative body mass' has been calculated as a percentage of mean values for a normal population (y) of given body height (x): men, y = −69.6 + 0.8x; women, y = −39.2 + 0.6x.

does not impair athletic performance in rowing, since the greater displacement of the boat resulting from an increase of body mass causes only a small increase in water resistance. The relative body mass (percentage of the predicted body mass; Wutscherk et al., 1988) can thus be used as a second criterion to characterize a somatotypic prediction for a particular endurance activity.

Effect of somatotypic characteristics on cardiovascular capacity

Endurance performance is affected not only by the capacity of the muscular system, but also by the systems supplying energy and removing endproducts. Davies (1978) proposed the relative maximal oxygen intake ($ml \cdot kg^{-1} \cdot min^{-1}$) as an indicator of cardiovascular performance, given that the $\dot{V}o_{2\,max}$ can also be viewed as 'a measure of aerobic energy transformation for a given time' (Neumann, 1981).

Following Wyndham (1971), the absolute maximal oxygen intake ($l \cdot min^{-1}$) is a linear function of body mass ($r = 0.76-0.96$; $p = 0.01$). Depending on somatotype, body masses (total body mass (BM), lean body mass (LBM) and muscle mass) show the closest correlation with $\dot{V}o_{2\,max}$ (equation 1). Body surface area (Fig. 4.3) and somatotype (equation 2) are, however, also differentiating values.

Table 4.2 Body height (BH), body mass (BM) and relative body mass (RBM) of competitors in the Olympic summer games of 1988.

Event	Finalists			Winners			Range of variation	
	BH (cm)	BM (kg)	RBM (%)	BH (cm)	BM (kg)	RBM (%)	BH (cm)	RBM (%)
Track and field								
Men								
800 m	184.4	69.6	89.3	186.0	72.0	90.9	178–193	85.2– 94.1
1500 m	177.3	63.0	87.0	167.0	53.0	82.8	165–186	82.8– 92.2
5000 m	177.3	62.9	87.1	175.0	63.0	89.5	169–184	85.2– 89.5
10 000 m	175.3	61.6	85.6	178.0	61.0	83.8	165–185	81.5– 89.8
Marathon	177.9	64.3	88.6	183.0	67.0	87.2	175–183	84.2– 92.3
3000 m*	180.0	67.9	91.2	174.0	62.0	89.1	174–188	86.5– 96.8
20 km (walking)	175.6	64.8	91.3	171.0	59.0	87.7	168–183	83.3–101.9
50 km (walking)	178.6	67.1	91.8	164.0	56.0	90.9	164–187	82.0–101.9
Women								
800 m	171.1	55.6	87.6	166.0	54.0	89.4	165–178	82.0– 92.7
1500 m	166.6	53.3	87.8	170.0	57.0	90.8	154–176	77.9– 92.9
3000 m	165.6	51.0	84.9	165.0	54.0	90.3	154–173	77.3– 92.1
10 000 m	163.4	46.6	80.1	154.0	41.0	77.1	154–172	73.0– 83.6
Marathon	162.0	47.6	82.1	157.0	44.0	80.0	147–170	76.2– 92.5
Freestyle swimming								
Men								
400 m	191.6	81.1	96.8	193.0	87.0	102.6	185–200	92.0–102.6
1500 m	190.8	82.3	97.6	181.0	74.0	98.4	181–200	92.0–102.6
Women								
400 m	174.5	61.6	93.8	166.0	44.0	74.5	166–181	74.5–101.7
800 m	175.4	63.0	95.1	166.0	44.0	74.5	166–187	74.5–101.7
Rowing								
Men								
Skiff	190.7	86.0	103.8	189.0	89.0	109.1	189–194	98.1–109.1
Double + four								
Without coxswain	193.2	92.5	108.9	—	—	—	188–200	95.9–115.3
With coxswain	193.8	92.9	109.0	—	—	—	182–205	97.4–121.3
Eight-oar	186.3	87.8	106.6	197.6	91.5	103.4	185–204	99.5–118.2
Women								
Skiff	174.3	71.0	108.6	181.0	75.0	108.1	168–181	107.4–110.4
Four with coxswain	181.3	77.9	111.9	184.0	79.5	111.6	172–186	106.3–116.4
Eight-oar	180.0	76.6	111.4	182.0	77.4	110.7	172–186	103.3–117.7
Cycling								
Men								
Road, single	178.3	73.6	101.0	182.0	82.0	107.9	170–196	94.7–107.9
Road, team	183.5	75.0	97.2	183.6	76.0	99.3	180–188	90.9–106.8
Women								
Road, single	166.9	59.4	97.5	168.0	61.0	99.0	162–175	92.0–100.0
Skiing†								
Men								
Northern	181.1	74.1	96.2	180.0	72.2	93.7	171–189	89.0–101.0
Biathlon	179.2	70.4	93.2	—	—	—	172–187	90.0– 98.0
Combination	174.7	65.5	91.3	—	—	—	170–182	87.0– 95.0
Women								
Northern	168.8	54.5	89.7	171.0	55.3	88.9	162–176	83.0– 96.0

* Steeplechase; † values of GDR national team.

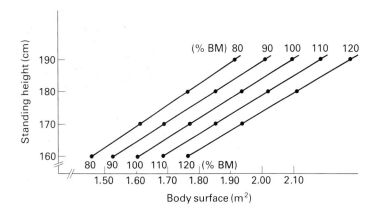

Fig. 4.3 The relationship of body surface area to standing height.

Men: $\dot{V}_{O_2\,max} = 0.042\,LBM + 0.579; r = 0.815$
        (LBM in kg)   (1)

Women: $\dot{V}_{O_2\,max} = 0.030\,LBM + 0.493; r = 0.493$
        (Taguchi, 1978)   (1)

Men: $\dot{V}_{O_2\,max}$ (ectomorph) $= 0.0819$
        BM $- 2.354; r = 0.95$ (BM in kg)   (2)
        $\dot{V}_{O_2\,max}$ (mesomorph) $= 0.0744$
        BM $- 1.579; r = 0.98$ (2)
        $\dot{V}_{O_2\,max}$ (endomorph) $= 0.0072$
        BM $- 2.901; r = 0.50$ (2)
        (Strydom, 1978)   (2)

There are also more or less tight relationships between various linear ($r = 0.22$; Strydom, 1978) and spatial ($r = 0.36-0.73$) measures and the percentage of body fat ($r = 0.26$; Mayhew & Gifford, 1975) and even the muscle fibre spectrum (slow-twitch fibres; $r = 0.67$; Bergh et al., 1978). The relationships between $\dot{V}_{O_2\,max}$ and body mass seem to be logically the most cogent, and effects upon endurance are lost if body mass is excluded (Kitagawa et al., 1978). However, this could be related to methodical insufficiencies, together with the typological and ethnic features of the population studied (Cureton, 1978). A lack of relationship to performance could also be explained by the fact that well trained athletes reach borderline values that differ little between heavy and light athletes, so that the best relationship between oxygen supply and supplied area occurs in competitors with the smallest body mass. Endurance athletes who are smaller have a much smaller body surface area, even if their

total body masses are equal in relation to their standing height (Fig. 4.3). Body surface area at a relative body mass of 80–120% ranges from 1.46 to 1.73 m^2 if the standing height is 160 cm, but it increases to 1.91 and 2.27 m^2 at 190 cm. These findings support the very low relative body masses observed in endurance athletes, and show the tendency of lower heights to enhance performance particularly in events where the projected body surface is a major competitive factor.

Effect of standing height on endurance

Increasing standing height on average increases: (a) the body mass, body surface area and body volume; and (b) the leverage of the muscles. Irrespective of whether the relationship between body mass and height is linear (Noack et al., 1985) or non-linear (Martirosov, 1982), there is agreement that the force relative to body mass becomes larger as body mass decreases. Endurance athletes have a below-average height to mass ratio; this characteristic can be seen for both men and women, for instance in the mean values for finalists and placed athletes in the Seoul summer Olympics (1988) (Figs 4.4a & b). The graphs also demonstrate that competitors in the strength- or power-endurance events can be separated from those contesting 'pure' endurance events, as would be predicted on theoretical grounds (see Fig. 4.2).

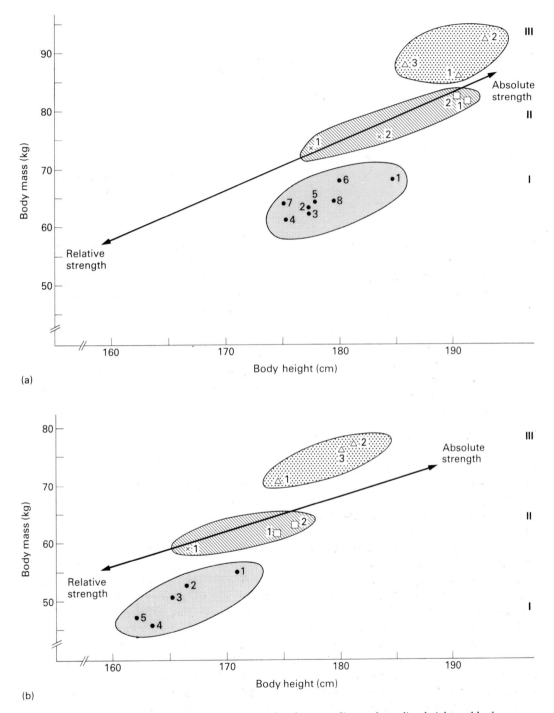

Fig. 4.4 Categories of endurance sport participants placed on coordinate of standing height and body mass: (a) men; (b) women. I, 'pure' endurance; II, 'speed' endurance; III, 'strength' endurance. ●, Track and field: 1, 800 m; 2, 1500 m; 3, 5000 m; 4, 10 000 m; 5, marathon; 6, 3000 m (steeplechase); 7, 20 km (walking); 8, 50 km (walking). ×, Cycling: 1, road race (single); 2, road race (team). □, Swimming: 1, 400 m (freestyle); 2, 1500 m (freestyle). △, Rowing: 1, skiff; 2, double skull and four skull (with and without coxswain); 3, eight-oar.

The advantage that tall athletes might have, particularly in track events, results from the greater leverage of long limbs. Assuming a constant applied force, longer levers allow a larger amplitude of movement (stride length), but also require a lower stride frequency for economical movement. Based on somatotypic characteristics, an athlete will achieve good or very good results by using a long stride length (SL), or a high stride frequency (SF) or by an optimal combination of the two. The average velocity depends on the product of $SL \times SF$ ($m \cdot s^{-1}$).

These factors explain why fatigue over a given training distance can be delayed by a greater motor efficiency attributable to a somatotypic advantage. In track sprinting, the relationship between anthropometric and stride characteristics has been demonstrated several times (Hoffmann, 1964; Wutscherk, 1977; Wutscherk & Tittel, 1982). Similar relationships can be assumed for middle and long-distance runners, although Alexander and Thiessen (1983) leave the choice of stride pattern to the runner. An analysis of female 400-metre runners has demonstrated that the better runners are indeed shorter (165.7 and 173.2 cm, respectively), but are also able to use their somatotypic characteristics to better advantage because of their greater strength, reaching longer stride lengths (1.84 and 1.74 m, respectively), without substantial reduction of stride frequencies (3.29 and 3.28 s^{-1}, respectively). Fatigue was delayed in the better runners, particularly during the last stage of the 400-metre race, because their stride lengths decreased by only a small extent. It seems advantageous for the runner to select an (optimal) stride length appropriate to body build. The blood lactate concentration rises more steeply with an excessive frequency of stride than with the use of longer strides.

Differentiation of body proportions among endurance athletes

There are almost no representative data on performance-determining body proportions in top-class endurance athletes. DeGaray et al. (1974) presented the last useful set of data on participants in the 1972 Olympic Summer Games. In later publications, such data have unfortunately been pooled without due reference to event or sport. That is why Table 4.2 includes anthropometric values for world-class former GDR athletes in the endurance sports mentioned.

Functionally the most important and interesting values are body measurements directly related to the motor process, as determinants of stride amplitude and frequency. In track events, the critical feature is leg length, or the lengths of the thigh and the leg (since both parameters contribute to the amplitude of movement, while thigh length has a negative correlation with limb frequency). In swimmers, the arm length influences propulsive leverage, as does leg length. In rowing and canoeing the sitting height (trunk length) is also important, in addition to the factors mentioned above.

Somatotype of endurance athletes

When evaluating these measurements, it does not seem to be useful to consider only proportional differences between sports, although statistical procedures support them (DeGaray et al., 1974). Carter et al. (1982) show somatotype ratings ranging from 7.1.1. through 4.4.4. to 1.1.7., with men situated in the mesomorph, extreme mesomorph or between endomorph and ectomorph ranges (mesomorph component = 1); however, such findings are not representative of women. Athletes are positioned in a much narrower spectrum than that provided by the overall scheme. The mean somatotypes of high-class endurance athletes (Olympic participants, and international top-class ranking members of the former GDR national team) have been relatively constant over the years. Figures 4.5a−e therefore present a stable impression of body form.

Two methods are currently used to determine somatotype: the Heath−Carter procedure and the Conrad method. Both procedures result in comparable findings, despite methodological

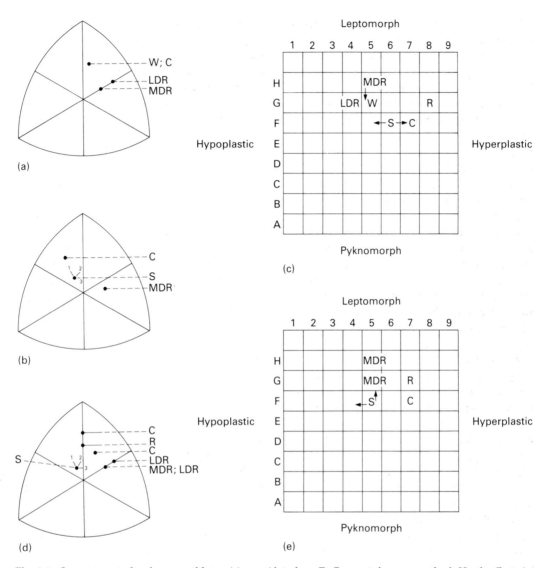

Fig. 4.5 Somatotypes of endurance athletes: (a) men (data from DeGaray *et al.*, 1974; method: Heath−Carter); (b) men (data from Tanner, 1964; method: Sheldon); (c) men (data from Wutscherk, 1981; method: Conrad); (d) women (data from DeGaray *et al.*, 1974; method: Heath−Carter); (e) women (data from Wutscherk, 1981; method: Conrad). C, Canoeing; LDR, long-distance running; MDR, middle-distance running; R, rowing; S, swimming (S₁, breast stroke; S₂, back stroke; S₃, freestyle); W, walking.

differences:

1 Athletes competing in 'pure' endurance events differ from those in strength-endurance events.

2 The former represent a medium type of body build, situated halfway between the meso-morph and the ectomorph pole on Heath−Carter's scheme, and expressed in Conrad's coordinate scheme by medium leptomorphy (metroplastic). Strength-endurance athletes, in contrast, are characterized by a strong mesomorphy.

3 In Conrad's scheme (1963), the somatotypes of male and female athletes correspond with each other for all endurance sports. In Heath and Carter's scheme (1967), the positions are different; only the swimmers from the two sexes have a similar body build.

Somatotypes can thus offer a first impression of predisposition towards specific sports or events. However, similar information can be deduced from the base data (for instance, standing height and relative body mass). The new understanding of sport type (Wutscherk, 1977; Wutscherk & Tittel, 1982) is no longer related simply to a certain phenotype, but reflects the way in which differences of body measurements affect function.

Summary

'Endurance' implies the relationship between the muscular strength required for a given sport and time. Somatotypic characteristics (body mass, fractional body masses, standing height and somatotype) are useful measures of such endurance. There are differences in optimal body mass between participants in various endurance events, shaping the athlete's phenotype markedly. From a functional point of view, body mass influences both muscular strength and gravitational forces. Endurance sports can be categorized by evaluating these differing effects. Data on participants at the 1988 Olympic summer games support the logical correctness of these deductions, demonstrating in particular that participants in endurance events, where total body mass must be supported against gravity, weigh very little. On the other hand, in endurance sports where gravity is partly or completely compensated, the body mass lies close to or even above average values. These are typically strength-requiring events, with a relatively short competitive duration. 'Relative body mass' (%) characterizes endurance well, although the muscle mass (which is highly correlated with total body mass) is the underlying structural factor.

Prolonged muscular exercise depends not only on the somatically non-quantifiable internal structure of the skeletal musculature, but also, more importantly, on the energy supply.

The $\dot{V}_{O_2 max}$ is a measure of maximal aerobic energy transformation that depends strongly on body dimensions. The closest relationships are with body masses, but standing height is also related, and the practical value of $\dot{V}_{O_2 max}$ is also affected by the relationships of body surface area to standing height. In 'pure' endurance events, medium or short height is an advantage. However, taller athletes gain from a greater leverage, allowing movements of greater amplitude, with a greater economy of action.

Despite differences of methodology, Heath–Carter (1967) and Conrad (1963) somatotyping lead to similar conclusions. Neither yields findings that contradict ideas deduced directly from measured data.

The physician who is caring for endurance athletes should monitor body masses, setting an optimal 'competitive weight', and optimizing this in terms of the relative proportions of muscle mass and fat mass.

References

Alexander, M.J.L. & Thiessen, P.J. (1983) The relationship between stride parameters and oxygen uptake in middle distance runners during a maximal treadmill test. *J. Hum. Mv. Studies* **9**, 105.

Bergh, U., Thorstensson, A.J. & Sjödin, B. (1978) Maximal oxygen uptake and muscle fiber types in trained and untrained humans. *Med. Sci. Sports* **10**, 151.

Carter, J.E.L., Hebbelinck, M. & de Garay, A. (1978) Anthropometric profiles of Olympic athletes at Mexico City. In: F. Landry & W.A.R. Orban (eds) *International Congress of Physical Activity Sciences: Biomechanics of Sports and Kinanthropometry*, Vol. 6, pp. 305–312. Symposia Specialists, Miami, Florida.

Carter, J.E.L., Aubry, S.P. & Sleet, D.A. (1982) Somatotypes of Montreal Olympic athletes. In: E. Jokl (ed.) *Medicine and Sport*, Vol. 16, pp. 53–80. Karger, Basel.

Conrad, K. (1963) *Der Konstitutionstypus*. Springer Verlag, Berlin.

Cureton, T.K. Jr. (1978) Physique, performance and oxygen intake capacity. In: F. Landry & W.A.R. Orban (eds) *International Congress of Physical Activity Sciences: Biomechanics of Sports and Kinanthropometry*, Vol. 6. pp. 623–633. Symposia Specialists, Miami, Florida.

Davies, C.T.M. (1978) A reference standard for

maximal aerobic power output during weight-supported work with the arms or legs. In: F. Landry & W.A.R. Orban (eds) *International Congress of Physical Activity Sciences: Biomechanics of Sports and Kinanthropometry*, Vol. 6, pp. 297–303. Symposia Specialists, Miami, Florida.

DeGaray, A.L., Levine, L. & Carter, J.E.L. (1974) *Genetic and Anthropological Studies of Olympic Athletes*. Academic Press, New York.

Grimm, H. (1966) *Grundriß der Konstitutionsbiologie und Anthropometrie*. Volk u.Gesundheit, Berlin.

Heath, B.H. & Carter, J.E.L. (1967) A modified somatotype method. *Am. J. Phys. Anthropol.* **27**, 57.

Hoffmann, K. (1964) Die Abhängigkeit der Schrittlänge und Schritt-frequenz von ausgewählten morphologischen Eigenschaften. *Kult. fiz.* **17**, 541.

Kitagawa, K., Yamamoto, K. & Miyashita, M. (1978) Maximal oxygen uptake, body composition and running performance in Japanese young adults of both sexes. In: F. Landry & W.A.R. Orban (eds) *International Congress of Physical Activity Sciences: Biomechanics of Sports and Kinanthropometry*, Vol. 6, pp. 553–561. Symposia Specialists, Miami, Florida.

Kohlrausch, W. (1927) Sporttypen. In: H. Rautmann (ed.) *Arzt und Skilauf*. Fischer, Jena.

Kunze, D., Hughes, P.G.R. & Tanner, J.M. (1976) *Anthropometrische Untersuchungen an Sportlern der XX Olympischen Spiele 1972 in München*. Gräfelfing.

Martirosov, E.G. (1982) *Metody issledovanija v sportivnoj antropologii*. Moskva.

Matiegka, J. (1921) The testing of physical efficiency. *Am. J. Phys. Anthropol.* **4**, 223.

Mayhew, J.L. & Gifford, B.P. (1975) Prediction of maximal oxygen intake in preadolescent boys from anthropometric parameters. *Res. Quart.* **46**, 302.

Neumann, G. (1981) *Ausgewählte sportmedizinische Beiträge zur Leistungssportentwicklung in der Sportartengruppe Ausdauer*. Dtsch. Hochsch. Körperkult., Leipzig.

Noack, R., Möhr, M. & Hust, L. (1985) Das wünschenswerte Körpergewicht. *Ernährungsforsch.* **30**, 144.

Ross, W.D. (1978) Kinanthropometry: an emerging scientific technology. In: F. Landry & W.A.R. Orban (eds) *International Congress of Physical Activity Sciences: Biomechanics of Sports and Kinanthropometry*, Vol. 6, pp. 269–282. Symposia Specialists, Miami, Florida.

Ross, W.D. & Wilson, N.C. (1974) A stratagem for proportional growth assessment. In: J. Borms & M. Hebbelinck (eds) *Children in Exercise*, pp. 169–182.

Stepnicka, J. (1981) Beziehungen zwischen den Somatotypen und der körperlichen Grundleistungsfähigkeit. *Med. Sport* **21**, 83.

Strydom, N.B. (1978) The relationship of maximum oxygen intake to gross body mass and somatotype. In: F. Landry & W.A.R. Orban (eds) *International Congress of Physical Activity Sciences: Exercise Physiology*, Vol. 4, pp. 571–580. Symposia Specialists, Miami, Florida.

Taguchi, S. (1978) Age and sex trends in aerobic capacity related to lean body mass of Japanese from childhood to maturity. In: F. Landry & W.A.R. Orban (eds) *International Congress of Physical Activity Sciences: Exercise Physiology*, Vol. 4, pp. 581–588. Symposia Specialists, Miami, Florida.

Tanner, J.M. (1964) *The Physique of the Olympic Athlete*. Allen & Unwin, London.

Thiess, G. & Schnabel, G. (1985) *Grundbegriffe des Trainings*. Sport-Verlag, Berlin.

Tittel, K. & Wutscherk, H. (1972) *Sportanthropometrie*. Barth, Leipzig.

Wutscherk, H. (1977) *Grundzüge der Methodologie der Sportanthropometrie*. D. Sc. Dissertation, University of Leipzig.

Wutscherk, H. (1981) *Grundlagen der Sportanthropometrie*. Dtsch. Hochsch. Körperkult., Leipzig.

Wutscherk, H. & Tittel, K. (1982) On the problem of the sports type. In: *Proceedings of the Second Anthropological Congress of Ales Hrdlicka*. Charls University, Prague.

Wutscherk, H., Schmidt, H. & Schulze, S. (1988) Zur Beurteilung der Körpermasse bei Kindern und Jugendlichen. *Med. Sport* **28**, 177.

Wyndham, G.H. (1971) The influence of body weight on energy expenditure during walking on a road and on a treadmill. *Int. Z. angew. Physiol.* **29**, 285.

Chapter 5

Cellular Metabolism and Endurance

JAN HENRIKSSON

The capacity of skeletal muscle cells for adaptation to changes in metabolic demand has been shown to be quite remarkable and it is a well known fact that endurance training induces marked adaptive changes in several structural components and metabolic variables in the engaged skeletal muscles. Among the observed changes with different training regimens are those involving the muscle's content of metabolic enzymes, the sensitivity to hormones and the composition of the contracting filaments. Other adaptations affect membrane transport processes and the muscular capillary network. Since these adaptive changes occur regularly in response to endurance training, these factors are likely to be important determinants of an individual's physical working capacity. The adaptive changes in metabolic enzymes and capillaries are among the most well described consequences of endurance training and are probably also among the most important ones for the muscle's capacity to perform prolonged work. This chapter is devoted to a closer look at the cellular adaptation to endurance training, particularly with regard to changes in these two variables.

How to determine the metabolic capacity of skeletal muscle

The introduction of the muscle biopsy procedure (Bergström, 1962), whereby small (10–100 mg) muscle pieces can be sampled, and the development of sensitive biochemical techniques have made it possible to estimate the capacity of different metabolic pathways in human muscle. Using micromethods, this can be done even at the single fibre level (Lowry & Passonneau, 1972). The most important metabolic pathways for energy delivery in exercising muscle are glycolysis/glycogenolysis, fatty acid oxidation, the citric acid cycle and the respiratory chain (for a detailed discussion see Chapter 23). The capacity of a metabolic pathway is limited mainly by the amount of pathway enzymes contained in the cell. In this context, some enzymes, the rate-limiting or flux-generating ones, are more important than others. Such an enzyme has low activity and constitutes a bottleneck in a pathway. Therefore, theoretically, an increased concentration of the rate-limiting enzyme with unchanged concentrations of the other pathway enzymes would be sufficient to increase the capacity of the entire metabolic pathway (see Newsholme & Leech, 1983). Generally, however, with a change in the capacity of a metabolic pathway, perhaps as a result of training or inactivity, the content of all enzymes, whether rate-limiting or not, changes in the same direction. This can be illustrated by the changes recorded in the anterior tibial muscle of the rabbit in response to chronic electrical stimulation. In this situation there is an almost identical decrease in all glycolytic and glycogenolytic enzymes, although only one, phosphofructokinase, is considered to be rate limiting (Figs 5.1 & 5.2). The reason for this is not entirely clear, but it may

Fig. 5.1 Enzyme changes induced by chronic electrical muscle stimulation. The rabbit anterior tibial muscle was stimulated at 10 impulses per second, 24 h a day, for different periods of time (from 3 days to 10 weeks). The figure depicts changes in the muscle content of three oxidative and two glycolytic enzymes. SDH (succinate dehydrogenase), CS (citrate synthase) and MDH (malate dehydrogenase) are enzymes in the citric acid cycle; LDH (lactate dehydrogenase) and PFK (6-phosphofructokinase) are involved in glycolysis. The value for unstimulated control muscles has been set at 100%. From Henriksson *et al.* (1986), modified with permission.

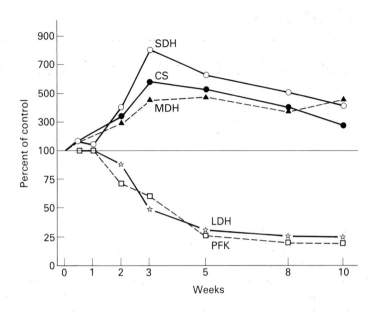

Fig. 5.2 Enzyme changes induced by chronic electrical muscle stimulation. HAD (3-hydroxyacyl coenzyme A dehydrogenase) represents the fat degradation (the fatty acid oxidation) system and phosphorylase and phosphoglucomutase represent glycolysis. The main function of the enzyme HK (hexokinase) is to make glucose, taken up from the blood, available to the muscle cell by channelling it into the glycolytic pathway. For further explanations, see the text to Fig. 5.1. From Henriksson *et al.* (1986), modified with permission.

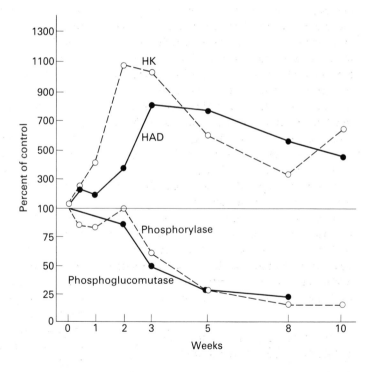

be that relatively constant proportions of the different enzymes in a certain metabolic pathway are necessary in order to maintain the metabolic equilibrium of a cell. It is therefore possible to obtain a good estimation of the cellular capacity of a specific metabolic pathway simply by measuring the content (maximal activity) of any one of its enzymes. The choice of enzymes for analyses is therefore largely dependent on the simplicity and speed of the available analytical methods. Below is a list of enzymes, the levels of which are commonly used as a measure of the capacity of their respective metabolic pathways: (i) *glycolysis*: phosphofructokinase (PFK), lactate dehydrogenase (LDH); (ii) *fatty acid oxidation*: 3-hydroxyacyl coenzyme A dehydrogenase (HAD); (iii) *citric acid cycle*: citrate synthase (CS), succinate dehydrogenase (SDH); and (iv) *respiratory chain*: cytochrome c oxidase. The location of these enzymes in the pathways is shown in Fig. 23.5.

The maximal adaptability of skeletal muscle — effects of chronic electrical stimulation

It is of considerable theoretical interest to know how skeletal muscle adapts to a maximal training stimulus. This knowledge can then be used as a frame of reference, against which the effects of, for instance, different endurance training regimens can be compared and evaluated. One way to obtain such information has been to subject a normally rather inactive muscle, such as the rabbit anterior tibial muscle, to chronic electrical stimulation. This can be done in a way that is essentially painless to the animal. During anaesthesia, a stimulator (of fingertip size) is implanted under aseptic conditions. When activated, it subjects the anterior tibial muscle to chronic stimulation via the common peroneal nerve. The stimulator is activated non-invasively by means of an electronic flashgun after the rabbit has been allowed to recover from the operation. When stimulating with a continuous train of pulses at a frequency of 10 Hz, as in most studies, there is a very small-amplitude oscillation of the hindpaw but without any observable effect on either the use of the limb in posture control and locomotion or the general wellbeing of the animal.

These investigations have revealed a quite remarkable capacity of skeletal muscle for adaptation to the extreme metabolic demand imposed by chronic stimulation. This response is therefore described in some detail before discussing the effects of more physiological endurance training regimens.

The rabbit anterior tibial muscle is predominantly a fast muscle, containing not more than 6% of slow-twitch fibres. However, the chronic stimulation programme results in a striking fibre-type transformation so that after stimulation durations of 5–6 weeks or more, the anterior tibial muscle contains only slow-twitch fibres. Simultaneously, the normally very fatiguable anterior tibial muscle becomes highly fatigue resistant. The increased endurance is most likely mainly a result of the pronounced enzyme and microcirculatory adaptation induced by chronic stimulation, but fibre-type transformation may also be of major importance in this respect. For a more detailed description of the effects of chronic stimulation on muscles, see reviews by Salmons and Henriksson (1981), Jolesz and Sreter (1981), and Pette (1984).

Enzyme adaptation

The stimulation-induced enzyme changes are summarized in Figs 5.1 and 5.2. Of all enzymes analysed, hexokinase shows the most rapid response to chronic stimulation. The main function of this enzyme is to channel (phosphorylate) glucose, taken up by muscle, into the muscle cell's glycolytic pathway. A hexokinase increase (which on chronic stimulation was 11-fold at its peak) is not normally seen in endurance training, but it illustrates the capacity of skeletal muscle to adapt rapidly to the use of blood glucose as the preferred energy substrate. The absence of a hexokinase increase on endurance training makes sense physiologically, since, with a large trained muscle mass, a large consumption of blood-derived glucose during exercise would rapidly override the capacity of the liver to replenish the consumed blood glucose.

The enzymes of the citric acid cycle and the fatty acid β-oxidation also display large increases on stimulation, but the increases occur somewhat later. In our investigations maximal changes (6–12-fold) were reached after 2–5 weeks. Thereafter the enzyme concentrations decreased somewhat before stabilizing at a lower level (Fig. 5.1). It is not known whether this two-phase pattern of change is specific for chronic stimulation or whether it may also occur with certain endurance training programmes. However, to date there has been no report that this occurs in response to endurance training in humans or in any other species. Instead, the glycolytic enzymes, as well as creatine kinase (i.e. enzymes supplying energy to the muscle during short-term, intense exercise), decrease drastically with chronic stimulation. After 2 months of continuous stimulation only one fifth of the initial glycolytic enzyme content remains in the anterior tibial muscle. On discontinuing stimulation, the enzymes whose activity had increased again decline towards the initial level, at first rapidly and later more slowly, and return to normal after 5–6 weeks. This is also true of the glycolytic enzymes,

which increase when stimulation is stopped, but with these enzymes normalization occurs more rectilinearly (Brown et al., 1989).

Figure 5.3 shows that the normally large variation in enzyme content among different fibres in the same muscle, and even between those of the same type, is reduced with chronic stimulation. No corresponding information is available with regard to the effect of endurance training, although some information can be found in Chi et al. (1983).

Other stimulation-induced changes

There is a doubling of the number of blood capillaries per unit muscle cross-sectional area, thus greatly improving the muscle's blood supply (Brown et al., 1976). The time-course of this change has not been studied in detail, but preliminary data indicate that it is roughly similar to that of the oxidative enzymes. Con-

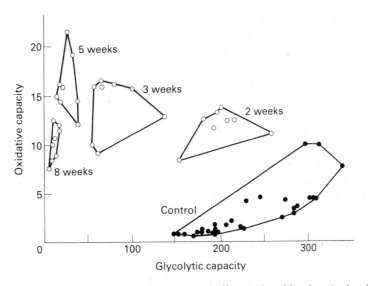

Fig. 5.3 Changes of enzyme activity in single skeletal muscle fibres induced by chronic electrical muscle stimulation. The anterior tibial muscle of the rabbit was stimulated as described in the text to Fig. 5.1. Single fibres were isolated by microdissection from muscles stimulated for different periods of time (2, 3, 5 and 8 weeks respectively) as well as from unstimulated control muscles. The fibres were subsequently analysed for two enzymes, citrate synthase, as a measure of the fibre's oxidative capacity, and fructose bisphosphatase, as a measure of its glycolytic capacity. Citrate synthase is a member of the citric acid cycle and fructose bisphosphatase catalyses the reversal of the 6-phosphofructokinase reaction in glycolysis. As is evident from the figure, all fibres in a normal unstimulated (control) muscle have a high content of glycolytic enzymes, whereas the content of oxidative enzymes varies 10-fold. The chronic stimulation induces a high oxidative capacity in all fibres, whereas the glycolytic capacity decreases to low levels. Units are mol (citrate synthase) or mmol (fructose bisphosphatase) kg^{-1} dry weight h^{-1} at 20°C. From Chi et al. (1986), with permission.

comitant with these changes there is, as mentioned above, a dramatic improvement in the muscle's endurance. In our investigations this variable has been measured as an index: the remaining muscle force following a 5-min protocol of intense muscle stimulation divided by the muscle force exerted during the first few contractions. This index increases from a normal value of 0.5 to 1.0 in muscle that has been continuously stimulated for 6 weeks. Following discontinuation of the chronic stimulation, the fatiguability again increases, the time needed for normalization (5–6 weeks) being similar to that of the metabolic enzymes and the capillary supply. An interesting general observation from these chronic stimulation experiments is that the different biochemical and morphological adaptations to chronic stimulation fit into a 'first in, last out' pattern for the response to stimulation and recovery. This means that the earlier the stage at which a parameter changes during the course of stimulation, the later the stage at which it returns to control levels during recovery. For further information on this, see Brown et al. (1989).

This summary of what is likely to be the maximal activity-induced adaptability of skeletal muscle will serve as a background to a description of the effect of endurance training on skeletal muscle characteristics.

Effects of endurance training on human muscle

Background

The first observations of the effects of endurance training on metabolic enzymes in skeletal muscle (rat) were made by Russian investigators in the 1950s, but a detailed investigation of these changes was first performed by Holloszy et al. (see Holloszy & Booth, 1976). That the capillary network of rat skeletal muscle was influenced by training had already been shown in 1937 by Petrén et al. The first human studies on muscle metabolic enzymes were published around 1970 (Varnauskas et al., 1970; Morgan et al., 1971). During the 1970s and

1980s improved methodology allowed more detailed studies both on humans and other species. For the human studies small muscle biopsy specimens (20–100 mg) were obtained, usually from the thigh muscle, but also from other muscles such as the gastrocnemius, deltoid and the triceps of the upper arm. In these studies different groups of individuals were compared, e.g. untrained persons vs. athletes in different sports, or, alternatively, a group of previously untrained individuals was studied repeatedly with muscle biopsies taken during a training period. In spite of the fact that different parts of the same muscle may often differ with regard to fibre-type composition, capillary density and enzyme content, the muscle biopsy technique has proved surprisingly useful for these studies. With this technique, even small changes may be detected, such as a change in enzyme content or capillary density of 15–20%, when a group of five or six subjects is studied with single biopsies before and after training. Generally, however, the biopsy technique is not sensitive enough to allow conclusions to be drawn from the analysis of a single sample. With several samples from the same muscle, the methodological error is markedly reduced.

Enzyme changes

An illustration of the effects of endurance training on human muscle is the observed differences between endurance athletes and untrained individuals (Fig. 5.4). With regard to oxidative enzymes (i.e. enzymes of fatty acid oxidation, the citric acid cycle and the respiratory chain), the contents are approximately three times higher in the trained thigh muscle of the athletes than in the thigh muscle of untrained individuals. With total inactivity, such as muscle encased in plaster after an injury, the oxidative enzyme contents decrease to 70–75% of the 'untrained level'. It can be speculated that lower levels than this would not be compatible with survival of the muscle cell. The maximal range of oxidative enzyme content in the human thigh muscle is therefore approximately fourfold, but it may be supposed that a

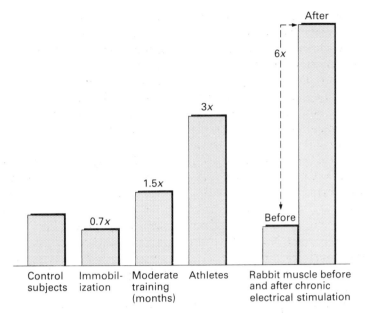

Fig. 5.4 Influence of physical fitness level on skeletal muscle oxidative capacity, measured as the content of citrate synthase. Muscle tissue from normal sedentary individuals has been compared to muscle subjected to encasement in plaster after injury or to 2−3 months of moderate endurance training as well as to values recorded in top-class cyclists and long-distance runners. As a further comparison, the corresponding values from the rabbit anterior tibial muscle before and after 3−5 weeks of chronic electrical stimulation are indicated on the right. (The human data have generously been placed at my disposal by Dr Eva Jansson, Department of Clinical Physiology, Karolinska Hospital, Stockholm, Sweden; the results regarding chronic stimulation are from Henriksson *et al.*, 1986.)

very long training time would be required for an individual to cover this whole range. A comparison with chronically stimulated rabbit muscle (Fig. 5.4) reveals that muscles of endurance athletes have approximately 40% lower levels of oxidative enzymes than these chronically stimulated muscles. The difference with respect to fat oxidation enzymes is somewhat higher. Ignoring possible differences between the rabbit and humans, this result may be taken to indicate that the trained muscles of our best endurance athletes have an oxidative capacity that is one half to two thirds of the theoretically attainable maximal level.

Another important question concerns the magnitude of the enzyme changes that can be attained with a few weeks or months of more moderate endurance training regimens. Here, information is available from a large number of investigations, in which different research groups have studied the effects of 2−3 months

of training on the oxidative enzyme content of leg or arm muscles. These studies have usually involved bouts of 30−60 min of exercise at intensities corresponding to 70−80% of $\dot{V}_{O_2 max}$, from three to five times per week. With a group of previously untrained individuals, the general finding is an approximately 40−50% increase in the content of oxidative enzymes in the trained muscles (Fig. 5.5). This increase occurs gradually over 6−8 weeks, with the most rapid change taking place during the first 3 weeks of training (see Saltin & Gollnick, 1983).

Importance of exercise intensity and duration of training

Data from experimental animals

A question of practical importance is the intensity and duration of training needed to obtain

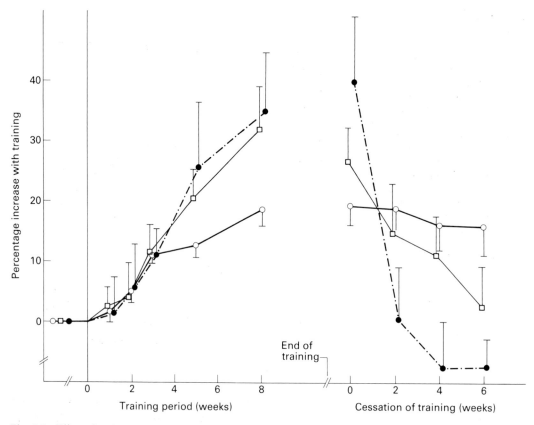

Fig. 5.5 Effect of endurance training on the content of oxidative enzymes in human skeletal muscle. A group of previously untrained subjects trained for 8–10 weeks on cycle ergometers (40 min·day^{-1}, 4 days per week; the rate of work corresponded to 80% of the maximal oxygen intake). Biopsy samples were obtained from the thigh muscle at different intervals during the training period as well as 2, 4 and 6 weeks after the cessation of training (after 8–10 weeks). The muscle samples were analysed for the oxidative enzymes succinate dehydrogenase (of the citric acid cycle) (□) and cytochrome c oxidase (the last enzyme of the respiratory chain) (●). In addition, the subjects' maximal oxygen intake was determined using the Douglas bag technique (○). It is noteworthy that, in the post-training period, the whole-body $\dot{V}o_{2\ max}$ is maintained significantly longer than the muscle oxidative enzyme content. From Henriksson & Reitman (1977), modified with permission.

optimal results with respect to enzyme adaptation. For an untrained but not inactive person, some increase in the muscle content of oxidative enzymes can be obtained by fairly light running (jogging), but the enzyme adaptation becomes much more marked if the training intensities are increased to power levels demanding 70–80% of the individual's $\dot{V}o_{2\ max}$. In theory, even higher training intensities would result in a further enhancement of the muscle's oxidative capacity, but in practical

terms this may not be so, because another important factor is the duration of the training bouts. There are no conclusive human data illustrating this interdependency between exercise intensity and duration, but interesting information can be obtained from a detailed study on the rat by Dudley and colleagues (1982). These authors subjected rats to training in the form of treadmill running 5 days per week for 2 months at varying speeds and daily training times (Fig. 5.6). The rats trained at six

Fig. 5.6 Effects of endurance training on the oxidative enzyme content of different muscles in the rat. The rats were trained on a treadmill 5 days per week for 2 months at varying running speeds (usually 45–60 min daily). The muscle content of cytochrome c, a respiratory chain component, was used as an indicator of muscle oxidative capacity. The three muscles studied were chosen to represent different fibre types: deep thigh muscle, fast-twitch oxidative glycolytic (type IIA) fibres (○); soleus muscle, slow-twitch (type I) fibres (●); and superficial thigh muscle, fast-twitch glycolytic (type IIB) fibres (■). The approximate percentage of the rat's maximal oxygen intake demanded at each speed is also indicated. From Dudley *et al.* (1982), modified with permission.

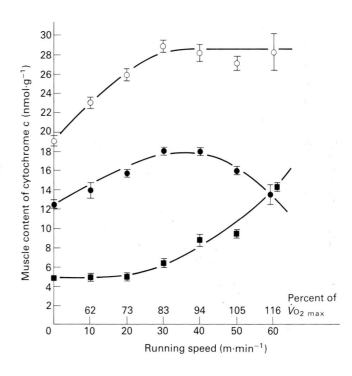

different running speeds, demanding approximately 60%, 70%, 80%, 95%, 105% and 115% of their maximal oxygen intake. At the two highest speeds, the exercise was performed intermittently. For each speed, the muscle enzyme adaptation increased with the duration of the daily exercise, but no additional training effect was noted when the daily duration exceeded 45–60 min. At the two highest speeds, the rats could tolerate exercise for only 30 and 15 min daily, but this was sufficient for marked training effects to occur. As might be expected, the initial period of the daily exercise bout gave the highest training effect per unit of training time, with successively smaller effects for the following periods.

Fibre-type differences

An interesting observation in the study by Dudley *et al.* (1982) was that the training response differed markedly between fibre types. For a training effect to occur in the fast glycolytic fibres (type IIB), the exercise intensity had to require at least 80% of the rat's $\dot{V}_{O_2\,max}$ (Fig. 5.6). Higher running speeds gave successively better training effects in this fibre type. On the contrary, for the fast oxidative glycolytic fibre type (IIA), the training effect increased with increasing speeds up to an intensity (speed) demanding 80% of $\dot{V}_{O_2\,max}$. Higher running speeds did not result in an enhanced training effect. The slow-twitch fibre type (type I) responded in yet another fashion. In this fibre type, the training effect increased up to a running speed demanding 95% of the $\dot{V}_{O_2\,max}$. Paradoxically, higher speeds than this resulted in a decreased training effect. These fibre-type-specific training effects are most likely to be explained by a specific recruitment pattern of different rat muscles during running. The deep part of the thigh muscle, which was the source of the IIA fibres in the cited study, is fully activated during running at 30 m·min^{-1}, and consequently this training speed results in a maximal training effect. The superficial part of the thigh muscle, which was the source of the IIB fibres, has a higher activation threshold. No training effect is therefore seen at low running speeds, but above the activation threshold there is a linear relationship between running speed and training effect. The soleus muscle, which contains exclusively slow-twitch (type I) fibres, is fully activated at 30 m·min^{-1}. Therefore, higher running speeds than this would not be expected to increase the training effect. There is, however, no obvious explanation of the finding in the study by Dudley *et al.* (1982) that higher running speeds than 30 m·min^{-1} resulted in a successively diminished training effect in this muscle.

Conclusions

Can these findings in the rat be used to predict effects of endurance training in humans? The answer is likely to be yes, provided that the different conditions in the two species are taken into account. One important difference is that, in the rat, the different fibre types are largely located in different muscles or in different parts of one muscle, whereas most human muscles are mixed muscles, with all fibre types occurring intermingled in a mosaic pattern. The procedure of using results from different muscles or muscle groups to illustrate the behaviour of a specific fibre type, as is often done especially in rodent studies, may not be entirely correct. The reason is that fibres of a specific type in one muscle often differ markedly from fibres of the same histochemical type located in another muscle. One example of this is the finding that slow-twitch (type I) fibres in the rabbit tibialis anterior muscle have approximately three times as high concentrations of both oxidative and glycolytic enzymes as fibres of the same type in the rabbit soleus muscle. Similarly, the content of glycolytic enzymes has been found to be twice as high in type IIB fibres of the rabbit psoas muscle as in type IIB fibres in the anterior tibial muscle (see Chi *et al.*, 1986).

Regardless of these precautions, the rat data clearly illustrate that knowledge of the fibre-type recruitment pattern during exercise is essential when trying to predict the effects of different training regimens. For humans, quite detailed information is available on cycle ergometer exercise at different power levels. It has been shown that, as in the rat, the slow-twitch (type I) muscle fibres are the first to be activated and are kept activated even at higher exercise intensities. With increasing rates of work there is a recruitment of the fast-twitch motor units, type IIA followed by type IIB. It is believed that fibres (motor units) of all types are recruited at exercise intensities demanding more than 80–85% of the $\dot{V}o_{2\,max}$. However, very strenuous exercise is probably required to activate maximally all the type IIB motor units in a given muscle (for references see Saltin & Gollnick, 1983).

This fibre-type recruitment pattern probably applies also to other activities, such as running. It may be, however, that the recruitment of high-threshold IIB units is less marked in running than in cycling, especially at high exercise intensities, when cycling may involve quite forceful pedalling. Training at an exercise intensity slightly above that resulting in a marked increase in the blood lactate concentration is generally sufficient for maximal recruitment of the muscle's slow-twitch (type I) fibres. There is, however, no evidence that more intense exercise would decrease the training effect in this fibre type as it did in the rat studies referred to above. A maximal training effect on the muscle's IIA and IIB fibres demands higher rates of work — how high may be dependent on the percentage fibre-type composition of the particular muscle. At high submaximal exercise intensities the recruitment of fast-twitch (type II) fibres, and thus probably also the training effect, is increased with long exercise durations and the resulting glycogen depletion of the slow-twitch fibres.

It may be concluded that for a large training effect per unit of training time, it is advisable to use high training intensities. With very heavy exercise, the duration of the exercise bouts may be insufficient, however, for an optimal training effect. The rat study by Dudley and colleagues, referred to above, gives some hints about the optimal balance between the intensity and duration of training but there are still insufficient human data available. The importance of this balance at the cellular level may be illustrated by the results of an investigation performed in our laboratory a few years ago. In this study two different training protocols were compared: (a) 72–79% of $\dot{V}o_{2\,max}$ 30 min daily; and (b) 100% of $\dot{V}o_{2\,max}$ performed as interval training with 4 min of exercise and 2 min of rest, five times daily. The training was performed on cycle ergometers during a period of 2 months, three times a week. The oxidative enzyme content of the thigh muscle (measured as the maximal activity of the enzyme succinate dehydrogenase, SDH) increased by approximately 25% with both training protocols. If, on the other hand, the SDH analysis was performed on a microscale on the different fibre types, there were clear differences between the two training groups. In the group training at the lower exercise intensity, SDH increased only in the slow-twitch type I fibres, whereas interval training at high exercise intensities resulted in an SDH increase mainly in the fast-twitch type II fibres (Henriksson & Reitman, 1976). These results stress the importance of training at the exercise intensity at which an improvement is most desirable.

Effect of endurance training on glycolytic enzymes, capillarization and fibre types

The muscle cell's content of glycolytic enzymes is not, or is only marginally, affected by endurance training programmes of 2–6 months' duration. The content of glycolytic enzymes is normally low in the skeletal muscles of endurance athletes, but this finding is entirely explained by the large percentage of slow-twitch fibres in their muscles. The content of glycolytic enzymes in this fibre type is normally only half of that in slow-twitch fibres. The mean glyco-

lytic enzyme level of athletes' slow-twitch or fast-twitch muscle fibres has thus been found to be normal, or even slightly enhanced (Chi et al., 1983; Essén-Gustavsson & Henriksson, 1984). This finding is in accord with what has been observed during chronic stimulation (see above), when there is a complete fibre-type transformation from fast-twitch glycolytic (type IIB) to slow-twitch (type I) fibres. In this situation the glycolytic enzyme content of the muscle is decreased to 20% of the initial level, a decrease which precisely reflects the large difference in glycolytic potential between fast-twitch glycolytic and slow-twitch fibres in the rabbit (Chi et al., 1986). It can therefore be concluded that the type of muscle fibre, based on its composition of myofibrillar proteins, is a strong determinant of its content of glycolytic enzymes. The same is not true of most of the oxidative enzymes, which change with training and inactivity completely independently of the specific myofibrillar protein isoforms of the fibre.

Skeletal muscle capillarization in humans is rapidly enhanced with endurance training, 2 months of training at high submaximal exercise intensities being sufficient to increase the total number of muscle capillaries by 50% (Andersen & Henriksson, 1977; Fig. 5.7). The difference between endurance athletes and untrained individuals with respect to the capillary count per muscle fibre (leg muscles) has been found to be two to threefold (Saltin & Gollnick, 1983). There is a lack of information about the extent to which capillary neoformation is dependent upon training intensity and duration. It is known, however, that less intense training regimens often result in oxidative enzyme increases without any change in capillarization.

When stains for myofibrillar adenosine triphosphatase (ATPase) have been used as the basis for fibre-type classification, most longitudinal studies in humans have failed to demonstrate an interconversion of fibre types (i.e. fast-twitch to slow-twitch) in response to endurance training. The stable nature of a muscle's fibre-type composition is further il-

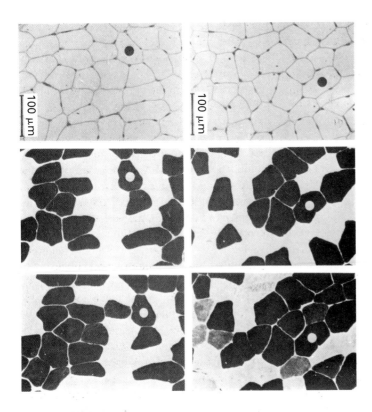

Fig. 5.7 A typical effect of 2 months of endurance training (identical to that described in Fig. 5.5) on capillary density in the human thigh muscle. The capillaries are seen in the upper stain as dark spots on the boundary between muscle fibres (amylase–periodic acid–Schiff staining). The histochemical type of the muscle fibres is indicated by the two lower stains. These are myofibrillar ATPase stains pretreated at different pHs (the middle stain at pH 4.3 and the lower one at pH 4.6). Slow-twitch (type I) fibres appear dark in both stains, while the fast-twitch oxidative glycolytic (type IIA) fibres appear light. Fast-twitch glycolytic (type IIB) fibres appear light in the middle stain but dark in the lower stain. From Andersen & Henriksson (1977b), with permission.

lustrated by the results of chronic stimulation studies in rabbits. Although in this situation there is a gradual and complete replacement of fast-twitch by slow-twitch fibres, quite long periods of chronic stimulation are required. The fibre-type changes are also the first to revert to normal when stimulation is discontinued (Brown *et al.*, 1989). On the basis of these findings, the high percentage of slow-twitch (type I) fibres in endurance athletes and the opposite finding in sprinters have therefore been ascribed to genetic factors (Komi *et al.*, 1976). Endurance training is known, however, to lead to a complete type transformation within the fast-twitch (type II) fibres from type IIB to type IIA (Andersen & Henriksson, 1977a; Jansson & Kaijser, 1977).

The concept that endurance training does not change the relative occurrence of fast-twitch and slow-twitch fibres has been challenged in recent years, however. It has been shown that:

1 Endurance training of long duration leads to the appearance of fibres intermediate between fast-twitch and slow-twitch.

2 The muscles of the dominant leg in different types of athletes, such as badminton players, contain a significantly increased percentage of slow-twitch fibres.

3 In several studies of detraining the percentage of fast-twitch muscle fibres increases.

It is therefore reasonable to conclude that extensive endurance training will result in an enhanced percentage of slow-twitch fibres. The extent to which this might occur still remains to be demonstrated (see Schantz, 1986).

Regression of the training-induced adaptation following discontinuation of training

An increase in the oxidative capacity of a muscle, induced by 2 months of endurance training, is lost in 4–6 weeks if the training is stopped (see Fig. 5.5). This loss of muscle oxidative enzymes occurs faster than the decrease in muscle capillarization (Schantz *et al.*, 1983) and in whole-body maximal oxygen intake (see Fig. 5.5). The time-course of the decrease in muscle oxidative enzyme content following cessation of training agrees well with that observed following cessation of chronic stimulation in the rabbit (see above). In the latter case, however, the restoration of muscle capillarization and the restoration of the oxidative enzyme content occur simultaneously. There has been only one detailed investigation of the enzyme changes that take place during the detraining of individuals who have undergone endurance training for several years (Chi *et al.*, 1983; very well trained, although not top, athletes). It was found that the oxidative capacity of the slow-twitch fibres rapidly decreased with detraining to the level found in untrained control subjects. Interestingly, however, the oxidative capacity of the fast-twitch fibres maintained an elevated level throughout the studied 12-week period of detraining. One theory put forward was that, due to prolonged endurance training, changes had occurred in the normal impulse pattern of fast motoneurons in the spinal cord.

Metabolic significance of the training-induced adaptation of skeletal muscle

After the cessation of chronic electrical stimulation, the restoration of a normal muscle oxidative enzyme content and capillarization follows a time-course similar to that of the normalization of muscle endurance. This indicates that the described adaptations are of importance for the muscle's capacity to perform prolonged exercise. This can be further illustrated by an investigation in which a group of subjects underwent one-leg endurance training on the cycle ergometer during 6 weeks. With one well trained leg (the level of succinate dehydrogenase being 25% higher than in the untrained leg), the subjects then performed two-leg endurance exercise at 70% of the $\dot{V}_{O_2 max}$, in which both legs performed ident-

ically. The energy metabolism of the two legs could be analysed and compared by means of arterial and venous catheterization and muscle biopsy analysis.

As illustrated in Fig. 5.8, there was a significantly smaller release of lactate from the trained leg than from the untrained one, and a significantly larger percentage of the energy output in the trained leg was derived from fat combustion. It is known from a large number of studies that, at the same absolute exercise intensity, trained individuals rely more on fat as an energy substrate than untrained individuals. This is the case despite the fact that, at a given rate of work, the plasma levels of free fatty acids are often lower in endurance-trained subjects (for a more detailed discussion see Holloszy, 1988). Taken together, the available evidence, including the result of the one-leg training study, indicates that the heavier reliance on fat in endurance-trained individuals must be explained to a large extent by local factors within the trained muscle. Such factors may be a larger utilization of intracellular or extracellular adipose tissue stores, but it is likely that the high content of mitochondrial oxidative enzymes is also important in this respect. This is supported by the results of a study in the rat in which it could be shown that the amount of glycogen (muscle plus liver) remaining after an endurance exercise test on a rodent treadmill was directly proportional to the muscle's content of oxidative enzymes (Fitts *et al.*, 1975). Figure 5.9 depicts a possible biochemical mechanism whereby a large concentration of oxidative enzymes (i.e. citric acid cycle and fat oxidation enzymes and respiratory chain components) leads to a situation in which a major part of the energy supply is derived from fat metabolism, a lower rate of lactate formation and sparing of muscle glycogen during exercise. The training-induced enhancement of muscle capillarization probably contributes to the metabolic adaptation seen in trained muscle. A conceivable mechanism for this effect might involve an augmented muscle supply of oxygen and fatty acids.

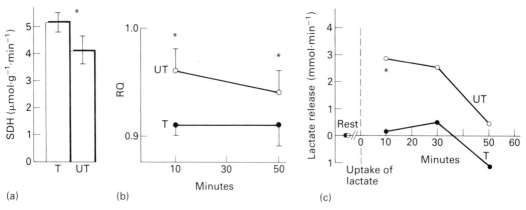

Fig. 5.8 Metabolic significance of the training-induced adaptation of human skeletal muscle. A group of subjects underwent one-leg endurance training on the cycle ergometer during 6 weeks. With one well trained (T) leg (the level of succinate dehydrogenase (SDH) being 25% higher than in the untrained leg, UT) (a), the subjects performed two-leg cycle ergometer exercise at 70% of the $\dot{V}_{O_2\,max}$ in which both legs performed identically. The energy metabolism of the two legs could be analysed and compared by means of arterial and venous catheterization and muscle biopsy analyses. The catheterization made possible measurements of the oxygen intake ($\dot{V}_{O_2}$) and the carbon dioxide production ($\dot{V}_{CO_2}$) of both legs separately. The $\dot{V}_{CO_2}/\dot{V}_{O_2}$ ratio, known as the respiratory quotient (RQ), indicates the relative contributions of carbohydrate and fat to the oxidative metabolism. Carbohydrate oxidation only would result in an RQ of 1.0, whereas an RQ of 0.7 indicates that fat is the sole source of energy. (b) indicates that fat is a more important energy source for the trained leg than for the untrained one (the RQ value being significantly lower for the trained leg). Accompanying the greater use of carbohydrates in the untrained leg, there is a larger formation and release of lactate (c). In the trained leg, the lactate release is low and at the end of the exercise bout there is even a tendency towards an uptake of lactate from the blood. *, $p < 0.05$ (significant difference between T and UT legs). From Henriksson (1977), modified with permission.

Possible mechanisms inducing the enzyme adaptation to training

The enzymes, as well as other protein molecules, have a limited lifespan. They are built up and degraded in a continuous cycle in which the biological half-life of many of the mitochondrial enzymes is about a week and that of the glycolytic enzymes is from one to a few days. Accordingly, the cellular content of a certain enzyme is the result of this balance between synthesis and degradation. It has been shown that changes in the rate of synthesis of enzyme proteins are the most important factor in explaining the enzyme changes resulting from chronic stimulation or training (Booth & Holloszy, 1977; Pette, 1984; Williams *et al.*, 1986). An interesting area of research now is to explore the biochemical mechanisms underlying the altered rate of enzyme synthesis, i.e. how is the information that there is a need for an increased amount of oxidative enzymes in the muscle cell transferred to the genes? Among suggested mediators are decreases in the concentration of adenosine triphosphate (ATP) or in other high-energy phosphate compounds; a decreased oxygen tension; an increased sympathoadrenal stimulation of the muscle cell; substances released from the motor nerve; and calcium-induced diacylglycerol release with subsequent activation of protein kinase C. The availability of advanced genetic techniques, as well as improved cell culture systems, has led to a renewed interest in this area of research and this will very likely lead to a better understanding of the mechanisms whereby the skeletal muscle cell adapts to different normal and pathological states.

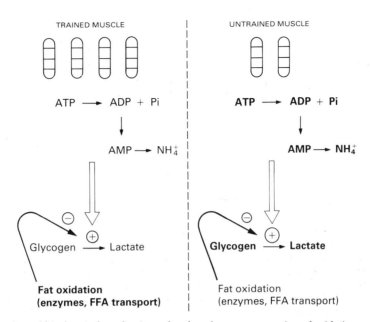

Fig. 5.9 A hypothetical biochemical mechanism whereby a large concentration of oxidative enzymes (i.e. citric acid cycle and fat oxidation enzymes and respiratory chain components) in trained muscle would lead to a greater reliance on fat metabolism, a lower rate of lactate formation, and sparing of muscle glycogen during exercise. The increased content of oxidative enzymes in trained skeletal muscle is explained to a large extent by a larger mitochondrial volume (volume fraction). In the figure this is indicated schematically with mitochondrial symbols. Suppose that, in the untrained muscle, there are only half as many enzyme molecules of the citric acid cycle and half as many components of the respiratory chain (which is a reasonable assumption, see Fig. 5.4). Owing to the lower enzymatic capacity and mitochondrial volume fraction of the untrained muscle, it follows that, at a given rate of work, i.e. at a given rate of oxygen uptake, each mitochondrial unit has to be activated twice as much in the untrained muscle as in the trained one. An important component of this activation is the increased levels of the degradation products of ATP (e.g. ADP), which are the result of muscle contractions. These levels must thus be stabilized at a higher level in the untrained muscle than in the trained muscle. However, in addition to stimulating mitochondrial respiration, these ATP degradation products are also powerful stimulators of the glycolytic pathway. This would lead to a higher glycolytic rate in untrained muscle, resulting in a greater lactate release and carbohydrate oxidation. The fat oxidation rate is higher in trained muscle, and the higher content of enzymes of fatty acid transport and oxidation is likely to contribute to this. An increased rate of fat oxidation leads to a more pronounced inhibition of glycolysis in the trained muscle than in the untrained muscle, where the rate of fat oxidation is lower. In concert, these factors lead to a sparing of glycogen during exercise in trained skeletal muscle. From Holloszy & Booth (1976).

Acknowledgments

The author's own cited work was supported by grants from the Swedish Medical Research Council, the Karolinska Institute, the Research Council of the Swedish Sports Federation and the National Institutes of Health (USA). The author wishes to express his appreciation to Ms Ulla Siltberg for her help in the preparation of the manuscript and to Ms Christina Henriksson and Ms Anne-Britt Olrog for drawing the illustrations.

References

Andersen, P. & Henriksson, J. (1977a) Training induced changes in the subgroups of human type II skeletal muscle fibres. *Acta Physiol. Scand.* **99**, 123–125.

Andersen, P. & Henriksson, J. (1977b) Capillary supply of the quadriceps femoris muscle of man: adaptive response to exercise. *J. Physiol.* **270**, 677–690.

Bergström, J. (1962) Muscle electrolytes in man. *Scand.*

J. Clin. Lab. Invest. **68** (Suppl.), 1–110.

Booth, F.W. & Holloszy, J.O. (1977) Cytochrome c turnover in rat skeletal muscles. *J. Biol. Chem.* **252**, 416–419.

Brown, J.M.C., Henriksson, J. & Salmons, S. (1989). Restoration of fast muscle characteristics following cessation of chronic stimulation:physiological, histochemical and metabolic changes during slow-to-fast transformation. *Proc. R. Soc. Lond. B* **235**, 321–346.

Brown, M.D., Cotter, M.A., Hudlicka, O. & Vrbová, G. (1976). The effects of different patterns of muscle activity on capillary density, mechanical properties and structure of slow and fast rabbit muscles. *Pflüg. Arch. Physiol.* **361**, 241–250.

Chi, M.M.-Y., Hintz, C., Coyle, E. *et al.* (1983) Effects of detraining on enzymes of energy metabolism in individual human muscle fibres. *Am. J. Physiol.* **244**, C276–C287.

Chi, M.M.-Y., Hintz, C.S. Henriksson, J. *et al.* (1986) Chronic stimulation of mammalian muscle: enzyme changes in individual fibres. *Am. J. Physiol.* **251** (*Cell Physiol.* **20**), C633–C642.

Dudley, G.A., Abraham, W.M. & Terjung, R.L. (1982) Influence of exercise intensity and duration on biochemical adaptations in skeletal muscle. *J. Appl. Physiol.* **53**, 844–850.

Essén-Gustavsson, B. & Henriksson, J. (1984) Enzyme levels in pools of microdissected human muscle fibres of identified type. Adaptive response to exercise. *Acta Physiol. Scand.* **120**, 505–515.

Fitts, R.H., Booth, F.W., Winder, W.W. & Holloszy, J.O. (1975) Skeletal muscle respiratory capacity, endurance and glycogen utilization. *Am. J. Physiol.* **228**, 1029–1033.

Henriksson, J. (1977) Training induced adaptation of skeletal muscle and metabolism during submaximal exercise. *J. Physiol.* **270**, 661–675.

Henriksson, J. & Reitman, J.S. (1976) Quantitative measures of enzyme activities in type I and type II muscle fibres of man after training. *Acta Physiol. Scand.* **97**, 392–397.

Henriksson, J. & Reitman, J.S. (1977) Time course of changes in human skeletal muscle succinate dehydrogenase and cytochrome oxidase activities and maximal oxygen uptake with physical activity and inactivity. *Acta Physiol. Scand.* **99**, 91–97.

Henriksson, J., Chi, M.M.-Y., Hintz, C.S. *et al.* (1986) Chronic stimulation of mammalian muscle: changes in enzymes of six metabolic pathways. *Am. J. Physiol.* **251** (*Cell Physiol.* **20**), C614–C632.

Holloszy, J.O. (1988) Metabolic consequences of endurance exercise training. In: Horton, E.S. & Terjung, R.L. (eds) *Exercise, Nutrition and Energy Metabolism*, pp. 116–131. Macmillan, New York.

Holloszy, J.O. & Booth, F.W. (1976) Biochemical adap-

tations to endurance exercise in muscle. *Annu. Rev. Physiol.* **38**, 273–291.

Jansson, E. & Kaijser, L. (1977) Muscle adaptation to extreme endurance training in man. *Acta Physiol. Scand.* **100**, 315–324.

Jolesz, F. & Sreter, F.A. (1981) Development, innervation, and activity-pattern induced changes in skeletal muscle. *Annu. Rev. Physiol.* **43**, 531–552.

Komi, P.V., Viitasalo, J.T., Havu, M., Thorstensson, A. & Karlsson, J. (1976) Physiological and structural performance capacity: effect of heredity. In: Komi, P.V. (ed.) *International Series of Biomechanics, Biomechanics V-A*, Vol. 1A, pp. 118–123. University Park Press, Baltimore.

Lowry, O.H. & Passonneau, J.V. (1972) *A Flexible System of Enzymatic Analysis.* Academic Press, New York.

Morgan, T.E., Cobb, L.A., Short, F.A., Ross, R. & Gunn, D.R. (1971) Effects of long-term exercise on human muscle mitochondria. In: Pernow, B. & Saltin, B. (eds) *Muscle Metabolism During Exercise*, pp. 87–95. Plenum Press, New York.

Newsholme, E. & Leech, A. (1983) *Biochemistry for the Medical Sciences*, pp. 38–42. John Wiley, Chichester.

Petrén, T., Sjöstrand, T. & Sylvén, B. (1937) Der Einfluss des Trainings auf die Häufigkeit der Capillaren in Herz- und Skeletmuskulatur. *Arbeitsphysiologie* **9**, 376–386.

Pette, D. (1984) Activity-induced fast to slow transitions in mammalian muscle. *Med. Sci. Sports Exerc.* **16**, 517–528.

Salmons, S. & Henriksson J. (1981) The adaptive response of skeletal muscle to increased use. *Muscle Nerve* **4**, 94–105.

Saltin, B. & Gollnick, P.D. (1983) Skeletal muscle adaptability: significance for metabolism and performance. In: Peachey, L.D. (ed.) *Handbook of Physiology. Skeletal Muscle*, Section 10, pp. 555–631. American Physiological Society, Bethesda, Maryland.

Schantz, P.G. (1986) Plasticity of human skeletal muscle. *Acta Physiol. Scand.* **128** (Suppl.), 558.

Schantz, P.G., Henriksson, J. & Jansson, E. (1983) Adaptation of human skeletal muscle to endurance training of long duration. *Clin. Physiol.* **3**, 141–151.

Varnauskas, E., Björntorp, P., Fahlén, M., Prerovsky, I. & Stenberg, J. (1970) Effects of physical training on exercise blood flow and enzymatic activity in skeletal muscle. *Cardiovasc. Res.* **4**, 418–422.

Williams, R.S., Salmons, S., Newsholme, E.A., Kaufman, R.E. & Mellor, J. (1986) Regulation of nuclear and mitochondrial expression by contractile activity in skeletal muscle. *J. Biol. Chem.* **261**, 376–380.

Chapter 6

The Pulmonary System and Endurance

JEROME A. DEMPSEY AND MURLI MANOHAR

The response of the lungs and chest wall to exercise of any duration aims at homoeostatic regulation of arterial blood gases for minimum physiological cost. During prolonged exercise, this control system faces the challenges of oxygenating and deacidifying markedly hypercapnic and hypoxaemic mixed venous blood, while maintaining a low pulmonary vascular resistance and minimizing the turnover of plasma water into the lung's interstitium in the face of a rising pulmonary blood flow. Furthermore, the chest muscles must generate and sustain intrathoracic pressures at levels which are a substantial fraction of maximum available pressures. Sufficient alveolar ventilation must be provided, without incurring muscular fatigue or requiring an inordinate blood flow to and energy utilization by the thoracic muscles. We outline here key pulmonary adaptations to prolonged exercise — their regulation, limitations and cost. A comprehensive review of this topic has been published recently (Dempsey *et al.*, 1988).

Ventilatory responses in a neutral environment

Effect of exercise intensity and duration

Several phases of the ventilatory response to exercise have been described. Hyperpnoea in the initial seconds of exercise is followed by a rise over $1-2$ min to a steady state. Thereafter, if the relative intensity of exercise is less than $40-50\%$ of maximal oxygen intake ($\dot{V}o_{2\,max}$), a true steady state prevails; respiratory minute ventilation ($\dot{V}e$), breathing frequency (f_B) and tidal volume (V_T) all remain constant, and arterial P_{CO_2}, pH and P_{O_2} also remain close to resting values. This response is observed in the healthy assembly-line worker, or the recreational hiker, cyclist or walker, all of whom are capable of sustaining this level of energy expenditure for at least 8 h and probably indefinitely without departing from a steady state of homoeostasis. As the relative intensity of exercise is increased, the threat to a steady state of ventilatory response increases. At work intensities requiring $60-80\%$ of $\dot{V}o_{2\,max}$, exercise for more than $5-10$ min leads to an upward 'drift' in breathing frequency and minute ventilation (Table 6.1). Arterial P_{CO_2} is reduced to a varying extent as exercise continues and, depending on the amount of metabolic acid production, arterial pH remains constant or shows a frankly alkaline shift. So a true steady state of ventilation and acid–base regulation no longer prevails. Nevertheless, reasonably fit subjects can tolerate such work rates for $1-3$ h. At a work intensity greater than $80-90\%$ of $\dot{V}o_{2\,max}$, marked tachypnoea, hyperpnoea and dyspnoea develop, together with progressive increases in $\dot{V}e$, arterial hydrogen ion concentration and circulating noradrenaline. The relative intensity at which these responses occur varies, and is undoubtedly dependent upon the individual's fitness level (Costill, 1970; Hanson *et al.*, 1982; Dempsey *et al.*, 1988).

61

Table 6.1 Selected respiratory responses during prolonged heavy exercise at $70-75\%$ of maximal oxygen intake (carbon dioxide output $3-3.5$ l·min^{-1}) in a neutral environment.

	Rest	Exercise 5–10 min	Exercise 60–90 min
$\dot{V}_E$ (l·min^{-1})	6	86	98
V_T (litres)	0.5	2.2	1.8
f_B min^{-1}	12	40	54
$V_D : V_T$	0.35	0.18	0.23
$\dot{V}_A$ (l·min^{-1})	4	71	75
Core temperature (°C)	37	37.5	39.5
Pa_{CO_2} (mmHg)	40	38	34
pHa	7.40	7.42	7.44
$A - aD_{O_2}$ (mmHg)	10	20	20
Pa_{O_2} (mmHg)	90	90	90
Ppa (mmHg)	15	30	20

The increase in breathing frequency with prolonged exercise is analogous to (and coincidental with) a cardiovascular drift. The ventilatory response is unusual in that humans commonly respond to chemical stimuli or submaximal exercise with an increase of tidal volume. During very heavy and maximal exercise, V_T commonly plateaus and f_B rises; this is associated with a V_T in excess of $60-65\%$ of vital capacity (VC), or an end-inspiratory lung volume greater than 90% of total lung capacity (TLC), and may well be related to pulmonary stretch receptor feedback (Dempsey et al., 1980; Scuirba et al., 1988). However, this explanation does not apply to the tachypnoea of long-term exercise, which commonly occurs at a tidal volume of less than $40-50\%$ VC. It is a highly inefficient response, because as frequency increases and tidal volume falls, the dead-space tidal volume ratio ($V_D : V_T$) rises, alveolar ventilation is reduced, and Pa_{CO_2} will rise. Thus to preserve $\dot{V}_A$, alveolar P_{O_2} and P_{CO_2} during long-term exercise, $\dot{V}_E$ must increase by $10-30\%$ (Table 6.1) This would not have been necessary had V_T increased rather than breathing frequency (Hanson et al., 1982). Mechanical efficiency suffers from this tachypnoeic response in two ways. First, flow rate and therefore flow resistive work must increase further, especially at these high flow rates, where the proportion of turbulent air flow is high. Second, the expiratory time is shortened, so that the expiratory flow rate may approach the limits of the maximum flow : volume loop. Both of these occurrences may cause the end-expiratory lung volume to rise, shortening inspiratory muscle length, jeopardizing optimal muscle tension development and increasing the metabolic cost of breathing (Sharratt et al., 1987; Henke et al., 1988). Why would the control system respond in this inefficient manner? The answer may be found in the underlying mechanisms of ventilatory control.

Possible causes of the tachypnoeic drift

A number of factors are potential contributors to the progressive hyperventilation of prolonged exercise. We view these as disturbing influences that override the usual, precise association of alveolar ventilation ($\dot{V}_A$) to carbon dioxide output ($\dot{V}_{CO_2}$) during exercise.

A compensatory response to metabolic acidosis may have contributed in a minor way to the observed hyperventilation, at least at the beginning of prolonged exercise. However, the predominant trend is towards an increase of alkalinity with time. The arterial hydrogen ion concentration is apparently determined by, rather than a determinant of, the hyperventilatory response.

If body temperature is increased by more

than 1.5°C by external heating (whether at rest or in exercise), this causes tachypnoeic hyperventilation (Peterson & Vejby-Christiansen, 1973; MacDougall *et al.*, 1974). Furthermore, skin cooling (which minimizes the normal rise in body temperature during prolonged exercise) reduces the time-dependent hyperventilatory response (MacDougall *et al.*, 1974; Dempsey *et al.*, 1975). During prolonged, heavy exercise, a significant ventilatory stimulus linked to accumulation of metabolic heat is indicated by the increases in core and blood temperatures, and by the dominant tachypnoeic breathing pattern. On the other hand, ventilatory drift is seen in prolonged exercise when the increase in core temperature is less than 1°C and apparently is insufficient to cause a hyperventilatory response (Martin *et al.*, 1981).

Long-term exercise, and especially road racing, causes marked increases in circulating noradrenaline, which is fairly well correlated with the time-course of ventilatory drift (Martin *et al.*, 1981; Hanson *et al.*, 1982). However, the relative importance of these humoral changes as ventilatory stimulants remains unclear, especially in normoxia.

Pulmonary congestion and increased pulmonary venous or lung interstitial fluid pressure are known to produce tachypnoeic responses, presumably via the activation of pulmonary vagal C-fibre endings (Paintal, 1973). In addition, respiratory muscle fatigue or impending fatigue leads to a tachypnoeic breathing pattern (Roussos & Moxham, 1986). These intriguing possibilities remain theoretical, because neither the accumulation of extravascular lung water nor the occurrence of respiratory muscle fatigue has been established during exercise of any type or duration.

The regulation of time-dependent tachypnoeic hyperventilation during prolonged exercise is multifaceted and thus very difficult to sort out. One intriguing and relatively unexplored cause may well be 'extra' stimuli to mechanically associated respiratory neurons with impending fatigue of the locomotor muscles — namely the stimulation of acid and temperature-sensitive non-

myelinated nerve fibres in working skeletal muscle and/or the recruitment of a 'descending' input to medullary respiratory neurons from higher locomotor areas of the central nervous system (Kaufman *et al.*, 1984; Dempsey *et al.*, 1985).

Alveolar to arterial oxygen transport and the gas exchange surface area

During prolonged heavy exercise at sea level (Dempsey *et al.*, 1988), the partial pressure of arterial oxygen (Pa_{O_2}) usually remains within 10 mmHg of resting values. The alveolar to arterial oxygen difference ($A-aD_{O_2}$) rises to 2–2.5 times resting levels. It remains constant throughout prolonged exercise, as PA_{O_2} and Pa_{O_2} both rise with the time-dependent increase in alveolar ventilation. Even highly trained athletes (who sometimes experience significant arterial hypoxaemia during short-term maximal or near-maximal exercise; Dempsey *et al.*, 1988), usually show normal oxygenation of arterial blood during heavy submaximal prolonged exercise (mainly because their level of hyperventilation is augmented in prolonged vs. short-term work). There are rare exceptions in whom Pa_{O_2} remains below 75 mmHg throughout prolonged work at 70–85% of $\dot{V}_{O_2 \, max}$ (Dempsey *et al.*, 1988).

So this evidence indicates, indirectly at least, that the diffusion surface area, the diffusion distance from the alveoli to the capillary red cells, the red cell transit time and the ventilation to perfusion distribution (the major determinants of $A-aD_{O_2}$) remain constant during prolonged exercise. None the less, this general index of gas exchange may not be sensitive enough to detect an accumulation of extravascular lung water or a narrowing or closure of small airways as suggested by some measurements made immediately after marathons and long-distance races. Immediately after endurance events, the residual lung volume increases significantly, the expiratory flow rate at low lung volumes is reduced, so-called airway 'closing capacity' increases, and the carbon monoxide membrane diffusing capacity (D_MCO) at a normal pulmonary capillary blood flow falls (Maron *et al.*, 1979; Miles *et al.*, 1986). These small but significant changes have all been interpreted to mean that some degree of pulmonary oedema has developed at the peribronchiolar and/or alveolar level, compressing small airways and impeding alveolar–capillary diffusion. At least theoretically, conditions may exist during very heavy short-term exercise, especially in the highly fit, where pulmonary blood flow increases to the point where the hydrostatic pressure at the alveolar–capillary membrane is sufficient for a progressive accumulation of extravascular lung water (that is, the fluid flux into the interstitial fluid space exceeds the lymphatic drainage; Younes *et al.*, 1987; Reeves *et al.*, 1989). Hyperventilation also increases fluid filtration at any given pulmonary capillary pressure (Younes & Bshouty, 1990). The potential for pulmonary oedema might be alleviated in prolonged exercise, because pulmonary arterial pressure falls progressively with the duration of exercise; there is significant pulmonary vasodilatation for a considerable time following prolonged exercise (Widimski *et al.*, 1963; Ekelund, 1967). The reason for these changes in the pulmonary vascular bed is not clear; they are suggestive of an exercise-induced vasodilatation of medial smooth muscle (as occurs in skeletal muscle), but available evidence points only to passive non-neural, non-humoral factors as important regulators of the pulmonary vasculature (Reeves *et al.*, 1989). These considerations are purely theoretical in lieu of definitive measures of extravascular lung water in exercise in humans (Gallagher *et al.*, 1988). Available evidence does not support a significant accumulation of extravascular lung water during prolonged heavy exercise in a healthy human.

Environmental factors affecting the pulmonary response to prolonged exercise

In competitive endurance races, the ventilatory and acid–base response remains much as outlined for laboratory conditions, at least when energy expenditure remains fairly constant. Hot and humid environments provoke an exaggerated tachypnoeic response. This has been shown by external heating of the skin during prolonged exercise in the laboratory (MacDougall *et al.*, 1974) and in two competitors on a hot humid day; the latter progressively fatigued during a road race, so that their running velocity and metabolic rate fell throughout most of the race (Hanson *et al.*, 1982). Lactic acid concentration also fell and arterial pH rose, but $\dot{V}_E$ was fairly well maintained, breathing frequency remained high, and $V_D : V_T$ rose throughout exercise. The partial pressure of carbon dioxide (Pa_{CO_2}) tended to be slightly elevated in these two subjects toward the end of the race. This ventilatory response, and especially the frequency response, bore little relationship to metabolic demand or chemoreceptor stimulation. The absence of any apparent teleological reason for the breathing pattern adopted in long-term work is even more perplexing. We mentioned above the inefficiency of gas exchange and the mechanical inefficiency caused by this pattern. In rare cases, a panting-like response occurs ($f_B > 80-90 \cdot \mathrm{min}^{-1}$ with a twofold rise of $V_D : V_T$ and some carbon dioxide retention). It is doubtful that this response contributes significantly to temperature regulation in the human brain, in contrast to non-sweating quadrupeds, such as the dog (Baker, 1979).

Prolonged exercise at high altitudes also exaggerates the hyperventilatory tachypnoeic drift and respiratory alkalosis both during acute exposure and after short-term acclimatization to altitudes above 3000 m (Dempsey *et al.*, 1977). A number of powerful synergistic ventilatory stimuli coexist under these conditions, namely exercise, hypoxaemia, increased circulating noradrenaline levels, elevated temperature and progressive locomotor muscle fatigue. Not uncommonly, dyspnoea develops because of: (i) the foreign sensations presented by an inability to entrain breathing and stride rate in the presence of 'extra' ventilatory stimuli; and

(ii) an extremely high work of breathing. Prolonged exercise often induces quite severe hyperventilation, resulting in a $Paco_2$ of $15-20$ mmHg at 4300 m. This in turn causes severe cerebral respiratory alkalosis and a reduced cerebral blood flow, which may be maintained throughout the exercise bout (Dempsey *et al.*, 1975). Pulmonary vasoconstriction would also be expected to cause persistent pulmonary hypertension during prolonged exercise at high altitude. This may occasionally precipitate cardiogenic pulmonary oedema in mountain climbers; however, pulmonary oedema has not been documented in a normal population during hypoxic exercise. In fact, the alveolar to arterial oxygen difference remains constant during prolonged heavy exercise in an acclimatized sojourner at altitudes of 3000 m, just as at sea level.

Prolonged competitive exercise may be complicated and potentially compromised by environmental pollutants. Ozone increases airway resistance and provokes rapid, shallow breathing (Adams *et al.*, 1981; Lauritzen & Adams, 1985). Because prolonging heavy work increases exposure, athletes in endurance competition may be affected most seriously.

Airway impedance may be affected by endurance exercise. Following short-term exercise the maximum flow rate at 50% of TLC (MEF_{50}) is increased, presumably via bronchiolar dilatation. Following a marathon run, MEF_{50} normally remains unchanged; however, following a run at subfreezing temperatures, a substantial *decrease* of MEF_{50} occurs (Mahler & Loke, 1981). One would expect this effect to be exaggerated in subjects whose airway smooth muscle is sensitive to bronchoprovocation.

Respiratory muscle fatigue during prolonged exercise

Do the diaphragm and/or other principal respiratory muscles become fatigued during prolonged exercise, generating less than the expected tension (or pressure) for a given nervous motor input? Certainly, the healthy human diaphragm can become fatigued, at least when one breathes at very high fractions of maximal occlusion pressure against an imposed external resistance (Roussos & Moxham, 1986). Moreover, the ventilatory requirements sustained over 3 h or more of exertion in the highly trained athlete are not trivial ($\dot{V}E$ $100-120$ l·min^{-1}), and they might require 'fatiguing' levels of pressure development by the diaphragm.

Utilization of respiratory muscles in exercise

All portions of the diaphragm and other respiratory muscles are heavily recruited during exercise, as indicated by measurements of muscle perfusion, pressure development and/or muscle electromyography. Evidence from microsphere studies in ponies at $\dot{V}o_{2\,max}$ indicates maximal vasodilatation in the diaphragm (local blood flow $300-350$ ml·min^{-1} 100 g^{-1} tissue) with more than 85% extraction of arterial oxygen content, at a time when significant vasodilator reserve remains in the exercising limb muscles (Manohar, 1986). Further, the diaphragm maintained high submaximal levels of perfusion and a 75% oxygen extraction throughout 30 min of exercise at 90% of maximal heart rate for this species (Fig. 6.1). In the human, the peak inspiratory pressure during tidal breathing commonly approaches only $45-65\%$ of the maximal volitional inspiratory pressure 'available' at the flow rate and lung volume achieved during short-term maximal exercise (LeBlanc *et al.*, 1988). However, the highly trained athlete often approaches the available capacity for inspiratory muscle pressure development during maximal exercise (Johnson *et al.*, 1990). Such mechanical parameters have not been measured during prolonged exercise but, given the hyperventilatory drift during very heavy endurance exercise, total ventilatory output and possibly inspiratory pressure development at $>85\%$ $\dot{V}o_{2\,max}$ may well approach that available during maximal short-term exercise.

Other inspiratory and expiratory muscles of

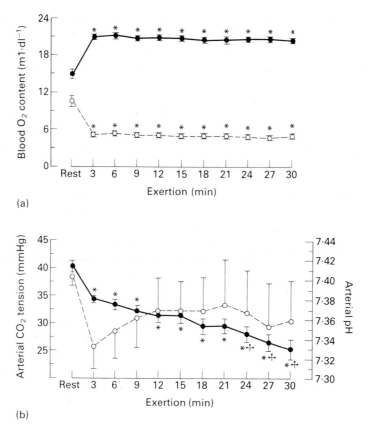

Fig. 6.1 Effects of long-term treadmill exercise to exhaustion in ponies at 90% of maximal heart rate on: (a) the oxygen content of arterial and diaphragmatic venous blood; and (b) arterial P_{CO_2} (●) and pH (○). Note the progressive hyperventilation and respiratory alkalosis in the face of a high, constant oxygen extraction and (presumably) a constant oxygen consumption of the diaphragm. Apparently, the substantial extrahyperventilation which developed over the course of exercise must have been produced via recruitment of respiratory muscles other than the diaphragm. From M. Manohar, unpublished observations on ponies. *, $p < 0.05$ versus rest; †, $p < 0.05$ versus all values between 3 and 15 min of exercise.

the rib cage and abdomen, usually considered 'accessory' muscles at rest, become highly active — phasically and tonically — during mild exercise (Henke *et al.*, 1988; Ainsworth *et al.*, 1989; Dempsey *et al.*, 1990a; Manohar, 1990). Mechanical consequences of this recruitment include: (a) a dual action for both locomotion and respiration; for example, in running, tonic abdominal muscle activity occurs over each combined respiratory and locomotory cycle; (b) the end-expiratory lung volume is reduced by activation of expiratory muscles, thereby placing the diaphragm at a

longer and more optimal length for tension generation; (c) the diaphragm operates more efficiently as a piston to increase rib cage volume, because both the abdominal wall and rib cage are stiffened; and (d) expiratory muscle pressure development increases progressively with increasing exercise up to (and sometimes beyond) the point where expiratory flow limitation occurs; thus maximum or near maximum use of the expiratory flow : volume loop is frequent during maximal exercise in the highly trained subject (Johnson *et al.*, 1990).

Estimates have been made of the energy and

blood flow requirements of this respiratory muscle recruitment. Microsphere studies of six inspiratory and expiratory muscles showed a cumulative blood flow which averaged 14−15% of the total cardiac output when ponies were performing maximal exercise (Manohar, 1990). While we cannot be certain that the action of these muscles is devoted entirely to producing the exercise hyperpnoea, none the less this quantity is indeed a substantial fraction of the total cardiac output to be directed to the musculature of the rib cage and abdominal wall. The situation may be somewhat analogous in the human. When the tidal pressure : volume loop breathing pattern and lung volumes achieved at $\dot{V}o_{2\,max}$ are mimicked in the resting subject, oxygen consumption increases to 9−14% of the total exercise oxygen consumption (Aaron et al., 1990). The cost is highest in those subjects who closely approximate their capacities for expiratory flow rate and inspiratory pressure development during maximal exercise.

Evidence for respiratory muscle fatigue

We have outlined above the substantial recruitment of respiratory muscles throughout prolonged heavy exercise. Is the related metabolic demand placed on the chest wall able to be met by bloodborne substances, or does anaerobic glycolysis occur in the diaphragm? If so, is glycolysis predictive of mechanical fatigue? This question has been addressed in several animal studies (Gorski et al., 1978; Moore & Gollnick 1982; Fregosi & Dempsey, 1986; Iannuzzo et al., 1987) and the implications have recently been summarized (Dempsey et al., 1988). The consensus is that: (a) the diaphragm utilizes its glycogen to some extent during some, but not all, types of prolonged exhausting exercise; and (b) that usage by the diaphragm is substantially less than that shown in limb muscles of similar mixed fibre type.

More recent work has utilized the arteriovenous differences across the diaphragm during prolonged strenuous exercise to exhaustion in the pony. These data show that the diaphragm effluent phrenic venous lactate and ammonia concentrations rise with, but never exceed, arterial concentrations during prolonged strenuous exercise (Fig. 6.2). While it is possible that the diaphragm may engage in simultaneous production and utilization of lactate, the fact that there was no net lactate production, even during strenuous exertion, makes the diaphragm uniquely different from skeletal muscle (which readily engages in lactate and ammonia production, the latter from deamination of adenine monophosphate (AMP) following the myokinase reaction: $2\ ADP \rightarrow ATP + AMP$). The exercising rat also shows increased diaphragmatic tissue lactate concentration in the absence of substantial glycogen depletion, a combination that probably reflects lactate uptake by the diaphragm (Fregosi & Dempsey, 1986). Similarly, there was no net lactate production by the diaphragm of awake sheep who experienced respiratory 'failure' (carbon dioxide retention) when subjected to severe inspiratory resistive loads for 30 min (Bazzy et al., 1989).

Thus, animal data suggest that the energy supplied to the diaphragm remains adequate and its metabolism continues to be principally aerobic during strenuous prolonged exercise. We caution, however, that the diaphragm probably becomes quite acidic during strenuous exercise, when one considers a fall in phrenic venous pH to near 6.9 (M. Manohar, unpublished data) and a fivefold increase in lactic concentration in the rat diaphragm at exhaustion (Fregosi & Dempsey, 1986). This cellular acidosis could conceivably depress the myofilaments and diminish calcium ion release by the sarcoplasmic reticulum in response to excitation (Fabiato & Fabiato, 1978).

We lack objective *neuromechanical evidence* as to whether prolonged strenuous exercise ever causes diaphragmatic fatigue. Volitional tests of peak inspiratory pressure, peak transdiaphragmatic pressure or maximum sustainable ventilation have been applied before and after exercise, with mixed results; but such tests cannot be adequately controlled, and are not

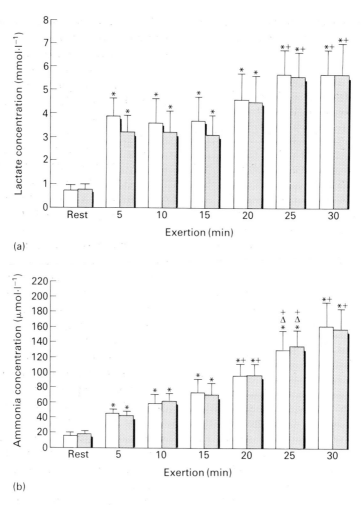

(a)

(b)

Fig. 6.2 (a) Arterial and phrenic venous lactate and (b) ammonia concentrations during exercise to exhaustion in ponies (see also Fig. 6.1). From Manohar & Hassan (in press). *, $p < 0.05$ from rest; +, $p < 0.05$ from all values between 3 and 15 min of exercise; Δ, $p < 0.05$ from previous exercise period.

sufficiently objective or independent of total body fatigue (Dempsey *et al.*, 1988). A change in the frequency spectrum of the diaphragmatic electromyogram is often cited as evidence of diaphragmatic fatigue during short-term exercise (Bye *et al.*, 1983); however, the validity of this index remains speculative. The diaphragmatic pressure response to supramaximal phrenic nerve stimulation provides objective evidence of diaphragmatic fatigue (Bellemare & Bigland-Ritchie, 1987). If muscle length is carefully controlled and the electrical stimulus to the muscle is standardized, phrenic stimulation offers an objective way of defining the effects of exercise on diaphragmatic mechanical output. No change in the diaphragmatic response to the supramaximal stimulus is seen following short-term exercise to maximum (Levine & Henson, 1988). Further, if a servo-ventilator is used to 'unload' the respiratory muscles during heavy or maximal exercise, there is no change in either ventilatory response or in $\dot{V}_{O_2\,max}$ (Gallagher & Younes, 1989). Such techniques should be applied further to endurance exercise, using a variety of subjects capable of sustaining varying levels of exercise and ventilatory response.

Does the pulmonary system limit performance in endurance exercise?

The ability of the pulmonary system to maintain arterial oxygen pressures is very rarely a threat to oxygen transport during prolonged heavy exercise in healthy persons at sea level. The alveolar to arterial oxygen pressure difference may widen substantially during prolonged heavy work, but the hyperventilatory response to submaximal work which can be maintained for 30 min or more increases alveolar oxygen pressure (and lowers $Paco_2$) sufficiently, so that arterial oxygen saturation and pH are almost always maintained near resting levels. The appropriate amount of ventilation (or hyperventilation) is carefully protected, even at a substantial metabolic cost. For example, during short-term maximal exercise, the highly fit subject reaches virtual mechanical limits to volume, flow rate and pressure development by the inspiratory muscles, and a substantial mechanical inefficiency is incurred. Nevertheless, alveolar hyperventilation is such that Pao_2 usually exceeds 115 mmHg and $Paco_2$ is in the 28–35 mmHg range except in cases of extreme flow limitation (Dempsey *et al.*, 1990b; Johnson *et al.*, 1990). Based on this same premise, we would speculate that even if the maximum available diaphragmatic pressure was actually achieved during the progressive hyperpnoea of prolonged heavy exercise, this would not lead to an inadequate alveolar hyperventilation; rather, accessory muscles would assist to allow development of an appropriate (total) inspiratory muscle pressure. While the ventilatory requirement of the very fit during short-term maximal exercise may occasionally exceed the maximum capability to develop an appropriate amount of alveolar ventilation, it is unlikely that this intensity of exercise could be maintained beyond a few minutes, even in the fittest of performers.

At the level of $\dot{V}o_2$ and $\dot{V}co_2$ achieved by untrained individuals during prolonged exercise, an adequate hyperventilatory response still occurs, even at altitudes of 3500–4000 m; but limitations of pulmonary diffusion lead to a time-dependent fall in arterial oxygen pressures and content, limiting systemic oxygen transport to the working muscles at a time when the muscle arteriovenous oxygen difference is near maximum (Dempsey *et al.*, 1977).

It is unlikely that sufficient pulmonary oedema develops during prolonged heavy exercise to affect pulmonary diffusion or ventilation to perfusion distribution significantly. However, pulmonary vascular (and possibly interstitial fluid) pressures in the lung may increase sufficiently to stimulate the pulmonary C-fibres and reflexes from the lung parenchyma and great vessels, contributing to locomotor muscle inhibition and fatigue (Paintal, 1973). Vagally dependent reflex inhibition of contracting skeletal muscle has been demonstrated in the anaesthetized dog, but we do not know to what extent these receptors might be stimulated and contribute to fatigue in heavy prolonged exercise. We would predict this to occur only in cases where a pulmonary blood flow of about 30 $l \cdot min^{-1}$ and a pulmonary arterial pressure of 30–35 mmHg could be sustained for long periods.

The only generally applicable respiratory limitation of endurance performance might be found in the metabolic cost of breathing. The blood flow and oxygen consumed by the respiratory muscles in heavy and maximum short-term exercise is 10–15% of total body values for normal, healthy young subjects. This same range of metabolic requirement for breathing is probably reached in prolonged, heavy exercise, at least in the highly fit performer who is capable of sustaining a high ventilation. Thus, the blood flow potentially 'stolen' by the respiratory muscles should be added to the more traditional considerations of the competition between skin blood flow (for temperature regulation) and limb locomotor muscle flow during prolonged endurance exercise. This competition may present extra-ordinary problems during prolonged heavy exercise in the heat, where the demand for both skin and respiratory muscle blood flow becomes substantial. An even greater problem may arise during long-term exercise in hypoxia, because the ventilatory demand is greater yet oxygen transport to the respiratory muscles is reduced by the arterial hypoxaemia. This may explain the increased glycogen utilization and greater lactate accumulation by the rat diaphragm during long-term exercise (Fregosi & Dempsey, 1986). Finally, a combination of reduced lung elastic recoil and a relatively high ventilatory requirement (Dempsey *et al.*, 1990b) may bring older endurance athletes very close to the mechanical limits for inspiratory and expiratory muscle pressure generation during prolonged exercise; sustaining this non-limiting ventilatory response would, at least theoretically, create substantial energy demands in older subjects during prolonged exercise.

Acknowledgments

We are indebted to Jennifer Thew for her excellent preparation of the manuscript. This work was supported by NHLBI and the USARDC.

References

Aaron, E., Johnson, B., Pegelow, D. & Dempsey, J. (1990) The oxygen cost of exercise hyperpnea: a limiting factor? *Am. Rev. Resp. Dis.* (in press).

Adams, W.C., Savin, W.M. & Christo, A.E. (1981) Detection of ozone toxicity during continuous exercise via the effective dose concept. *J. Appl. Physiol.* **51**, 415–422.

Ainsworth, D.M., Smith, C.A., Eicker, S.W., Henderson, K.S. & Dempsey, J.A. (1989) The effects of locomotion on respiratory muscle activity in the awake dog. *Respir. Physiol.* **78**, 145–162.

Baker, M.A. (1979) A brain cooling system in mammals. *Sci. Am.* **240**, 130–139.

Bazzy, A.R., Pang, L.M., Akabas, S.R. & Haddad, G.G. (1989). O_2 metabolism of the sheep diaphragm during flow resistive loaded breathing. *J. Appl. Physiol.* **66**, 2305–2311.

Bellemare, F. & Bigland-Ritchie, B. (1987) Assessment of human diaphragm strength and activation using phrenic nerve stimulation. *Resp. Physiol.* **58**, 263–277.

Bye, P.T.P., Farkas, G.A . & Roussos, C. (1983) Respiratory factors limiting exercise. *Ann. Rev. Physiol.* **45**, 439–451.

Costill, D. (1970) Metabolic responses during distance running. *J. Appl. Physiol.* **28**, 251–255.

Dempsey, J.A., Aaron, E. & Martin, B.J. (1988) Pulmonary function and prolonged exercise. In: Lamb, D.R. & Murray, R. (eds) *Perspectives in Exercise. Science and Sports Medicine, Vol. 1. Prolonged Exercise*, pp. 75–119. Benchmark Press, Indianapolis.

Dempsey, J.A., Gledhill, N., Reddan, W.G., Forster, H.V., Hanson, P.G. & Claremont, A.D. (1977) Pulmonary adaptation to exercise: effects of exercise type and duration, chronic hypoxia and physical training. *Ann. N.Y. Acad. Sci.* **301**, 243–261.

Dempsey, J.A., Johnson, B.D. & Bayly, W.M. (1990a) Constraints on the ventilatory response to maximum exercise in health. In: Sutton, J.R., Coates, G. & Remmers, J.E. (eds) *Hypoxia: The Adaptations*, pp. 178–181. B.C. Decker, Burlington, Ontario.

Dempsey, J.A., Johnson, B.D. & Saupe, K.W. (1990b) Adaptations and limitations in the pulmonary system during exercise. *Chest* **97** (3), 81–86S.

Dempsey, J.A., Thomson, J.M., Aleander, S.C., Forster, H.V. & Chosy, L.W. (1975) Respiratory influences on acid–base status and their effects on O_2 transport during prolonged muscular work. In: Howald, H. & Poortmans, J.R. (eds) *Metabolic Adaptation to Prolonged Physical Exercise*. Proceedings of the 2nd International Symposium on Biochemistry of Exercise, No. 7, pp. 56–64. Birkhauser Verlag, Basel.

Dempsey, J.A., Vidruk, E.H. & Mastenbrook, S.M. (1980) Pulmonary control systems in exercise. *Fed. Proc.* **39**, 1498–1505.

Dempsey, J.A., Vidruk, E.H. & Mitchell, G.S. (1985) Pulmonary control systems in exercise: update. *Fed. Proc.* **44**, 2260–2270.

Ekelund, L.G. (1967) Circulatory and respiratory adaptation during prolonged exercise of moderate intensity in the sitting position. *Acta. Physiol. Scand.* **69**, 327–340.

Fabiato, A. & Fabiato, F. (1978) Effects of pH on the myofilaments and the sarcoplasmic reticulum of skinned cells from cardiac and skeletal muscles. *J. Physiol. (Lond.)* **276**, 233–255.

Fregosi, R. & Dempsey, J.A. (1986) Effects of exercise in normoxia and acute hypoxia on respiratory muscle metabolities. *J. Appl. Physiol.* **60**, 1274–1283.

Gallagher, C.G., Huda, W., Rigby, M., Greenberg, D. & Younes, M. (1988) Lack of radiographic evidence of interstitial pulmonary edema after maximal exercise in normal subjects. *Am. Rev. Respir. Dis.* **137**, 474–476.

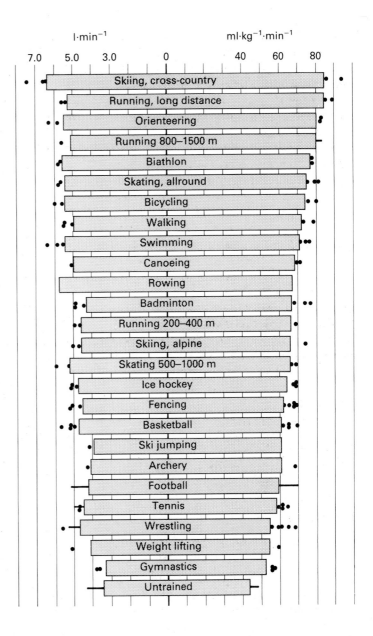

Fig. 7.2 Maximal oxygen uptakes in top Swedish male athletes. From Åstrand & Rodahl (1986), with permission. Dots show values above the mean, lines show range above the mean.

amount of oxygen in the blood (arterial oxygen content) and the litres of blood pumped per minute (cardiac output) are both important for delivery of oxygen to the tissues, so the amount of oxygen transported can be assessed by considering the product of these two measurements, known as the systemic oxygen transport. The value of systemic oxygen transport is closely correlated to maximal oxygen intake across a wide range of values. This is illustrated in Fig. 7.4 which is drawn from data observed while breathing air, when approximately 15% of the haemoglobin was bound by carbon monoxide, and while breathing gas with high oxygen content.

The oxygen content in normal men is usually around 200 ml·l^{-1} arterial blood and changes in content are usually modest or nil during exer-

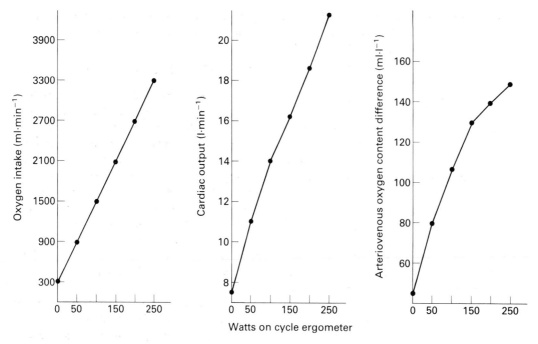

Fig. 7.3 Adjustments of oxygen intake, cardiac output and arteriovenous oxygen content differences at varying levels of power production.

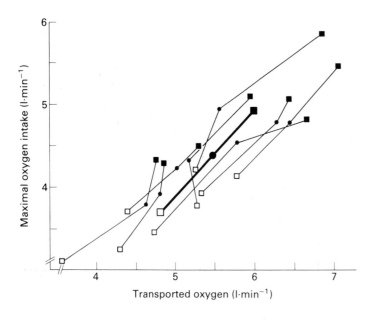

Fig. 7.4 Maximal oxygen uptake at various levels of transported oxygen. ■, High oxygen level; □, carboxy haemoglobin level, ●, control. The heavy central line connects the three mean values. From Astrand & Rodahl (1986), with permission.

cise and training. Consequently, variations in maximal oxygen transport are most related to maximal cardiac output. Hence let us consider the factors that regulate cardiac output.

Regulation of cardiac output

Cardiac output can be expressed mathematically as heart rate multiplied by stroke volume. It follows that maximal cardiac output could potentially be altered by changes in either maximal heart rate or maximal stroke volume.

Regulation of maximal heart rate

Increases in heart rate during exercise are due to both sympathetic nervous system activity and withdrawal of parasympathetic nervous tone (Ekblöm *et al.*, 1973). There is no known intervention that will increase the maximal exercise heart rate of normal individuals while maintaining normal sinus rhythm. However, the maximal heart rate can be slowed by blocking the autonomic nervous system with propranolol (Fig. 7.5). This manoeuvre has little or no effect on maximal oxygen intake. Failure of maximal oxygen intake to fall with a slower

peak heart rate strongly suggests that maximal stroke volume has considerable reserve.

Regulation of stroke volume

The stroke volume of the heart is determined by a number of factors including the filling pressure of the left ventricle and contractility. The factors that regulate the vigour of contraction are multiple and complex and are difficult to describe briefly. However, contractility is a term that is used to express the vigour of contraction, and we use it while recognizing that no single measurement expresses all aspects of myocardial performance. The relationship between stroke volume and filling pressure can be understood by examining Fig. 7.6.

As end-diastolic volume increases, the stroke volume increases. End-diastolic volume is determined by the pressures in the venous system, which in turn are functions of blood volume and size and compliance of the vascular bed. However, the ventricular response is also dependent upon the state of the contractile elements of the myocardium, so that the vigour of contraction, known as contractility, can vary.

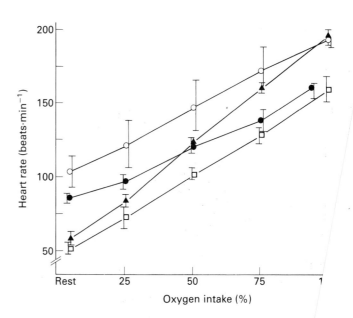

Fig. 7.5 Heart rate during exercise in control state and during autonomic blockade with atropine and/ or propranolol. ○, Atropine; □, propranolol; ●, atropine plus propranolol; ▲, control. From Ekblöm *et al.* (1973), with permission.

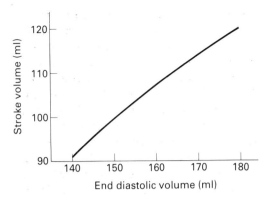

Fig. 7.6 Starling curve showing increasing stroke volume with increasing ventricular diastolic volumes.

Inotropic agents such as isoprenaline lead to increased contractility, and heart disease can decrease contractility. It is obvious that in the presence of disease, the ventricle is very limited

and even at very high levels of filling pressures, maximal exercise cardiac output remains low (Fig. 7.7).

The customary marker for myocardial contractility is the ejection fraction, the quotient of stroke volume divided by end-diastolic volume and expressed as a percentage. The ejection fraction has not been found to be greater in athletes compared with normals (Gilbert et al., 1977). However, there are important differences in myocardial structure. The hearts of athletes are larger and have a greater volume and wall thickness (Bar-Shlomo et al., 1982). Because this increased size is accompanied by normal ejection fractions, it follows that the capacity to eject blood must be increased in the athletic individual. The hearts of sprinters are smaller in both size and volume, so their overall capacity to pump blood is less than that of endurance athletes.

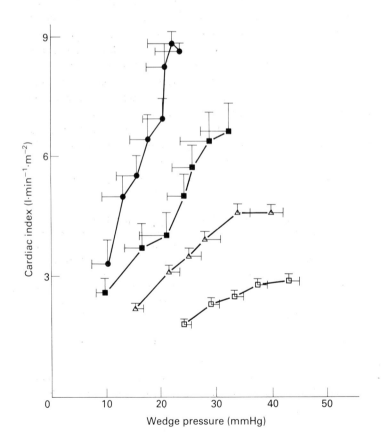

Fig. 7.7 Response of cardiac output and pulmonary capillary wedge pressure to increasing work rates in patients with congestive heart failure, in four categories of maximal oxygen intake (ml·min^{-1}·kg^{-1}): ●, > 20; ■, 15–20; △, 10–14; □, < 10. From Weber & Janicki (1985), with permission.

Effects of physical training

What is the contribution of exercise training to endurance performance? It seems likely that a major consequence of exercise conditioning is to increase maximal stroke volume and cardiac output. Part of this is due to an increase in blood volume (Saltin et al., 1968); part may be due to an increase in myocardial contractility, so far demonstrated to occur only in experimental animals (Scheuer, 1973).

To what extent are the high values of maximal oxygen intake in endurance athletes achieved by training, and how much is bestowed by heredity? Clearly, both are important. The maximal oxygen intake rarely increases from sedentary to maximal training effect by more than 50% and the gain is usually 25–30%. This suggests that the basic capabilities of individuals are fixed at birth, although training will maximize the potential of each.

Age also influences the values of maximal physical performance. After reaching a peak value at around 20 years of age, a gradual decline occurs so that at 65 years of age, the maximal oxygen intake is 70% of the value noted at 25 years of age. With regular physical training, there is a lessening but not an elimination of the reduction due to ageing. Ageing may cause quantitative differences in the method of adjustment of the cardiovascular system to exercise conditioning (Table 7.1).

Training of young individuals seems to lead to an increase in maximal oxygen intake due to both widening of maximal arteriovenous oxygen content difference and increase in maximal cardiac output (Hartley et al., 1969). On the other hand almost all of the increase in maximal oxygen intake which occurs in middle-aged individuals can be explained by an increase in maximal cardiac output. This apparent difference may be explainable by the greater responsiveness of the younger individuals when distributing blood to the exercising tissues.

Cardiac output as a limiting factor for $\dot{V}O_{2\ max}$

An important physiological question is whether maximal oxygen intake is determined by central or peripheral factors. If it were primarily central, improving cardiac output would increase maximal oxygen intake. If it were primarily peripheral, then changes in cardiac output would have little effect.

Observing changes in the central and peripheral circulation with exercise conditioning, when maximal oxygen intake increases, have been of little help. This is because the increase in maximal cardiac output is accompanied by an increased oxidative capacity of the skeletal muscles (Holloszy & Booth, 1976), suggesting

Table 7.1 Comparison of circulatory variables during maximal exercise in young and middle-aged men.

	Age (years)	Oxygen intake (l·min^{-1})	Cardiac output (l·min^{-1})	Heart rate (beats·min^{-1})	Stroke volume (ml)	Arteriovenous oxygen content difference (ml·dl^{-1})
Young men (n = 17)	23	3.11	21.5	196	110	14.4
Percentage change*		+15	+8	−3	+11	+8
Middle-aged men (n = 13)	47	2.68	18.7	182	103	14.4
Percentage change*		+14	+13	−3	+16	+1

These data have been collected from several studies in the literature for the young group, referenced in Hartley et al. (1969).
*, after training.

that both central and peripheral factors contribute.

The close correlation between systemic oxygen transport and maximal oxygen intake is strong circumstantial evidence that the body will use all of the oxygen that can reach the exercising muscles. If the systemic oxygen transport is increased by infusion of blood (Ekblöm et al., 1975) or by hyperbaric oxygen breathing (Fagraeus, 1974) the maximal oxygen intake increases. These experiments strongly suggest that the muscles are capable of using more oxygen than can be delivered by the normal cardiovascular system.

Since oxygen content is usually fixed during exercise, muscle blood flow would seem likely to determine maximal systemic oxygen transport. Could it be that the muscles have a vasculature that only permits a certain maximal blood flow? In such an event, not cardiac output but vascular conductance in the skeletal muscles would determine maximal oxygen transport and hence maximal oxygen uptake.

Saltin (1986) has estimated that the potential of human skeletal muscle to accommodate blood flow is $2-2.5 \, l \cdot kg^{-1} \cdot min^{-1}$ in normoxia. During maximal exercise, the muscle oxygen intake would be expected to be $0.35 \, l \cdot min^{-1} \cdot kg^{-1}$. As pointed out by Saltin and emphasized later by Åstrand (1988), a person with a total skeletal muscle mass of 30 kg could accommodate a blood flow of $60-70 \, l \cdot min^{-1}$. This is of course far higher than the maximal values of $35 \, l \cdot min^{-1}$ observed in athletes for cardiac output. This suggests that maximal vascular conductance is not the limiting factor for maximal oxygen uptake.

Studying the effects of increasing maximal cardiac output on the maximal oxygen intake is difficult. One might expect the maximal cardiac output to be higher when using all 30 kg of muscles than when doing treadmill exercise. In fact, adding arms to leg exercise has little incremental effect on maximal oxygen intake. Also when one-legged exercise is converted to two-legged exercise, the blood flow actually decreases in the original exercising leg. This

suggests that more vascular beds can be opened up than can be supplied by cardiac output, and that pressure is defended by baroreflex vasoconstriction.

So how much muscle mass can the central circulation perfuse? Saltin's data suggest that about 8 kg can be accommodated in a normal person. Activation of more than this amount will result in vasoconstriction, so that the overall cardiac output will remain fixed. The preponderance of data seem to indicate that the central circulation is the limiting factor for maximal oxygen intake in that skeletal muscles could use more oxygen and more blood flow, if available. However, issues of distribution of blood flow and factors regulating local cellular metabolism have not been completely excluded as contributors.

Certainly, local changes in the muscle are important for endurance performance. However, it seems likely that these changes are most important for submaximal endurance exercise. The duration of activity which can be sustained is greater and the rate of lactate accumulation is less in trained compared with untrained individuals. This is true for both absolute and relative (percentage of maximal) work rates (also see Chapter 22).

Summary

For activities that last for more than a few minutes, energy is derived mostly from aerobic metabolic sources which depend on an adequate supply of oxygen. This oxygen is supplied by the cardiovascular system and hence the ability of individuals to perform endurance exercise is dependent upon the ability to deliver blood to exercising muscles. Maximal oxygen intakes are consistently high in athletes whose events last for more than a few minutes. The high values are accompanied by large cardiac outputs. Because increasing oxygen delivery can increase maximal oxygen intake, it would appear that in athletes the maximal oxygen intake is largely limited by the maximal cardiac output. This ability is heavily influenced by genetic factors, but can be increased by regular physical training.

References

Åstrand, P.-O. (1988) From exercise physiology to preventive medicine. *Ann. Clin. Res.* **20**, 10–17.

Åstrand, P.-O. & Rodahl, K. (1986) *Textbook of Work Physiology*, 3rd edn. McGraw-Hill, New York.

Bar-Shlomo, B.-Z., Druck, M.N. & Morch, J.E. (1982) Left ventricular function in trained and untrained healthy subjects. *Circulation* **65**, 484–488.

Ekblöm, B., Huot, R., Stein, E.M. & Thorstensson, A.T. (1975) Effect of changes in arterial oxygen content on circulation and physical performance. *J. Appl. Physiol.* **39**, 71–79.

Ekblöm, B., Kilbom, A. & Soltysiak, J. (1973) Physical training, bradycardia, and autonomic nervous system. *Scand. J. Clin. Lab. Invest.* **32**, 251–256.

Fagraeus, L. (1974) Cardiorespiratory and metabolic functions during exercise in hyperbaric environment. *Acta Physiol. Scand.* **414** (Suppl.), 1–10.

Gilbert, C.A., Nutter, D.O., Felner, J.M., Perkins, J.V., Heymsfield, S.B. & Schlant, R.G. (1977) Echocardiographic study of cardiac dimensions and function in the endurance-trained athlete. *Am. J. Cardiol.* **40**, 528–533.

Hartley, L.H., Grimby, G., Kilböm, Å. *et al.* (1969) Cardiac output during submaximal and maximal exercise in middle-aged man before and after physical conditioning. *Scand. J. Clin. Lab. Invest.* **24**, 335–344.

Holloszy, J.O. & Booth, F.W. (1976) Biochemical adaptations to endurance exercise in muscle. *Ann. Rev. Physiol.* **18**, 273–277.

Saltin, B. (1986) Physiological adaptation to physical conditioning. In: Åstrand, P.-O. & Grimby, G. (eds) *Acta Med. Scand.* Symposium Series No. 2, pp. 11–24. Almqvist & Wiksell International, Stockholm.

Saltin, B., Blomqvist, G., Mitchell, J.H., Johnson, R.L., Wildenthal, K. & Chapman, C. (1968) Response to exercise after bed rest and training. *Circulation* **7** (Suppl.), 1–78.

Scheuer, J. (1973) Physical training and intrinsic cardiac adaptations. *Circulation* **47**, 677–687.

Weber, K.T. & Janicki, J.S. (1985) Pathophysiologic responses to exercise in patients with congestive heart failure. *Heart Failure* **1**, 131–139.

Chapter 8

Peripheral Circulation and Endurance

ROY J. SHEPHARD AND MICHAEL J. PLYLEY

Introduction

The primary functions of the cardiovascular system are to maintain an adequate supply of oxygen and essential nutrients to the cells of the various body organs in proportion to their individual needs, to deliver hormonal messengers to various target tissues, and to provide a means for the removal of metabolic byproducts, including heat, thereby assuring homoeostasis in the various tissues of the body.

During brief bouts of exercise, temporary departures from homoeostasis are tolerated, but this becomes progressively less practical as the duration of activity is increased; thus, with the type of pursuits considered in this volume, blood flow must meet the metabolic demands of the active tissues. With vigorous endurance exercise, the oxygen consumption of the skeletal muscle is increased 10–20-fold. Because the arterial oxygen content remains essentially constant from rest to maximal exercise (see Chapter 6), the additional oxygen requirements of steady state activity must be met by some combination of an increase of total cardiac output and a redistribution of flow from the less active to the more active tissues (Table 8.1).

Control of peripheral blood flow

The rate of blood flow through a vessel is directly proportional to the pressure gradient, and is inversely proportional to the vascular resistance. Customarily, this relationship is re-arranged and is solved for resistance. In terms of the cardiovascular system as a whole, the relationship becomes:

$$\text{Total peripheral resistance} = \frac{\text{Pressure gradient}}{\text{Cardiac output}}$$

where the pressure gradient is measured as the difference between the mean arterial pressure and the mean venous blood pressure. Since right atrial pressure is essentially zero in the healthy individual, the pressure gradient becomes equal to the mean arterial blood pressure. Therefore, under resting conditions, the total peripheral resistance (TPR) in the normal person is of the order of 15–18 peripheral resistance units (PRU) that is [80 + 0.33 (120 −80) mmHg/5.5 l·min^{-1}], 17 mmHg·l^{-1}·min^{-1}, or 17 PRU).

Factors influencing vascular resistance include blood viscosity and vascular geometry (that is, the length and radius of the vessel). The fundamental law describing the relationships between pressure and the various factors determining resistance to flow was derived experimentally by Poiseuille:

$$\text{Flow} = \frac{(\text{Pressure gradient}) \; \pi r^4}{8l\eta}$$

where r is the radius of a vessel, l is its length, and η the viscosity of blood.

While this relationship was intended to describe non-pulsatile flow in inelastic tubes of

80

Table 8.1 Distribution of cardiac output to various vascular regions during progressive exercise to maximum aerobic power. Modified from Vander *et al.* (1985).

Vascular region	Cardiac output (ml·min^{-1})			
	At rest (6%)	Light exercise (30%)	Heavy exercise (75%)	Maximal exercise (100%)
Cardiac output	6000	12 000	24 000	30 000
Cerebral	720 (12%)	720 (6%)	720 (3%)	720 (2%)
Myocardial	240 (4%)	480 (4%)	960 (4%)	1200 (4%)
Muscle	1260 (21%)	5760 (48%)	17 280 (72%)	26 400 (88%)
Renal	1320 (22%)	1200 (10%)	720 (3%)	300 (1%)
Hepatosplanchnic	1560 (26%)	1440 (12%)	960 (4%)	300 (1%)
Skin	540 (9%)	1920 (16%)	2640 (11%)	900 (3%)
Other	360 (6%)	480 (4%)	720 (3%)	180 (1%)

uniform diameter, it serves to highlight the relative importance of the various factors that determine human blood flow. Most of the factors involved in this equation are commonsense. However, the dependence of flow upon the fourth power of the radius is less expected. An effect of cross-sectional area, or r^2, might have been anticipated in terms of vessel size. The dependence on r^4 has important implications with regard to the control of blood flow. Those vessels with the greatest capacity to alter their radius become the ultimate site for the control of flow. A twofold change of diameter in such vessels will change blood flow by a factor of 16. The cross-sectional structure of the various components of the cardiovascular system (Table 8.2) is such that vessels with the greatest amount of smooth muscle and the lowest vessel diameter to wall thickness ratio, the key essentials in altering vascular size, are the arterioles and the precapillary sphincters, although there may also be some regulation of flow through the larger arteries, due mainly to an endothelium-mediated, flow-dependent vasodilatation, and myogenic autoregulation (Bassenge & Münzel, 1988).

The factors that normally determine arteriolar diameter can be categorized as neural, humoral and chemical (Table 8.3). Vessel length and blood viscosity do not usually vary to any great extent. In clinical situations such as coronary or peripheral vascular arteriosclerosis, the critical site of narrowing may be shifted from the arterioles to larger vessels; however, the r^4 relationship is preserved, so that an atherosclerotic plaque must block more than 70% of the arterial lumen before there is a substantial decrease of blood flow distal to the lesion. The viscosity of the blood is related to the red cell count in a complex, non-linear manner. Blood doping and increases of red cell count attributable to training, high altitude exposure, or steroid abuse all increase the viscosity of the blood. However, few endurance athletes would normally reach a level of polycythaemia where the increase of red cell count is having a substantial impact upon peripheral blood flow.

A further factor that can limit muscle blood flow is a direct compression of the main arterial supply by the intramuscular pressure developed during contraction. This factor first comes into play when muscles are exerting more than 15% of their maximal voluntary force, and vascular occlusion is likely to be complete at 60−70% of maximal voluntary force. During rhythmic endurance exercise, the muscle force is usually only a small fraction of maximal effort, but partial occlusion can develop, for example, when a distance cyclist is developing additional force on the pedals during the ascent

Table 8.2 Vascular geometry and anatomical structure (presented as relative amounts of tissue*) of the various components of the cardiovascular system. Modified from Burton (1975) and Rushmer (1976).

	Vascular component							
	Aorta	Artery	Arteriole	Precapillary sphincter	Capillary	Venule	Vein	Vena cava
Vascular geometry								
Vessel diameter	25 mm	4 mm	30 μm	35 μm	8 μm	20 μm	5 mm	30 mm
Wall thickness	2 mm	1 mm	20 μm	30 μm	1 μm	2 μm	0.5 μm	1.5 μm
Diameter : wall thickness	12.5	4	1.5	1.2	8	10	10	20
Vascular structure								
Endothelium	M	M	M	H	M	M	M	M
Elastic tissue	VH	H	M	L	NA	NA	M	M
Smooth muscle	M	VH	H	H	NA	NA	M	H
Fibrous tissue	H	M	M	L	NA	L	M	H

* VH, very high; H, high; M, medium; L, low; NA, not a component in the vessel wall.

Table 8.3 Factors involved in the extrinsic and local control of blood flow. Modified from Fox (1984).

Agent/factor	Source	Vascular action	Comments
Neural			
α-adrenergic	Sympathetic nerves	Vasoconstriction	Occurs in all blood vessels except those of the cerebral circulation
Cholinergic	Sympathetic nerves	Vasodilatation	Occurs only in the blood vessels of skeletal muscle
Cholinergic	Parasympathetic nerves	Vasodilatation	Occurs in the blood vessels of the gastrointestinal tract and external genitalia
Humoral			
Noradrenaline	Adrenal medulla	Vasoconstriction	Interacts with α-adrenergic receptors in vascular smooth muscle
Adrenaline	Adrenal medulla	Vasoconstriction	Interacts with α-adrenergic receptors in vascular smooth muscle
Adrenaline	Adrenal medulla	Vasodilatation	Interacts with β_2-adrenergic receptors in vascular smooth muscle of heart and skeletal muscle
Angiotensin II	Blood plasma	Vasoconstriction	Produced from angiotensin by the action of renin, an enzyme produced by the kidneys, and made active from angiotensin I by a converting enzyme; important in the maintenance of salt balance
Vasopressin	Neurohypophysis	Vasoconstriction	Important in the maintenance of fluid balance
Local			
Myogenic	Intravascular blood pressure	Vasoconstriction	Stretching of the vessel wall results in a reflex contraction of the vascular smooth muscle; assures a relatively constant rate of blood flow to an organ when blood pressure varies widely (termed autoregulation)
Metabolic	Oxygen, carbon dioxide, hydrogen ions, adenosine, potassium, other metabolic byproducts, osmolarity	Vasodilatation	Changes in the concentration of certain constituents and metabolic byproducts in the milieu of the cell acts directly to produce a relaxation of the vascular smooth muscle
Other factors	Histamines	Vasodilatation	Released locally following injury or allergic reactions
	Prostaglandins	Vasodilatation	Mechanism not well understood
	Bradykinin	Vasodilatation	Released by the sweat glands
	Heat	Vasodilatation	Used therapeutically; after cold is removed, there is a reflex vasodilatation termed reactive hyperaemia
	Cold	Vasoconstriction	

of a steep hill. Finally, account must be taken of body posture. When the legs are below heart level, as in running or cycling, the hydrostatic pressure is increased in both the arteries and the veins, but the 'muscle pump' is apparently able to counteract the hydrostatic increment of venous pressure, allowing a greater maximal perfusion of the leg muscles (Folkow et al., 1971).

Neural control of blood flow

The neural regulation of arteriolar size occurs mainly through the sympathetic nervous system; control lies in the medulla. Four main areas have been identified: the cardioacceleratory and cardioinhibitory centres directing cardiac function, and the pressor and depressor areas regulating vascular function. In most vascular beds (the cerebral circulation being the exception), sympathetic regulation of vessel size occurs by way of vasoconstrictor fibres and the chemical mediator noradrenaline. The latter acts to produce a contraction (vasoconstriction) via α-receptors in the smooth muscle component of the vascular wall. In some species, a second set of sympathetic nerve fibres produces skeletal muscle vasodilatation via the mediator acetylcholine, but the presence of such fibres has not yet been confirmed in humans. In situations of flight, fright or fight, activation of the sympathetic nervous system causes both a generalized vasoconstriction in most regions of the cardiovascular system and vasodilatation in the active skeletal muscles.

At rest, the smooth muscle in a vessel wall receives a steady discharge from the sympathetic fibres. It is therefore normally in a state of slight vasoconstriction (termed basal tone). In this way, vasodilatation can also be achieved by withdrawing the basal sympathetic neural activity.

Humoral control of blood flow

In addition to neural reflexes, arteriolar radius is influenced by a number of humoral agents

(Table 8.3), the two most active agents during exercise being the noradrenaline and adrenaline that are released as a result of sympathetic discharge to the adrenal medulla. The noradrenaline released in this way acts in a similar fashion to that released by the sympathetic nerve fibres, serving as a vasoconstrictor through the α-receptors in the vessel wall. Adrenaline exerts two opposing actions, depending on the receptor(s) with which the hormone interacts. It induces a vasoconstriction when acting upon the α-receptors, but if it acts upon β$_2$-receptors a relaxation (vasodilatation) of the vessel wall is produced. In most tissues of the body, the blood vessels are supplied with α-receptors (the cerebral circulation is an exception), but only the smooth muscle of vessels supplying the heart and skeletal muscles contains β$_2$-receptors.

Other hormones that serve as potent vasoactive agents include angiotensin II, important in maintaining a proper salt balance (and therefore indirectly involved in fluid balance) and vasopressin (actively involved in maintaining fluid homeostasis).

Local control of blood flow

The vascular control system would be incomplete if total control resided with 'central command', since the real needs of individual tissues might not be satisfied. The vascular system thus relies on an ever-present interplay between central control (represented by the nervous system and tasked with the maintenance of arterial blood pressure) and local control (tasked with assuring an optimal distribution of the available blood flow to the various tissues according to their individual needs). During endurance exercise, the central command is typically directed to a maintenance or even a progressive increase of mean blood pressure; this is achieved by a decrease of blood flow to the viscera, the inactive muscles and (as the circulating blood volume is reduced by exudation of fluid into the extracellular space), a progressive cutaneous vasoconstriction. However, flow to the active muscles is augmented by local control mechanisms (particularly a decrease of oxygen partial pressure and a leakage of potassium ions from the working muscles). Given that the resting cardiac output is about 5.5 l·min^{-1}, and the maximum cardiac output ranges from 35 l·min^{-1} in a well trained young male endurance athlete to 20 l·min^{-1} in a sedentary 65-year-old man, the ability to redirect flow from inactive to active tissues can make only a moderate contribution to endurance performance.

The blood flow to the skin can vary from about 0.5 to 6.0 l·min^{-1}, depending on the environmental temperature. It is less clear whether the increase of cutaneous blood flow induced by a hot environment steals cardiac output from the working muscles, or (by reducing cardiac afterload) allows the subject to develop a larger peak cardiac output.

If effort is prolonged, and the subject becomes dehydrated, central homeostatic mechanisms begin to fail (see section on circulatory drift below). Ultimately, the blood pressure falls, with impaired consciousness and fainting. Impairment of blood flow to the kidneys may lead to anuria and renal failure, while impairment of blood flow to the adrenal glands can progress to adrenal shock. Such situations are particularly likely when a prolonged race is held on a hot afternoon (see Chapter 42). Cutaneous blood flow can of itself be reduced by 3–5 l·min^{-1}, and an ability to dissipate heat with a smaller flow of blood to the skin (for instance, by greater sweating and thus a lower skin temperature) can thus serve to augment a prolonged endurance performance.

The blood flow to the limb muscles can have a substantial impact upon body heat loss during an endurance pursuit such as long-distance swimming. If the vessels are constricted, the muscles provide a useful supplement to the insulation provided by subcutaneous fat, but if the blood flow to the limbs is augmented by physical activity the extra loss of heat may more than outweigh the added heat production by the local muscles.

Peripheral versus central limitation of endurance performance

Physiologists have debated for more than 30 years whether endurance performance is limited by central or by peripheral factors (Shephard, 1977; 1982, see Chapter 3). Three main arguments have been advanced in favour of a central limitation of oxygen transport and thus endurance performance:

1 A theoretical analysis of the partial pressure gradients shows that the main decrease of oxygen partial pressure occurs between the pulmonary capillaries and the muscle capillaries. By analogy with a linked system of electrical conductances, this implies that the main impedance to oxygen transport resides in the pumping ability of the heart (Shephard, 1977). We may note that this is not an absolute proof. Arguably, the pumping ability of the heart is limited by a poor preload, associated with poor peripheral venous tone, and thus a pooling of blood in the legs. Likewise, function could be limited if a poor local perfusion of the working muscle led to a large increase of systemic blood pressure, with an increase of after-loading that limited cardiac pumping.

2 An empirical comparison of various large muscle tasks shows that the oxygen transport developed during uphill treadmill running can be only marginally augmented by the addition of a second form of activity (for example, the handling of a ski pole while striding on the treadmill). However, if performance were limited by either peripheral blood flow or the enzyme activity of the muscles, one would anticipate that an increase in the volume of active muscle would increase peak oxygen transport (Shephard, 1977; 1982).

3 Measurements of peak local muscle blood flow suggest that the vascular conductance per unit of tissue is such that if all of the muscles were vasodilated, the available peripheral conductance would far exceed the pumping ability of the heart (Andersen and Saltin, 1985; Reading et al., 1990).

While these seem strong arguments, they

have not convinced all of those who favour peripheral hypotheses such as external compression of the muscle vessels by the contracting muscle, an inadequate anatomical development or functional dilatation of the capillary bed, a lack of oxygen transport and enzymic mechanisms within the active muscles, or loss of fluid into the extracellular space and relaxed veins.

Proof of a peripheral limitation has sometimes been sought in an increased arteriovenous oxygen difference subsequent to training. Many studies of coronary rehabilitation, for example, have found that in the first few months following a myocardial infarction oxygen transport is augmented by a widening of arteriovenous oxygen difference rather than an increase of cardiac output (Paterson et al., 1979). Peripheralists have argued that, initially, either the capillary supply or the enzyme activity in the working muscles was inadequate for aerobic demand, and that development of such systems was responsible for the training-induced increase of maximal oxygen intake. However, such an analysis ignores the point that the arteriovenous difference has usually been measured between arterial and mixed venous blood, rather than between the arterial system and the venules draining the working muscles. Blood specimens taken from the veins of working muscle are almost completely oxygen depleted before any special training begins (Saltin, 1973), and the widened average arteriovenous difference of a trained subject is arising largely because of a redistribution of blood to vascular beds where a larger proportion of the oxygen is being extracted.

In terms of the importance of central and peripheral factors, much presumably depends upon the volume of muscle that is required to perform a given sport. If most of the large muscles of the body are active, then any limitation of oxygen transport is likely to be central in nature, but if the performance draws heavily upon a few small muscle groups, then a peripheral limitation of function becomes increasingly likely (LeJemtel et al., 1986; Shephard

et al., 1988). The matter is nevertheless important to resolve, because very different training tactics are demanded to counter the various potential limitations of aerobic function.

Measurement of peripheral blood flow

Under resting conditions, it is relatively easy to measure limb blood flow by venous occlusion plethysmography (Brodie & Russell, 1905), using either traditional water-filled systems or simpler capacitance (Dresler et al., 1987) and strain-gauge systems (Whitney, 1953). The last approach measures changes in limb dimensions as the increased impedance of a rubber or silicone tube filled with mercury or a gallium—indium alloy. One important advantage of the strain gauge approach is that the limb can be exposed to the air, and that the temperature of the part is thus not predetermined by that of the flow-measuring chamber. On the other hand, it is necessary to assume that the limb is cylindrical, data are only obtained for a narrow cross-section of the limb (Anderson et al., 1983), and the impedance of the measuring gauge may be affected by a change of limb temperature during exercise (Hokanson et al., 1975).

Flow data have traditionally been expressed per 100 ml of limb volume. The main component of blood flow to the hand and the foot is skin flow. Measurements of the extremities have thus been considered as representative of the cutaneous circulation. In contrast, the flow to the forearm, calf or thigh depends largely upon muscle perfusion, particularly if the precaution is taken to exclude flow from the hand or foot by the fitting of a high pressure cuff at the wrist or ankle. In some instances, the local volume of muscle has been estimated by anthropometric techniques (Savard et al., 1977; Andersen & Saltin, 1985; Rowell et al., 1986; Reading et al., 1990), with the flow rates being expressed per 100 ml muscle, or of active muscle. More specialized techniques are needed to measure the other elements of peripheral blood flow shown in Table 8.4 (Wade & Bishop, 1962; Shephard,

Table 8.4 Distribution of blood flow at rest and during maximal aerobic exercise in an 80-kg athlete.

Region of body	Mass of tissue (kg)	Blood flow at rest			Blood flow during exercise		
		ml·min^{-1}	ml·min^{-1}· 100 g^{-1} tissue	Percentage of cardiac output	ml·min^{-1}	ml·min^{-1}· 100 g tissue	Percentage of cardiac output
Lungs	1.2	6000	600	100	30 000	2500	100
Brain	1.6	840	53	14	840	53	3
Myocardium	0.4	240	60	4	1 200	300	4
Hepatosplanchnic	4.1	1680	41	28	450	11	1
Kidneys	0.4	1380	345	23	360	90	1
Muscle	34.7	1200	4	20	26 400	76	88
Skin*	2.2	480	22	8	600	27	2
Other	35.4	180	c. 1	3	150	c. 1	1

* At an ambient temperature of 25°C.

1982). Because the flow to these regions is rarely measured in athletes, we shall not discuss such techniques in any detail.

Venous occlusion plethysmography is not practical during most types of exercise because of the encumbrance of the measuring equipment. Data can only be collected within a few seconds of ceasing activity, backward extrapolation being needed to estimate flows during exercise, but unfortunately perfusion drops by as much as 50% within 10 s of ceasing exercise (Walløe & Wesche, 1988). The options during exercise include the transport of heat away from a heated thermocouple (Hensel et al., 1954), thermodilution (Andersen & Saltin, 1985; LeJemtel et al., 1986), pulsed Doppler techniques (Walløe & Wesche, 1988), the infusion of indocyanine green dye (Jorfeldt, 1988), the removal of radioisotopes such as sodium, or the washout of inert gases such as xenon or acetylene from intramuscular depots (Clausen, 1973; Grönlund et al., 1989) and (in animals) the use of microspheres (Cerretelli et al., 1984). While the washout of ^{133}xenon has become quite popular in recent years, it underestimates actual flow rates by up to 50% (Cerretelli et al., 1986).

Blood flow during exercise

The resting blood flow of muscle is no more than $2-4$ ml·min^{-1}·100 ml^{-1} of limb volume, but during vigorous endurance exercise, a flow of $60-100$ ml·min^{-1}·100 ml^{-1} of limb volume is common. Maximal flow rates of $250-400$ ml·min^{-1}·100 g^{-1} of muscle have been described in both dogs (Stainsby & Andrew, 1988) and humans (Rowell et al., 1986; Rowell, 1988). The flow seems to be determined largely by local metabolic rate, although there is also a pharmacological reserve, since higher flow rates than those seen in maximal effort can be induced by infusions of adenosine (Barclay, 1988). Flow rates also depend on fibre composition, and a positive correlation has been shown between vastus lateralis flow and the percentage of slow-twitch fibres in that muscle (Frisk-

Holmberg et al., 1981). Possibly, training may lead to a redistribution of intramuscular blood flow between slow- and fast-twitch fibres (Terjung et al., 1988). If the muscle effort during rhythmic exercise exceeds $15-20\%$ of maximal voluntary force, an oscillatory pattern of flow is observed, values being higher during relaxation than during contraction (Barcroft & Dornhorst, 1949). While not proof of a causal relationship, maximal oxygen intake is inversely related to systemic vascular resistance (Clausen, 1976). Likewise, local measures of vascular conductance made during exercise of a small muscle group show a rather consistent relationship to the overall peak oxygen transport during a large muscle activity such as treadmill running (Fig. 8.1). Snell et al. (1987) found a higher correlation between the two variables in trained than in untrained subjects ($r = 0.81$ and 0.45 respectively). The intervening factor linking the two variables is probably the ability to induce vasodilatation in the skeletal musculature, although it is less clear whether there is a functional or a structural difference of

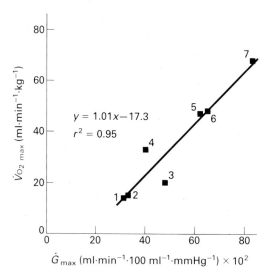

Fig. 8.1 Scatterplot of literature values for aerobic power as a function of vascular conductance in several subject groups. 1, 3, Goodman et al. (1990); 2, Yancy et al. (1988); 4, 6, Reading et al. (1990); 5, 7, Snell et al. (1987).

vascular conductance between endurance athletes, sedentary subjects and patients with cardiovascular disease (LeJemtel *et al.*, 1986; Yancy *et al.*, 1988). In congestive heart failure, at least, there is evidence that central regulatory mechanisms restrict flow to the exercising limbs in order to maintain a necessary minimum blood flow to non-exercising regions of the body (Sullivan *et al.*, 1989). Likewise, for a given systemic blood pressure, the local blood flow is greater during one-legged than during two-legged exercise, suggesting that during normal two-legged exercise vasoconstrictor activity is invoked to conserve flow to non-exercising regions (Clausen, 1977; Klausen *et al.*, 1982). Such local vasoregulation contributes to the limb-specific nature of flow enhancement after endurance training.

The number of capillaries per muscle fibre appears to be somewhat greater in a well trained subject than in a sedentary individual (see below), but the arrangement of the capillaries is complex (Plyley & Groom, 1975), and the greater capillary number may do no more than compensate for a longer oxygen diffusion path through the hypertrophied fibres of a well trained subject. Sinoway *et al.* (1987) demonstrated that local muscular training could induce a greater blood flow in the dominant forearm, independent of any changes in aerobic power; they speculated that there might be an increased capillarization of the trained arm, or a unilateral modification of sympathetic tone. On the other hand, at any given absolute work rate, the blood flow tends to be lower in the well trained athlete, because of a better capillary supply to the active fibres (Ozolin, 1986).

If the pursuit involves either repeated isometric activity (for example, the handgrip of a tennis player), or very vigorous rhythmic contractions at a substantial fraction of the peak local muscle force, then flow to the muscle group in question is likely to be impeded by the rising intramuscular pressure. Peripheral chemoreceptors are stimulated by substances such as substance P and somatostatin (Kaufman *et al.*, 1988), and there is a substantial rise of systemic blood pressure in an attempt to restore perfusion of the part. The endurance athlete normally seeks to operate at an intensity of effort where perfusion can match demand, so that the various disadvantages of anaerobic metabolism are avoided, at least until the final stages of a competition. Studies of xenon clearance (Clausen, 1973) have demonstrated that the quadriceps blood flow of the cyclist decreases if effort exceeds 75% of maximal aerobic power, and in the dog gastrocnemius flow also levels off before maximal effort is attained (Cerretelli *et al.*, 1986; Musch, 1988). Thus, when healthy young adults participate in a marathon run it has been estimated that effort is held to about 75% of maximal oxygen intake (Costill, 1972), although postcoronary patients (who begin with a much smaller aerobic power) may utilize as much as 80–85% of their peak aerobic power (Kavanagh *et al.*, 1977). Isometric activity in one region can also influence rhythmic exercise elsewhere. Thus, the rise of blood pressure invoked by a gripping of the handlebars could, at least in theory, increase the blood flow to the legs of a cyclist who was tiring.

The blood flow to non-exercising muscles is decreased during endurance exercise, despite a normal or an increased mean systemic blood pressure (Bevegard & Shepherd, 1967). Reports that the reduction of flow is less in trained subjects (Ozolin, 1986) probably reflect largely the lesser relative workload to which trained individuals are exposed in a standard laboratory test.

Coronary circulation

The coronary circulation is unusual in that oxygen extraction is almost complete even under resting conditions. The work of the myocardium is increased up to fivefold during vigorous endurance exercise, and the greater oxygen demand can thus only be satisfied by an increase of perfusion pressure (normally a minor response) or a substantial vasodilatation that allows a matching increase of blood flow (see Table 8.1).

The healthy athlete is able to augment coronary blood flow by the required fivefold margin, but difficulties can arise in two groups of competitors. Occasional young athletes have a restriction of perfusion associated with an anomalous origin of the coronary vessels, while Masters' competitors may have a partial blockage of the coronary vessels caused by atherosclerotic lesions. A recent study by Kavanagh *et al.* (1989) suggested that the proportion of older men showing electrocardiographic evidence of myocardial ischaemia during maximal aerobic exercise was similar in Masters' competitors and in the general population.

Pulmonary circulation

The pulmonary circulation must accommodate the entire cardiac output. It also has a substantial capacity, and can thus provide a useful reserve of blood, modulating preloading of the left ventricle. Finally, because of blood storage, substantial numbers of leucocytes are sequestered in the pulmonary circulation, and their release by an exercise-induced increase of cardiac output can lead to a substantial leucocytosis in peripheral venous blood.

Under resting conditions, pressures in the pulmonary circuit are low (pulmonary arterial pressures typically being 25/10 mmHg). There is a potential for about a threefold increase of blood flow by vasodilatation, without increase of intravascular pressures. However, if the cardiac output is increased sixfold, as can occur in a top endurance performer during all-out effort, then pulmonary arterial pressures rise. There have been suggestions that this could induce pulmonary oedema during events such as a triathlon, although in events of shorter duration a pulmonary exudation of fluid appears unlikely (see Chapter 41). A second consequence of the augmented pressure is that the speed of blood flow through the pulmonary circuit is increased. Under resting conditions, there is a virtual equilibrium between alveolar gas and pulmonary capillary blood, but this equilibrium is challenged in the top endurance athlete who can develop an extremely large peak pulmonary flow.

Because of the low resting pressures, alveolar gas pressures in the apex of the lung exceed intravascular pressures throughout most of the respiratory cycle, and the apical region is not perfused. Because vigorous aerobic exercise increases intravascular pressures, it facilitates perfusion of the upper part of the lungs, improving the match between alveolar ventilation and perfusion and increasing the effective alveolar surface for the exchange of respiratory gases (West, 1977).

Visceral blood flow

Viscera such as the kidneys and the liver have a large blood flow under resting conditions (see Table 8.1), with a correspondingly limited extraction of oxygen from the circulating blood. The reason is that the main function of the regional blood flow is the transport of metabolites and excretory products rather than carbon dioxide and oxygen.

When endurance exercise is performed under hot conditions, there is a dramatic reduction of visceral flow, sometimes to as little as one third of the resting value, with a corresponding increase of oxygen extraction. This change contributes to a broadening of the average arteriovenous oxygen difference (Wade & Bishop, 1962; Rowell, 1986). The excretory functions of the kidneys are temporarily curtailed, and a steep rise in the serum concentration of such substances as urea is observed over the course of a marathon run (Kavanagh *et al.*, 1977).

The circulatory failure associated with heat stress leads to a particularly drastic reduction in blood flow to the viscera, sometimes with pathological consequences including renal damage (manifested as haematuria, proteinuria and anuria) and adrenal shock.

Animal studies (Musch *et al.*, 1987) suggest that the ability to decrease regional flow to the intestines, spleen, liver, adrenal glands and kidneys is increased by training.

Cutaneous blood flow

If a subject is resting in a very warm environment, the blood flow to the skin can rise to $5-6$ $l \cdot min^{-1}$. The main function of the local circulation is the transport of heat, rather than carbon dioxide and oxygen, and, as in the viscera, only a small fraction of the available oxygen is extracted from the arterial blood.

When endurance exercise is performed in a warm environment, internal heat production is increased, and provided that the ceiling of cardiac output is not reached, cutaneous vasodilatation continues. However, if the circulation begins to fail through a combination of excessive vasodilatation and fluid loss in sweating, there may be a cutaneous vasoconstriction, and if competitive participation is continued, there is then a risk of serious hyperthermia (see Chapter 42).

When endurance exercise is performed in a cold environment, the peripheral blood flow is reduced, in an attempt to conserve body heat. The constriction of both the arterioles and the peripheral veins increases both the preloading and the after-loading of the heart. In a well trained individual, this may lead to a small increase of aerobic power (Bryan, 1967), but in an older individual the resultant increase of cardiac work rate may precipitate a bout of angina. When exercising in the cold, the muscle temperature is lower than when in a temperate environment (the opposite of a 'warm-up'), with an increase of local tissue viscosity, a deterioration of performance and an increased risk of musculoskeletal injuries. Cutaneous vasoconstriction leads to a numbing of the extremities, with a clumsiness that impedes fine movements. The function of the sensory nerves is also impaired, decreasing the feedback of information to coordinating centres in the brain, increasing clumsiness and the risk of injury. If the cold is more severe, a paralysis of the vasoconstrictor nerves may occur, leading to a 'hunting' reaction, periods of paradoxical vasodilatation and rewarming of the extremities alternating with bouts of vasoconstriction and cooling. The rewarming may be misinterpreted by a subject who is already confused by central hypothermia and hypoglycaemia, and on occasion the sensation of warmth has caused undressing, sometimes confused with a sexual assault (Wedin, 1976). With yet more severe cooling, local tissue temperatures drop below a critical value of from -1 to $-2°C$, with resultant freezing or frostbite (see Chapter 42). At this stage, all of the extremities have an extremely low blood flow, and if rewarming is attempted too quickly the restoration of blood flow may transfer heat to the cold limbs, with a further disastrous drop in core temperature.

Cerebral circulation

The cerebral circulation is unique in that it is relatively devoid of vasomotor function. Flow to the region (see Table 8.1) is determined largely by the mean systemic blood pressure, and for this reason the main pressure-regulating sensors are situated in the root of the neck.

Moderate endurance exercise leads to a progressive increase of systolic blood pressure and little change of diastolic pressure, so that there is a tendency to increase of cerebral blood flow. Gerontologists have argued that this may be one of the factors improving the apparent intelligence of older individuals who participate regularly in endurance exercise.

However, if exercise is pursued to exhaustion, particularly on a very hot day, the systemic blood pressure begins to fall, and there is an associated decrease of cerebral blood flow, leading to an impairment of consciousness. The subject may give a confused response to questioning, may make technical mistakes (for instance, the marathon runner who turns in the wrong direction on entering the stadium), and is more liable to accidents carrying a risk of physical injury. The decrease of blood flow to the motor cortex and cerebellum also leads to a deterioration of coordination and postural control, with an inefficient, staggering gait progressing to final collapse.

Animals such as greyhounds have continued to run on the treadmill until they die from circulatory failure, and the human athlete is perhaps fortunate that collapse from the upright posture puts an end to excessive circulatory demand. Recovery is usually rapid when lying down, because venous return from the legs is facilitated, while a lower blood pressure is needed to perfuse the brain.

Capillary bed

The number of patent capillaries increases dramatically during endurance exercise, reaching a maximum in the range of 380–2340 vessels per mm^2, compared with about 200 per mm^2 at rest (Honig et al., 1970; Plyley & Groom, 1975). Early studies found little difference of counts between slow- and fast-twitch muscle, but more recent reports have suggested that muscle fibres with a high rate of aerobic metabolism have a larger array of capillaries than anaerobic fibres (Hudlická, 1985). The capillary : fibre ratio is also increased by aerobic training (Brodal et al., 1977; Klausen et al., 1981; Plyley, 1990), by chronic electrical stimulation of muscle and by vasodilating drugs (Hudlická, 1985). There is no evidence that endurance athletes have abused such drugs to date. Training apparently has a selective effect, increasing peak blood flow to slow-twitch but not to fast-twitch fibres (Mackie & Terjung, 1983).

During exercise, the local distribution of blood flow within a muscle depends upon the pattern of fibre recruitment. With the moderate pace of the endurance runner, the primary recruitment is of slow-twitch fibres, and the capillary flow is directed selectively to such fibres (Armstrong & Laughlin, 1985). The highest local flow rate is associated with fast-twitch oxidative fibres (almost 400 ml·min^{-1}·100 g^{-1} of tissue; Armstrong & Laughlin, 1983; Laughlin & Korthuis, 1987). Estimates made in conscious animals yield much higher peak flow rates than measurements on isolated muscle preparations, possibly because the rhythmic muscle contractions contribute to the flow process (Armstrong, 1988).

Venous circulation

The peripheral veins of the endurance athlete have received relatively little study. However, they contain about two thirds of the total blood volume, and are thus of considerable importance to overall circulatory function. Radionuclide technology has in recent years facilitated measurement of venous volumes and capacity (Clements et al., 1981).

Rhythmic muscle contraction against the venous valves plays a large part in assuring an adequate return of blood to the heart, particularly in the seated or upright position. The wheelchair competitor with paralysed lower limbs, or the Masters' athlete with compromised valves and varicosities, thus faces a substantial handicap in most sports except swimming (where a combination of horizontal posture and water pressure offers an alternative means for venous return).

Early tests of fitness such as the Crampton index emphasized that a normal athlete with a good level of endurance fitness had an enhanced ability to increase the tone of the leg veins on moving from the horizontal to a vertical position. The fit athlete is also able to sustain a greater venous tone in the face of a high environmental temperature (which normally causes a relaxation of the peripheral veins). However, the extent of such changes in venous capacitance is still debated, and Hainsworth (1986) has suggested that a variation of some 300 ml is possible, due largely to adjustments in the splanchnic reservoirs.

Training induces a small increase of blood volume, and thus preloading of the heart (Saltin et al., 1968). Some of the gains in performance from blood doping may reflect an increase of preloading, rather than an increase of haemoglobin level.

Circulatory drift

If endurance exercise is continued for more than a few minutes, a progressive 'circulatory drift' occurs (Saltin, 1964). This is shown by a gradual increase of heart rate and at least a matching decrease in stroke volume (Goodman et al., 1989). Among factors contributing to the phenomenon, we may note a progressive increase of core temperature (and thus a tendency to cutaneous vasodilatation), an increase of circulating catecholamines, a progressive dehydration due to sweating and other sources of water loss, and an exudation of fluid into the tissues.

The last mechanism has particular relevance to the present chapter. Under resting conditions, the balance of hydrostatic and osmotic pressures is such that there is an egress of fluid from the capillaries into the muscles at the arterial end of the circulation, with a roughly equivalent pressure gradient assuring resorption of fluid at the venous end of the circuit. However, during exercise, there tends to be a leakage of protein from the capillaries into the extracellular space, disturbing the balance of osmotic pressures, while local vasodilatation induced by a combination of exercise and heat also increases the hydrostatic pressure, favouring the leakage of fluid into the tissues. In consequence, there may be a 5–10% decrease of blood volume in the first few minutes of exercise.

The impact of such leakage upon aerobic performance was studied by Pirnay et al. (1970). Brief exposure to a very hot environment had no influence upon maximal oxygen intake, but performance was depressed by 30 min or more of exposure because such a leakage of fluid had occurred.

The leakage of fluid in itself is self-limiting, since it leads to a rise of intramuscular pressure, restoring the hydrostatic gradient that encourages resorption of fluid. However, the decrease of blood volume has an adverse effect upon performance unless it is made good by an appropriate ingestion of fluid.

References

Andersen, P. & Saltin, B. (1985) Maximal perfusion of skeletal muscle in man. *J. Physiol.* **366**, 233–249.

Anderson, F.A., Penney, B.C. & Wheeler, H.B. (1983) Non-invasive quantification of the degree of venous outflow obstruction in the extremities by means of venous occlusion plethysmography. *Advances in Bioengineering*, ASME Annual Winter Meeting, Boston, Massachusetts.

Armstrong, R.B. (1988) Magnitude and distribution of muscle blood flow in conscious animals during locomotory exercise. *Med. Sci. Sports Exerc.* **20**, S119–S123.

Armstrong, R.B. & Laughlin, M.H. (1983) Blood flows within and among rat muscles as a function of time during high speed treadmill exercise. *J. Physiol.* **344**, 189–208.

Armstrong, R.B. & Laughlin, M.H. (1985) Metabolic indicators of fibre recruitment in mammalian muscles during locomotion. *J. Exp. Biol.* **115**, 201–213.

Barclay, J.K. (1988) Physiological determinants of Q_{max} in contracting canine skeletal muscle in situ. *Med. Sci. Sports Exerc.* **20**, S113–S118.

Barcroft, J. & Dornhorst, A.C. (1949) Blood flow through the human calf during rhythmic exercise. *J. Physiol.* **109**, 402–411.

Bassenge, E. & Münzel, T. (1988) Consideration of conduit and resistance vessels in regulation of blood flow. *Am. J. Cardiol.* **62**, 40E–44E.

Bevegard, B.S. & Shepherd, J.T. (1967) Regulation of the circulation during exercise in man. *Physiol. Rev.* **47**, 178–213.

Brodal, P., Ingjer, F. & Hermansen, L. (1977) Capillary supply of skeletal muscle fibres in untrained and endurance trained men. *Am. J. Physiol.* **232**, H705–H712.

Brodie, T.E. & Russell, A.E. (1905) On the determination of the rate of blood flow through an organ. *J. Physiol.* **32**, 47P.

Bryan, A.C. (1967) Commentary. *Can. Med. Assoc. J.* **96**, 804.

Burton, A.C. (1975) *Physiology and Biophysics of the Circulation*. Year Book Publishers, Chicago.

Cerretelli, P., Marconi, C., Pendergast, D., Meyer, M., Heisler, N. & Piiper, J. (1984) Blood flow in exercising muscles by xenon clearance and by microsphere trapping. *J. Appl. Physiol.* **56**, 24–30.

Cerretelli, P., Pendergast, D., Marconi, C. & Piiper, J. (1986) Blood flow in exercising muscle. *Int. J. Sports Med.* **7**, 29–33.

Clausen, J.P. (1973) Muscle blood flow during exercise and its significance for maximal performance. In: Keul J. (ed.) *Limiting Factors of Human Performance*, pp. 253–266. G. Thieme, Stuttgart.

Clausen, J.P. (1976) Circulatory adjustments to dynamic exercise and effect of physical training in normal subjects and in patients with coronary artery disease. *Progr. Cardiovasc. Dis.* **18**, 459–495.

Clausen, J.P. (1977) Effect of physical training on cardiovascular adjustments to exercise in man. *Physiol. Rev.* **57**, 779–815.

Clements, I.P., Strelow, D.A., Becker, G.P., Vlietstra, R.E. & Brown, M.L. (1981) Radionuclide evaluation of peripheral circulatory dynamics: new clinical application of blood pool scintigraphy for measuring limb venous volume, capacity and blood flow. *Am. Heart J.* **102**, 980–983.

Costill, D.L. (1972) Physiology of marathon running. *J.A.M.A.* **221**, 1024–1029.

Dresler, C.M., Jeevanandam, M. & Brennan, M.F. (1987) Extremity blood flow in man: comparison between strain gauge and capacitance plethysmography. *Surgery* **101**, 35–39.

Folkow, B., Haglund, U., Jodal, M. & Lundren, O. (1971) Blood flow in the calf muscle of man during heavy rhythmic exercise. *Acta Physiol. Scand.* **81**, 157–163.

Fox, S.I. (1984) *Human Physiology.* W.C. Brown Publishing, Dubuque, Iowa.

Frisk-Holmberg, M., Jorfeldt, L., Juhlin-Dannfelt, A. & Karlsson, J. (1981) Leg blood flow during exercise in man in relation to muscle fibre composition. *Acta Physiol. Scand.* **112**, 339–342.

Goodman, J., Lapade, A. & Liu, P. (1989) Effects of prolonged exercise on left ventricular function. *Can. J. Sport Sci.* **14**, 113P (abstract).

Goodman, J., Reading, J., Plyley, M.J., McLaughlin, P.R., Floras, J. & Shephard, R.J. (1990) Peripheral vascular conductance and exercise capacity in sedentary, endurance trained and chronic heart failure subjects. *J. Am. Coll. Cardiol.* **15**, 238A (abstract).

Grönlund, J., Malvin, G.M. & Hlastala, M.P. (1989) Estimation of blood flow distribution in skeletal muscle from inert gas washout. *J. Appl. Physiol.* **66**, 1942–1955.

Hainsworth, R. (1986) Vascular capacitance: its control and importance. *Rev. Physiol. Biochem. Pharmacol.* **105**, 102–264.

Hensel, H., Ruef, J. & Golenhofen, K. (1954) Fortlaufende Registrierung der Muskeldurchblutung am Menschen mit einer Calorimetersonde. *Pflüg. Archiv.* **259**, 267–280.

Hokanson, D.E., Sumner, D.S. & Strandne, D.E. (1975) An electrically calibrated plethysmograph for direct measurement of limb blood flow. *IEEE Trans. Biomed. Eng.* **22**, 25–29.

Honig, C.R., Frierson, J.L. & Patterson, J.L. (1970) Comparison of neural controls of resistance and capillary density in resting muscle. *J. Physiol.* **218**, 937–942.

Hudlická, O. (1985) Development and adaptability of microvasculature in skeletal muscle. *J. Exp. Biol.* **115**, 215–228.

Jorfeldt, L.S. (1988) Measurement of skeletal muscle blood flow in humans: plethysmographic, bolus and continuous infusion techniques. *Am. J. Cardiol.* **62**, 25E–29E.

Kaufman, M.P., Rotto, D.M. & Rybicki, K.J. (1988) Pressor reflex response to static muscular contraction: its afferent arm and possible neurotransmitters. *Am. J. Cardiol.* **62**, 58E–62E.

Kavanagh, T., Mertens, D.J., Matosevic, V., Shephard, R.J. & Evans, B. (1989) Health and aging of Masters athletes. *Clin. Sports Med.* **1**, 72–88.

Kavanagh, T., Shephard, R.J. & Kennedy, J. (1977) Characteristics of post-coronary marathon runners. *Ann. N.Y. Acad. Sci.* **301**, 455–465.

Klausen, K., Andersen, L.B. & Pelle, J. (1981) Adaptive changes in work capacity, skeletal muscle capillarization and enzyme levels during training and detraining. *Acta Physiol. Scand.* **113**, 9–16.

Klausen, K., Secher, N.H., Clausen, J.P., Hartling, O. & Trap-Jensen, J. (1982) Central and regional adaptations to one-leg training. *J. Appl. Physiol.* **52**, 976–983.

Laughlin, M.H. & Korthuis, R.J. (1987) Control of muscle blood flow during sustained physiological exercise. *Can. J. Sport Sci.* **12** (Suppl. 1), 77S–88S.

LeJemtel, T.H., Maskin, C.S., Lucido, D. & Chadwicj, B.J. (1986) Failure to augment maximal limb blood flow in response to one-leg versus two-leg exercise in patients with severe heart failure. *Circulation* **74**, 245–251.

Mackie, B.G. & Terjung, R.L. (1983) Influence of training on blood flow to different skeletal muscle fibre types. *J. Appl. Physiol.* **55**, 1072–1078.

Musch, T.I. (1988) Skeletal muscle blood flow in exercising dogs. *Med. Sci. Sports Exerc.* **20**, S104–S108.

Musch, T.I., Haidet, G.C., Ordway, G.A., Longhurst, J.C. & Mitchell, J.H. (1987) Training effects on regional blood flow response to maximal exercise in foxhounds. *J. Appl. Physiol.* **62**, 1724–1732.

Ozolin, P. (1986) Blood flow in the extremities of athletes. *Int. J. Sports Med.* **7**, 117–122.

Paterson, D.H., Shephard, R.J., Cunningham, D., Jones, N.L. & Andrew, G. (1979) Effects of physical training upon cardiovascular function following myocardial infarction. *J. Appl. Physiol.* **47**, 482–489.

Pirnay, F., Deroanne, R. & Petit, J.M. (1970) Maximal oxygen consumption in a hot environment. *J. Appl. Physiol.* **28**, 642–645.

Plyley, M.J. (1990) Fine-tuning muscle capillary supply for maximum exercise performance. *Perspect. Cardiol.* **6**, 25–34.

Plyley, M.J. & Groom, C. (1975) Geometrical distribution of capillaries in mammalian striated muscle. *Am. J. Physiol.* **228**, 1376–1383.

Reading, J., Goodman, J., Plyley, M., Liu, P., McLaughlin, P.R. & Shephard, R.J. (1990) Calf vascular conductance in sedentary and endurance trained men. *Can. J. Sport Sci.* **14**, 134P (abstract).

Rowell, L.B. (1986) *Human Circulation During Physical*

Stress. Oxford University Press, New York.

Rowell, L.B. (1988) Muscle blood flow in humans: how high can it go? *Med. Sci. Sports Exerc.* **20**, S97–S103.

Rowell, L.B., Saltin, B., Kiens, B. & Christensen, N.J. (1986) Is peak quadriceps flow in humans even higher during exercise with hypoxia? *Am. J. Physiol.* **251**, H1038–H1044.

Rushmer, R.F. (1976) *Cardiovascular Dynamics*. W.B. Saunders, Toronto.

Saltin, B. (1964) Aerobic work capacity and circulation at exercise in man. With special reference to the effect of prolonged exercise and/or heat exposure. *Acta Physiol. Scand.* **62** (Suppl. 230), 1–52.

Saltin, B. (1973) Oxygen transport by the circulatory system during exercise in man. In: Keul, J. (ed.) *Limiting Factors of Physical Performance*, pp. 235–252. Thieme, Stuttgart.

Saltin, B., Blomqvist, G., Mitchell, J.H., Johnson, R.L., Wildenthal, K. & Chapman, C.B. (1968) Response to exercise after bed rest and after training. *Circulation* **38** (Suppl. 7) 1–78.

Savard, G., Kiens, B. & Saltin, B. (1987) Limb blood flow in prolonged exercise: magnitude and implication for cardiovascular control during muscular work in man. *Can. J. Sport Sci.* **12** (Suppl. 1), 89S–101S.

Shephard, R.J. (1977) *Endurance Fitness*, 2nd edn. University of Toronto Press, Toronto.

Shephard, R.J. (1982) *Physiology and Biochemistry of Exercise*. Praeger Publishing, New York.

Shephard, R.J., Vandewalle, H., Bouhlel, E. & Monod, H. (1988) Muscle mass as a factor limiting physical work. *J. Appl. Physiol.* **64**, 1472–1479.

Sinoway, L.I., Sheberger, J., Wilson, J., McLaughlin, D., Musch, T. & Zelis, R. (1987) A 30-day forearm work protocol increases maximal forearm blood flow. *J. Appl. Physiol.* **62**, 1063–1067.

Snell, P.G., Martin, W.H., Buckey, J.C. & Blomqvist, C.G. (1987) Maximal vascular leg conductance in trained and untrained men. *J. Appl. Physiol.* **62**, 606–610.

Stainsby, W.N. & Andrew, G.M. (1988) Maximal blood flow and power output of dog muscle *in situ*. *Med. Sci. Sports Exerc.* **20**, S109–S112.

Sullivan, M.J., Knight, J.D., Higginbotham, M.B. & Conn, F.R. (1989) Relation between central and peripheral hemodynamics during exercise in patients with chronic heart failure. *Circulation* **80**, 769–781.

Terjung, R.L., Mathien, G.M., Erney, T.P. & Ogilvie, R.W. (1988) Peripheral adaptations to low blood flow in muscle during exercise. *Am. J. Cardiol.* **62**, 15E–19E.

Vander, A.J., Sherman, W.J. & Luciano, D.S. (1985) *Human Physiology: The Mechanisms of Body Function*, 4th edn. McGraw Hill, Toronto.

Wade, O.L. & Bishop, J.M. (1962) *Cardiac Output and Regional Blood Flow*. Blackwell Scientific Publications, Oxford.

Walløe, L. & Wesche, J. (1988) The course and magnitude of blood flow changes in the human quadriceps muscles during and following rhythmic exercise. *J. Physiol.* **405**, 257–273.

Wedin, B. (1976) Cases of paradoxical undressing by people exposed to severe hypothermia. In: Shephard R.J. & Itoh, S. (eds) *Circumpolar Health*, pp. 61–71. University of Toronto Press, Toronto.

West, J.B. (1977) Blood flow. In: West, J.B. (ed.) *Regional Differences in the Lung*, pp. 85–165. Academic Press, New York.

Whitney, R.J. (1953) The measurement of volume changes in human limbs. *J. Physiol.* **121**, 1–27.

Yancy, C.W., Vissing, S., Buckey, J.C., Bellomo, J.F., Firth, B.G. & Blomqvist, C.G. (1988) Maximal conductance versus maximal oxygen uptake in patients with congestive heart failure. *J. Am. Coll. Cardiol.* **11**, 72A (abstract).

Chapter 9

Central Nervous Influence on Fatigue

NIELS H. SECHER

Introduction

Achievement in sports depends on the skill and training of the athlete as reflected by muscle strength and maximal oxygen intake (Secher, 1983). The results are at the same time modulated by psychological factors, for example endurance is enhanced by payment (Asmussen, 1979). An uncomfortable situation may, on the other hand, impose a hindrance to expression of the physiological capability of the individual or team. This is taken into consideration in the soccer cups by letting goals scored on the foreign field count twice those scored at home. These conflicting psychological influences on performance have been described by the 'inverted U hypothesis' (Kerr, 1985).

Lack of motivation will reduce performance but it is not clear how the central nervous system may exert a negative influence on performance despite a strong personal motivation. In this chapter some observations on muscle fatigue of apparently central nervous origin are reviewed and an attempt is made to point to relevant neurophysiological control mechanisms. Little or no attention is given to motivation and situations where the athlete is disturbed, and performance thereby blunders. The focus is on the somewhat paradoxical hypothesis that a negative central influence may exist despite the subject's full motivation and concentration on the requested task. Such fatigue is named *central inhibition*. Arousal is the term used to describe an upgrade of the

central nervous system by non-specific stimuli leading to central 'disinhibition' and, experimentally, the result of *diverting activities*.

Central command

It has not been possible to find a quantitative measure of the central nervous system's commanding role in exercise. The physiological variable closest to 'central command' may be the change in regional cerebral blood flow which occurs in association with thinking (Roland & Friberg, 1985). Still the increase in cerebral blood flow is the same during light and intense dynamic exercise and is thereby independent of central command (Thomas *et al.*, 1989). Even intense static contractions are not associated with an increase in cerebral blood flow as a whole (Roberts *et al.*, 1990) and only a small bilateral increase in the motor-sensory area takes place at a low level in the brain (Friedman *et al.*, 1989). It is worth noting that these increases depend on afferent rather than efferent neuronal activity, as they are eliminated by peripheral nerve blockade. During movement, a large contralateral increase in cerebral blood flow appears in the corresponding motor-sensory cortex at a high level in the brain. As this increase in regional cerebral blood flow is attenuated but not reversed to the resting value by peripheral nerve blockade, it might reflect an increase in both efferent and afferent neuronal activity.

In animals, neural activity in the basal ganglia

and cerebellum precedes activity in the cerebral motor cortex and the resulting muscle activity. It may be that activity in the basal ganglia is involved in the planning of slow movement, while the role of the cerebellum is to plan mainly fast movement, with the activity in the motor cortex related to the force generated rather than the type of movement performed (Evarts, 1973). Yet the role of central nervous activity in fatigue is not known and it may be felt that the incorporation of the central nervous system in explanations of fatigue resembles the use of a black box encompassing findings that do not fit into a hypothesis which can be more rigorously tested. Indeed, the existence of central inhibition has been denied, but mainly by exclusion. If fatigue appears to be of central origin, the contraction is taken to be less than 'maximal' and the subject is familiarized with the experimental set-up, or the experimental situation is arranged so as to attenuate central fatigue, for example by allowing visual feedback (Bigland-Ritchie, 1981). Yet, despite the lack of an expression of the central nervous system's involvement in exercise, experiments may be designed indirectly to demonstrate central nervous effects on fatigue (Asmussen, 1979; Secher, 1987) as well as on other physiological variables related to circulatory, ventilatory and hormonal control during exercise (Leonard et al., 1985; Galbo et al., 1990).

Central inhibition

Experimentally, a role for the central nervous system in fatigue becomes relevant when differing performances are noticed in nearly identical situations where muscle biochemistry is likely to be the same. Mosso investigated fatigue during repeated contractions of the middle finger of one hand (Asmussen, 1979). In one experiment his professor was studied before and after his inaugural lecture at the university of Sienna in 1892. After the lecture the amount of work he could perform increased by 45%, suggesting that the mental stress before the lecture had decreased performance.

Open versus closed eyes

It has been shown that fatigue is more pronounced during both dynamic (Asmussen, 1979) and static (Secher, 1987) muscle contractions when they are performed with closed as opposed to open eyes. Furthermore, during repeated maximal voluntary (static) contractions (MVCs) fatigue is paradoxically enhanced when the subject concentrates on performing the MVC as opposed to situations when motivation appears to be low. Exhaustion may be reached with little more than 100 MVCs, while under other circumstances more than 1000 MVCs can be carried out. For example, if the subject is disturbed because the door to the experimental room is opened, fatigue apparently disappears.

Role of the experimenters

Fatigue during repeated MVC has been compared in situations where the experimenters are present or the subjects perform the MVCs on their own (Rube & Secher, 1981). Invariably, strength decreases more (approximately 22% during 150 MVCs) when the experimenters are present than when the subjects are on their own (approximately 8%), despite the fact that the initial strength is the same (Fig. 9.1). In further support of the hypothesis that fatigue during repeated MVC is largely due to central inhibition is the finding that the electromyographic activity decreases in parallel with strength, and the ratio between electromyographic activity and force remains constant.

Electrical stimulation

A third experimental approach has been to compare fatigue during voluntary contractions with fatigue developed during electrically induced muscle contractions. In such experiments Ikai et al. (1967) found that fatigue during repeated MVC was more profound than that seen during electrically induced muscle contractions. This difference appeared despite the fact that the electrically induced contractions were

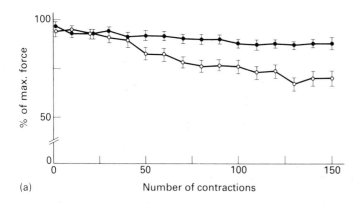

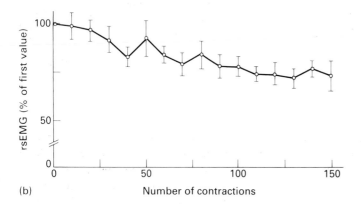

Fig. 9.1 Fatigue during repeated maximal voluntary leg contractions. ○, Contractions performed with the experimenters present; ●, contractions performed with the subjects on their own (a). Also shown (b) is the electromyographic activity during contractions performed while the experimenters were present. From Rube & Secher (1981).

stronger than the subjects' voluntary strength. The result contrasts with the experience of other investigators (Bigland-Ritchie, 1981; MacLaren *et al.*, 1989) who also studied the adductor pollicis muscle but used sustained contractions. Only during sustained contractions of the quadriceps muscle did Bigland-Ritchie (1981) note that some subjects developed a more pronounced fatigue during voluntary effort than during short, electrically-induced muscle contractions interrupting the maintained effort. This means that, at least in some situations, differences in fatigue appear that can be taken to reflect central inhibition. In studies where no difference in fatigue has been observed following voluntary and electrically induced muscle contractions, the subjects appear to be thoroughly familiarized with the experimental set-up.

Effect of training on central factors in fatigue

In athletics it is of key interest to know how training affects fatigue. Fatigue during repeated one-leg as well as two-leg extension has been followed after one-leg and two-leg static training (Rube & Secher, 1991; Fig. 9.2). Fatigue during repeated one-leg MVC is reduced after one-leg training, as is fatigue during two-leg MVC after two-leg training (Fig. 9.3). More surprisingly, one-leg training does not affect fatigue during two-leg MVC and, likewise, two-leg training does not affect fatigue during repeated one-leg MVC. After training a greater degree of fatigue remains (approximately 12%) than when the subjects are on their own (8%; see Fig. 9.1), suggesting that even in subjects who are thoroughly familiarized with the

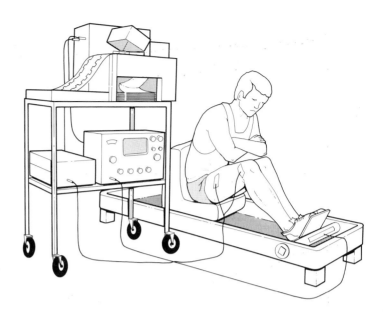

Fig. 9.2 Experimental set-up for the measurement of leg strength. From Rube & Secher (1991).

specific type of exercise, an unusual environment (as exemplified by the presence of the experimenters) imposes central inhibition. In addition, when only a small change in the type of exercise performed is introduced, as exemplified by the use of one or both legs, a pronounced central inhibition is re-established.

Diverting activities

Setchenow's phenomenon

In 1903 Setchenow made the observation that after exhaustive sawing he recovered faster if he exercised with the other arm than if he relaxed (Asmussen, 1979). This fatigue-reducing effect of a diverting activity has been called *Setchenow's phenomenon*. Later studies have used other types of diverting activity in pauses between work bouts. They include dynamic as well as static muscle contractions. It has been speculated that the enhanced recovery caused by diverting activities is due to an increase in blood flow to the exercised muscle, although such an increase has not been reported (Asmussen, 1979). Moreover, the activity per-

formed to enhance recovery does not have to be physical exercise. Mental activity such as problem-solving or just opening the eyes at the point of exhaustion (but not closing the eyes if exhaustion is reached with open eyes) increases performance (Fig. 9.4d). Taken together, these findings suggest that the recovery role played by diverting activities is within the central nervous system and, conversely, that the fatigue that can be eliminated is due to central inhibition.

Pattern of human muscle contractions

Normal contractions

In order to evaluate further the events taking place during repeated MVC, their configuration has been followed (Secher, 1987). During light, graded contractions the rate of rise in tension is usually low and the tension that is developed can be maintained (Fig. 9.4a). With increasing contraction intensity, the rate of rise in tension also increases. If emphasis is placed only on performing a MVC, the rate of rise in tension is usually comparatively low and if the subject is

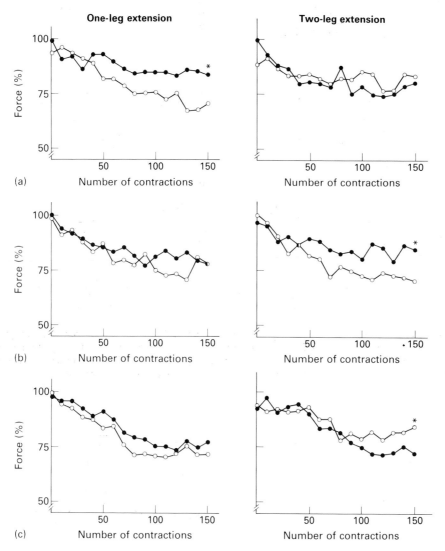

Fig. 9.3 Fatigue during repeated maximal voluntary one-leg (left hand side) and two-leg (right hand side) extension before (○) and after (●) training. (a) One-leg training; (b) two-leg training; (c) control group of subjects. *, $p < 0.05$ (comparison between values before and after training). From Rube & Secher (1991).

asked not only to perform a MVC but also to perform it as fast as possible, the rate of rise in tension increases.

During rapid MVCs, two contraction maxima may appear, separated by a notch in the contraction curve after approximately 0.4–0.5 s (Figs 9.4 & 9.5). The two relative maxima may represent the involvement of different muscle fibres, because they can be blocked separately by the neuromuscular blocking agents decamethonium and tubocurarine (Secher *et al.*, 1978; 1981; Fig. 9.5), which have a preference for fast-twitch and slow-twitch muscle fibres, respectively. Accordingly, the electromyographic activity at the onset of the contraction is severely affected by decamethonium, while

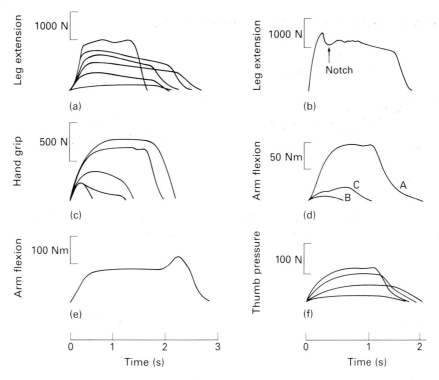

Fig. 9.4 Superimposed force recordings: (a) graded submaximal and maximal leg contractions; (b) rapid leg maximal voluntary contraction (MVC); (c) repeated hand grip MVCs; (d) repeated arm MVC performed with a blindfold (A and B) and after the blindfold was removed (C); (e) arm MVC with superimposed 'extra' force during an MVC; (f) repeated finger MVCs performed during ischaemia. From Secher (1987).

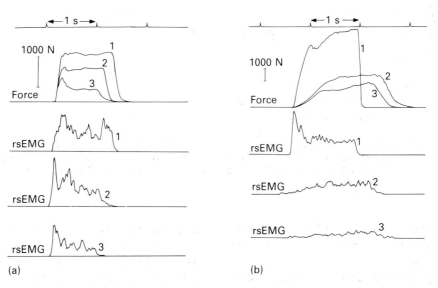

Fig. 9.5 Three superimposed force recordings from rapid leg maximal voluntary contractions and the corresponding rectified electromyograms (rsEMG). (a) Control contraction and two degrees of partial curarization. (b) Control contraction and two degrees of partial neuromuscular blockade with decamethonium. From Secher (1987).

tubocurarine mainly affects the latter part of the electromyogram. Two similar contraction patterns can also be described in the weak MVC of patients with sequelae from poliomyelitis (which affect the motoneurons at random). As during partial curarization, intended rapid MVCs show an early maximum, as well as a large electromyographic activity at the onset of the contraction. Conversely, if the patient is unable to develop a high rate of rise in tension, the electromyographic activity is of the same size throughout the MVC (Secher, 1987).

In accordance with the observation that a rapid MVC consists of two separate contraction elements (Fig. 9.6) is the finding that the two contraction elements may be added not only in the beginning of the contraction in order to increase the rate of rise in tension, but also later on giving rise to a sudden increase in strength of up to 20% for a duration of about 0.5 s (Secher *et al.*, 1978; Secher, 1987; see Fig. 9.4e). Similarly, during a sustained MVC with partial curarization (and in patients with myasthenia gravis), but not during partial neuromuscular blockade with decamethonium, short-lasting bouts of 'extra' strength can easily be demonstrated if the effort is renewed (Secher *et al.*, 1978; Leonard *et al.*, 1985).

Fatigue

Repeated MVCs are likewise associated with two different contraction patterns. If peripheral fatigue is emphasized by the use of an arterial tourniquet, the contraction pattern becomes slow and enduring, and thus resembles the contraction pattern developed during low intensity, graded contractions and MVCs performed during partial neuromuscular blockade with decamethonium (see Fig. 9.4f) (Secher, 1987). However, with no hindrance to the circulation, repeated MVC resembles the contraction pattern developed during partial curarization (see Fig. 9.4c). Exhaustion is reached at a characteristic point where the 'tail' of the contraction curve disappears and the MVC has a duration

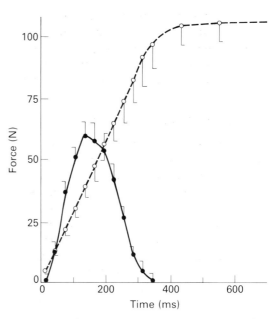

Fig. 9.6 Separation of rapid maximal voluntary finger muscle contractions (MVC) into a 'tonic' and 'phasic' component which can be manipulated independently by fatigue, neuromuscular blocking agents and neuromuscular diseases (see text). Values are means and standard errors of the mean. The separation is based on a straight line from the starting point of the contraction curve to the notch. (see Fig. 9.4b) (N. Rube & N.H. Secher, unpublished data). The straight line (○) corresponds to the rate of rise in tension during ordinary MVCs. Only during rapid MVCs is the part of the contraction curve to the left of this line added (●). The phasic component, therefore, has a higher innervation threshold than the tonic component. Central inhibition and arousal affect mainly the tonic part of the contraction. Training may have two effects: one is to increase the size of the tonic element by reducing central inhibition; the other is to make motor units that were previously phasically active respond tonically.

of only about 0.5 s. If this point is reached after only a few contractions (100−150 MVCs), there is little reduction in the rate of rise of tension (see Fig. 9.4c). On the other hand if it takes 1000 or more MVCs to reach exhaustion, the rate of rise in tension is severely reduced (see Fig. 9.4d).

Figure 9.4d exemplifies the effect of opening the eyes after exhaustion is reached with closed eyes. Not only does opening of the eyes cause the contraction to become stronger, but it also becomes more enduring by regaining its tail, which is lost again if the MVCs are continued until exhaustion is reached with the eyes open.

Neurophysiological model

Although the experimental background is far from adequate, it is tempting to point out some neurophysiological findings which may be of relevance for central inhibition and arousal. Patterns of human voluntary contractions are not easily translated into an understanding of how motor units are recruited. Yet their patterns may be described in terms which closely resemble those used for describing the electromyographic recordings of single motor units in humans. Slow-twitch muscle fibres are recruited at low contraction intensities and are continuously firing, while fast-twitch fibres are recruited at a high innervation threshold and fire intermittently (Freund, 1983). The motor units with the highest firing frequencies cease to fire tonically, but they can still be brought to discharge phasically during a sustained effort.

From the electromyographic recording of motor units it is derived that the latter part of the contraction curve is dominated by the contribution of slow-twitch muscle fibres; accordingly, the nervous influence on fatigue would affect these fibres. In agreement with this concept is the resemblance between the contraction pattern developed during repeated MVC and partial curarization affecting mainly slow-twitch muscle fibres. In other words it seems as if central inhibition causes a restraint on the ability to use some, and ultimately all, slow-twitch muscle fibres. Conversely, diverting activities and training may have the effect of minimizing this restraint when exercising at maximal intensity.

Recruitment of motor units

Only during lengthening contractions has a selective recruitment of high-threshold motor units been demonstrated in humans by electromyographic techniques (Nardone et al., 1989). The suggestion that subjects may not be able to use all of their slow-twitch muscle fibres during repeated MVC is therefore in contrast to the current concepts on how muscle fibres are recruited. The current thinking is based on an 'orderly recruitment' of motor units, also called the 'size principle' from the work of Henneman (1957). Experimentally, the size principle is based mainly on reflex recruitment of motor units, but it is also widely applicable to human voluntary contractions (Freund, 1983). The work of Henneman and coworkers, however, justifies only the conclusion that among a population of motoneurons activated through a given afferent input, the sequence of recruitment is determined by the size of the motor units (Kots, 1977).

Muscle fibre size

With intense strength-training, as in weightlifting, fast-twitch muscle fibres hypertrophy (Edström & Ekblom, 1972) and selective glycogen depletion of fast-twitch (type IIb) fibres takes place during intense static as well as dynamic exercise (Secher & Jensen, 1976). If the slow-twitch motor units were always recruited when the fast-twitch motor units were engaged in exercise, it would be expected that both fibre types would show hypertrophy. This is the case when movement is more 'automated' but still strength-demanding, as in rowing (Larsson & Forsberg, 1980). Thus selective hypertrophy of fast-twitch muscle fibres takes place during fast maximal contractions, and only during fast contractions is strength correlated to the area of muscle occupied by fast-twitch muscle fibres (Thorstensson, 1988).

Corticospinal influence

Exercise is associated with activity in the motor-sensory cortex, possibly including commanding signals through the pyramidal tract. The increase in cerebral blood flow in this area is more pronounced during exercise with the left hand than with the dominant right hand (Halsey *et al.*, 1979). With this background it may be speculated that part of the neurophysiological element in training involves a reduced cortical representation of the work performed. Such an effect would be advantageous as some cortical neurons possess an inhibitory influence on the motoneurons innervating slow-twitch muscle fibres in addition to their excitation of motoneurons innervating fast-twitch fibres (Granit, 1970). This is reflected during reflex activation of human motor units, in that the voluntary 'gain' is 700–800% for fast-twitch motor units (the medial gastrocnemius), but is almost non-existent for slow-twitch motor units (the soleus) (Kots, 1977).

The rubrospinal system

With the complexity of the central nervous system, other possible controlling pathways should be considered, such as the phylogenetically older rubrospinal system. However, even activity in the rubrospinal system involves an inhibition of motoneurons innervating slow-twitch muscle fibres in addition to its excitatory effect on motoneurons innervating fast-twitch fibres (Burke *et al.*, 1970). This implies that a discrepancy exists between the orderly recruitment normally exercised in humans and the neurophysiological possibilities allowed by the most obvious commanding pathways. One possible explanation of this discrepancy is the use of γ-motoneurons, as suggested by Merton (1953) and later modified to involve parallel α- and γ-innervation of motoneurons (Vallbo, 1971). In this scheme, γ-motoneuron innervation stimulates reflex recruitment of the α-motoneurons due to their innervation of muscle spindles and thereby activation of I_a afferents (which, in turn, innervate the α-motoneurons; Fig. 9.7).

α–γ configuration

If the role of the γ-loop is not simply to adjust the length of the muscle spindle during contractions, then indirect innervation of the α-motoneurons could explain variations in muscle strength. Using the scheme outlined in Fig. 9.7, submaximal contractions, and even maximal contractions for which the subject is trained, may be accomplished by a dominance of γ innervation and thus reflex excitation of the α-motoneuron. Therefore, during increasing contraction intensity, muscle fibres are recruited in an orderly fashion. When the subject makes a rapid maximal contraction, motor units with apparently phasic activity are recruited through direct α-motoneuron innervation.

During rapid maximal contractions, parallel innervation through the γ-loop would prevent the inhibitory influence exerted by command signals directly innervating the α-motoneurons belonging to slow-twitch motor units (Fig. 9.8). However, in situations where the subject is untrained, especially with repeated maximal effort, direct α-motoneuron innervation may become increasingly important, with associated maintenance of rate of rise in tension at the expense of endurance. Ultimately, a point is reached where only bursts of approximately 0.5 s in duration can be performed, as the γ-loop becomes inoperative. Conversely, with diverting activities and training, parallel innervation of the α-motoneurons through the γ-loop is re-established. In fact, training increases the responsiveness of the γ-loop (Hutton, 1988). Alternatively, training may develop other commanding pathways so that muscle contractions can be maintained with little or no inhibition of motoneurons. In this respect Grimby *et al.* (1981) reported that the period over which motor units can be brought to respond tonically increases with training.

Conclusion

Mental training is an integral part of an athlete's routine. In a classical sense, this type of training involves learning the discipline in question. In addition, observations on fatigue during maximal exercise suggest that trained subjects

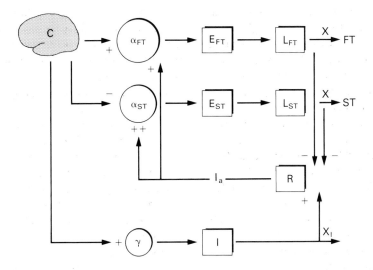

Fig. 9.7 α—γ configuration of muscle control (Houk, 1972), modified to distinguish between innervation of slow-twitch and fast-twitch muscle fibres. C, command signal; α and γ, extrafusal and intrafusal motoneurons, respectively; E, the characteristics of the extrafusal muscle fibres, separated into slow-twitch (ST) and fast-twitch (FT) fibres. They produce a force exerted on a load (L) resulting in a shortening of the muscle fibres (X). I refers to the γ configuration which controls intrafusal shortening (X_I). R represents the muscle spindle receptors resulting in a signal transmitted in I_a afferents and exciting mainly the α-motoneurons of the slow-twitch motor units. +, positive; −, negative influence. For an anatomical presentation of the muscle spindle, see Tittel (1988).

are able to use their muscles to an extent for which the untrained do not have competence due to central inhibition. However, central inhibition may be established even in well trained individuals following only small changes in the environment. Although force in many endurance sports is far below MVC, these observations indicate that athletes should familiarize themselves thoroughly with every aspect of the environment in which they are going to compete.

References

Asmussen, E. (1979) Muscle fatigue. *Med. Sci. Sports* **11**, 313−321.

Bigland-Ritchie, B. (1981) EMG/force relations and fatigue of human voluntary contractions. *Exerc. Sports Sci. Rev.* **9**, 75−117.

Burke, R.E., Jankowska, E. & Bruggencate, G. Ten (1970) A comparison of peripheral and rubrospinal synaptic input to slow and fast twitch motor units of triceps surae. *J. Physiol. (Lond.)* **207**, 709−732.

Edström, L. & Ekblom, B. (1972) Differences in sizes of red and white muscle fibres in vastus lateralis of musculus quadriceps femoris of normal individuals and athletes. Relation to physical performance. *Scand. J. Clin. Lab. Invest.* **30**, 175−181.

Evarts, E.V. (1973) Brain mechanisms in movement. *Sci. Am.* **229**, 96−103.

Freund, H.-J. (1983) Motor unit and muscle activity in voluntary motor control. *Physiol. Rev.* **63**, 387−436.

Friedman, D.B., Friberg, L., Mitchell, J.H. & Secher, N.H. (1989) Regional cerebral blood flow during isometric handgrip contractions. *Clin. Res.* **37**, 260A.

Galbo, H., Kjær, M., Mikines, K.J. *et al.* (1990) Hormonal adaptation to physical activity. In: Bouchard, C., Shephard, R.J., Sutton, J.R., Stephens, T. & McPherson, B.D. (eds) *Exercise, Fitness and Health*, pp. 259−263. Human Kinetics, Champaign, Illinois.

Granit, R. (1970) *The Basis of Motor Control.* Academic Press, London.

Grimby, L. Hannerz, J. & Hedman, B. (1981) The fatigue and voluntary discharge properties of single motor units in man. *J. Physiol. (Lond.)* **316**, 545−554.

Halsey, J.H., Blauenstein, U.W., Wilson, E.M. & Wills, E.H. (1979) Regional cerebral blood flow comparison of right and left hand movement. *Neurology* **29**, 21−28.

Henneman, E. (1957) Relationship between size of neurons and their susceptibility to discharge.

Science **126**, 1345.

Houk, J.C. (1972) The phylogeny of muscular control configurations. In: Drischel, H. & Dettmar, P. (eds) *Biocybernetics IV*, pp. 125–144. Fischer, Jena.

Hutton, R.S. (1988) The central nervous system. In: Dirix, A., Knuttgen, H.G. & Tittel, K. (eds) *The Olympic Book of Sports Medicine*, Vol. 1, pp. 69–79. Blackwell Scientific Publications, Oxford.

Ikai, M., Yabe, K. & Ishii, K. (1967) Muskelkraft und muskuläre Ermüdung bei willkürlichen Anspannung und elektrischer Reizung des Muskels. *Sportarzt Sportmed.* **5**, 197–211.

Kerr, J.H. (1985) The experience of arousal: a new basis for studying arousal effects in sports. *J. Sports Sci.* **3**, 169–179.

Kots, Y.M. (1977) *The Organization of Voluntary Movement*. Plenum Press, New York.

Larsson, L. & Forsberg, A. (1980) Morphological muscle characteristics in rowers. *Can. J. Appl. Sports Sci.* **5**, 239–244.

Leonard, B., Mitchell, J.H., Mizuno, M., Rube, N., Saltin, B. & Secher, N.H. (1985) Partial neuromuscular blockade and cardiovascular responses to static exercise in man. *J. Physiol. (Lond.)* **359**, 365–379.

MacLaren, D.P., Gibson, H., Parry-Billings, M. & Edwards, R.H.T. (1989) A review of metabolic and physiological factors in fatigue. *Exerc. Sports Sci. Rev.* **17**, 29–66.

Merton, P.A. (1953) Speculations on the servo-control of movement. In: J.L. Malcolm & J.A.B. Gray (eds) *CIBA Foundation Symposium. The Spinal Cord*, pp. 247–260. Churchill Livingstone, London.

Nardone, A., Romano, C. & Schieppati, M. (1989) Selective recruitment of high-threshold human motor units during voluntary isotonic lengthening of active muscles. *J. Physiol. (Lond.)* **409**, 451–471.

Roberts, H., Schroeder, T., Secher, N.H. & Mitchell, J.H. (1990) Cerebral blood flow during static exercise in man. *J. Appl. Physiol.* **68**, 2358–2361.

Roland, P.E. & Friberg, L. (1985) Localization of cortical areas activated by thinking. *J. Neurophysiol.*

53, 1219–1243.

Rube, N. & Secher, N.H. (1981) Paradoxical influence of encouragement on muscle fatigue. *Eur. J. Appl. Physiol.* **46**, 1–7.

Rube, N. & Secher, N.H. (1991) Effect of training on central factors following two- and one-leg static exercise in man. *Acta Physiol. Scand.* **141**, 87–95.

Secher, N.H. (1983) The physiology of rowing. *J. Sports Sci.* **1**, 23–53.

Secher, N.H. (1987) Motor unit recruitment. A pharmacological approach. *Med. Sports Sci.* **26**, 152–162.

Secher, N.H. & Jensen, E.N. (1976) Glycogen depletion pattern in types I, IIa and type IIb muscle fibres during maximal voluntary static and dynamic exercise. *Acta Physiol. Scand.* **440** (Suppl.), 174.

Secher, N.H., Rørsgaard, S. & Secher, O. (1978) Contralateral influence on recruitment of curarized muscle fibres during maximal voluntary extension of the legs. *Acta Physiol. Scand.* **103**, 456–462.

Secher, N.H., Rube, N. & Molbech, S. (1981) The voluntary muscle contraction pattern in man. In: de Potter, J.C. (ed.) *Adapted Physical Activities*, pp. 225–236. Editions de l'Université de Bruxelles, Brussels.

Thomas, S.N., Schroeder, T., Secher, N.H. & Mitchell, J.H. (1989) Cerebral blood flow during submaximal and maximal dynamic exercise in humans. *J. Appl. Physiol.* **67**, 744–748.

Thorstensson, A. (1988) Speed and acceleration. In Dirix, A., Knuttgen H.G. & Tittel K. (eds) *The Olympic Book of Sports Medicine*, Vol. 1, pp. 218–229. Blackwell Scientific Publications, Oxford.

Tittel, K. (1988) Coordination and balance. In: Dirix, A., Knuttgen, H.G. & Tittel, K. (eds) *The Olympic Book of Sports Medicine*, Vol. 1, pp. 194–211. Blackwell Scientific Publications, Oxford.

Vallbo, Å.B. (1971) Muscle spindle response at the onset of isometric voluntary contractions in man. Time difference between fusimotor and skeletomotor effects. *J. Physiol. (Lond.)* **318**, 405–431.

Chapter 10

Muscular Factors in Endurance

HENRY GIBSON AND RICHARD H.T. EDWARDS

The ability to resist fatigue, often referred to as endurance, is most important for maintaining a physical activity whether in sports or everyday life. Fatigue of muscle is defined as a failure to maintain force or power output, the cause and characteristics of which vary according to the nature of the activity performed (Edwards, 1981). The changes in muscle that accompany activity are not all detrimental; while some processes result in loss of force others act to offset these changes (Jones, 1981; Gibson *et al.*, 1988).

It has long been realized that muscle contraction involves a series of steps from the brain to the contractile machinery itself (Fig. 10.1). Each of these has been separately analysed in different physiological systems, ranging from whole animal preparations to isolated cells or subcellular fractions. However, the study of all these controlling steps in humans has its practical and ethical limitations. Despite these problems, there is a distinct advantage in studying humans in that any findings are instantly applicable to the whole integrated system. In view of the complexities of the central nervous components that influence endurance, which are considered in Chapter 9, this chapter will be confined only to those changes that occur within the muscle itself. Much work has generally been directed to exploring the two principal causes of force loss: the electrophysiological aspects of contraction (resulting in fatigue as impaired neuromuscular transmission or excitation propagation along

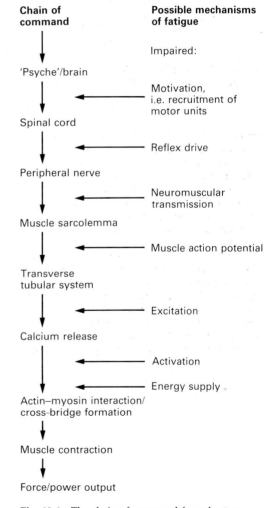

Fig. 10.1 The chain of command for voluntary contractions and the major possible causes for fatigue. From Edwards (1983).

the sarcolemmal membrane) and metabolic factors associated with or causing fatigue. The former mechanisms are considered in detail here. The metabolic changes in the muscle are important because depletion of phosphocreatine, adenosine triphosphate (ATP) or glucose/glycogen, or accumulation of metabolic byproducts in the myoplasm can impair the function of the contractile elements. The biochemical correlates of endurance are discussed further in Chapters 5, 11 and 12.

For practical reasons, largely to avoid movement artefacts, many studies in humans have been carried out using isometric contractions. The stimulated human muscle contraction model has yielded much information of the changes in muscle during activity. The significance of the changes observed will be presented with particular reference to the way in which they may combine to influence the time-course of a prolonged contraction.

Investigation of muscle performance in humans

Studies of voluntary and electrically stimulated contractions of human muscle have long been used in the investigation of muscular performance (Waller, 1891; Mosso, 1915; Merton, 1954).

Electrical stimulation of muscle via the motor nerve trunk (Merton, 1954; Stephens & Taylor, 1972) or via intramuscular motor end-nerves by percutaneous stimulation (Edwards et al., 1977b) allows the contractile properties of human muscle to be studied in a way that is directly comparable to that used when examining the function of isolated muscle preparations (Fig. 10.2). Stimulation techniques for the investigation of human muscle function and fatigue have been applied to a wide range of muscles including adductor pollicis (Merton, 1954), first dorsal interosseus (Bigland-Ritchie et al., 1982), quadriceps (Edwards et al., 1977b), anterior tibialis (Vandervoort et al., 1983), triceps surae (Hughson et al., 1987), biceps brachialis (Jones & Newham, 1989), sterno-

mastoid (Moxham et al., 1980) and diaphragm (Bellemare & Bigland-Ritchie, 1987). However, it is not possible to excite large muscle groups such as quadriceps completely by percutaneous stimulation, in view of the high voltages required and the potential discomfort or injury that may be induced. Although maximal stimulated force cannot be obtained in this way, it is still possible to construct frequency:force curves (see below) and determine other physiological characteristics such as contraction and relaxation rates. Direct stimulation of muscle is not often performed because very high voltages (up to 1000 V or more) are required (Hill et al., 1979) and tetanic contractions are not possible. Force measurements using strain gauges (Merton, 1954; Edwards et al., 1977b) and other physiological variables such as relaxation rate (Wiles & Edwards, 1982a), metabolic heat production (Wiles & Edwards, 1982b) and electromyography, have contributed to a greater understanding of the electrical and metabolic factors underlying muscular performance.

Changes during stimulated activity

The frequency dependence of the force generated in isometric contractions of human muscle has now been established as an investigative procedure (Edwards et al., 1977b). Tetanic electrical stimulation of muscle with various frequency trains of impulses via the motor nerve trunk or via intramuscular motor end-nerves by percutaneous stimulation allows the recording of the 'programmed stimulation electromyogram' (PSEM) (Fig. 10.3a). Unlike voluntary contractions, tetanic supramaximal stimulation is synchronous and all motor units are recruited. Consequently at low stimulation frequencies, where fusion is incomplete, force development is small, whereas with increasing frequency fusion is more evident, resulting in still greater force generation (Fig. 10.4). The frequency dependence of fatigue can be demonstrated when such computer-controlled contractions are made to form a train. Using this approach it can be shown that at high fre-

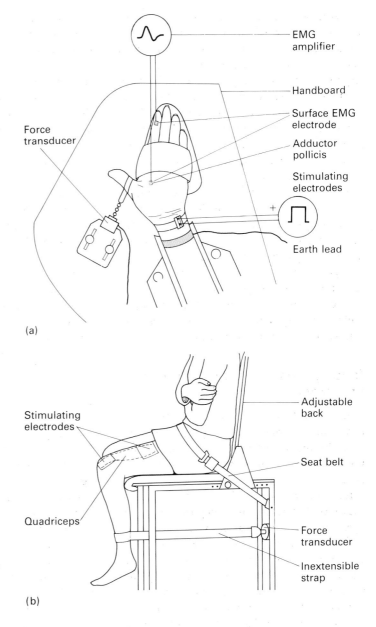

EMG
amplifier

Handboard

Surface EMG
electrode

Adductor
pollicis

Stimulating
electrodes

Earth lead

Force
transducer

(a)

Adjustable
back

Seat belt

Force
transducer

Inextensible
strap

Stimulating
electrodes

Quadriceps

(b)

Fig. 10.2 Excitation of muscle contraction by indirect stimulation of: (a) adductor pollicis via the motor nerve; and (b) quadriceps via percutaneous stimulation of the motor endplate.

quencies (80–100 Hz) force is maintained for only a few seconds, whereas at a lower frequency of 20 Hz, force may be maintained for 60 s or longer (Jones *et al.*, 1979). From this came the recognition of different mechanisms of fatigue resulting from 'high' and 'low' frequency stimulation.

High frequency stimulation

HIGH FREQUENCY FATIGUE (HFF)

In association with a rapid decline in force, there is a concomitant decline in the surface evoked action potential amplitude and a

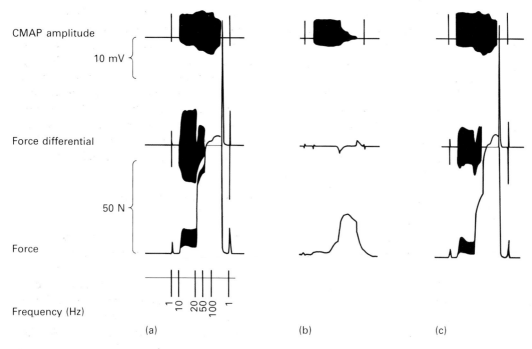

Fig. 10.3 Programmed stimulation electromyograms of adductor pollicis in one subject: (a) fresh muscle; (b) fatigued muscle; and (c) after 15 min recovery. Note the development of low frequency fatigue, evident as a reduction of low frequency force after recovery. CMAP, compound muscle action potential.

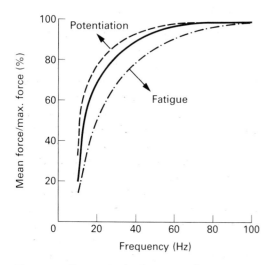

Fig. 10.4 Changes in the frequency–force curve with fatigue. Note the shift of the curve to the right as a result of the fall in the ratio of low to high frequency stimulated force, and the shift to the left as a result of an increase in force at low stimulation frequency (potentiation).

slowing in conduction velocity. Recovery occurs rapidly on reducing the frequency of stimulation (Jones *et al.*, 1979); this suggests that the cause of this type of fatigue is electrical rather than metabolic, in view of the relatively slow time course of recovery of metabolic factors. The first possible site of failure is the neuromuscular junction (Krnjevic & Miledi, 1958), but it is now realized that this does not make the most important contribution to fatigue in voluntary contractions. This was demonstrated by Bigland-Ritchie *et al.* (1982) who showed no loss of excitation of the evoked action potential superimposed on a maximal voluntary contraction during the first 60 s of activity. It is probable that the loss of force and change in electrical properties seen during high frequency stimulation is due to alterations in ionic composition across the sarcolemmal and t-tubular membranes as a consequence of electrical activity. Several studies in isolated muscle preparations (Krnjevic & Miledi, 1958; Bigland-Ritchie et al., 1979; Jones et al., 1979; Jeul, 1988) and theoretical calculations (Adrian & Peachey, 1973) suggest that accumulation of K^+ in the extracellular space or a reduction of intracellular Na^+ at high stimulation frequencies leads to the decline in action potential amplitude and slowing of action potential conduction velocity. Marked changes of transmembrane Na^+ and K^+ concentrations have also been reported during exhaustive dynamic exercise in humans (Vyskocil et al., 1983; Sjogaard et al., 1985; Medbo & Sejersted, 1990) in which the interstitial K^+ concentration measured with intramuscular electrodes and the plasma K^+ concentration have each been reported to increase to $8-9$ mmol·l^{-1}. Furthermore, recent studies have shown that isolated fast-twitch muscle fibres incubated with 15 mmol·l^{-1} of K^+ are rendered totally inexcitable, with a doubling in conduction time at concentrations of 10 mmol·l^{-1} (Jeul, 1988). Clearly, extracellular K^+ accumulation is a most important contributor to the force and excitation loss observed in human muscle fatigue.

HIGH FREQUENCY SAFETY FACTOR

The importance of HFF during voluntary muscular contraction is probably not significant since it is unlikely that high tetanic rates or motoneuron discharge rates are ever achieved except during the initial stages of a contraction (Desmedt & Godaux, 1977) or in brief ballistic contractions. Nevertheless, recent studies have revealed that high frequency stimulated force may initially be maintained despite severe excitation failure, indicating the operation of a 'safety factor' (Gibson et al., 1988). The decline in excitation probably leads to a reduction in Ca^{2+} release per impulse which would be predicted to lead to a fall in force, but at high stimulation frequencies it is likely that myoplasmic calcium levels remain sufficiently high to sustain activation of the contractile apparatus.

The physiological significance of a safety factor at high frequencies is probably limited to ballistic types of activity, since it is only in the brief initial phase of contraction that the benefit can occur before loss of excitation supervenes. This latter point may be a distinct disadvantage if fatigue limits motor performance which is dependent on the rate of development of force. This will depend on which muscle fibre types are recruited and on their metabolic demand; a high power output will require a high stimulation rate and a high degree of ATP utilization.

Low frequency stimulation

One of the most striking features of low frequency compared with high frequency stimulation is the marked increase in work × time (area under the force curve) that can be obtained. However, this occurs at a cost of lower force generation than that produced with high frequency stimulation. Several mechanical changes occur which may in part explain the prolonged maintenance of force in addition to a marked preservation of excitation. These factors are considered below.

SLOWING OF RELAXATION

Relaxation of muscle contraction force after a tetanus follows a well defined time-course, approximating a single exponential during the later phase. A two- to threefold prolongation of the half-time of this latter phase occurs as a result of fatiguing voluntary contractions (Edwards et al., 1972). Slowing of relaxation has long been recognized as a feature of prolonged muscular activity (Mosso, 1915; Feng, 1931). Its effect is to potentiate the frequency : force curve at low frequencies, as a consequence of increasing fusion of tetani owing to a smaller reduction in force between stimuli (Fig. 10.4).

The rate of relaxation following contraction may be dependent on the rate of removal of Ca^{2+} from the myoplasm (Cannell, 1986) or the dissociation of cross-bridges (Edwards et al., 1975). Under anaerobic conditions no recovery of relaxation occurs, suggesting a metabolic basis to the slowing of relaxation.

When circulation is restored to muscle, the recovery of relaxation has a half-time of about 60 s (Wiles & Edwards, 1982a), a time-course similar to that of phosphocreatine recovery (Harris *et al.*, 1976). Clearly, energy is required for the relaxation process. However, metabolic acidosis has also been proposed to play a critical role (Sahlin, 1983) and it has recently been suggested that two processes — one H^+ dependent, the other H^+ independent — are involved (Cady *et al.*, 1989). The generation of metabolites may also lead to a reduction in the free energy for hydrolysis of ATP that is necessary for relaxation (Dawson *et al.*, 1980). As yet, the precise mechanisms that lead to slowing of relaxation have not been resolved.

POTENTIATION OF FORCE

Potentiation of twitch force is a further mechanical change associated with muscle contraction which may contribute to resisting fatigue (Green, 1986). Potentiation of twitch force has long been identified during low frequency (2–3 Hz) stimulated contractions ('staircase' potentiation) in both human and rodent muscle (Desmedt & Hainaut, 1968; Krarup, 1981) and following brief tetanic stimulation (Takamori *et al.*, 1971; Blinks *et al.*, 1978). Twitch potentiation also occurs after short (5–10 s) maximal voluntary contractions (Belanger & Quinlan, 1982), presumably as a result of preceding endogenous tetanic stimulated activation. Decay of this type of potentiation may take several minutes.

Low frequency force potentiation is observed immediately following brief high frequency stimulated activity (Gibson *et al.*, 1988). It is unclear whether similar mechanisms to twitch potentiation are responsible for this form of potentiation, and studies of the decay kinetics may give a clue to this phenomenon. Nevertheless, it may be speculated that during voluntary activity, twitch and low frequency potentiation act over and above slowing of relaxation rate to maintain force. Indeed, there is evidence to suggest that brief bursts of high

frequency motor unit discharges (50 Hz) occur in the first dorsal interosseus (De Luca *et al.*, 1982) and that these become more pronounced as fatigue ensues (Oldham, 1987), thereby promoting potentiating mechanisms. The requirement of such a mechanism in type I fibres may be unnecessary in view of their high degree of fatigue resistance, long contraction times and fusion at lower discharge rates.

FATIGUE AT LOW STIMULATION FREQUENCY

This form of fatigue can be demonstrated following a series of contractions made under anaerobic conditions (Edwards *et al.*, 1977a) and also following specific forms of voluntary dynamic contraction (Edwards *et al.*, 1977a; Davies & White, 1981; 1982). Low frequency fatigue (LFF) is characterized by a selective loss of force without loss of excitation after several hours of low frequency stimulation (Fig. 10.3b & c). This suggests that the cause of LFF is further down the chain of command, in a failure of excitation–contraction coupling (Edwards, 1981; see Fig. 10.2). LFF may be due in part to a reduction in Ca^{2+} release, possibly owing to impaired transmission of excitation in the transverse tubular system. LFF is not simply due to lactate and proton accumulation as a consequence of muscular activity, since it may be demonstrated in individuals with a variety of metabolic defects which influence energy exchanges and lactate production, for example McArdle's disease (Wiles *et al.*, 1981).

The comparatively slow recovery of low frequency stimulated force after exercise (a day or more; Edwards *et al.*, 1977a) could indicate that LFF is due to structural damage of the sarcoplasmic reticulum or tubular system. The observation that LFF is more pronounced following eccentric contractions (Newham *et al.*, 1983) would appear to support this hypothesis.

The effect of this type of fatigue is to move the steep part of the force–frequency curve to the right. Since it is likely that the firing frequency for voluntary contractions in everyday life activities is in the range of 5–30 Hz (Bellemare *et al.*, 1983), this type of fatigue may result in a significant force reduction unless a compensatory increase in firing frequency can be achieved or there is a concomitant recruitment of further motor units in parallel.

The post-tetanic behaviour of muscle minimizes the progress of low frequency fatigue during short-term repetitive activity (Green & Jones, 1989). Thus, as LFF develops, loss of force is reduced by potentiating mechanisms. It is unlikely that slowing of relaxation ameliorates LFF during such activity, owing to its recovery without restoration in force.

Interrelation of fatigue-resisting mechanisms

During prolonged voluntary effort a reduction in motor unit discharge rate accompanies the slowing of relaxation rate described above (Bigland-Ritchie *et al.*, 1983; Marsden *et al.*, 1983). This process has been described as the muscle's 'natural wisdom' (Marsden *et al.*, 1983) and it may serve as a mechanism protecting against excitation failure at the neuromuscular junction or at the excitable membranes of the muscle cell (Jones & Edwards, 1986). The high frequency safety factor and low frequency potentiating mechanisms may additionally act during activity, their relative contributions being summarized as shown in Fig. 10.5. This figure illustrates that the contribution of the high frequency safety factor is limited to periods of high frequency activity, where maximal force is generated, whereas the contribution of potentiation is limited to periods of low frequency activity. The usefulness of these mechanisms is not without cost, however, owing to the curvilinear relation of excitation frequency to force and the relation of force to endurance as described by Rohmert's curve (Rohmert, 1960). Thus, although high forces are developed with high excitation rates, maintenance of force is short lived, whereas at low excitation rates the benefit of prolonged maintenance of force is limited by the low level of

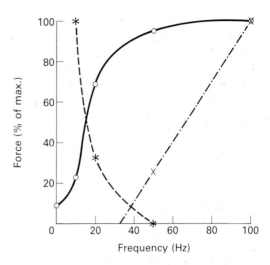

Fig. 10.5 Frequency dependence of the contribution of the high frequency safety factor (x) and low frequency potentiating mechanisms (*) during stimulated activity. Low frequency potentiating mechanisms may be of greatest importance during low frequency activity, but the benefits gained may be small in view of the low force (o) achieved. Conversely, at high stimulation frequency, despite the high forces achieved, the contribution of the high frequency safety factor may be short lived owing to rapid fatigue at such high frequencies.

force that is developed. These observations may have important practical implications in functional electrical stimulation.

Conclusions

Clearly, the limitation of muscle endurance is dependent on many factors, both deleterious and advantageous. No single factor can be uniquely identified with endurance. Alteration of excitation, slowing of relaxation and changes in contractile characteristics can all be seen separately or in combination, their contributions depending on the nature of the contraction performed. The chemical and electrical limits to continued contractile activity have been vigorously debated over the years (Ciba Foundation Symposium, 1981). Models may be constructed to account for changes in the single muscle cell, but it must be remembered that the events occurring in one cell at any one time may not be duplicated in another cell of the same muscle. Moreover, the conclusions drawn from the studies described may not necessarily apply to activities in which muscle length alters, as in most everyday activities. The concepts described cannot be claimed to have direct relevance to athletic performance, since this is a function of careful tuning by the body, integrating skill and coordination of muscle function, with cardiovascular, respiratory and central control factors all contributing to minimize the tendency to fatigue.

References

Adrian, R.H. & Peachey, L.D. (1973) Reconstruction of the action potential of frog sartorius muscle. *J. Physiol.* **235**, 103−131.

Belanger, A.Y. & Quinlan, J. (1982) Muscle function studies in human plantar−flexor and dorsi-flexor muscles. *Can. J. Neurol. Sci.* **9**, 358−359.

Bellemare, F. & Bigland-Ritchie, B. (1987) Central components of diaphragmatic fatigue assessed by phrenic nerve stimulation. *J. Appl. Physiol.* **62**, 1307−1316.

Bellemare, F., Woods, J.J., Johansson, R. & Bigland-Ritchie, B. (1983) Motor-unit discharge rates in maximal voluntary contractions of three human muscles. *J. Neurophysiol.* **50**, 1380−1392.

Bigland-Ritchie, B., Johansson, R., Lippold, O.C.J., Smith, S. & Woods, J.J. (1983) Changes in motoneuron firing rates during sustained maximal voluntary contractions. *J. Physiol.* **340**, 335−346.

Bigland-Ritchie, B., Jones, D.A. & Woods, J.J. (1979) Excitation frequency and muscle fatigue. Electrical responses during human sustained and stimulated contractions. *Exp. Physiol.* **64**, 414−427.

Bigland-Ritchie, B., Kakula, C.B., Lippold, O.C.J. & Woods, J.J. (1982) The absence of neuromuscular transmission failure in sustained maximal voluntary contractions. *J. Physiol.* **330**, 265−278.

Blinks, J.R., Rudel, R. & Taylor S.R. (1978) Calcium transients in isolated amphibian skeletal muscle fibres; detection with aequorin. *J. Physiol.* **277**, 291−323.

Cady, E.B., Jones, D.A., Lynn, J. & Newham, D.J. (1989) Changes in force and intracellular metabolites during fatigue of human skeletal muscle. *J. Physiol.* **418**, 311−325.

Cannell, M.B. (1986) Effect of tetanus duration on the free calcium during the relaxation of frog skeletal muscle fibres. *J. Physiol.* **376**, 203−218.

Ciba Foundation Symposium 82 (1981) In: Porter, R. & Whelan, J. (eds) *Human Muscle Fatigue: Physiological Mechanisms*. Pitman Medical, London.

Davies, C.T.M. & White, M.J. (1981) Muscle weakness following eccentric work in man. *Pflügers Arch.* **392**, 168−171.

Davies, C.T.M. & White, M.J. (1982) Muscle weakness following dynamic exercise in humans. *J. Appl. Physiol.* **53**, 236−241.

Dawson, M.J., Gadian, D.G. & Wilkie, D.R. (1980) Mechanical relaxation rate and metabolism studied in fatiguing muscle by phosphorous nuclear magnetic resonance. *J. Physiol.* **299**, 465−484.

De Luca, C.J., LeFever, R.S., McCue, M.P. & Xenakis, A.P. (1982) Control scheme governing concurrently active human motor units during voluntary contractions. *J. Physiol.* **329**, 129−142.

Desmedt, J.E. & Godaux, E. (1977) Ballistic contractions in man: characteristic recruitment pattern of single motor units of the tibialis anterior muscle. *J. Physiol.* **264**, 673−693.

Desmedt, J.E. & Hainaut, K. (1968) Kinetics of myofilament activation in potentiated contraction: staircase phenomenon in human skeletal muscle. *Nature* **217**, 529−532.

Edwards, R.H.T. (1981) Human muscle function and fatigue. In: Porter, R. & Whelan, J. (eds) *Human Muscle Fatigue: Physiological Mechanisms*, Ciba Foundation Symposium 82, pp. 1−18. Pitman Medical, London.

Edwards, R.H.T. (1983) Biochemical basis of fatigue. In: Knuttgen, H.G. (ed.) *Biochemistry of Exercise*, pp. 3−28. Human Kinetics, Champaign, Illinois.

Edwards, R.H.T., Hill, D.K. & Jones, D.A. (1972) Effect of fatigue on the time course of relaxation of skeletal muscle in man. *J. Physiol.* **227**, 26−27P.

Edwards, R.H.T., Hill, D.K. & Jones, D.A. (1975) Metabolic changes associated with the slowing of relaxation in fatigued mouse muscle. *J. Physiol.* **251**, 287−301.

Edwards, R.H.T., Hill, D.K., Jones, D.A. & Merton, P.A. (1977a) Fatigue of long duration in human skeletal muscle after exercise. *J. Physiol.* **272**, 769−778.

Edwards, R.H.T., Young, A., Hosking, G.P. & Jones, D.A. (1977b) Human skeletal muscle function: description of tests and normal values. *Clin. Sci. Mol. Med.* **52**, 283−290.

Feng, T.P. (1931) The heat−tension ratio in prolonged tetanic contractions. *Proc. R. Soc. Lond. Biol.* **108**, 522−537.

Green, H.J. (1986) Muscle power: fibre type recruitment, metabolism and fatigue. In: Jones, N.L., McCartney, N. & McComas, A.J. (eds) *Human Muscle Power*, pp. 65−79. Human Kinetics, Champaign, Illinois.

Green, H.J. & Jones, S.R. (1989) Does post-tetanic

potentiation compensate for low frequency fatigue? *Clin. Physiol.* **9**, 499–514.

Gibson, H., Cooper, R.G., Stokes, M.J. & Edwards, R.H.T. (1988) Mechanisms resisting fatigue in isometrically contracting human skeletal muscle. *Q. J. Exp. Physiol.* **73**, 903–914.

Harris, R.C., Edwards, R.H.T., Hultman, E. & Nordesjø, L.-O. (1976) The time course of phosphorylcreatine resynthesis during recovery of the quadriceps in man. *Eur. J. Physiol.* **367**, 137–142.

Hill, D.K., McDonnell, M.J. & Merton, P.A. (1979) Direct stimulation of the adductor pollicis in man. *J. Physiol.* **300**, 2–3P.

Hughson, R.L., Green, H.J., Alway, S.E., Patla, A.E. & Frank, J.S. (1987) The effects of β-blockade on electrically stimulated contraction in fatigued human triceps surae muscle. *Clin. Physiol.* **7**, 133–150.

Jeul, C. (1988) Muscle action potential propagation velocity changes during activity. *Muscle Nerve* **11**, 714–719.

Jones, D.A. (1981) Muscle fatigue due to changes beyond the neuromuscular junction. In: Porter, R. & Whelan, J. (eds) *Human Muscle Fatigue: Physiological Mechanisms*, Ciba Foundation Symposium 82, pp. 178–197. Pitman Medical, London.

Jones, D.A. & Edwards, R.H.T. (1986) Muscle strength and metabolism. In: Dimitrijevic, M., Kakulas, B. & Vrbova, G. (eds) *Recent Achievements in Restorative Neurology* 2: *Progressive Neuromuscular Diseases*, pp. 123–138. Karger, Basel.

Jones, D.A. & Newham, D.J. (1989) Human muscle fatigue: effects of muscle length during isometric contractions. *J. Physiol.* **409**, 16P.

Jones, D.A., Bigland-Ritchie, B. & Edwards, R.H.T. (1979) Excitation frequency and muscle fatigue: mechanical responses during voluntary and stimulated contractions. *Exp. Neurol.* **64**, 401–413.

Krarup, C. (1981) Enhancement and diminution of mechanical tension evoked by staircase and by tetanus in rat muscle. *J. Physiol.* **311**, 355–372.

Krnjevik, L. & Miledi, R. (1958) Failure of neuromuscular propagation in rats. *J. Physiol.* **140**, 440–461.

Marsden, C.D., Meadows, J.C. & Merton, P.A. (1983) 'Muscular wisdom' that minimizes fatigue during prolonged effort in man: peak rates of motoneuron discharge and slowing of discharge during fatigue. In: Desmedt, J.E. (ed.) *Motor Control Mechanisms in Health and Disease*, pp. 169–211. Raven Press, New York.

Medbo, J.I. & Sejersted, O.M. (1990) Plasma potassium changes with high intensity exercise. *J. Physiol.* **421**, 105–122.

Merton, P.A. (1954) Voluntary strength and fatigue. *J.*

Physiol. **123**, 553–564.

Mosso, A. (1915) *Fatigue*, 3rd edn (translated by Drummond, M. & Drummond, W.G.). Allen & Unwin, London.

Moxham, J., Wiles, C.M., Newham, D. & Edwards, R.H.T. (1980) Sternomastoid muscle function and fatigue in man. *Clin. Sci.* **59**, 463–468.

Newham, D.J., McPhail, G., Mills, K.R. & Edwards, R.H.T. (1983) Ultrastructural changes after concentric and eccentric contractions of human muscle. *J. Neurol. Sci.* **61**, 102–122.

Oldham, J.A. (1987) *Rehabilitation of Skeletal Muscle in the Arthritic Hand*. PhD thesis, University of Liverpool.

Rohmert, W. (1960) Emittlung von Erholungspausen für statische Arbeit des Menschen. *Int. Archiv. ange. Physiol.* **18**, 123–164.

Sahlin, K. (1983) Effects of acidosis on energy metabolism and force generation in skeletal muscle. In: Knuttgen, H.G. & Vogel, H. (eds) *Biochemistry of Exercise*, pp. 151–160. Human Kinetics, Champaign, Illinois.

Sjogaard, G., Adams, R.P. & Saltin, B. (1985) Water and ion shifts in skeletal muscle of humans with intense dynamic knee extension. *Am. J. Physiol.* **248**, R190–R196.

Stephens, J.A. & Taylor, A. (1972) Fatigue of maintained voluntary muscle contraction in man. *J. Physiol.* **220**, 1–18.

Takamori, M., Gutmann, L. & Shane, S.R. (1971) Contractile properties of human skeletal muscle. *Arch. Neurol.* **25**, 535–546.

Vandervoort, A.A., Quinlan, J. & McComas, A.J. (1983) Twitch potentiation after voluntary contraction. *Exp. Neurol.* **81**, 141–152.

Vyskocil, F., Hnik, P., Rehfelat, H., Vejsada, R. & Ujec, E. (1983) The measurement K^{+e} concentration changes in human muscles during volitional contractions. *Pflügers Arch.* **399**, 235–237.

Waller, A.D. (1891) The sense of effort: an objective study. *Brain* **14**, 179–249.

Wiles, C.M. & Edwards, R.H.T. (1982a) The effect of temperature, ischaemia and contractile activity on the relaxation rate of human muscle. *Clin. Physiol.* **2**, 485–497.

Wiles, C.M. & Edwards, R.H.T. (1982b) Metabolic heat production in isometric ischaemic contractions of human adductor pollicis. *Clin. Physiol.* **2**, 499–512.

Wiles, C.M., Jones, D.A. & Edwards, R.H.T. (1981) Fatigue in human metabolic myopathy. In: Porter, R. & Whelan, J. (eds) *Human Muscle Fatigue: Physiological Mechanisms*, Ciba Foundation Symposium 82, pp. 264–283. Pitman Medical, London.

Chapter 11

Endocrine Factors in Endurance

HENRIK GALBO

Introduction

The autonomic nervous system, which is not influenced by the will, and hormones secreted into the blood by endocrine glands serve to regulate and coordinate body functions during the varying internal and external conditions of daily life. It is not possible to separate the nervous and endocrine control systems sharply (Galbo, 1986). This chapter deals with the general response of autonomic neuroendocrine systems to exercise and with their role in the regulation of metabolism and water and electrolyte balance. Autonomic neuroendocrine mechanisms are also involved in cardiovascular, thermoregulatory and pulmonary adaptations to exercise, and these aspects are discussed in other chapters.

The autonomic nervous system has two divisions called the sympathetic (or adrenergic) and the parasympathetic, respectively. The two divisions have opposing effects, and during exercise the balance is changed in favour of sympathetic predominance. Sympathetic nerves spread from the spinal cord to the heart and liver, to smooth muscle (e.g. in blood vessels), to fat, and to endocrine and exocrine glandular cells all over the body (Fig. 11.1). The major signal transmitter released from sympathetic nerve endings at the target cells is noradrenaline (norepinephrine). On top of the kidneys lie the adrenal glands, the central part of which — the adrenal medulla — consists of modified sympathetic nerve cells specialized

for releasing methylated noradrenaline, i.e. adrenaline (epinephrine), directly into the blood stream (Fig. 11.1). The sympathetic nervous system also influences the secretion of other hormones. The pancreas is a gland which lies beneath the stomach and secretes insulin and glucagon. Insulin secretion is inhibited by sympathetic nerve activity (Fig. 11.1). Furthermore, in response to adrenergic stimulation the kidneys secrete an enzyme, renin, which gives rise to production of a peptide, angiotensin-2, from a protein in the blood. Angiotensin-2, in turn, stimulates the secretion of the hormone aldosterone from the adrenal cortex (Fig. 11.1).

In addition to sympathetic control, subordinate endocrine glands are regulated by hormones secreted from the pituitary gland. This gland lies underneath the brain and secretes, for example, adrenocorticotrophic hormone (ACTH), which stimulates the secretion of cortisol from the adrenal cortex (Fig. 11.1). Both sympathetic activity and pituitary secretion are influenced by higher integrating neural centres in the brain (e.g. the hypothalamus).

Endocrine regulation of metabolism in exercise

Energy for muscular contraction is delivered by splitting of the compound adenosine triphosphate (ATP). During prolonged exercise ATP is produced in the exercising muscles by oxidation of carbohydrate and lipid. These fuels are stored as the high molecular weight compounds gly-

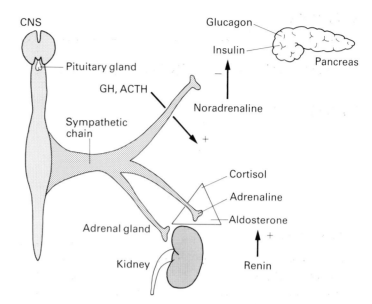

Fig. 11.1 A simplified scheme of the autonomic neuroendocrine system. ACTH, adrenocorticotrophic hormone; CNS, central nervous system; GH, growth hormone.

cogen and triglyceride, both within the muscles and in extramuscular depots. During exercise, liver glycogen is broken down to glucose, which is transported by the blood to working muscle. In parallel, triglyceride is broken down to free fatty acids and glycerol in fat tissue, and the free fatty acids are transported to muscle. Changes in autonomic neuroendocrine activity are responsible for the mobilization of extramuscular fuels in favour of the working muscles. Mobilization of intramuscular fuel stores can be elicited by contractions *per se*, but it is enhanced by neuroendocrine mechanisms, which are essentially the same as those involved in mobilization of extramuscular fuel stores.

Mobilization of glycogen by glycogenolysis, as well as mobilization of triglyceride by lipolysis, is inhibited by insulin. In contrast these processes are stimulated by sympathetic nervous activity and by several counter-regulatory hormones that oppose the action of insulin. Examples of the latter are adrenaline, glucagon, cortisol, the pituitary hormones growth hormone and ACTH. During exercise, sympathetic nervous activity is increased and so is the secretion and, in turn, plasma concentrations

of all counter-regulatory hormones (Figs 11.2–11.5) (Galbo, 1983; 1985; 1986). On the other hand, the secretion and plasma concentration of insulin are decreased during exercise (Fig. 11.2) (Galbo, 1983; 1985; 1986). Thus, fuel mobilization is enhanced during exercise by a concerted increase in activating factors and a decrease in the only inhibiting factor; one steps on the accelerator while releasing the brake.

The evidence that the described neuroendocrine setting explains fuel mobilization in exercise has come from experiments interfering with the various components by pharmacological blockade of hormone receptors, by pharmacological or surgical suppression of endocrine secretion, and by exogenous hormone administration (Galbo, 1983; 1985). It seems that the exercise-induced increase in symphoadrenomedullary activity is of primary importance, acting directly on intra- and extramuscular fuel stores as well as indirectly via the adrenergic inhibition of insulin secretion.

Considering the well known fact that insulin increases the glucose uptake in muscle, it may seem surprising that muscle glucose intake is increased during exercise even though

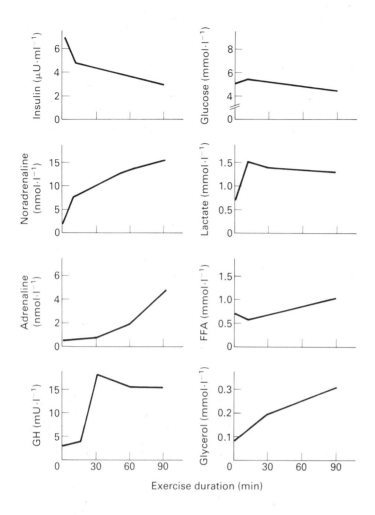

Fig. 11.2 Typical changes in concentrations of hormones and substrates in plasma during exercise at 60–70% of $V_{O_2\,max}$ in the overnight fasted state. FFA, free fatty acids; GH, growth hormone.

the insulin concentration in plasma is decreased. However, muscle contractions *per se* enhance muscle glucose intake by mechanisms that are independent of insulin. This fact, as well as inhibition of lipolysis, implies that muscle glucose intake increases inappropriately during exercise, if the insulin concentration does not decrease below basal levels. This may happen if food is ingested within the last 2 h before exercise. The accelerated muscular glucose intake from plasma may, together with insulin-mediated inhibition of hepatic glucose production, result in development of hypoglycaemia and acute impairment of the function of the central nervous system.

Endocrine factors influencing body fluids and electrolytes in exercise

Exercise causes production of heat in the working muscles. If the exercise intensity is more than very mild the heat is removed from the body predominantly by evaporation of sweat. The evaporative water loss through the airways is also increased during exercise due to the increase in ventilation and body temperature. These external fluid losses as well as transcapillary filtration in working muscles cause a fall in plasma volume. Because sweat and expired water contain less sodium chloride than plasma, the osmolality of body fluids increases

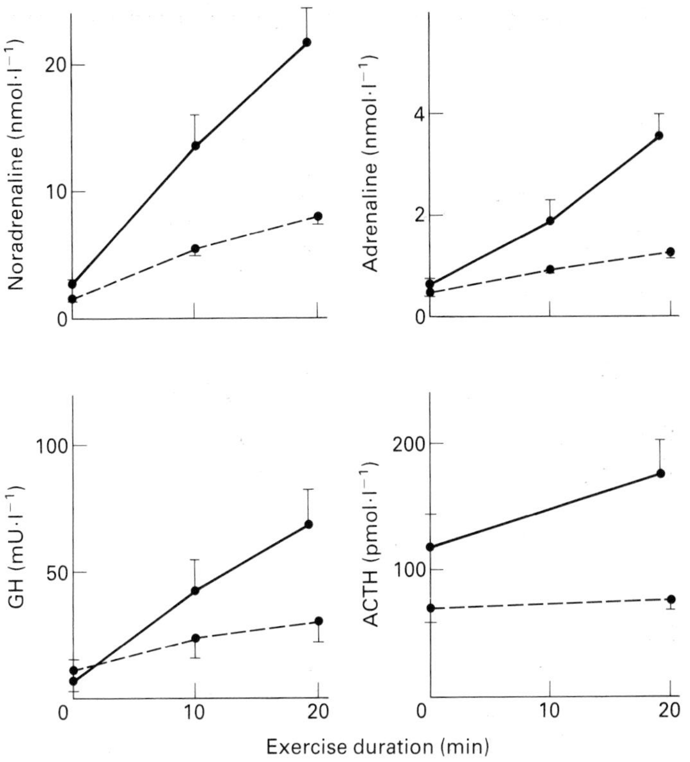

Fig. 11.3 Hormone concentrations in plasma in seven trained (– – –) and seven untrained (——) subjects exercising at 210 W on a cycle ergometer. Values are means ± s.e. ACTH, adrenocorticotrophic hormone; GH, growth hormone. From Kjær *et al.* (1988).

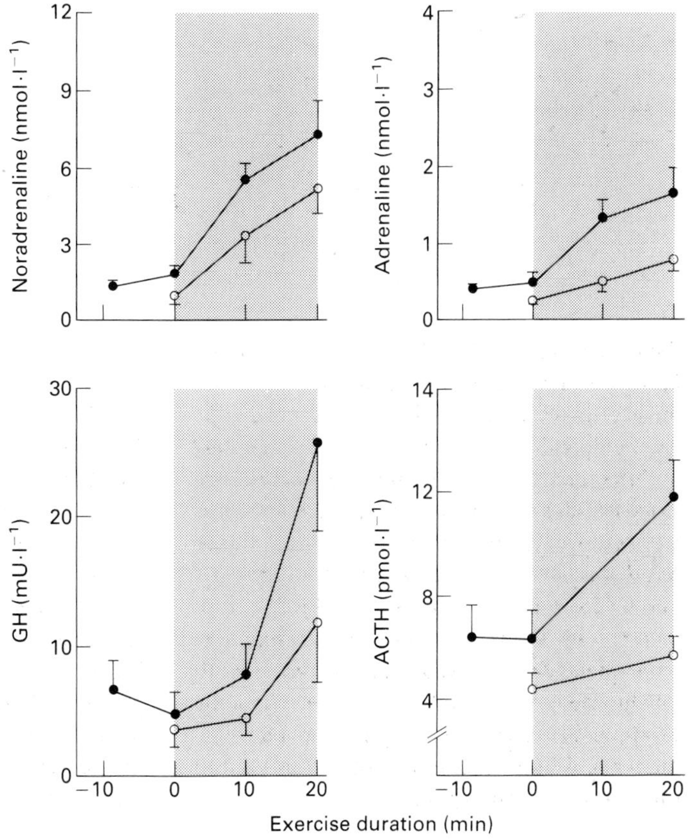

Fig. 11.4 Effect of partial neuromuscular blockade with curare (●) on hormone concentrations in plasma measured at rest and during semisupine exercise (□) at 150 W on a cycle ergometer in seven subjects. ○, Control subjects. Values are means ± s.e. Curare was administered after the −10 min blood sample had been drawn. ACTH, adrenocorticotrophic hormone; GH, growth hormone. From Kjær *et al.* (1987).

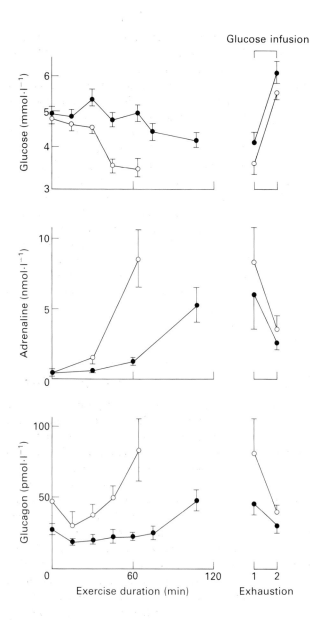

Fig. 11.5 Effect of preceding diet on plasma concentrations of glucose, adrenaline and glucagon during running at 70% $V_{O_2 max}$. At exhaustion the seven subjects were encouraged to run for 10 min more, while glucose was infused. Values are means ± s.e. ●, Carbohydrate; ○, fat. From Galbo (1983).

during exercise. A relatively marked increase in plasma potassium concentration may be seen because potassium leaks out of muscle in response to depolarization.

Sympathetic activity is heavily engaged in water and electrolyte shifts in exercise. Thus increased activity in the sympathetic nerves to sweat glands is responsible for the increase in sweat production, which is necessary for thermoregulation. At the same time sympath-

etic activity reduces the deleterious effects of sweat loss on cardiovascular function by reducing renal losses of sodium chloride and water. This happens by direct intrarenal adrenergic mechanisms (Galbo, 1983) as well as indirectly by adrenergic release of renin from the kidneys (see Fig. 11.1) (Galbo, 1986; Sutton *et al.*, 1990). Renin increases the plasma concentration of angiotensin-2 and, in turn, of aldosterone and antidiuretic hormone (ADH).

Aldosterone from the adrenal cortex (see Fig. 11.1) and ADH secreted from the pituitary gland reduce sodium and water excretion in the kidneys. During exercise, aldosterone secretion is also enhanced by the increases in ACTH and potassium. The increase in ADH is enhanced by the increase in plasma osmolality, and increases in both aldosterone and ADH are favoured by reductions in plasma volume.

The tendency to hyperkalaemia during exercise is counteracted by a direct adrenergic enhancement of potassium uptake in muscle, as well as by increased excretion of potassium in urine, sweat and saliva caused by increased aldosterone levels. In recent years a peptide hormone, atrial natriuretic factor (ANF), which, at least in pharmacological concentrations, enhances renal sodium excretion, has been described. The concentration of ANF increases in exercise, but the significance of this finding is not understood.

High osmolality, angiotensin and low plasma volume provoke thirst. The combination of thirst and the above described exercise-activated mechanisms reducing renal sodium and water excretion, may account for the increase in plasma volume which takes place during training (Galbo, 1983; Sutton *et al.*, 1990). The red blood cell mass may also increase during training, probably primarily as a result of bone marrow stimulation by the hormone erythropoietin. Erythropoietin is produced predominantly in the kidneys, and during exercise increased release is probably caused by adrenergic mechanisms.

Endogenous opioid peptides

A single bout of exercise may increase the pain threshold, relieve anger, depression and anxiety, and even cause euphoria (the 'runner's high'). These effects are similar to those of morphine. Accordingly, it has been proposed that they result from release of endogenous substances which bind to the same receptors as morphine. Such substances, endogenous opioid peptides (EOPs), are found in several

areas within the brain, but are also found outside the brain; for example, the EOP most familiar to the layperson, β-endorphin, is secreted from the pituitary gland. In accordance with the postulated role for EOPs in exercise, EOP concentrations in plasma may increase with exercise (Galbo, 1986; Sutton *et al.*, 1990). However, the effects of exercise on pain perception and mood would be explained only by changes in opioid activity within the central nervous system. So far such changes have not been clearly documented. Furthermore, abolition of EOP effects by pharmacological receptor blockade has failed to impair the morphine-like action of exercise. The conclusion is that the reputation of β-endorphin and other EOPs among exercise enthusiasts is based on myth rather than facts (Galbo, 1986; Sutton *et al.*, 1990).

Regulation of autonomic neuroendocrine activity in exercise

Accumulating evidence suggests that during exercise control of the neuroendocrine system is exerted along the same lines as control of circulation and respiration. Feedforward as well as feedback mechanisms are involved in regulation. It is believed that, from the onset of exercise, impulses from motor centres radiate within the brain ('central command') as well as through afferent nerves from recruited muscles to higher endocrine centres, eliciting a work rate-dependent increase in sympatho-adrenomedullary activity and in the release of some pituitary hormones (e.g. ACTH, growth hormone, β-endorphin, ADH). These responses control the changes in secretion of subordinate endocrine cells; for example, ACTH stimulates cortisol secretion and sympathoadrenomedullary activity depresses insulin secretion while stimulating the renin–angiotensin–aldosterone–ADH system (Galbo, 1983). The rapid onset of the hormonal changes means that the need for endocrine adjustments is, so to speak, anticipated. The primary setting depends on the state of the organism, for instance, as regards nutrition, training, phase of menstrual cycle and state of health (Galbo, 1983; 1986; Sutton *et al.*, 1990). Training diminishes the hormonal response to a given work rate (see Fig. 11.3), reflecting the fact that the hormonal response to exercise is more closely related to relative work rate (% $\dot{V}\text{O}_{2\,max}$) than to work rate expressed in absolute terms. During continued exercise the hormonal changes may be gradually intensified due to feedback from receptors sensing changes in the internal milieu, for example in metabolic variables, intravascular volume, pressure, osmolality and temperature.

The most direct evidence in favour of immediate activation of endocrine centres from motor centres has come from studies involving partial neuromuscular blockade with tubocurarine (Kjær *et al.*, 1987). Tubocurarine weakens the muscles and probably makes higher motor centre activity necessary to elicit a given absolute work intensity. In agreement with this suggestion, subjects in experiments with blockade had a higher perceived exertion for a given absolute work rate than did those in experiments without blockade. The higher motor centre activity during curarization was accompanied by exaggerated exercise responses of catecholamines and pituitary hormones, indicating that motor centre activity stimulates endocrine changes directly (see Fig. 11.4). The exaggerated hormonal changes in tubocurarine compared with control experiments were accompanied by a more rapid increase in hepatic glucose production and enhanced lipolysis in exercise (Kjær *et al.*, 1987). The interpretation of these findings in humans is supported by the fact that in paralysed cats electrical stimulation of subthalamic motor centres elicits a hormonal response similar to that seen in exercise and, in addition, an increase in glucose production (Vissing *et al.*, 1989).

The view that afferent nervous feedback from working muscle influences the hormonal changes in exercise has been confirmed in studies showing diminished responses of ACTH and β-endorphin to submaximal cycling during epidural anaesthesia of the thin afferent nerve fibres from the lower part of the body (Kjær *et al.*, 1989). Furthermore, we have recently found in cats that electrical stimulation of afferent nerves from muscles increases the levels of ACTH, β-endorphin and glucose in the blood and decreases insulin concentrations (J. Vissing *et al.*, unpublished results).

During exercise, the most important metabolic error signal is a decrease in glucose availability. The existence of the glucose feedback mechanism has been shown most clearly in experiments with different diets (Fig. 11.5) (Galbo, 1983). After 4 days of a diet rich in fat, the plasma glucose concentration declined more rapidly during prolonged running than it did after intake of a diet rich in carbohydrate. A close correlation was seen between the decrease in plasma glucose and the increase in adrenaline and glucagon levels, the hormonal responses to exercise being enhanced in fat compared with carbohydrate experiments. Furthermore, when late during exercise in both experiments plasma glucose concentrations were restored to preexercise levels by glucose infusion, concentrations of adrenaline and glucagon decreased markedly. Considering that a decrease in plasma glucose reflects a need for substrate supply to the working muscles, and that the hormonal changes elicited by this decrease can meet the substrate demand, the depicted feedback mechanism is very appropriate.

Training-induced adaptations within the autonomic neuroendocrine system

The adrenal medulla

Endocrine adaptations to training, for example the diminished hormonal response to a given work rate (see Fig. 11.3), may reflect that the signals influencing autonomic neuroendocrine activity are modified during training. However, illustrating the profound influence that regularly repeated exercise has on the body, training may also change the secretory capacity of the endocrine glands. Thus prolonged endurance training increases the adrenal medullary secretory capacity, and causes a 'sports adrenal medulla'. This is indicated by an exaggerated adrenaline response by athletes to various stimuli, e.g. hypoglycaemia, hypoxia, hypercapnia, glucagon, caffeine and maximum exercise, as well as by an increase in size of the adrenal medulla with training in rats (Stallknecht *et al.*, 1990). Taking into account the various effects of adrenaline, e.g. enhancement of mental alertness and of contractility in heart and skeletal muscle, it is clear that a high capacity to secrete adrenaline represents an advantage in competitive sports. It is also interesting to note that the capacity to secrete adrenaline normally diminishes with age. So, training causes biological rejuvenation of the adrenal medullary secretory capacity, as it does of the capacity of heart and skeletal muscle.

The pancreatic β-cells

Studies with infusion of glucose (Fig. 11.6) and arginine (Dela *et al.*, 1990) indicate that the capacity of athletes to secrete insulin is diminished by training. Conversely, the capacity is increased by inactivity, as indicated by studies

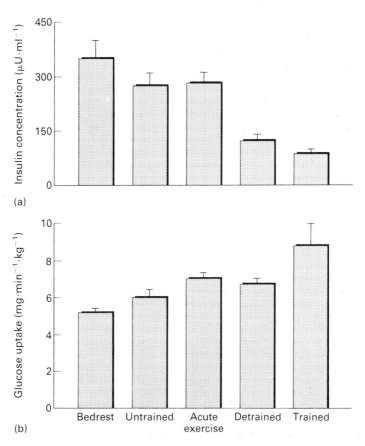

Fig. 11.6   Effect of preceding level of physical activity on pancreatic β-cell function and insulin sensitivity. (a) Insulin concentrations during steady state glucose infusion (20 mmol·l^{-1}); (b) glucose uptake from plasma during steady state insulin infusion (40 μU·ml^{-1}). Values are means ± s.e. obtained from six to seven subjects. Untrained subjects were studied without and with 1 h of prior exercise at 60% $\dot{V}$O$_{2\,max}$ as well as after 7 days of bedrest. Trained subjects were studied both 15 h and 5 days after last exercise bout. From Mikines *et al.* (1989a; 1989b).

of detraining and bedrest (Fig. 11.6). The diminished capacity of athletes to secrete insulin in physically active subjects is justified by training-induced adaptations in target cells, resulting in a lower need for insulin to handle a given carbohydrate load. As shown in Fig. 11.6, an inverse relationship exists over a wide range of daily activity levels between the β-cell response to glucose and the effect of insulin. Recent studies have indicated that the adaptations in secretion and action of insulin induced by physical training are accurately matched to the increase in fuel turnover, which accompanies the training regimen: during ordinary living conditions trained subjects have the same overall responses of insulin secretion and plasma glucose concentrations as in untrained subjects despite a higher carbohydrate intake (Dela et al., 1991). This means that during training adaptations in β-cells and insulin-sensitive tissues allow the necessary increase in food intake without potentially harmful hyperglycaemia, hyperinsulinaemia and overloading of β-cells.

Gonadal function

Neither women nor men show changes in plasma concentrations of the pituitary gonadotrophins, follicle stimulating hormone (FSH) and luteinizing hormone (LH) in response to a single bout of exercise (Galbo, 1986; Sutton et al., 1990). Nevertheless, an early increase in the plasma concentrations of gonadal hormones may take place due to haemoconcentration and decreased hormone clearance, and this phase may be succeeded by a decrease below basal levels as a result of diminished hormone secretion.

Physical training may disturb hypothalamic function and provoke hypothalamic hypogonadotrophic hypogonadism (Galbo, 1986; Sutton et al., 1990). In women this may be accompanied by menstrual irregularities including delayed menarche, luteal phase shortening and anovulatory cycles, oligomenorrhoea and amenorrhoea. Altered menstrual cycle

function may be seen during all kinds of endurance training, but the prevalence of amenorrhoea is higher in runners than in swimmers and cyclists. The risk of developing menstrual irregularities increases with the amount of training, and is increased in girls with late menarche, in girls who start training before menarche and in very lean females. In men suppression of both testosterone levels and spermatogenesis may be seen with intense training.

Because a very high level of daily physical activity is not compatible with pregnancy and parental care, it may be argued that the severe hypogonadism sometimes occurring in intensively training women is appropriate. However, it is accompanied by bone loss and an increased risk of fractures (Sutton et al., 1990). Accordingly, training-induced hypogonadism should be regarded as an overuse injury and should be treated by a reduction in the amount of training. Although in trained animals even atrophy of ovaries has been found, training-induced menstrual dysfunction is reversible, hormone levels and menstrual cycles returning to normal when exercise is reduced (Galbo, 1986; see also Chapter 34).

Exercise in endocrine diseases

Diabetics produce no insulin (type 1) or an insufficient amount of insulin (type 2). Type 1 diabetics are treated with insulin injections. This means that in contrast to healthy subjects, in whom the plasma insulin concentration is automatically adjusted to any work rate, the diabetic has to carry out work under the influence of a given amount of insulin that they have injected. Therefore, they usually have either too much or too little insulin in their plasma. A high level of insulin may result in hypoglycaemia due to inhibition of hepatic glucose production and enhancement of glucose uptake in muscle. The decrease in blood glucose is accelerated because contractions *per se* enhance muscular glucose uptake. On the other hand, a relatively low level of insulin may result in hyperglycaemia and ketoacidosis due to exaggerated mobilization of glucose and free fatty acids and to inhibited glucose uptake in muscle. These changes are accelerated by the exercise-induced increases in counter-regulatory (insulin antagonistic) hormones. Thus exercise renders the regulation of type 1 diabetes difficult (Galbo, 1988). Moreover, after 10–20 years of diabetes, complications (atherosclerosis, cardiomyopathy, retinopathy, nephropathy and neuropathy) may develop increasing the risk of serious troubles in response to exercise (e.g. myocardial infarction or arrhythmias, blindness and wounds on the feet).

Type 1 diabetics ought to have regular medical examinations to be advised about how much exercise they can tolerate. Furthermore, they should be taught how to imitate the normal response to exercise by reducing their insulin dose immediately before exercise. Nowadays, diabetics can easily measure their own blood glucose concentration and from such measurements they can determine the amount and timing of insulin and food intake to match the exercise to be carried out.

In type 2 diabetics a certain insulin secretory capacity remains, and in principle their insulin secretion changes with needs as it does in normal persons. Accordingly, they do not run the same metabolic risks with exercise as type 1 diabetics (Galbo, 1988). Furthermore, they are more likely to benefit metabolically from exercise, because they are often overweight, and exercise-induced weight reduction will lower their blood glucose profile. However, type 2 diabetics also need regular medical examinations to detect long-term complications, which may necessitate adjustment of their training regimen. Moreover, if physically active type 2 diabetics are treated with drugs which stimulate the secretion and effect of insulin, the medication may have to be adjusted to avoid hypoglycaemia.

Both patients with hyperfunction and those with hypofunction of the thyroid gland (*thyrotoxicosis* and *myxoedema*, respectively) have a decreased work capacity. Compared with healthy subjects, both groups of patients have a lower cardiac ejection fraction during exercise, and the reduced myocardial contractility does not become normal until such patients have been made euthyroid by adequate drug treatment over several months. They should not embark on an exercise programme before this time. Furthermore, patients who have been hypothyroid should have exercise electrocardiography performed before physical training, because they are prone to accelerated atherosclerosis. The same is true for patients who have had hyperfunction of the adrenal cortex (*Cushing's disease*).

Hormone doping

Administration of hormones or their analogues in substituting doses is good medical practice if endogenous hormone secretion is irreversibly impaired (e.g. provision of insulin to diabetics, thyroxine in myxoedema, anabolic steroids to eunuchs, erythropoietin in severe kidney disease). However, because hormones are potent substances which may influence exercise performance, they have also been administered in supraphysiological doses to athletes during training periods and at competitions. For example, gonadotrophins that stimulate male gonadal hormone (testosterone) production (LH and human chorionic gonadotrophin), testosterone and its analogues (anabolic steroids) as well as growth hormone have been used to stimulate muscle growth. Erythropoietin is used to increase blood volume, and amphetamine to mimic the effects of adrenaline. Thyroxine is used to decrease body fat. However, the fact that hormone treatment of healthy subjects may have serious side-effects makes the use of hormones in sports not only ethically, but also medically, unacceptable.

Acknowledgments

The author received financial support from the Danish Medical Research Council (12-9360).

References

Dela, F., Mikines, K.J., Tronier, B. & Galbo, H. (1990) Diminished arginine-stimulated insulin secretion in trained men. *J. Appl. Physiol.* **69**, 261–267.

Dela, F., Mikines, K.J., von Linstow, M. & Galbo, H. (1991) Effect of training on response to a glucose load adjusted for daily carbohydrate intake. *Am. J. Physiol.* **260**, E14–E20.

Galbo, H. (1983) *Hormonal and Metabolic Adaptation to Exercise*. Thieme-Stratton, Stuttgart.

Galbo, H. (1985) The hormonal response to exercise. *Proc. Nutr. Soc.* **44**, 257–266.

Galbo, H. (1986) Autonomic neuroendocrine responses to exercise. *Scand. J. Sports Sci.* **8**, 3–17.

Galbo, H. (1988) Diabetes and exercise. *Scand. J. Sports Sci.* **10**, 89–95.

Kjær, M., Bangsbo, J., Lortie, G. & Galbo, H. (1988) Hormonal response to exercise in humans: influence of hypoxia and physical training. *Am. J. Physiol.* **254**, R197–R203.

Kjær, M., Secher, N.H., Bach, F. & Galbo, H. (1987) Role of motor center activity for hormonal changes and substrate mobilization in humans. *Am. J. Physiol.* **253**, R687–R695.

Kjær, M., Secher, N.H., Bach, F.W., Sheikh, S. & Galbo, H. (1989) Hormonal and metabolic responses to exercise in humans: effect of sensory nervous blockade. *Am. J. Physiol.* **257**, E95–E101.

Mikines, K.J., Sonne, B., Farrell, P.A. & Galbo, H. (1989a) Effect of training on the dose–response relationship for insulin action in men. *J. Appl. Physiol.* **66**, 695–703.

Mikines, K.J., Sonne, B., Tronier, B. & Galbo, H. (1989b) Effects of training and detraining on dose–response relationship between glucose and insulin secretion. *Am. J. Physiol.* **256**, E588–E596.

Stallknecht, B., Kjær, M., Mikines, K.J. *et al.* (1990) Diminished epinephrine response to hypoglycemia despite enlarged adrenal medulla in trained rats. *Am. J. Physiol.* **259**, R998–R1003.

Sutton, J.R., Farrell, P.A. & Harber, V.J. (1990) Hormonal adaptation to physical activity. In Bouchard, C., Shephard, R.J., Stephens, T., Sutton, J.R. McPherson, D.D. (eds) *Exercise, Fitness and Health*, pp. 259–263. Human Kinetics, Champaign, Illinois.

Vissing, J., Iwamoto, G.A. Rybicki, K.J., Galbo, H. & Mitchell, J.H. (1989) Mobilization of glucoregulatory hormones and glucose by hypothalamic locomotor centers. *Am. J. Physiol.* **257**, E722–E728.

Chapter 12

Food Stores and Energy Reserves

ERIC HULTMAN AND PAUL L. GREENHAFF

Introduction

The relationship between diet and exercise has been of scientific interest for over 150 years, but it is during the past 25 years that the most significant findings have been made. In 1842 von Liebig suggested that protein was the main energy substrate during exercise. However, towards the end of the nineteenth century and in the early 1900s a number of authors reported independently that fat and carbohydrate were the principal fuels for muscle contraction. In 1939, a major step forward was achieved when Christensen and Hansen demonstrated that during moderately intense exercise the contribution of fat to total energy production was increased as exercise was continued. Furthermore, if a high carbohydrate/low fat diet was consumed for the days preceding exercise, exercise capacity was nearly doubled. When a low carbohydrate/high fat diet was consumed before exercise, exercise capacity was reduced by 30%.

With the advent of muscle and liver biopsy techniques in the mid-1960s and early 1970s, it became possible to investigate at close hand the relationship between diet and substrate utilization during exercise. The introduction of these techniques had a profound effect upon the growth of exercise biochemistry and physiology as a scientific discipline.

Energy substrates and their availability

The mechanisms of muscle contraction and relaxation are fuelled exclusively by adenosine triphosphate (ATP). The availability of ATP to skeletal muscle is, however, relatively small (approximately 5.5 mmol·kg^{-1}) and therefore it is continually resynthesized from its breakdown products ADP and P$_i$. The energy for ATP resynthesis is derived from both aerobic and anaerobic processes. Aerobic resynthesis is achieved by the oxidation of glucose derived from muscle and liver glycogen stores, of fat, derived from circulating free fatty acids and intramuscular triglyceride stores, and to a lesser extent of protein. Anaerobic resynthesis of ATP occurs when the ATP requirement for a specific task cannot be met solely by aerobic metabolism and is achieved by the degradation of phosphocreatine to creatine and of glucose to lactate. Per glucose unit, the total capacity of anaerobic metabolism to resynthesize ATP is relatively small in comparison with aerobic metabolism (1:13); however, the potential rate of resynthesis is far greater for anaerobic metabolism.

Of the three available energy substrates, fat is the most abundant in humans and is comprised almost exclusively of triglycerides which are stored mainly in adipose tissue. The mobilization of adipose tissue, which is under fine hormonal control, results in the breakdown of triglycerides and the release of free fatty acids from adipose tissue into the circulation. The low concentration ($0.3-2.0$ mmol·l^{-1}) and short half-life (less than 2 min) of circulating free fatty acids demonstrate that they are rapidly utilized as a fuel source. The remainder of the body's fat stores are represented by circulating esterified fat and intramuscular triglycerides, both of which are of minor importance to energy production compared with adipose tissue.

In comparison with fat, the stores of carbohydrate available to humans for ATP resynthesis are minute, amounting to only 2% of the total energy available from fat. Skeletal muscle provides the major store of carbohydrate in humans (about 350 g), in the form of glycogen. However, during a normal working day the muscle glycogen store is not usually utilized. This is in contrast to the other main carbohydrate store, liver glycogen, which may fluctuate from about 150 g to practically zero. The liver provides the only store of carbohydrate that can be mobilized and released, in the form of glucose, for use by other tissues; it can be totally replenished only by dietary carbohydrate intake. Hepatic glucose formation from gluconeogenic substrates (lactate, amino acids and glycerol) taken up from the circulation amounts to about 80 g·day^{-1}.

Like fat, protein is widely available for use as an energy substrate. However, no specific stores of protein for use as energy substrate exist in the body. If energy intake is unrestricted, protein (amino acid) oxidation will provide about 2% of the total energy requirement during exercise, increasing to a maximum of 10% during prolonged exercise when the carbohydrate stores are exhausted. Possible sources of amino acids for energy production include the free amino acid pool in muscle and plasma and those released during normal protein catabolism. There is no evidence to suggest that contractile protein is utilized for energy production during exercise.

Availability and utilization of energy substrates during exercise

The relative contribution of carbohydrate, fat and protein to energy production during exercise is dependent on a number of factors.

Exercise intensity

At exercise intensities of 50% $\dot{V}o_{2\,max}$ and below, the oxidation of fat is the principal source of energy production in humans. The mobilization of free fatty acids from adipose tissue is under fine hormonal control, and during prolonged exercise at moderate intensities the hormonal milieu stimulates lipolysis. The increase in availability of free fatty acids is matched by a parallel increase in their uptake and oxidation in the muscle.

At work rates above 60% $\dot{V}o_{2\,max}$ there is an almost linear relationship between exercise intensity and the rate of muscle glycogen utilization (Fig. 12.1). As the work rate approaches 100% $\dot{V}o_{2\,max}$ and above, muscle glycogen utilization and phosphocreatine degradation become primarily responsible for energy pro-

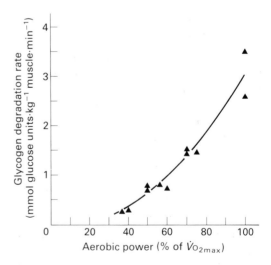

Fig. 12.1 Rate of muscle glycogen degradation during cycle exercise performed at different work intensities. From Hultman (1971).

duction. Glycogen utilization rates have been shown to approach 35 mmol·kg^{-1}·min^{-1} during maximal sprint exercise. At work rates ranging from 50–80% $\dot{V}o_{2\,max}$, complete oxidation is the principal fate of the glycogen utilized. However, at higher exercise intensities anaerobic metabolism accounts for the majority of the glycogen degradation. In situations where muscle glycogen is the main energy substrate utilized, with the exception of very high intensity exercise, its availability will be the principal determinant of exercise capacity. It is now known that low muscle glycogen availability will directly impair muscle ATP resynthesis during prolonged moderately intense exercise. For exercise to be continued beyond the point of muscle glycogen depletion, the exercise intensity must be lowered, thereby reducing the energy demand and enabling free fatty acids and blood glucose to provide a greater proportion of the energy requirement.

As already stated, protein utilization makes only a small contribution to total energy production during exercise. However, it has been demonstrated that there is a positive relationship between the rate of protein oxidation and exercise intensity.

Exercise duration

In the late 1930s it was shown for the first time that during low to moderate intensity exercise the contribution of fat to energy production increased with time (Christensen & Hansen, 1939). This is due to an alteration in the availability of both fat and carbohydrate during prolonged exercise. For example, during the first 40 min of prolonged exercise at 40% $\dot{V}o_{2\,max}$, about 35% of the total energy production is derived from oxidation of free fatty acids; towards the end of exercise, when the availability of carbohydrate is limited, the figure increases to about 60%. The relationship between the availability of muscle carbohydrate and exercise duration was investigated in the late 1960s. In one experiment 10 subjects per-

formed intermittent cycle exercise to exhaustion at a work rate equivalent to 80% $\dot{V}o_{2\,max}$. The analysis of muscle biopsy samples obtained during the study revealed a progressive decline in muscle glycogen content with time (Fig. 12.2). The point of exhaustion coincided with the point of muscle glycogen depletion. Table 12.1 shows that, in comparison with fat, the body's store of carbohydrate is very limited. If energy production was dependent upon the carbohydrate store alone, the élite marathon runner would be exhausted after approximately 90 min of exercise. As the world record for the marathon is close to 130 min this clearly exemplifies the importance of the integration of carbohydrate and lipid metabolism during exercise.

During prolonged exercise glucose output from the liver provides a significant contribution to total energy production and eventually results in the depletion of hepatic glycogen

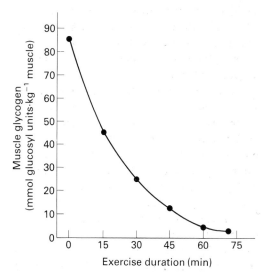

Fig. 12.2 Decline in glycogen content of the quadriceps femoris muscle during cycle exercise at a work rate equivalent to 80% $\dot{V}o_{2\,max}$. Each point represents the mean value for 10 subjects. On all occasions exercise was continued to the point of exhaustion which coincided with the point of glycogen depletion. From Bergström & Hultman (1967).

Table 12.1 Availability of fat and carbohydrate in humans. From Newsholme & Leech (1983).

Tissue fuel store	Approximate total fuel reserve		Estimated time for which a single substrate alone could provide energy if completely oxidized	
	g	kJ	Days of walking[†]	Minutes of marathon running[‡]
Triglyceride (adipose tissue)	9000	337 000	10.8	4018
Liver glycogen	90	1 500	0.05	18
Muscle glycogen	350	6 000	0.20	71
Blood and extracellular glucose	30	320	0.01	4

[*] Assumes average person has a bodymass of 65 kg of which 9 kg is triglyceride.
[†] Assumes average person (65 kg) walking at 6.4 km·h^{-1} expends 31 248 kJ·day^{-1}.
[‡] Assumes energy expenditure of 85 kJ·min^{-1}.

stores. At a work rate of 45% $\dot{V}o_{2\,max}$ hepatic glucose release can provide almost 25% of the total energy requirement, but this declines to about 10% at an intensity of 70% $\dot{V}o_{2\,max}$. The level of circulating glucose is finely regulated during exercise and under normal circumstances hepatic output matches tissue demand. However, towards the end of prolonged exercise, when the availability of muscle glycogen is low and the dependence upon blood glucose for energy production is increased, depletion of hepatic glycogen stores may lead to the development of hypoglycaemia, resulting in dysfunction of the central nervous system and/or muscle fatigue.

Diet

Due to the abundance of fat stores and the lack of capacity to store protein in humans, the immediate purpose of food intake is to maintain the body's carbohydrate stores.

Diet alone has little influence upon normal muscle glycogen levels (Fig. 12.3). However, if the muscle glycogen stores are depleted by exercise, the composition of subsequent dietary intake will have a marked effect upon muscle glycogen availability. A carbohydrate-free diet

or starvation following muscle glycogen depletion results in a slow rate of glycogen resynthesis; after 7 days levels are still lower than normal (Fig. 12.4). Conversely, a carbohydrate-rich diet will result in rapid muscle glycogen resynthesis, achieving levels far in excess of

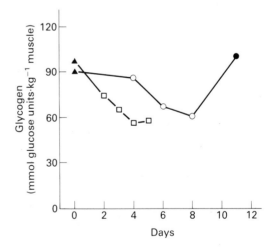

Fig. 12.3 Glycogen content of the quadriceps femoris muscle after a normal diet (▲), during 5 days of fasting (□), during 8 days of low dietary carbohydrate intake (○), and following 3 days of high dietary carbohydrate intake (●). From Hultman & Bergström (1967).

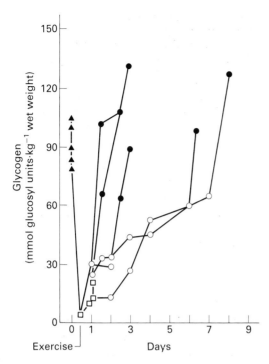

Fig. 12.4 Muscle glycogen content of the quadriceps femoris muscle before and after prolonged exercise and dietary manipulation. Measurements were made before exercise following the mixed diet (▲) and during 1 day of fasting (□), during 6 days of low carbohydrate intake (○), and during 2 days of high carbohydrate intake (●) following exercise. From Hultman & Bergström (1967).

those normally found at rest (Fig. 12.5). Furthermore, if the high carbohydrate diet is preceded by 3 days of low carbohydrate intake, muscle glycogen levels may be elevated even further. As Fig. 12.5 demonstrates, this 'supercompensation phenomenon' is restricted to the exercised muscles and although the majority of the resynthesis takes place in the first 24 h of high carbohydrate intake, it is not complete until after 3–4 days.

As already stated, liver glycogen stores are known to fluctuate widely, even at rest. Liver biopsy samples taken in the postprandial state show a continuous decrease in glycogen content at a rate of 0.3 mmol glucose units·min^{-1}·kg^{-1} liver. When food restriction is maintained, depletion of hepatic stores will occur within 24 h. Furthermore, continued starvation or a carbohydrate-free diet produces no change in liver glycogen levels, despite an increased delivery of gluconeogenic substrates to the liver. Blood glucose levels, however, are maintained. When a high carbohydrate diet is consumed, a supercompensation will occur as in muscle, and the response will be complete within 24 h (Fig. 12.6).

It is clear that under normal dietary conditions the availability of carbohydrate stores influences the pattern of substrate utilization during exercise. As muscle carbohydrate availability is reduced, energy production becomes increasingly dependent upon the oxidation of fat and to a lesser extent protein. If the energy demand cannot be met by these two substrates, the exercise intensity must be reduced for exercise to continue. However, even when the availability of muscle glycogen is not reduced, consumption of a high fat diet before exercise will reduce carbohydrate utilization and increase fat oxidation, even at exercise intensities where muscle glycogen is the principal energy substrate used. The change in the relative contribution of fat and carbohydrate to energy production is achieved by an increased utilization of free fatty acids and a corresponding decrease in muscle glycogen degradation. Conversely, following muscle glycogen supercompensation by diet and exercise manipulation, there is an increase in the rate of glycogen degradation and a concomitant decrease in fat oxidation. The mechanism(s) by which dietary manipulation influences the integration of carbohydrate and fat metabolism is not clearly understood, but is most likely related to dietary-induced hormonal changes.

Surprisingly, protein oxidation is also influenced by substrate availability. Both glucose infusion and a high muscle glycogen content have been shown to reduce leucine oxidation during exercise. Furthermore, an increase in the availability of free fatty acids is known to have the opposite effect.

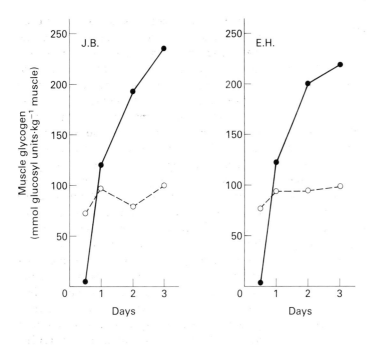

Fig. 12.5 Glycogen content of the quadriceps femoris muscle from previously inactive (○) and previously active (●) muscle of two subjects. Biopsies were obtained immediately after one-legged cycle exercise and during the subsequent 3 days of high dietary carbohydrate intake. From Bergström & Hultman (1966).

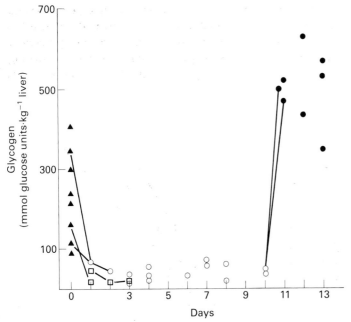

Fig. 12.6 Glycogen content of liver biopsy samples obtained after a mixed diet (▲), during 3 days of fasting (□), during 10 days of low dietary carbohydrate intake (○), and during 3 days of high dietary carbohydrate intake (●). From Nilsson & Hultman (1973).

Training status

The effects of muscle fibre composition and training frequency and intensity are of great importance to the availability of energy sub-strate and its utilization during exercise. However, to discuss the physiological effects of training upon energy metabolism is beyond the scope of this chapter and for this reason the topic will receive no further consideration.

Influence of diet on exercise performance

Because fat oxidation provides the majority of the energy requirement during low intensity exercise, the influence of diet upon the performance of prolonged activity has received relatively little attention. On a weight-for-weight basis, it is known that fat is approximately five times more efficient than carbohydrate as a storage fuel. However, in order to avoid hypoglycaemia during this type of exercise liver glucose output must be maintained constant. For these reasons, dietary intake has been of interest to military personnel involved in long-term activity. In one particular study, five subjects walked about 40 km·day^{-1} for 4 days, during which time the carbohydrate intake constituted only about 3% of their total energy intake. Although the utilization of fat was increased during the exercise, at no point was hypoglycaemia reported and all subjects completed the exercise task. It would appear that, as under resting conditions, liver gluconeogenesis can match the carbohydrate demands of this type of exercise.

At work rates above 60% $\dot{V}_{O_2\,max}$, muscle glycogen is the primary energy substrate utilized. When muscle glycogen levels are altered by using a mixture of dietary and exercise manipulation, a very close relationship is found between exercise capacity and the pre-exercise muscle glycogen content (Fig. 12.7). It is known that during competitive endurance racing, a decrease in running speed coincides with a fall in muscle glycogen below approximately 17 mmol·kg^{-1} wet weight. Therefore, if prerace muscle glycogen levels are elevated above normal a decrease in running speed can be avoided. Conversely, should dietary carbohydrate intake be insufficient to maintain muscle glycogen levels during training, subsequent race performance is likely to be impaired. For these reasons, carbohydrate loading has become popular among individuals competing in endurance-type events. It has been suggested that exercise capacity may be further enhanced if, in addition to glycogen stores, the availability of fat is increased immediately before exercise, thereby promoting oxidation of free fatty acids during exercise and 'sparing' muscle glycogen. It is advisable to practise any

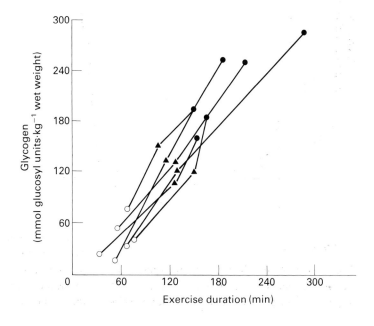

Fig. 12.7 Relationship between the pre-exercise glycogen content of the quadriceps femoris muscle and cycle exercise time to exhaustion at a power equivalent to 75% $\dot{V}_{O_2\,max}$. Each subject exercised to exhaustion on three occasions over 10 days: first, after 3 days of mixed dietary intake (▲); again after 3 days of low dietary carbohydrate intake (○); and finally after 3 days of high dietary carbohydrate intake (●). From Bergström *et al.* (1967).

regimen of dietary manipulation in training before applying it to competition. Extreme manipulation of dietary intake may lead to gastrointestinal upsets. In particular, the increase in muscle water content associated with muscle glycogen loading (300 ml water for each 100 g glycogen stored) and the diuretic effect of pre-exercise caffeine ingestion, in an attempt to stimulate lipolysis, may cause some discomfort.

The influence of dietary manipulation upon the performance of very high intensity exercise has not been extensively studied and is still open to some debate. It is clear that during short-term maximal exercise (close to 100% $\dot{V}o_{2\,max}$) fatigue is closely related to the onset of lactic acidosis and the disruption of high energy phosphate metabolism. However, these mechanisms may not totally explain the development of fatigue. It is generally considered that at high work rates glycogen availability will not limit performance because levels are still high at the point of fatigue. However, a number of studies have reported a positive correlation between muscle glycogen availability and high intensity exercise performance. Clearly more research is required. Most studies to date have involved the analysis of whole muscle glycogen levels. Because type II muscle fibres are primarily used during this type of exercise, the data obtained from whole muscle analysis may be misleading. Histochemical analysis of single muscle fibres has been performed after exercise, but the results are at best only semiquantitative. Despite this, it has been suggested that selective depletion of glycogen in type II muscle fibres may be responsible for fatigue at high exercise intensities.

Carbohydrate intake immediately before and during exercise

The ingestion of carbohydrate 1.5−2 h before exercise will ensure that liver glycogen levels are 'optimal'. Until recently, however, it had been considered that the ingestion of carbohydrate before exercise might be detrimental to exercise performance. The beneficial effect of replenishing liver glycogen stores may be offset by pre-exercise carbohydrate ingestion which increases the rate of carbohydrate utilization and decreases release of free fatty acids from adipose tissue during exercise due to increased blood levels of insulin.

It is generally accepted that the ingestion of carbohydrate during exercise will delay the development of fatigue. Glucose ingestion maintains carbohydrate oxidation towards the end of exercise, when the availability of muscle and liver glycogen is low and glucose uptake by muscle is increased. Without glucose ingestion, carbohydrate stores will become totally depleted, plasma glucose levels will fall and, as a consequence, both central nervous system and muscle metabolism will be disrupted. Fluid balance as well as carbohydrate availability influence exercise capacity during highly prolonged activity, and recent evidence has suggested that weak glucose/electrolyte solutions will be most beneficial to exercise performance by promoting both intestinal carbohydrate and fluid absorption. (See Chapter 30.)

Conclusion

Muscle ATP resynthesis is primarily dependent upon the utilization of the body's fat and carbohydrate stores. Due to the limited availability of the latter it is essential that carbohydrate and fat metabolism are integrated during exercise.

The near linear relationship between exercise intensity and carbohydrate utilization makes work rate an important determinant of exercise capacity. At the point of glycogen depletion, fatigue will occur unless the exercise intensity is reduced, enabling fat oxidation to provide a greater proportion of the energy requirement.

During low to moderately intense exercise (30−85% $\dot{V}o_{2\,max}$) the contribution of fat to energy production increases with time, thereby reducing dependence on the decreasing carbohydrate stores. Ultimately, however, muscle and liver glycogen depletion will occur, resulting in the development of fatigue.

A mixture of diet and exercise manipulation can have a marked effect upon both the availability and utilization of carbohydrate and fat during exercise. It has been shown repeatedly that a dietary-induced elevation of pre-exercise muscle and liver glycogen stores will increase exercise capacity during prolonged exercise (and possibly also during high intensity exercise) by delaying the onset of muscle glycogen depletion. Supercompensation of muscle and liver glycogen stores will require 3 days and 1 day of high carbohydrate intake, respectively. If the pre-exercise availability of free fatty acids is increased, the exercise capacity may be further enhanced during prolonged exercise because the contribution of carbohydrate to energy production is reduced.

It is not clear whether the ingestion of carbohydrate shortly before exercise will enhance subsequent exercise performance. However, it is generally accepted that carbohydrate intake during prolonged exercise will offset the development of fatigue. It is suggested that carbohydrate ingestion should take place towards the end of exercise when the body's stores of carbohydrate are close to depletion, thereby facilitating fat utilization during the early stages of exercise. Recent evidence suggests that consumption of weak glucose/electrolyte solutions will ensure optimal work performance by promoting both carbohydrate and fluid absorption.

References

Bergström, J., Hermansen, L., Hultman, E. & Saltin, B. (1967) Diet, muscle glycogen and physical performance. *Acta Physiol. Scand.* **71**, 140−150.

Bergström, J. & Hultman, E. (1966) Muscle glycogen synthesis after exercise: an enhancing factor localized to the muscle cells in man. *Nature* **210**, 309−310.

Bergström, J. & Hultman, E. (1967) A study of the glycogen metabolism during exercise in man. *Scand. J. Clin. Lab. Invest.* **19**, 218−228.

Christensen, E.H. & Hansen, O. (1939) Arbeitsfähigkeit und Ernährung. *Skand. Arch. Physiol.* **81**, 160−171.

Hultman, E. (1971) Muscle glycogen store and prolonged exercise. In: Shephard, R.J. (ed.) *Frontiers of Fitness*, pp. 30−42. C.C. Thomas, Springfield, Illinois.

Hultman, E. & Bergström, J. (1967) Muscle glycogen synthesis in relation to diet studied in normal subjects. *Acta Med. Scand.* **182**, 109−117.

Liebig, J. von (1842) *Animal Chemistry or Organic Chemistry in its Application to Physiology and Pathology*. Taylor & Walton, London.

Newsholme, E.A. & Leech, A.R. (1983) *Biochemistry for the Medical Sciences*. John Wiley, Chichester.

Nilsson, L. H:son, & Hultman, E. (1973) Liver glycogen in man − the effect of total starvation or a carbohydrate-poor diet followed by carbohydrate refeeding. *Scand. J. Clin. Lab. Invest.* **32**, 325−330.

Selected reading

Fox, E.L. (1983) *Sports Physiology*. CBS Publishing, New York.

Hultman, E. (1989) Nutritional effects on work performance. *Am. J. Clin. Nutr.* **49**, 949−957.

Hultman, E. & Harris, R.C. (1988) Carbohydrate metabolism. In: Poortmans, J.R. (ed.) *Medicine and Sports Science. Principles of Exercise Biochemistry*, Vol. 27, pp. 78−119. Karger, Basel.

Hultman, E. & Spriet, L.L. (1988) Dietary intake prior to and during exercise. In: Horton, E.S. & Terjung, R.L. (eds) *Exercise, Nutrition and Energy Metabolism*, pp. 132−149. Macmillan, New York.

Part 2b

Psychological Aspects of Endurance Performance

Chapter 13

Psychological Aspects of Endurance Performance

PATRICK J. O'CONNOR

Introduction

One of the most gruelling tests of human athletic endurance is the Tour de France bicycling race. In 1989, for example, the event covered a total of 3252 km (2025 miles) in 23 days including climbs through both the Pyrenees and the Alps. Greg LeMond won the 1989 Tour, finishing just 8 s ahead of two-time winner Laurent Fignon. LeMond's achievement was highlighted by his extraordinary performance on the last day of the race. The final stage, covering 24.5 km (15.2 miles), was considered to be too short by professional cycling standards for LeMond to make up the 50 s by which he trailed the leader Fignon. Despite the improbability of the task, LeMond won by cycling at an average speed of $54.6 \, km \cdot h^{-1}$ (34 m.p.h.), the fastest average speed ever recorded during a time trial in the 76-year history of the Tour de France.

Individuals such as Greg LeMond possess unique physical characteristics which allow them to excel as endurance athletes. However, many of the physiological characteristics known to be important contributors to above-average endurance performance (for example, maximal oxygen intake) have also been shown to be relatively homogeneous within groups of élite endurance athletes. Thus, attempts at predicting endurance performance in élite athletes solely on the basis of physiological variables have been generally unsuccessful (Shephard, 1980). As a consequence, it is often suggested that psychological factors play an important role in the achievement of outstanding endurance performance.

Athletes, coaches, journalists and scientists frequently attribute peak, as well as poor, performances to psychological variables such as concentration or motivation. For example, consider the following quotations concerning Greg LeMond's performance in the 1989 Tour de France (Swift, 1989):

> He had already decided he didn't want aides in his support vehicle to tell him his splits or how he was faring in relation to Fignon. That would only detract from his concentration (p. 71),

and LeMond himself recalled:

> I kept thinking about how I almost quit two months ago, and what a good thing it was that I never give up early (p. 72).

Anecdotal reports such as these illustrate and propagate the belief that endurance performance can be greatly influenced by psychological factors. There is, however, a paucity of scientific evidence documenting a beneficial impact of psychological interventions on the physical performance of athletes.

The purpose of this chapter is to summarize those aspects of the research literature regarding psychological aspects of athletic performance. More specifically, the focus will be on investigations that have examined athletes who compete in endurance sports such as bicycling, distance running, rowing and swimming. Although this chapter concentrates on variables that are typically classified as psychological in nature, most of these variables are more accurately described as psychobiological. In other words, an assumption is being made that the mind and body are inseparable. This position not only has longstanding philosophical and theoretical support, but it also possesses empirical support in the exercise sciences. For example, in investigations where both psychological and biological measurements have been made in athletes for the purpose of predicting endurance performance, a psychobiological approach has been shown to be more efficacious than predictions based on either psychological or biological assessments alone (Morgan, 1973).

Psychological characteristics of endurance athletes

A number of reports have described psychological characteristics of different groups of endurance athletes using standardized psychometric instruments. The resultant psychological profiles have been compared with profiles of athletes who are not engaged in endurance sports as well as to normative data from the population at large. The main findings of this research are summarized below.

Psychometric traits

A number of traits, or enduring features of personality, such as extroversion and neuroticism, have been evaluated in endurance athletes. As a group, endurance athletes have repeatedly been shown to fall within the normal range on trait personality measures (Morgan, 1980; Morgan et al., 1988). At the same time, there is a tendency for samples of athletes in general to be characterized by extroversion and emotional stability (i.e. the opposite of neuroticism) in comparison with published norms. In other words, there appears to be a consistent pattern of personality traits in endurance, as well as in other athletes, but it is not extreme in relation to the population norms.

Mood states

Endurance athletes have consistently been found to possess healthier mood state profiles when compared with the general population (Morgan, 1985). Using a standard measure of mood called the 'profile of mood states', groups of élite distance runners, rowers, wrestlers and cyclists have repeatedly been shown to be characterized by lower levels of tension, depression, anger, fatigue and confusion, as well as by greater vigour when compared with population norms. This mood profile has been referred to as the 'iceberg' profile (Morgan, 1985), and it is depicted in Fig. 13.1.

Although groups of endurance athletes are typically characterized by a more positive mood state in comparison with the general population, this does not mean that individual athletes are immune from affective disturbances. The prevalence of clinical anxiety and depressive disorders in groups of endurance athletes has been found to be approximately 10% (Morgan et al., 1987a; 1987b), and this is comparable with the prevalence rate for these disorders in the general population.

Endurance athletes are required to cope not only with the stressors of daily living but also with the rigours of physical training, and there is clear evidence that the training process itself can have adverse psychological consequences. For example, in response to a 1–3-week bout of training involving repeated high intensity workouts of long duration (a process known as overtraining), female and male endurance athletes have been found to exhibit significant mood disturbances (Morgan et al., 1987a; O'Connor et al., 1989). Anger, anxiety and depression levels, for example, are increased during periods of overtraining. During subsequent periods of light or moderate training mood states return toward the baseline level, which is typically lower (i.e. healthier) than that observed for non-athletes. A comprehensive overview of the relationship between changes in training and alterations in mood has been published previously (Morgan et al.,

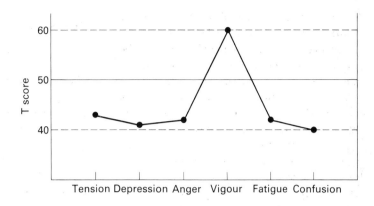

Fig. 13.1 The 'iceberg' profile. From Morgan *et al.* (1987).

1987a). The practical importance of this relationship is that the monitoring of mood states may prove to be a useful way, especially when accompanied by physiological monitoring, to titrate training loads in order to prevent decrements in endurance performance ('staleness') which can occur as a result of overtraining.

A mental health model of performance

Much of the data concerning the psychological characteristics of endurance athletes can be summarized by a model concerning the relationship between mental health and athletic performance which has been proposed by Morgan (1985). The model stipulates that success in sport is inversely correlated with psychopathology. A comprehensive summary of the empirical basis for the model is beyond the scope of this chapter, but is available elsewhere (Morgan, 1985). The model posits that athletes with positive mental health (operationalized using a variety of state and trait measures) will be able to achieve better performances than athletes with poor mental health such as those who are pathologically neurotic or who are suffering from clinically significant depression.

Figure 13.2 presents a modified version of the mental health model which has been adapted to describe only the relationship between psychopathology and endurance performance. In examining Fig. 13.2, it is important

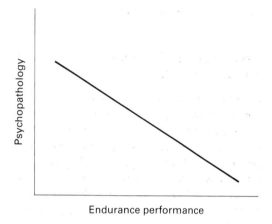

Fig. 13.2 Depiction of a hypothesized relationship between psychopathology and endurance performance. From Morgan (1985).

to realize that the *x*- and *y*-axes do *not* represent a single, specific measure of either psychopathology or endurance performance. Instead, a hypothesized relationship is depicted, based on the results of a number of studies in which both endurance performance and psychometric variables have been assessed simultaneously.

The effectiveness of the mental health model of athletic performance has been demonstrated in a number of studies. Candidates for the 1974 US heavyweight rowing team, for example, completed a battery of psychometric instruments, and the data were then used to predict which athletes would or would not make the team (Morgan, 1985). Those with positive mental health profiles were predicted to make the team, and those possessing less positive mental health were predicted not to make the team. The predictions were made in a blind fashion, i.e. the investigators were not involved in the decision to keep or cut the athletes. Based on this psychological model alone, correct predictions were made in 72% (41/57) of cases.

A more recent study conducted with élite US male distance runners (Morgan *et al.*, 1988) provides further support for the efficacy of the mental health model as a means of predicting endurance performance. It was found that state and trait measures accounted for a statistically significant percentage of the variance (45%; $p < 0.05$) in 10 000 m run performance. It is notable that a psychological model accounted for a large percentage of the variance in endurance performance, but it is emphasized that the mental health model is conservative; when psychological variables are combined with biological variables an even better prediction of endurance performance may be achieved.

Precompetition states and endurance performance

Psychologists have directed a substantial amount of attention to explaining the relationship between anxiety (or arousal) and performance (Hackfort & Spielberger, 1989). Most of this research has been conducted using novel motor tasks in laboratory settings, with the implied assumption that these findings can be generalized to the performance of well learned, large muscle tasks of the type typically performed by endurance athletes. Only a few investigations have actually assessed arousal states in endurance performers. In contrast to investigations examining the learning of motor skills, research involving athletes as test subjects has not compellingly demonstrated either a linear or curvilinear relationship between precompetition arousal and endurance performance.

Elite female and male distance runners have reported experiencing elevated arousal levels before competition (Morgan *et al.*, 1987b; 1988). In these same studies, however, it was also found that the mean precompetition arousal level was similar before personal best, personal worst and usual performance conditions. Based on these data, and in contrast with popular beliefs, it appears that *groups* of élite distance runners are neither uniformly relaxed nor aroused before a personal best performance. These findings suggest that a relationship between precompetition anxiety and endurance performance, if one exists at all, may be different for each *individual*.

The idea that anxiety is related to athletic performance on an individual but not a group level was first advanced by the Soviet researcher, Yuri Hanin (Hanin, 1986). Based on extensive testing of Soviet athletes, Hanin contended that each individual athlete had a narrow range of anxiety within which superior performances were generally achieved. This range was called the 'zone of optimal function'. However, the *absolute* precompetition anxiety level for any individual might be either low, moderate or high, even within a given event. Hanin's idea has recently been confirmed in part by workers in the US who have used endurance athletes as test subjects (Raglin *et al.*, 1990). While this individualized approach to preperformance anxiety is perhaps the most significant conceptual advance in this area in years, experiments demonstrating a causal link between anxiety and endurance performance within individuals have yet to be conducted.

Psychological concomitants of endurance performance

The characteristics of endurance athletes which have been described up to this point represent psychological factors observed in athletes before competition. Psychological functioning *during* exercise can also be of crucial importance in achieving above-average endurance performance. For instance, it makes intuitive sense that an individual who has a high capability for tolerating pain during exercise should have an advantage, in terms of athletic endurance performance, over individuals with a low tolerance for pain. Pain tolerance, cognitions and the perception of effort can all be classified as salient psychological concomitants of endurance exercise. Because the topic of perceived exertion is covered separately in Chapter 31 the present section will focus on pain tolerance and cognitive strategies.

At the outset it should be recognized that pain tolerance and cognitive strategies are not entirely separate entities. This can be illustrated by the following quotation from Greg LeMond, who compares the pain he experienced after being shot in a near fatal hunting accident to the pain he feels while cycling. The implication is that the cognitive strategy may increase his pain tolerance during exercise (Swift, 1989):

> You think you are used to pain on your bike, but that's not pain. The suffering you felt on your bike is nothing compared to real pain. I think of that sometimes when I ride (p. 58).

Pain tolerance

There is a widespread belief that willingness to tolerate pain is essential to outstanding endurance performance. Perhaps because this idea seems so obvious, relatively few experimental investigations have studied pain tolerance in samples of athletes. Ryan and his colleagues (Ryan & Kovacic, 1966; Ryan & Foster, 1967) conducted pioneering work in this area by demonstrating that contact and endurance athletes possessed significantly greater pain tolerance than non-athletes or athletes participating in non-contact sports such as tennis.

More recently, the observations made by Ryan's group have been replicated and extended by Scott and Gijsbers (1981), who found that pain tolerance was greater in national class swimmers ($n = 30$) than in less competitive, club swimmers ($n = 30$) or in non-competitive recreational athletes ($n = 30$). In this study, the pain stimulus involved inflating a standard sphygmomanometer to 100 mmHg above the subject's systolic blood pressure and then ischaemia was produced by the individuals opening and closing their hands at a rate of once per second. Differences in pain tolerance were observed among the three groups, despite finding no differences in pain threshold (i.e. the latency from the initiation of the pain stimulus to the first report of it being perceived as painful). In addition, the national class swimmers were studied longitudinally and it was demonstrated that pain tolerance increased significantly during heavy training and returned to baseline after the training had returned to a relatively low level. Scott and Gijsbers (1981) concluded: 'The origins of the enhanced pain tolerances of the competitive swimmers would seem to lie in their systematic exposure to brief periods of intense pain' (p. 91).

Pain variables are also influenced *during* acute bouts of exercise. Kemppainen et al. (1985) found that both sensitivity to pain and pain threshold were increased during cycle ergometry, and these dependent variables were related to exercise intensity in a dose-dependent fashion. The mechanisms by which pain might be modulated during exercise are at this point not clear. It has been reported, based on a double-blind, placebo-controlled investigation (Pauley et al., 1989), that the injection of the opiate antagonist naloxone before a bout of maximal running increased the perception of muscle pain during exercise. These data suggest that increases in endogenous opiates during exercise may act to reduce the perception of pain. Along a different line of research, however, a number of investigators (for example, Morgan & Horstman, 1978) have reported that selected psychological states and traits, such as anxiety and extroversion, are significantly related to the perception of pain. This last observation emphasizes that alterations in the perception of pain as a consequence of either acute or chronic exercise are probably multifactorial. Thus, it is likely that modulations in pain represent a complex psychobiological process involving both opioid and non-opioid pathways (Watkins & Mayer, 1982).

Cognitive strategies

Endurance athletes have reported using a number of different cognitive strategies in order to minimize pain and thereby attempt to maximize performance. Non-élite distance runners use elaborate thought patterns during marathon races; for instance, one runner relived his entire academic career from grade school through an advanced degree during marathons (Morgan, 1978). This type of cognitive strategy has been classified as 'dissociation', because the athlete's thoughts become separated from the activity being performed. A dissociative cognitive strategy has also been demonstrated as empirically effective in improving endurance performance in normal adult males (Morgan et al., 1983).

Elite female and male distance runners, however, have reported that during both competitive performances and high intensity training sessions they predominantly use a cognitive strategy which has been termed 'association' (Morgan & Pollock, 1977; Morgan et al., 1987b; 1988). As a group, these athletes pay close attention to what they are doing when working hard, and dissociate at lower exercise intensities. By carefully monitoring their mechanics, breathing, sensations of fatigue and pain levels during races, élite endurance athletes are presumably able to attain the fastest possible pace that can be achieved over an extended period of time. Thus, the élite and the non-élite distance runner appear to use different cognitive strategies in an attempt to reach the same end of maximizing endurance performance.

This does not imply that non-élite athletes can become élite athletes by changing their cognitions during exercise. It is entirely possible that élite athletes associate because they can 'afford' to pay attention to bodily signals of distress. Put another way, it may be that élite athletes elect to associate during heavy exercise because they possess unique physiological characteristics enabling them to do so. Individuals who do not have the physiological characteristics of an élite endurance athlete may not have the 'luxury' of using an associative cognitive strategy during intense exercise. Additionally, élite endurance athletes do not rely solely on association. For example, 22% of élite female distance runners also use dissociation during competition (Morgan et al., 1987a). This type of flexible approach might involve association during the first three quarters of a race followed by dissociation in order to block out intense pain in the later portion of the competition. Nevertheless, there is a need for further research examining the idea of using cognitive strategies to optimize endurance performance.

Summary

The study of human endurance has frequently focused on the importance of selected physiological variables in achieving high-level athletic performance, while the unexplained variance in performance has often been attributed to unmeasured 'psychological factors'. Increasingly, however, attention is being given to measuring aspects of endurance performance which can be labelled as psychological in nature. This chapter has summarized briefly what is currently known about the psychology of endurance performance, and at the same time has emphasized that endurance performance is neither psychological nor biological, but rather, psychobiological. Indeed, it is predicted that only when the links between the mind and body are elucidated will a complete understanding of endurance performance be obtained.

References

Hackfort, D. & Spielberger, C.D. (1989) *Anxiety in Sports: An International Perspective*. Hemisphere, Washington D.C..

Hanin, Y.L. (1986) State—trait anxiety research on sports in the USSR. In: Spielberger, C.D. & Diaz-Guerrero, R. (eds) *Cross-Cultural Anxiety*, pp. 45—64. Hemisphere, Washington D.C..

Kemppainen, P., Pertovaara, A., Huopaniemi, T., Johansson, G. & Karonen, S.L. (1985) Modification of dental pain and cutaneous thermal sensitivity by physical exercise in man. *Brain Res.* **360**, 33–40.

Morgan, W.P. (1973) Efficacy of psychobiologic inquiry in the exercise and sport sciences. *Quest* **20**, 39–47.

Morgan, W.P. (1978) Mind of the marathoner. *Psychol. Today* **11**, 38–49.

Morgan, W.P. (1980) The trait psychology controversy. *Res. Q. Exerc. Sport* **50**, 385–427.

Morgan, W.P. (1985) Selected psychological factors limiting performance: a mental health model. In: Clarke, D.H. & Eckert, H.M. (eds) *Limits of Human Performance*, pp. 70–80. Human Kinetics, Champaign, Illinois.

Morgan, W.P., Brown, D.R., Raglin, J.S., O'Connor, P.J. & Ellickson, K.A. (1987a) Psychological monitoring of overtraining and staleness. *Br. J. Sports Med.* **21**, 107–114.

Morgan, W.P. & Horstman, D.H. (1978) Psychometric correlates of pain perception. *Percept. Mot. Skills* **47**, 27–39.

Morgan, W.P., Horstman, D.H., Cymerman, A. & Stokes, J. (1983) Facilitation of physical performance by means of a cognitive strategy. *Cognit. Ther. Res.* **7**, 251–264.

Morgan, W.P., O'Connor, P.J., Ellickson, K.A. & Bradley, P.W. (1988) Personality structure, mood states, and performance in elite male distance runners. *Int. J. Sport Psychol.* **19**, 247–263.

Morgan, W.P., O'Connor, P.J., Sparling, P.B. & Pate, R.R. (1987b) Psychological characterization of the elite female distance runner. *Int. J. Sports Med.* **8** (Suppl. 2), 124–131.

Morgan, W.P. & Pollock, M.L. (1977) Psychological characterization of the elite distance runner. *Ann. N. Y. Acad. Sci.* **301**, 383–403.

O'Connor, P.J., Morgan, W.P., Raglin, J.S., Barksdale, C.M. & Kalin, N.H. (1989) Mood state and salivary cortisol levels following overtraining in female swimmers. *Psychoneuroendocrinology* **14**, 303–310.

Pauley, P.F., Thorholl, J.F., Nielsen, U. *et al.* (1989) Opioid involvement in the perception of pain due to endurance exercise in trained man. *Jpn. J. Physiol.* **39**, 67–74.

Raglin, J.S., Morgan, W.P. & Wise, K.J. (1990) Precompetition anxiety and performance in female high school swimmers: a test of optimal function theory. *Int. J. Sports Med.* **11**, 171–175.

Ryan, E.D. & Foster, R. (1967). Athletic participation and perceptual augmentation and reduction. *J. Pers. Soc. Psychol.* **6**, 472–476.

Ryan, E.D. & Kovacic, C.R. (1966) Pain tolerance and athletic participation. *Percept. Mot. Skills* **22**, 383–390.

Scott, V. & Gijsbers, K. (1981) Pain perception in competitive swimmers. *Br. Med. J.* **283**, 91–93.

Shephard, R.J. (1980) What can the applied physiologist predict from his data? *J. Sports Med.* **20**, 297–308.

Swift, E.M. (1989) LeGrand LeMond. *Sports Illustrated* **71**, 54–72.

Watkins, L.R. & Mayer, D.J. (1982) Organization of endogenous opiate and nonopiate pain control systems. *Science* **216**, 1185–1192.

Part 2c

Genetic Determinants of Endurance Performance

Chapter 14

Genetic Determinants of Endurance Performance

CLAUDE BOUCHARD

Introduction

Genes play a critical role in human motor performance, be it a very simple motor task accomplished in daily life or a complex sport skill executed by an élite performer. This is also true of human performance in endurance sports. It should not be surprising that the genes are so much involved, as their function is to provide the coded information serving as the template for the synthesis of the various classes of protein. And contractile, transport, enzymatic, immune, hormonal, cytoskeletal and other kinds of proteins are the essence of life and adaptive mechanisms.

The fundamental question is not whether the genes are important determinants of the potential to perform endurance activities, but rather if there are inherited differences in the genome that account for some of the commonly observed variations in endurance performance, and, if so, what are they? For our purpose, it will suffice to distinguish two types of genetic variation. First, variations are found in the DNA sequences coding for proteins. When DNA base-pair differences in the exon, or coding region, of a gene translate into a change in the amino acid composition of the encoded protein, the biological activity of that particular protein as well as its interactions with other molecules or cellular constituents may be affected. For example, a person may have a gene producing an enzyme with above average activity. This is one type of inherited variation

that may have implications for endurance activities. Second, DNA base differences can be found outside the exon(s) of a gene, in the intron(s) and the flanking regions of the same gene on a given chromosome. This type of DNA variant will not affect the amino acid composition of the protein encoded by that particular gene, but it may alter the expression of the gene permanently or under specific tissue or cellular conditions. For example, the characteristics of myocardial genes may facilitate training hypertrophy in a given individual. Such genomic variants may have a considerable impact on endurance performance, particularly in terms of the response to training.

Research into the effects of protein and DNA variations on sport performance in general, and endurance performance in particular, is still in its infancy. However, in spite of our lack of data at the molecular level, much has been learned during the past decade or so at the quantitative and epidemiological genetic level. Progress has been made concerning the heritability of performance and some of its transmission features across generations. New data have also been generated about the role of the genotype in the response to regular training. Currently available evidence concerning these two important issues will be briefly reviewed, with a focus on endurance performance and its biological determinants. Then, current knowledge concerning the genetic markers of performance will be summarized.

Heritability of endurance performance

In this section, we would like to deal with the following questions. Is there a familial concentration for indicators of the capacity to perform aerobic activities? What is the relative contribution of the estimated genetic effect (heritability) to the total population variation for the same phenotypes (a phenotype being the measured trait of interest; in the present context, an indicator of endurance performance or of a performance determinant)? Do we have evidence for a stronger maternal or paternal influence in the transmission pattern? The data available are typically based on maximal oxygen intake ($\dot{V}o_{2\,max}$), submaximal power output (for example, the physical working capacity (PWC) at a heart rate of 150 beats per minute), or the total work output in a 90 min endurance test, the last being most relevant to this book. A limited amount of research has also dealt with some of the determinants of endurance performance such as heart size, skeletal muscle and adipose tissue metabolism as well as substrate oxidation. We have reviewed this field in greater detail elsewhere (Bouchard & Malina, 1983; Bouchard & Lortie, 1984; Bouchard, 1986).

Familial resemblance

One approach allowing assessment of the importance of familial resemblance in the phenotypes contributing to endurance performance is to compare the variance between families or sibships to that observed within nuclear families or sibships. To reach a meaningful answer, one must control for relevant concomitant variables such as age, gender, body mass and body composition. Aerobic power seems to be characterized by a significant familial resemblance (Montoye & Gayle, 1978; Lortie et al., 1982; Lesage et al., 1985). Thus, the ratio of the between-nuclear families to the within-families variance of $\dot{V}o_{2\,max}$ expressed either per kg of body mass or per kg of fat-free mass

reaches about 1.3. On the other hand, the same ratio for between-sibships to within-sibships (which include only biological brothers and sisters) attains about 1.5. These ratios are known to be statistically significant.

When similar analyses are performed with submaximal power output data ($PWC \cdot kg^{-1}$) gathered on siblings by adoption or by descent (Bouchard et al., 1984), the between to within variance ratio reaches 1.4 for the adoptive sibships but 1.8 for the biological sibs. The ratios become 1.4 and 2.5, respectively, when PWC is expressed on a per kg of fat-free mass basis. These observations suggest that even though one finds a familial concentration of individual differences in measures of aerobic performance, the familial resemblance is caused not only by the genes shared by family members but also by common familial environmental conditions. This conclusion is supported by the significant husband/wife correlations for $\dot{V}o_{2\,max}$ and PWC_{150}, whether expressed on a per kg of mass or a per kg of fat-free mass basis. However, significant spouse correlations can be caused not only by shared cohabitational conditions but also by positive assortative mating for aerobic activities.

Heritability

Three kinds of data are currently available to estimate the size of the genetic effect relative to the total phenotypic variance adjusted for the proper concomitants (Bouchard et al., 1990). First, there are family studies of $\dot{V}o_{2\,max}$, the most important of which is probably that of Lesage et al. (1985). The results of that study suggest that the heritability of $\dot{V}o_{2\,max}$ per kg of mass or per kg of fat-free mass is 10–20% of the age- and gender-adjusted phenotypic variance.

Second, there are data from several twin studies. They have yielded inconsistent results, with heritability estimates ranging from almost zero to more than 90% of the phenotypic variance (Klissouras, 1971; Howald, 1976; Bouchard & Malina, 1983). Such discrepancies are associated with small sample sizes, as well as with improper analytical strategies including inadequate controls over concomitant variables. We have recently attempted to overcome these limitations in a more extensive research involving 27 pairs of brothers, 33 pairs of dizygotic twins and 53 pairs of monozygotic twins (Bouchard et al., 1986a). Heritability reached about 40% for $\dot{V}O_{2\,max}$ per kg of mass, but only about 10% for $\dot{V}O_{2\,max}$ per kg of fat-free mass using the twin data alone. However, considering the higher correlation found in dizygotic twins (intraclass = 0.51) in comparison to the brothers (intraclass = 0.41), we hypothesized that the 40% estimate was inflated by common environmental factors, and that the true heritability of $\dot{V}O_{2\,max}$ per kg of mass was more likely to be about 25% of the adjusted phenotypic variance. The total work output during a 90 min maximal cycle ergometer test was also measured in 31 pairs of dizygotic and 33 pairs of monozygotic twins. Heritability for this test of endurance performance reached 60% when performance was expressed on a per kg basis.

Third, extensive data on relatives by descent or by adoption were available for PWC_{150}. A total of nine different kinds of relative were identified among 1630 subjects living in 375 households (Bouchard et al., 1984; Pérusse et al., 1987). Using a path analysis procedure, we found that about 80% of the age- and gender- adjusted variance in PWC_{150} per kg of mass was associated with non-transmissible effects, leaving about 20% attributable to cultural and lifestyle inheritance. No genetic effect could be found for submaximal power output after controlling for age, gender and body mass. A transmission effect of similar magnitude (about 28%) was obtained for submaximal steptest scores in a study of 9986 subjects visited in the Canada Fitness Survey (Pérusse et al., 1988).

Maternal and paternal effects

There is a paucity of data on this issue. One familial study has suggested that a specific maternal effect was likely present for $\dot{V}O_{2\,max}$ per kg of mass or per kg of fat-free mass (Lesage et al., 1985). This was prompted by the observation that correlations reached 0.20 and above in pairs of mother–child, but were about zero in father–child. In contrast, no maternal effect was found in studies dealing with submaximal power output (Pérusse et al., 1987; 1988). There is also no evidence for an effect limited to one gender (boys or girls) in the transmission from parents to offspring.

Heritability of major determinants

Individual differences in heart size and stroke volume are important determinants of aerobic performance involving large muscle masses. Several twin studies have examined the heritability of echographic heart size (Adams et al., 1985; Fagard et al., 1987). None of these studies suggested a large genetic effect on heart dimensions, once body mass had been taken into consideration. Our own study encompassing several kinds of relatives by descent or by adoption suggests that the heritability of the various heart dimensions is small but significant after adjusting data for age, gender, body mass and level of habitual physical activity. Maximal oxygen pulse is sometimes used as a simple estimate of the maximal stroke volume. We have reported that the heritability of maximal oxygen pulse, adjusted for the proper concomitants, is about 50% (Bouchard et al., 1986a).

The ability of the skeletal muscle tissue to utilize oxygen and to oxidize lipid substrates represents other determinants of endurance performance. We have investigated the histochemical and biochemical characteristics of that tissue, using data obtained through biopsy of the vastus lateralis muscle in 32 pairs of brothers, 26 pairs of dizygotic and 35 pairs of monozygotic twins (Bouchard et al., 1986b). The heritability for the fibre-type distribution and fibre areas was non-significant. The heritability of the maximal activity of key regulatory enzymes of glycogen breakdown (phosphofructokinase) and substrate oxidation (oxoglutarate dehydrogenase) reached about 25–50% of the corresponding age- and gender-adjusted phenotypic variance. In this context, black people from western and central African countries less frequently exhibited the skeletal muscle characteristics associated with a high oxidative metabolism when compared with matched Canadian white subjects of French descent (Ama *et al.*, 1986). The ultrastructural features of skeletal muscle were studied in 11 monozygotic and six dizygotic twin-pairs (Howald, 1976). No genetic effect could be detected for mitochondrial density, the ratio of mitochondrial volume of myofibril volume, or other mitochondrial characteristics.

Individual differences in the respiratory exchange ratio during submaximal exercise were characterized by a significant genetic effect (Bouchard *et al.*, 1989b). This would seem to reflect an inherited tendency for some individuals to oxidize more lipid than carbohydrate substrates under similar conditions. Unpublished studies from our laboratory based on respiratory quotient data indicate that a significant genetic component to preferential lipid oxidation is observed at rest and under various nutritional and exercise challenges. This may have considerable importance for endurance performance. Moreover, twin studies have

shown a significant heritable component in the lipolytic capacity of the collagenase-isolated adipocytes and for the enzymatic synthesis of lipids as well as the capacity to store lipids in adipose tissue (Bouchard, 1985).

A summary of current knowledge about familial resemblance, heritability and specific maternal or paternal effects upon endurance performance phenotypes and some of their determinants is presented in Table 14.1. More research is needed to fill the gaps shown in the table and clarify trends that are at times based on very limited data.

Genotype and the response to training

From the above, one can conclude that inheritance makes only a minor contribution to the variations in the various phenotypes of endurance performance and some of their determinants among sedentary individuals. However, the subjects measured have been mainly sedentary and thus unchallenged by the demands of regular, intense and sustained exercise. Under such circumstances, individual differences are little influenced by DNA variants that affect gene expression, as opposed to a situation when people are under the stress of large increases in

Table 14.1 Summary of the evidence for familial resemblance and for a maternal or a paternal effect, as well as for the approximate heritability level, in various phenotypes of endurance performance and some of their determinants.

Phenotype	Familial concentration	Heritability	Maternal or paternal effect
Submaximal power output	+	No	No
90-min performance	++	++	Unknown
$\dot{V}o_{2\,max}$	+	+	Slight maternal
Heart size	++	+	No
Stroke volume*	++	++	Unknown
Muscle fibre composition	++	+	Unknown
Muscle oxidative potential	++	+	Unknown
Lipid substrate oxidation	++	+	Unknown
Lipid mobilization	++	++	Unknown

* Estimated from maximal oxygen pulse.
+, Significant familial concentration or heritability; ++, very significant familial concentration or heritability.

metabolic rate. Thus, it would seem quite reasonable to suggest that genetic differences may become more striking when sedentary subjects are exposed to regular exercise (Bouchard, 1986).

Research has amply demonstrated that aerobic performance, stroke volume, skeletal muscle oxidative capacity and lipid oxidation are phenotypes that can adapt to training. For instance, the $\dot{V}o_{2\,max}$ of sedentary persons increases by about 20–30% after a few months of training. The skeletal muscle oxidative potential can easily increase by 50% with training and, at times, it may even double. However, if one is to consider a role for the genotype in such responses to training, there must be evidence of individual differences in trainability. There is now considerable support for this concept (Bouchard, 1986; Bouchard et al., 1988a). Some indications about the extent of individual differences in the response of $\dot{V}o_{2\,max}$ to training are given in Table 14.2. The same training programme may result in almost no change in $\dot{V}o_{2\,max}$ for some subjects, while others gain as much as 1 litre of oxygen uptake. Such differences in trainability cannot be attributed to age (all subjects were young adults, 17–29 years of age) or gender (all males). The initial (pretraining) level of fitness accounted for about 25% of the variance in the response of $\dot{V}o_{2\,max}$ to the programme; the lower the initial $\dot{V}o_{2\,max}$ the greater the increase with training.

What is the main cause of the individuality in the response to training? We believe that it has to do with as yet undetermined genetic characteristics. To test this hypothesis, we have now performed four different training studies with pairs of monozygotic twins, the rationale being that the response pattern can be observed for individuals having the same genotype (within pairs) and for subjects with differing genetic characteristics (between pairs). We are convinced that the individuality in trainability of phenotypes governing endurance performance is highly familial and primarily genetically determined. Table 14.3 summarizes some of the evidence pertaining to the trainability of $\dot{V}o_{2\,max}$. There is about six to nine times more variance between genotypes than within genotypes in the response of $\dot{V}o_{2\,max}$ to standardized training conditions. The fourth experiment along these lines, as yet unpublished, is not included in the table. It was, however, the most stringent of all the studies: we controlled seven male monozygous twin-pairs, 24 hours a day, over a period of 4 months. Energy intake, composition of diet, twice daily exercise periods, and other aspects of lifestyle were all standardized. We again found differences in the response of $\dot{V}o_{2\,max}$, and similar evidence to the previous studies indicating a within-pair resemblance in trainability. The similarity of the training response among members of the same monozygotic pair is illustrated in

Table 14.2 $\dot{V}o_{2\,max}$ before training and the response to training in young adult males from two different studies*.

Subjects	Pretraining $\dot{V}o_{2\,max}$		Changes in $\dot{V}o_{2\,max}$			
	Mean	s.d.	Mean	s.d.	Minimum	Maximum
Quebec ($n = 17$)[†]	2.9	0.42	0.63	0.25	0.13	1.03
Arizona ($n = 29$)[‡]	3.4	0.57	0.42	0.22	0.06	0.95

* From C. Bouchard et al. (unpublished data) and J.S. Skinner et al. (unpublished data); all values are in litres of $\dot{V}o_2$ per minute.
[†] Subjects were trained for 20 weeks following the procedures described by Lortie et al. (1984).
[‡] Subjects were trained for 12 weeks, three times per week, 40 min per session, at onset of blood lactate accumulation (about 70–77% of $\dot{V}o_{2\,max}$).

Table 14.3 Effects of training on maximal oxygen intake in monozygotic twins and twin resemblance in training response. From Bouchard *et al.* (1990).

Experiments	Effect of training (F ratio)	F ratio of between- to within-pair variances in response	Intrapair resemblance in response
Endurance training (16 pairs)*	45.6[‡]	5.8[‡]	0.71[‡]
Endurance and intermittent training (26 pairs)[†]	105.9[‡]	9.4[‡]	0.81[‡]

* Data in litres of oxygen per min were adjusted for pretraining value and gender. From studies reported by Prud'Homme *et al.* (1984) and Hamel *et al.* (1986).
[†] Data in litres of oxygen per min were adjusted for pretraining value, gender and training programme. From studies reported by Prud'Homme *et al.* (1984), Hamel *et al.* (1986) and Boulay *et al.* (1986).
[‡] $p < 0.001$.

Fig. 14.1. In this case, 10 pairs of monozygotic twins were subjected to a fully standardized and laboratory controlled training programme for 20 weeks, and gains of absolute $\dot{V}_{O_2\,max}$

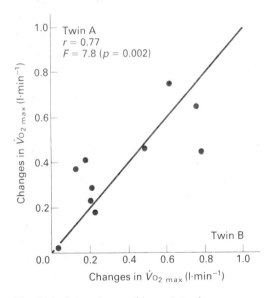

Fig. 14.1 Intrapair resemblance (intraclass coefficient) in 10 pairs of monozygotic twins for training changes in $\dot{V}_{O_2\,max}$ (litres of oxygen per min) after 20 weeks of endurance training. Constructed from the original data of Prud'Homme *et al.* (1984).

showed almost eight times more variance between pairs than within pairs.

The total work output during a 90 min maximal cycle ergometer test was also monitored before and after 15 weeks of training in a study involving six pairs of monozygotic twins (Hamel *et al.*, 1986). A highly significant within-pair resemblance in response was observed, the ratio of between-pairs to within-pairs variances being about 11, and the intraclass coefficient for twin resemblance in response reaching 0.83. We have also reported evidence of a familial resemblance in the training response of some cardiac dimensions (Landry *et al.*, 1985) and several enzyme markers of skeletal muscle oxidative metabolism (Hamel *et al.*, 1986; Simoneau *et al.*, 1986). Similarly, maximal oxygen pulse is characterized by a significant within-pair resemblance in training response, with a variance ratio of about 6 and an intrapair resemblance of 0.70 (Prud'Homme *et al.*, 1984; Bouchard *et al.*, 1990) (Fig. 14.2).

All the above studies strongly suggest that undetermined genetic characteristics contribute to individuality in response to a laboratory controlled exercise-training programme. Table 14.4 summarizes the evidence for such genetic effects for aerobic performance phenotypes and their determinants.

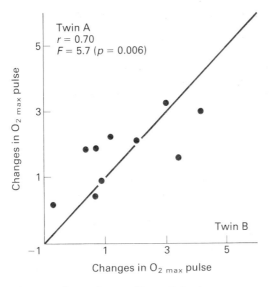

Twin A
$r = 0.70$
$F = 5.7 \ (p = 0.006)$

Fig. 14.2 Intrapair resemblance (intraclass coefficient) in 10 pairs of monozygotic twins for training changes in maximal oxygen pulse ($\dot{V}_{O_2 max}$/ maximal heart rate) after 20 weeks of endurance training (data are millilitres of oxygen per heart beat). Constructed from the original data of Prud'Homme *et al.* (1984).

Table 14.4 Importance of the between-genotypes variance with respect to the within-genotype variance in the phenotypic response to training. The evidence is summarized in terms of F ratios of the two variance components*.

Phenotype	Approximate F ratio
Submaximal power output[†]	2–4
90-min performance	10–12
$\dot{V}_{O_2 max}$	6–9
Heart size	Undetermined
Stroke volume[‡]	6–10
Muscle fibre composition	1–2
Muscle oxidative potential	2–5
Lipid substrate oxidation	2–5
Lipid mobilization	5–10

* Summary based on several studies reported from our laboratory.
† Physical working capacity phenotypes or ventilatory threshold data
‡ Estimated from maximal oxygen pulse.

Genetic markers and aerobic performance

There are strong indications that the level of heritability of aerobic performance phenotypes and their most important determinants is rather low, while the role of undetermined genetic elements in trainability is quite striking. Thus, attempts to identify genetic markers are more likely to succeed when using the magnitude of the response to training as the phenotype of interest, rather than the individual differences seen in the sedentary population. None the less, we have been investigating the problem with batteries of genetic markers, using three different strategies: (i) to discriminate between endurance-trained élite athletes and matched sedentary controls; (ii) to account for the individual differences in aerobic performance among sedentary subjects; and (iii) to predict the pattern of response to aerobic training. In each case, we are including in the battery of genetic markers: (i) genetic variants in gene products such as enzymes, red blood cell antigens, human leucocyte antigen (HLA) system specificities at class I and II loci, and others; (ii) restriction fragment length polymorphism (RFLP) for a variety of candidate genes encoded in the nuclear DNA; and (iii) RFLPs in mitochondrial DNA.

We have previously shown that red blood cell antigen and enzyme polymorphisms were not associated with the status of élite athletes in endurance events (Chagnon *et al.*, 1984; Couture *et al.*, 1986). Moreover, the 11 enzymes of the glycolytic pathway and the nine enzymes of the tricarboxylic acid cycle of the skeletal muscle did not exhibit any charge variants in a large sample of subjects, thus supporting the notion that variations in the coding sequences of these genes are unlikely to account for the individuality of aerobic performance or trainability (Marcotte *et al*,. 1987; Bouchard *et al.*, 1988b).

However, in a sample of 295 sedentary young adult males and females, muscle biopsies were obtained from the vastus lateralis and proteins were fractionated by a thin-layer isoelectro-focusing technique (Bouchard *et al.*, 1989a). Six individuals exhibited a muscle creatine kinase (CK) enzyme variant, while 21 were heterozygotes for a variant of the adenylate kinase-1 (AK1) enzyme. In the same population, four alleles (variant forms of the gene) and seven phenotypes were recovered for the phosphoglucomutase-1 (PGM1) enzyme (C. Bouchard *et al.*, unpublished results). No significant relationships were found between CK, AK1 and PGM1 classes and the untrained $\dot{V}_{O_2 max}$ per kg of body mass. The relationships between variants of these three proteins and the response of $\dot{V}_{O_2 max}$ to training were considered in a sample of 72 young adults trained in our laboratory. The training response in litres of oxygen was adjusted for the pretraining level, gender differences and type of training programme (there were three different programmes, lasting from 15 to 20 weeks). The associations between the enzyme markers and the adjusted $\dot{V}_{O_2 max}$ response to training are described in Table 14.5. CK and AK1 each accounted only for about 1% of the variance in trainability, but PGM1 was associated with 6% of the individual differences in the responder status (C. Bouchard *et al.*, unpublished results). If 75% of the variance in trainability of $\dot{V}_{O_2 max}$ is related to undetermined genetic elements, the contribution of these three enzyme loci remains small, but that of PGM1 cannot be considered negligible. Indeed, it is unlikely that a single gene locus (or a few loci) or a given DNA variant (or a few polymorphic sequences for that matter) will be sufficient to define the responder status, considering the enormous complexity of the $\dot{V}_{O_2 max}$ phenotype. One must also recognize that for genetic (e.g. linkage) or physiological reasons, the CK, AK1 and PGM1 variant loci may be only surrogate markers of an association with the responder status, and the true determinants may lie with other genes or gene products.

We have considered the relationships between the A, B and C loci of the HLA system and the adjusted $\dot{V}_{O_2 max}$ response to training

Table 14.5 Effect of three muscle enzyme markers on the adjusted $\dot{V}_{O_2 max}$ response to training.*

Gene	$R^2 \times 100$
Creatine kinase	1
Adenylate kinase-1	1
Phosphoglucomutase-1	6

* Based on $\dot{V}_{O_2 max}$ changes (litres of oxygen) in 72 secondary subjects submitted to training for 15–20 weeks; data adjusted for gender, pretraining level and training programmes. The effect was quantified with correlation techniques using two genotypes each for creatine kinase and adenylate kinase-1, and seven genotypes for phosphoglucomutase-1.

in the same sample of 72 sedentary subjects (L. Pérusse *et al.*, unpublished results). A total of 19 HLA alleles could be tested, and none exhibited a consistent pattern of association with the responder status. Given the extensive polymorphism at these loci of the HLA system, a fully satisfactory test of the association would require an enormous traning experiment with hundreds of subjects.

The study of DNA sequence variations and their associations with trainability is still in its infancy. In one recently completed experiment, we looked into sequence polymorphism, using a human cDNA probe for the CK gene and two restriction enzymes (NcoI and TaqI). Each enzyme defined two different polymorphisms, each with two alleles of different length (Dionne *et al.*, 1991a). The relationships between the DNA fragment length genotypes and the response to training were generally negligible (Dionne & Bouchard, 1990). There was perhaps one exception to the above, as the three homozygotes for a 3.4 kb fragment defined by NcoI gained significantly more (0.8 litre of oxygen) than 39 other male control subjects with a fragment length of 2.5 kb (a mean increase of about 0.5 litres of oxygen).

On the other hand, we are particularly interested in the mitochondrial DNA, because of the apparent maternal effect on $\dot{V}_{O_2 max}$ that we reported above. Mitochondrial DNA is a closed, circular molecule of 16 569 base-pairs that codes for 13 of the 67 polypeptides involved in the respiratory chain and oxidative phosphorylation, plus transfer and ribosomal RNAs. It is a small genome that is transmitted following a maternal mode of inheritance. In one recent study, mitochondrial DNA sequence variation was investigated using the RFLP technology in sedentary subjects submitted to endurance training in two different laboratories. About 3% of the mitochondrial genome was screened for DNA variants, using a battery of 22 restriction enzymes. Multiple DNA variants were detected with 15 of these enzymes. The sequence polymorphism was weakly related to individual differences in pretraining $\dot{V}o_{2\,max}$ (Dionne *et al.*, 1991b). For instance, carriers of three different RFLPs (three subjects in each case) had a significantly higher $\dot{V}o_{2\,max}$ per kg of body mass in the sedentary state than control subjects. On the other hand, three low responders to training had a sequence variation in the subunit 5 of the mitochondrial NADH dehydrogenase gene detected with HincII. Their response to training (gain of 0.28 litres of oxygen) was significantly less than the other individuals (gain of 0.50 litres of oxygen) even when taking into account the initial level of $\dot{V}o_{2\,max}$. This is an issue that clearly deserves further research, using other restriction enzymes and perhaps other strategies.

Genetic research and endurance sports

We are beginning to understand the genetic epidemiology of endurance performance phenotypes. More importantly, we now understand that there are non-responders, low responders and high responders to prolonged endurance training and that the responder status runs in family lines and is probably determined by genetic characteristics (Bouchard, 1986). However, the nature of these genetic elements remains largely unknown. It will take several further years of research before the genetic basis of endurance performance

and trainability is clearly understood. Promising candidate genes can be tested, as probes are available for a good number of them. In the event that the relevant genetic elements turn out to be beyond a large battery of candidate genes, anonymous DNA probes could also be used. Definitive investigations will have to incorporate a large number of genetic markers. In order to cover the entire human genome adequately, it will be necessary to use aerobic metabolism and endurance performance phenotypes, as well as examining the response to training for these phenotypes and their determinants in a large number of families whose members will have been submitted to the same testing and training protocols. This strategy will make possible the detection of unknown gene loci or DNA sequences, by analysis of linkages which may impact on endurance performance or trainability.

The combination of genetic methods and the tools of molecular biology offers great opportunities for understanding the genetic and molecular basis of endurance performance and trainability. The increase of knowledge in this area should have considerable impact on sport and the Olympic Movement itself. Fundamental ethical questions will arise and the ensuing long and complex debate will touch upon the fundamental values of the Olympic Movement. Understanding the genetics and molecular biology of performance and trainability will alter screening procedures for talented individuals (infants will eventually be targeted), their evolution in sports clubs and sports governing bodies, training methods and surveillance, rules governing competitions and eligibility, especially at the élite level, and other dimensions of the sports pyramid. A positive step in preparing for these challenges would be for all involved (including coaches, sports administrators, members of sports governing bodies, sport scientists and sport physicians) to become acquainted with the fundamentals of genetics, molecular biology, sociobiology and ethics. The future will be interesting and challenging, and not only for sport geneticists!

References

Adams, T.D., Yanowitz, F.G., Fisher, A.G. *et al.* (1985) Heritability of cardiac size: an echocardiographic and electrocardiographic study of monozygotic and dizygotic twins. *Circulation* **71**, 39–44.

Ama, P.F.M., Simoneau, J.A., Boulay, M.R., Serresse, O., Thériault, G., Bouchard, C. (1986) Skeletal muscle characteristics in sedentary Black and Caucasian males. *J. Appl. Physiol.* **61**, 1758–1761.

Bouchard, C. (1985) Inheritance of fat distribution and adipose tissue metabolism. In: Vague, J., Björntorp, P., Guy-Grand, B., Rebuffé-Scrive, M. & Vague, P. (eds) *Metabolic Complications of Human Obesities*, pp. 87–96. Elsevier, Amsterdam.

Bouchard, C. (1986) Genetics of aerobic power and capacity. In: Malina, R.M. & Bouchard, C. (eds) *Sport and Human Genetics*, pp. 59–88. Human Kinetics, Champaign, Illinois.

Bouchard, C., Boulay, M.R., Dionne, F.T., Pérusse, L., Thibault, M.C. & Simoneau, J.A. (1990) Genotype, aerobic performance and response to training. In: Beunen, G., Ghesquière, J., Reybrouck T., Claessens, A.L. (eds) *Children and Exercise XIV*, Band 4 Schriftenreihe der Hamburg-Mannheimer-Stiftung für Informationsmedizin, Enke Verlag.

Bouchard, C., Boulay, M.R., Simoneau, J.A., Lortie, G. & Pérusse, L. (1988a) Heredity and trainability of aerobic and anaerobic performances. An update. *Sports Med.* **5**, 69–73.

Bouchard, C., Chagnon, M., Thibault, M.C. *et al.* (1989a) Muscle genetic variants and relationship with performance and trainability. *Med. Sci. Sports Exerc.* **21**, 71–77.

Bouchard, C., Chagnon, M., Thibault, M.C., Boulay, M.R., Marcotte, M. & Simoneau, J.A. (1988b) Absence of charge variants in human skeletal muscle enzymes of the glycolytic pathway. *Hum. Genet.* **78**, 100.

Bouchard, C., Lesage, R., Lortie, G. *et al.* (1986a) Aerobic performance in brothers, dizygotic and monozygotic twins. *Med. Sci. Sports Exerc.* **18**, 639–646.

Bouchard, C. & Lortie, G. (1984) Heredity and endurance performance. *Sports Med.* **1**, 38–64.

Bouchard, C., Lortie, G., Simoneau, J.A., Leblanc, C., Thériault, G. & Tremblay, A. (1984) Submaximal power output in adopted and biological siblings. *Ann. Hum. Biol.* **11**, 303–309.

Bouchard, C. & Malina, R.M. (1983) Genetics of physiological fitness and motor performance. *Exerc. Sport Sci. Rev.* **11**, 306–339.

Bouchard, C., Simoneau, J.A., Lortie G., Boulay, M.R., Marcotte, M. & Thibault, M.C. (1986b) Genetic effects in human skeletal muscle fiber type distribution and enzyme activities. *Can. J. Physiol.*

Pharmacol. **64**, 1245–1251.

Bouchard, C., Tremblay, A., Nadeau, A. *et al.* (1989b) Genetic effect in resting and exercise metabolic rates. *Metabolism* **38**(4), 364–370.

Boulay, M.R., Lortie, G., Simoneau, J.A. & Bouchard, C. (1986) Sensitivity of maximal aerobic power and capacity to anaerobic training is partly genotype dependent. In: Malina, R.M. & Bouchard, C. (eds) *Sport and Human Genetics*, pp. 173–182. Human Kinetics, Champaign, Illinois.

Chagnon, Y.C., Allard, C. & Bouchard, C. (1984) Red blood cell genetic variation in Olympic endurance athletes. *J. Sport Sci.* **2**, 121–129.

Couture, L., Chagnon, M., Allard, C. & Bouchard, C. (1986) More on red blood cell genetic variation in Olympic athletes. *Can. J. Appl. Sport Sci.* **11**, 16–18.

Dionne, F.T. & Bouchard, C. (1990) Muscle creatine kinase: protein and DNA sequence variations and trainability of $\dot{V}o_{2\,max}$. *Med. Sci. Sports Exerc.* **22**, 57 (abstract).

Dionne, F.T., Turcotte, L., Grondin, J., Thibault, M.C. & Bouchard, C. (1991a) NcoI RFLP in human brain creatine kinase gene (CKBB). *Nucl. Acids. Res.* **19**, 195.

Dionne, F.T., Turcotte, L., Thibault, M.C., Boulay, M.R., Skinner, J.S. & Bouchard, C. (1991b) Mitochondrial DNA sequence polymorphism, $\dot{V}o_{2\,max}$, and response to endurance training. *Med. Sci. Sports Exerc.* **23**, 177–185.

Fagard, R., Van Den Brocke, C., Bielen, E. & Amery, A. (1987) Maximum oxygen uptake and cardiac size and function in twins. *Am. J. Cardiol.* **60**, 1362–1367.

Hamel, P., Simoneau, J.A., Lortie, G., Boulay, M.R. & Bouchard, C. (1986) Heredity and muscle adaptation to endurance training. *Med. Sci. Sports Exerc.* **18**, 690–696.

Howald, H. (1976) Ultrastructure and biochemical function of skeletal muscle in twins. *Ann. Hum. Biol.* **3**, 455–462.

Klissouras, V. (1971) Heritability of adaptive variation. *J. Appl. Physiol.* **31**, 338–344.

Landry, F., Bouchard, C. & Dumesnil, J. (1985) Cardiac dimension changes with endurance training: indications of a genotype dependency. *J. Am. Med. Assoc.* **5**, 77–80.

Lesage, R., Simoneau, J.A., Jobin, J., Leblanc, J. & Bouchard, C. (1985) Familial resemblance in maximal heart rate, blood lactate and aerobic power. *Hum. Hered.* **35**, 182–189.

Lortie, G., Bouchard, C., Leblanc, C. *et al.* (1982) Familial similarity in aerobic power. *Hum. Biol.* **54**, 801–812.

Lortie, G., Simoneau, J.A., Hamel, P., Boulay, M.R., Landry, F. & Bouchard, C. (1984) Responses of maximal aerobic power and capacity to aerobic training. *Int. J. Sports Med.* **5**, 232–236.

Marcotte, M., Chagnon, M., Côté, C., Thibault, M.C., Boulay, M.R. & Bouchard, C. (1987) Lack of genetic polymorphism in human skeletal muscle enzymes of the tricarboxylic acid cycle. *Hum. Genet.* **77**, 200.

Montoye, H.J. & Gayle, R. (1978) Familial relationships in maximal oxygen uptake. *Hum. Biol.* **50**, 241–249.

Pérusse, L., Leblanc, C. & Bouchard, C. (1988) Intergeneration transmission of physical fitness in the Canadian population. *Can. J. Sport Sci.* **13**(1), 8–14.

Pérusse, L., Lortie, G., Leblanc, C., Tremblay, A., Thériault, G. & Bouchard, C. (1987) Genetic and environmental sources of variation in physical fitness. *Ann. Hum. Biol.* **14**, 425–434.

Prud'Homme, D., Bouchard, C., Leblanc, C., Landry, F. & Fontaine, E. (1984) Sensitivity of maximal aerobic power to training is genotype-dependent. *Med. Sci. Sports Exerc.* **16**, 489–493.

Simoneau, J.A., Lortie, G., Boulay, M.R., Marcotte, M., Thibault, M.C. & Bouchard, C. (1986) Inheritance of human skeletal muscle and anaerobic capacity adaptation to high-intensity intermittent training. *Int. J. Sports Med.* **7**, 167–171.

Part 2d

Physical Limitations of Endurance Performance

Chapter 15

Mechanical Constraints upon Endurance Performance

EDWARD C. FREDERICK

Role of mechanical and biomechanical constraints

Human endurance is strongly affected by a number of biomechanical and mechanical factors. One might even say that the challenge of endurance performance can be reduced to a single pair of linked objectives: to minimize the mechanical power requirements needed to maintain movement while minimizing the expenditure of metabolic power. Biomechanics affects the relationship between mechanical and metabolic power requirements in many ways. The breadth of this influence can be seen most easily by first looking at the mechanical constraints on endurance performance. Along the way we will examine examples of strategies for minimizing mechanical constraints. Constraints can also be overcome or reduced in influence biomechanically, and in another section we will review the biomechanical factors that affect the economy of movement.

Factors constraining movement

Figure 15.1 outlines the major mechanical constraints on performance in endurance sports. Although this is by no means a complete listing or necessarily a correct taxonomy, it does enumerate the major factors. It is useful when considering these mechanical constraints to observe that there is much overlap and interdependence among these various factors. For example, most of the equations that describe

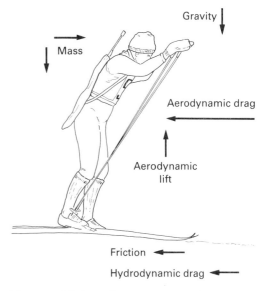

Fig. 15.1 Mechanical constraints on endurance performance. The Olympic biathlete (cross-country skiing and shooting) provides a good example of how physical constraints affect endurance performance. Gravity affects many factors but is especially important when climbing and descending hills. Sliding friction limiting ski glide is the next most significant factor. Aerodynamic and hydrodynamic drag (the ski glides on a layer of melted water) slows the biathlete, and the effects of mass are especially apparent in carrying the 5-kg mass of the rifle. The additional constraint of centripetal force is greatest on downhill, turning sections of the race course. In addition, lift, especially aerodynamic, can affect biathlon performance, although to a much lesser degree than the other factors. In rowing and other endurance water sports hydrodynamic lift can play a role in performance.

163

these constraints, such as frictional, centripetal, aerodynamic and hydrodynamic forces, have a gravitational acceleration term and/or a mass term. In fact, any one of these constraints seldom has an opportunity to work independently of the other factors.

Gravity

The most prevalent constraint on performance is gravity. It has a direct effect as well as a myriad of indirect effects. Without gravity, for example, a single long jump would continue on to infinity, provided nothing got in the way. The force due to terrestrial gravity (F_G, sometimes abbreviated as G) is described by a simple equation:

$$F_G \propto m'm \cdot r^{-2}$$

where m' and m are the masses of the earth and the object (e.g. an athlete) respectively, and r is the distance between the centres of mass of the earth and the object, i.e. the earth's radius. From this equation, F_G is an inverse squared function of the earth's radius, directly proportional to the mass of the object.

In discussing gravity as a practical matter, we are more directly concerned with the acceleration due to gravity (g). The quantity g is found from the equation $F_G = m \cdot g$, which describes the gravitational force acting on a particular object with a mass m. Scientists often define $g = 9.806$ m·s^{-2} but it is important to remember that this is an approximation. In fact, g varies with latitude and altitude above sea level because of variations in r. At 90° north latitude (North Pole) g is approximately 9.832, decreasing to 9.819 at 60° latitude, 9.806 at 45°; and 9.780 on the equator at zero latitude.

This is mainly due to the fact the earth is not spherical, but rather exhibits a progressively greater thickening of its crust on approaching the equator. The earth's average radius is some 32 km greater at the equator, and an altitude above sea level can exaggerate that effect even further. Quito, Ecuador, is a place where high altitude and low latitude conspire to minimize gravity.

The difference in gravitational forces acting on an athlete and the implements and equipment of sport can be significant at extreme latitudes. For example, F_G would be about 0.4% greater in Oslo, Norway than in Quito. In athletic events dominated by gravity such as shot-putting or downhill skiing, this effect can have negative or positive consequences proportional to differences in gravity's influence. A speed skier competing in Oslo would have a terminal velocity 0.2% greater, if we account for gravity-influenced wind and snow drag changes, than under the same conditions near Quito. On the other hand, a world-class shot putter would be able to put the shot 8 cm further in Quito because of the reduced gravity. Although these effects are small, they can be significant in world-calibre performances, where records are often improved by fractions of a percentage. Endurance sports like the 1-hour bicycling event also benefit from the lesser wind drag of reduced gravity.

Mass and mechanical work

Although we intuitively connect mass with weight, the force due to gravity, they are different quantities. Weight is a force equal to $m \cdot g$ where m is the mass of the body or object. Much confusion is generated by the use of pounds, a unit of weight in the Imperial system, and the frequent conversion of pounds to kilograms, a unit of mass. Although 2.204 624 pounds can equal the weight of a 1-kg mass (9.806 65 N), it does so only if g equals 9.806 65 m·s^{-2} (which it approximates at most moderate latitudes and altitudes). However, this is not always the case, and it perpetuates a misunderstanding, that weight and mass are the same quantity. In the Imperial system the unit of mass is the slug.

Although mass and gravity can conspire to limit human performance in many ways, mass is a unique property that can constrain sports performance independent of gravity. Kinetic energy changes, for example, are very costly from a biomechanical and metabolic standpoint and they are unaffected by gravity. Carrying added mass on the extremities, for example, where they undergo great changes in horizontal velocity during cyclic motions such as the foot makes in running, is costly because of the kinetic energy involved.

In running, the foot accelerates to about twice the average speed of the body during the swing phase and then slows to zero velocity at foot contact. The cost of accelerating and decelerating an added mass carried on the foot is a function of kinetic energy changes.

$$\text{Energy}_{kinetic} = 0.5 \cdot m \cdot v^2$$

The work due to changes in horizontal velocity during a complete stride can be estimated by:

$$\text{Work}_{horizontal} = 0.5 \cdot m \cdot (v_{max}^2 - v_{min}^2)$$

where v_{max} and v_{min} are maximum and minimum velocity. The fact that this is a squared function explains why this work alone accounts for such a high proportion (about 80%) of the added cost of carrying weight on the feet (Frederick, 1983). Most of the remainder of the cost is related to the lifting of the foot plus weight to a height of about 50 cm during the stride cycle. The cost due to vertical work has a gravity component, and it is described by the equation:

$$\text{Work}_{vertical} = m \cdot g \cdot h$$

where h is the height to which the mass is raised. This is the work required to lift a mass against the force of gravity, and it is a major component of the work required in sports where large masses are lifted, as in road cycling and cross-country skiing where a significant proportion of race time is spent climbing hills.

Mass also enters into the work required to perform rotational movements. The equation for rotational work:

$$\text{Work}_{rotational} = 0.5 \cdot I \cdot \omega^2$$

includes angular velocity ω, and the mass moment of inertia, I, a measure of a body's resistance to accelerated angular motion about an axis. The moment of inertia is a function of both the mass and the square of the distance of the centre of mass from the axis of rotation. The rotational component of carrying weight on the foot while running is relatively small, but in sports where motion has more of a cyclic rotational component, the cost due to rotational work can be quite high. For example, the added cost of heavier bicycle pedals (which rotate about 100 times a minute at a distance of about 18 cm from the bottom bracket axis) is considerable.

The costs of rotational and horizontal movements are thus dependent on mass, independent of gravity, and squared functions of the velocity changes involved. Such costs would be the same even in zero g, explaining, in part, why the metabolic costs of locomotion in the reduced gravity of space can be so high.

The effects of mass have far reaching and complex effects on performance. Table 15.1 lists some of the areas of study of performance enhancement in which mass plays a critical role.

Mass and gravity are the major constraints on sports movements, and efforts to reduce mass lower the mechanical power requirements needed to sustain movement in a number of ways. In our discussion of additional constraints, these factors will continue to demonstrate their importance.

Frictional force

Friction enters into the performance equation for a number of sports, either as an aid or an impediment to performance. A runner, for example, requires high friction between shoe and track surface to accelerate from the start, but cyclists and skiers go to great extremes to minimize friction because it is a factor limiting their performance.

The frictional force resisting the sliding of an object is described by the relationship:

$$F_g = \mu N \text{ [friction]}$$

Table 15.1   Areas of study incorporating mass as a major variable.

Load carriage factors
   Mass, distribution of mass, velocity changes,
     displacement of mass
Friction
Scale effects
   Metabolic consequences
   Speed
   Kinetic and kinematic effects
Energy cost studies, running, walking,
    cycling, skiing
Ground reaction forces
   Body mass
   Effective mass

---

where N is the *normal* force, perpendicular to the surface (equal to $m \cdot g$), and μ is the coefficient of friction, a dimensionless quantity that equals the ratio between the normal and horizontal force. A μ of 0.6, for example, means that a horizontal force equal to 60% of the normal force must be applied to cause the object to slide. Typical values of μ are 0.6–0.8 for most sport shoes, but values greater than 1.0 have been measured for cleated shoes which interlock with the playing surface.

When the body is on a slope of angle α, the frictional force is a function of the angle of the slope:

$$F_g = \mu \cdot m \cdot g \cdot \cos\alpha$$

This is particularly illuminating, for example, in skiing where the frictional force resisting sliding and thus slowing the skier decreases at steeper slopes, even if the frictional coefficient remains the same.

Various coefficients of resistance or friction can be determined experimentally to help understand how performance in various sports is affected. All are essentially ratios between forces normal to the movement and forces in the direction of movement. In skiing, sliding friction is important and coefficients of sliding friction around 0.05 are typical between ski bottom and snow. Cyclists, on the other hand, are more concerned with rolling friction and

rolling resistance. A soft tyre deforms more and interacts with unevenness in the road surface, creating a resistance to the rolling of the tyre.

Rolling resistance or the force required to overcome rolling resistance is found from the equation:

$$F_r = \mu_r \cdot N \text{ [rolling resistance]}$$

Whitt and Wilson (1985) have shown that the coefficient of rolling resistance can be viewed in practical terms via the empirically derived relationship for bicycle wheels:

$$\mu_r \cong 0.07 \cdot L_M / 2 \cdot r$$

where μ_r is the coefficient of rolling resistance for a bicycle wheel, $2 \cdot r$ is the diameter of the inflated wheel, and L_M is the maximum length of the loaded wheel's footprint. Larger diameter wheels pumped up to higher pressures lower L_M, reduce μ_r, and therefore lower rolling resistance. Rolling resistance is estimated by multiplying μ_r by the load on the wheel.

Rolling resistance is, practically speaking and at normal cycling speeds, only partially dependent on speed (Kyle, 1986). A typical rolling resistance for a 27″ (68.5 cm) racing bicycle wheel would be about 3.0 N ($\mu_r = 0.005$ on a smooth road surface) for a rider + cycle weighing 600 N pedalling at normal racing speeds. Although there are certainly benefits to reducing the μ_r of bicycle wheels, as with all other sports where velocity is high, drag forces most often present the greatest constraint to performance.

Drag forces

Athletes moving through fluids such as air or water must do work to overcome drag forces. Although the physics of aerodynamics and hydrodynamics can be quite complex, in the simplest sense athletes must do work to displace the mass of these fluids. The drag force which they are working against can be estimated using the following basic equation:

$$D = 1/2 \cdot \rho \cdot A \cdot C_D \cdot V^2$$

where ρ is fluid density, A is cross-sectional or projected area, C_D is the drag coefficient, and V^2 is the athlete's relative velocity squared. This squared function of velocity results in one of the most significant impediments to endurance performance. Cyclists racing at speeds over 30 km·h^{-1} expend more than 50% of their metabolic energy just to overcome wind resistance, and wind resistance accounts for over 80% of the resisting forces constraining performance.

Typical values for the parameters in the drag equation in air are $\rho = 1.25$ kg·m^{-3}; $A = 0.55$ m^2 for a runner, or 0.33 m^2 for a racing cyclist; and $C_D = 0.9$ for a typical cyclist or runner. In water, the fluid density is much greater, by three orders of magnitude, and, although the cross-sectional area of a human swimmer or a rowing shell is much smaller (in the order of 0.1 m^2), skin-friction drag, which depends more on the total surface of contact than the cross-sectional area, becomes more significant and imposes a severe constraint on performance.

The drag coefficient is determined experimentally but is dependent on a dimensionless quantity, the Reynold's number, which in turn depends on velocity and temperature, as well as the size and shape of the object. The relationship between the drag coefficient and the Reynold's number is non-linear, and there are discontinuities in this relationship which have significant effects on performance. For example, for particular objects there are certain ranges of velocity where the drag coefficient declines dramatically. This creates the counterintuitive situation where speeding up to reach a critical velocity actually results in a lower drag force.

It is possible to reduce drag significantly by following some relatively simple recommendations. Chester Kyle and his colleagues have shown that runners and cyclists can reduce drag as much as 10% by choosing equipment and clothing wisely, and by up to 40% by drafting, i.e. following closely behind another rider (Kyle, 1986; Kyle & Caiozzi, 1986).

Factors which can be modified or selected to reduce the drag force are shown in Table 15.2.

Table 15.2 Factors that reduce drag force.

Factor	Modifications that reduce drag
ρ	Higher temperatures, higher absolute humidity, increased altitude, decreased barometric pressure
A	Reduce projected area
C_D	Streamlining, higher temperatures, change of Reynold's number (shape, velocity, temperature)
V	Minimize velocity changes to minimize average velocity

Similar strategies are pursued hydrodynamically, although the greater influence of skin-friction drag leads toward additional solutions which affect boundary layer conditions over the surface — such as moulding tiny grooves in boat hulls to reduce skin-friction drag.

Centripetal force

Moving in a circuit, such as around a track, introduces another constraint in the form of centripetal force. This force acts at the surface and toward the centre of rotation of the circuit. A cyclist negotiating a turn, for example, will experience a tendency for the bike, at the point where the tyres meet the road, to move toward the axis of the radius of the turn. Leaning into the turn will offset that centripetal force. It is described by the equation:

$$F_c = m \cdot \omega^2 \cdot r = m \cdot V^2/r \text{ [centripetal force]}$$

where r is the radius of the circle defined by the arc traversed; ω^2 is the angular velocity squared (in radians per second); m is mass; and V^2 is tangential velocity squared. Note once again the squared function. As the rotational velocity increases, centripetal force increases as the square of the increased velocity. Compensation for this phenomenon is achieved through the design of equipment, and by learning proper techniques that minimize the biomechanical cost of overcoming this constraint.

Summary

Athletes, coaches and sports scientists must work within mechanical constraints. If endurance is to be improved by mechanical means, it will be achieved by affecting one or more of these constraints. For example, the bicyclist who assumes a tucked position, drafts a competitor and wears a drag-reducing helmet and body suit is trying to reduce aerodynamic constraints. Rolling friction may also be reduced by using high pressure tyres with a smooth and narrow tread. Gravity and mass constraints are diminished by using lightweight components, and the toppling effect of centripetal forces is decreased by leaning into turns. All of these examples address mechanical constraints in a way that reduces physical power requirements, and thus decrease the metabolic power required to pedal at a given speed. Bicycling becomes energetically more economical and endurance performance is enhanced when these factors are taken into account.

Frederick (1983) has reviewed extrinsic mechanical aids to performance which operate by affecting one or more of these constraints. His review cites a number of documented aids to performance including: selecting appropriate environmental conditions (e.g. lower gravity and air density); wearing aerodynamically designed clothing and light and resilient footwear; rowing in smooth and correctly shaped racing shells; and running on surfaces of properly tuned compliance and correctly banked turns. In endurance sports, there is a potential to improve performance by 1 to 15%. It is important to remember, however, that there are other biomechanical factors that also influence economy, and they do not always operate directly on mechanical constraints. There may also be gains of mechanical efficiency, as discussed in Chapter 17.

References

Frederick, E.C. (1983) Extrinsic biomechanical aids. In: Williams, M. (ed.) *Ergogenic Aids in Sport*, pp. 323–339. Human Kinetics, Champaign, Illinois.

Kyle, C.R. (1986) Mechanical factors affecting the speed of a cycle. In: Burke, E. (ed.) *Science of Cycling*, pp. 123–136. Human Kinetics, Champaign, Illinois.

Kyle, C.R. & Caiozzo, V.J. (1986) The effect of athletic clothing aerodynamics upon running speed. *Med. Sci. Sport Exerc.* **18**, 509–515.

Whitt, F.R. & Wilson, D.G. (1985) *Bicycling Science*, 2nd edn. MIT Press, Cambridge, Massachusetts.

Chapter 16

Heat Exchange in Hot and Cold Environments

ETHAN R. NADEL

Introduction

Fatigue is defined in the simplest terms as the inability to maintain power output, or the inability to maintain a given muscular tension over time (Edwards, 1981). The fatigue that develops during the maximal voluntary contraction of a muscle has a different cause from that which develops during repeated moderate contractions, and both differ from the fatigue that occurs while performing prolonged exercise in hot or cold environments. Ultimately, all physical forms of fatigue during exercise are the consequence of the inability to generate energy at a rate sufficient to meet the energy requirements in contracting skeletal muscle. This chapter examines how an early onset of fatigue occurs in a hot or cold environment, thereby limiting endurance performance.

One definition of fatigue during prolonged exercise (for example, a loss of pace during a marathon race) is that the metabolic cost of maintaining a constant pace becomes greater than that which can be sustained entirely by aerobic means (that is, there is an increasing reliance on anaerobic energy production as time progresses, which would occur as the cost of exercise approached maximal aerobic power). To accept this view, we need to accept the notion that the maximal aerobic power is not a constant, but depends upon numerous factors, many of which vary during prolonged exercise, especially in extreme environmental temperatures. A rearrangement of the Fick equation reveals that maximal aerobic power can change over time if any of its component factors vary:

$$\dot{V}O_{2\,max} = [HR_{max}]\,[SV_{max}]\,[(a\text{-}v)O_{2\,max}]$$

where:

$\dot{V}O_{2\,max}$ = maximal aerobic power, (ml $O_2 \cdot min^{-1}$)

HR_{max} = maximal heart rate (beats·min^{-1})

SV_{max} = maximal cardiac stroke volume (ml blood per beat)

$(a\text{-}v)O_{2\,max}$ = maximal oxygen extraction, (ml $O_2 \cdot ml^{-1}$ blood)

Thus, any decrease in HR_{max}, SV_{max} or $(a\text{-}v)O_{2\,max}$ during prolonged exercise will, by definition, decrease $\dot{V}O_{2\,max}$, and therefore will ultimately decrease performance. To provide one example, SV is a function of cardiac filling pressure, according to Starling's law of the heart. An acute reduction in blood volume or an acute increase in the volume of blood residing in the periphery below heart level, such as will occur during exercise in the heat, should decrease the maximal cardiac filling pressure, SV_{max} and therefore $\dot{V}O_{2\,max}$. Alternatively, anything that acutely reduces the average arteriovenous oxygen difference, for example a redistribution of blood flow away from muscle, will also decrease $\dot{V}O_{2\,max}$. Excessive body heating or cooling during exercise will affect the determinants of $\dot{V}O_{2\,max}$ and thus will bring about an early onset of fatigue. How these changes occur is described in the following pages.

Heat exchanges in the body

During exercise, the oxidation rate of fuels in skeletal muscle increases dramatically in order to provide the energy necessary for the contraction and relaxation processes. The oxygen intake of skeletal muscle can increase from about 1.5 ml·kg^{-1}·min^{-1} in the resting state to as much as 150 ml·kg^{-1}·min^{-1} during intensive exercise. Ultimately, all of the energy released from the muscle during physical activity appears as heat. In a sedentary person, the whole body heat production is about 70 W. During moderately intensive exercise, the rate of heat production may exceed 1000 W and such values can be sustained throughout prolonged activity such as a marathon run. A thermal load of this magnitude would raise the body core temperature by 1°C every 5–8 min if there were no changes in the body's heat dissipation mechanisms, and exercise would be limited to less than 20 min before fatigue would occur from the effects of hyperthermia. In fact, moderately intensive physical activity can usually continue for more than 20 min, because of the effectiveness of the body's regulatory systems which act to alter rates of heat and mass transfer in response to specific stimuli.

At the onset of exercise, the rate of muscle heat production is a function of exercise intensity. At this instant, the rate of heat production exceeds the rate of heat dissipation from the muscle and a high rate of muscle heat storage develops, with an increase in muscle temperature. Saltin *et al.* (1968) have shown, by use of indwelling thermocouples, that the rate of temperature increase in the belly of the quadriceps muscle group approximates 1.0°C per minute during the initial transient of high intensity cycle ergometer exercise. This rate of heat storage cannot persist for very long, because the muscle machinery would then be inactivated by the effects of hyperthermia within 10 min. The measurements of Saltin *et al.* (1968) illustrate this point very well.

The primary means by which heat is removed from the muscle during exercise is by convective transfer to the blood stream. The rate of heat transfer is proportional to the product of the local blood flow and the temperature difference between the arterial blood and muscle. Before the onset of exercise, the rates of muscle metabolism and blood flow are low and the temperature of the arterial blood, about 37°C, is higher than muscle temperature, 33–35°C. Because heat flows down a temperature gradient, the resting heat transfer rate is low, due to the low rate of blood flow, and occurs from the arterial blood to the muscle. During the initial transient of exercise, the muscle blood flow rate increases as a consequence of neural and local influences, and the temperature gradient between arterial blood and muscle reverses, as the muscle temperature increases rapidly. Within several minutes after the onset of exercise, muscle blood flow attains a new, elevated plateau, proportional to the rate of energy metabolism and up to 30 times greater than that observed at rest. Heat is transferred down the temperature gradient from the warmer muscle to the blood during its passage through the muscle capillaries and the heat is then removed from the muscle by convective venous return to the body core. As the heat transfer rate increases to balance local heat production, the rate of heat storage in the muscle becomes negligible; muscle temperature thus plateaus at an elevated value as long as exercise persists and as long as there is no barrier preventing heat dissipation from the body to the environment.

Most of the heat generated in the contracting skeletal muscles is transferred to the body core via the venous return. Once this occurs, the body core temperature begins to rise, triggering reflexes that promote increased transfer of heat from the core to the skin and from the skin to the environment, thereby slowing and/or stopping the rate of rise of core temperature. The rate of heat transfer from the body core to the skin is determined by variables similar to those that determine the rate of heat transfer from muscle to core; that is, the temperature difference between the tissues, in this case the core and skin, and the rate of blood flow, in this case the skin blood flow. The overall conductance of heat to the skin is the sum of a fixed conductance, heat transfer by passive conduction from the core to the skin through inactive muscle and subcutaneous fat, and a variable conductance, heat transfer by convection in the blood as it flows from the body core to the skin. The skin blood flow is under physiological control and for the most part it determines changes in the flow of heat from the core to the skin. During exercise in the heat, skin blood flow can be as much as 20 times greater than during resting exposure to a cold environment, when the skin is maximally vasoconstricted. Thus, the ability to vasodilate the skin serves as one of the body's primary defences against overheating. However, it should not be forgotten that the net heat transfer rate from the core to the skin is the product of the rate of skin blood flow and the temperature difference between the core and the skin; thus, a high skin blood flow may not be sufficient to prevent the sequestration of heat in the body core during exercise on a hot, humid day when the skin temperature rises continuously due to an inability to evaporate sweat.

A fraction of the internally produced heat is transferred directly to the environment during exercise. Mitchell *et al.* (1972) quantified the rate of heat transfer from the respiratory tract by convection and evaporation at different intensities of exercise, demonstrating that the rate of respiratory heat loss is primarily a function of the rate of pulmonary ventilation. While this route of heat loss is small relative to the body's capacity for heat loss, it can be important during exercise in the cold, when heat conservation is the goal. A second means for heat transfer from the body core directly to the environment occurs when external work is performed. For example, when one pedals against a fixed resistance on a cycle ergometer, external work can be measured as the heat produced from the friction of the belt against the flywheel. When running on the level, external work is performed when one lifts the body off

the ground, but this work is recovered when one absorbs the impact as one lands back on the ground, and no net work occurs as a consequence.

Heat transfers from the body

Figure 16.1 illustrates the routes of heat transfer from the body core to the environment and the important factors that determine the transfer rates. Heat is transferred from the skin to the environment by convection, radiation and evaporation. The rates of heat transfer from the skin to the environment by convection and radiation are functions of the heat transfer coefficients (h_r and h_c) and the temperature differences between the skin and the environment; these rates of transfer are under physiological control only in so far as the changes in skin blood flow determine changes in the average temperature of the skin. Both h_r and h_c depend on the body surface area available for exchange with the environment. The value of h_r is constant, but the value of h_c varies directly with the air velocity (Nishi & Gagge, 1970) and differs dramatically between air and water environments (Rapp, 1971; Nadel *et al.*, 1974). The combined coefficient can vary fivefold between resting conditions in still air and when running on a breezy day, and therefore the rate of heat transfer by convection varies accordingly. However, on a very hot day, when the difference between the skin and ambient temperature is small, the ability to transfer heat from the skin to the environment is likewise small and of minimal importance in dissipating the thermal load of exercise.

The primary means by which humans are able to eliminate the thermal load of exercise, especially when exercise is performed in the heat, is via evaporation of sweat from the skin surface. The rate of evaporation is dependent upon the evaporative heat transfer coefficient, h_e, and the water vapour pressure gradient between the skin and the environment. The value of h_e depends on the air velocity in a similar fashion to the value of h_c (where $h_e =$

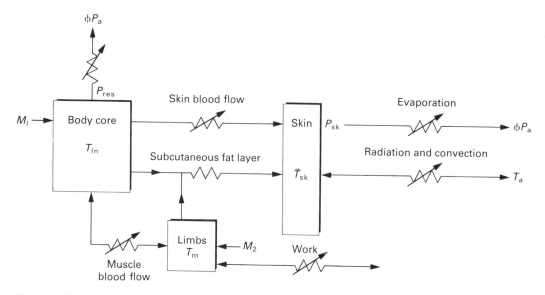

Fig. 16.1 Routes of heat transfer from the body core to the environment and the important factors that determine transfer rates. M, metabolic rate (M_1, at rest; M_2, during exercise); P, pressure; T, temperature.

2.2 h_c). The water vapour pressure of the skin is principally a function of the sweating rate, and thus under physiological control. A change of state from the liquid to the gaseous phase requires energy. Each gram of water evaporated from the skin surface removes about 2.5 kJ from the body. The sweat glands of a fit person can deliver sweat to the skin surface at rates up to about 30 g·min^{-1}, so nearly all of the heat produced during heavy exercise could be dissipated by evaporation in ideal conditions. The efficiency of the evaporative route of heat transfer is dependent upon both physiological and environmental factors. If the environmental humidity is high, the skin-to-environment water vapour pressure gradient cannot be elevated to a great extent and the evaporative rate will accordingly be low. This explains why excessive hyperthermia is inevitable during prolonged exercise on a hot, humid day. The rate of heat transfer by convection and radiation is low, due to the small skin-to-environment temperature gradient; the heat transfer rate by evaporation is likewise low, due to the small skin-to-environment water vapour pressure gradient. Thus, in the presence of a high rate of

heat production and a low rate of heat dissipation, heat is stored in the body and a progressive hyperthermia ensues.

With a knowledge of the heat transfer coefficients, and how they vary in different conditions, it becomes possible to predict, or at least anticipate the magnitude of change in internal body temperature during exercise at given intensities for different durations and in varying environmental conditions. This knowledge is important for the athlete, because the inability to maintain an optimal body temperature during exercise reduces performance, or results in an early onset of fatigue. To understand the means by which performance is affected by body temperature, it is necessary first to understand the physiology of temperature regulation.

Physiology of temperature regulation

All mammals have specialized thermosensitive nerve endings, within the central nervous system and over the skin surface, that relay information about the thermal status at these sites to a thermoregulatory centre, which also resides within the central nervous system. The thermal sensors on the skin serve to provide information about ambient temperature and, indirectly, the rate of heat transfer from the skin to the environment, and thus act as an early warning system in conditions of rapid changes in environmental temperature. The central thermosensors monitor the body core temperature and are especially important during exercise, one of the few naturally occurring conditions in which body core temperature is driven upward, and during immersion in cold water, one of the few naturally occurring conditions in which body core temperature is driven downward.

The primary effector organs that enable humans to modify the rates of heat transfer from the body core to the environment are the smooth muscles that control skin arteriolar resistance, and thereby heat conductance from the core to the skin, and the sweat glands, which secrete an ultrafiltrate of plasma on to the skin surface and thereby provide the substrate for evaporative cooling of the skin. In cases of excessive body cooling, skeletal muscles can act to produce heat above that generated by the basal metabolism by undergoing involuntary shivering contractions.

The central nervous system integrating centre for temperature regulation lies in the preoptic anterior hypothalamus. This centre can be thought of as constantly evaluating the thermal information from thermal receptors, comparing this information with an idealized thermal state and, in conditions in which these are not the same, directing changes in efferent activity that modify heat transfer to restore the ideal thermal state.

With this background it becomes easy to describe the thermoregulatory events that occur during exercise. As heat is transferred from the contracting muscles to the body core during the first minutes of exercise, body core temperature rises and the thermoreceptors in the hypothalamus increase their activity in response to the increase in local temperature. The hypothalamic integration centre determines that there is an error between the actual and ideal thermal states, and therefore increases efferent nervous system activity to the organs of heat dissipation. As the body core temperature rises, the threshold temperatures for skin vasodilatation and sweating are exceeded and the skin blood flow and sweating rates increase in proportion to the increase in body core temperature (Nadel *et al.*, 1971; Wenger *et al.*, 1975). Increases in the rate of heat transfer from the body core to the environment in response to a rising body core temperature cause an attenuation in the rate of rise of body core temperature. When the elevated rate of heat transfer from the body balances the rate of heat production in the body, the rate of heat storage becomes zero. The body core temperature remains elevated at the new steady state level until some new perturbation occurs. These events are depicted in Fig. 16.2 and described in more detail by Stitt (1979).

It is important to realize that the new steady state body core temperature is not regulated at its elevated level but has merely attained that elevated level as a consequence of: (i) the temporary imbalance between the rates of heat production in the body and heat dissipation from the body; and (ii) the 'quickness' of the heat dissipation response to the increase in body core temperature. Physical training induces an increase in the sensitivity of the sweating rate/internal temperature relationship, as well as a decrease in the internal temperature threshold for sweating (Nadel *et al.*, 1974); it thus provides for the attainment of the new, elevated steady state internal temperature at a lower level than when in the untrained state. This results in a somewhat greater margin of safety between the operating and limiting temperatures, as well as placing a lower demand on the peripheral circulation during exercise.

Exercise in the heat

The ability to deliver an adequate blood flow to the contracting skeletal muscles and to the skin

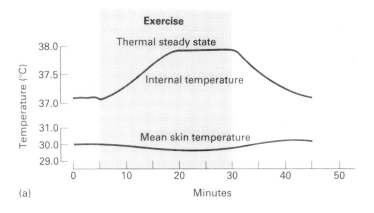

(a)

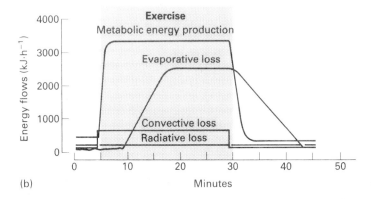

(b)

Fig. 16.2 Changes in (a) body temperature and (b) energy (heat) flows during exercise. A thermal steady state occurs when the rate of heat loss balances the rate of heat production. The absolute rise in internal temperature depends on the 'quickness' of the heat loss response.

in conditions in which both require a high flow rate, such as during prolonged heavy exercise in a warm or humid environment, depends largely on the body's ability to maintain an adequate central blood volume, which in turn provides for the maintenance of an adequate cardiac filling pressure and stroke volume. During mild intensity exercise or during exercise in a cool environment, the heart has no difficulty in providing an adequate output to meet the demands of both muscle and skin (Rowell *et al.*, 1966; Nadel *et al.*, 1979). During the former condition, the muscle blood flow requirement is relatively low and the heart meets the combined demand easily. In a cool environment the demand by the thermoregulatory system for blood flow to the skin is modest, and again the combined blood flow requirement is easily met by the heart. However, during moderately heavy exercise in a warm environment, the demands from skin and muscle become great and the ability of the heart to meet the high demand becomes increasingly compromised. Accompanying an increased skin blood flow is an increased blood volume in the capacious skin veins below the level of the heart; this reduces the central blood volume, the cardiac filling pressure and therefore the cardiac stroke volume. The effect is magnified when internal temperature is high (Fig. 16.3). While the muscle pump serves to aid the return of blood to the heart in such circumstances, the first reflex line of defence against a falling central venous pressure appears to be an increase in forearm vascular resistance (Johnson *et al.*, 1974; Tripathi *et al.*, 1989), which serves to reduce the volume of blood in the dependent veins. As the regulated arterial pressure decreases when the uncompensated fall in central venous pressure be-

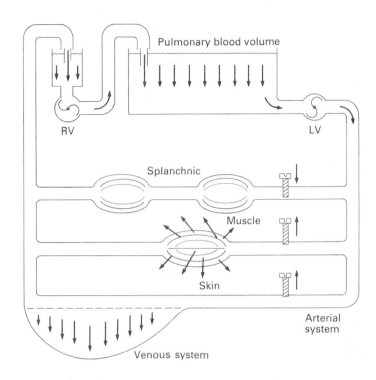

Pulmonary blood volume

RV

LV

Splanchnic

Muscle

Skin

Arterial system

Venous system

Fig. 16.3 Schematic representation of the factors associated with the pooling of blood in veins below heart level. LV, left ventricle; RV, right ventricle.

comes even greater, cardioacceleration occurs and compensates for the decrease in cardiac stroke volume, restoring cardiac output and arterial blood pressure if the exercise is conducted in the semirecumbent position (Nadel *et al.*, 1979), but not in the upright position (when the hydrostatic pressure head is greater; Rowell *et al.*, 1966). In the upright position, when the effects of gravity on a dilated cutaneous circulation are greatest, a heart rate increase of 20 beats·min^{-1} could not compensate for the decreased cardiac stroke volume; the cardiac output was found to be about 1.5 l·min^{-1} less during heavy exercise in the heat than during comparable exercise in a cool environment (Rowell *et al.*, 1966), despite a major redistribution of blood flow away from relatively inactive organs (Rowell *et al.*, 1965). Maximal cardiac stroke volume ought to be decreased as well in the latter condition (Rowell, 1983), and thus $\dot{V}_{O_2\,max}$, and performance, should be reduced by the same proportion.

Prolonged exercise in the heat presents a more complex problem for the body. Not only

is the ability to maintain an adequate cardiac stroke volume during exercise threatened by the displacement of a portion of the blood volume toward the periphery, but the continuous loss of body water due to the production and subsequent evaporation of sweat also decreases the body water content, including the water content of the intravascular compartment. In such conditions, a relative restriction in cutaneous blood flow occurs (Brengelmann *et al.*, 1977), presumably in response to a low pressure stimulus on the filling side of the heart. At the point of relative vasoconstriction in the skin, the progressive fall in cardiac stroke volume ceases (Nadel *et al.*, 1979). The consequence of a relative restriction in skin blood flow during prolonged exercise in the heat is that the optimal rate of heat transfer cannot occur. In our 1979 study, the exercising volunteer subjects continued to store heat at a rate of 0.1°C per minute, a storage that would limit exercise due to hyperthermia if continued for too long.

The more serious effects of prolonged exercise in the heat occur due to the progressive hypovolaemia accompanying dehydration. In actuality, the intravascular fluid compartment is defended reasonably well during dehydration, as the hyperosmolality that occurs as water leaves the vascular compartment tends to draw water in from the interstitial and intracellular fluid compartments (Nose *et al.*, 1988). None the less, hypovolaemia induces an upward shift in the internal temperature threshold for cutaneous vasodilation and a reduction in the maximal cutaneous blood flow (Nadel *et al.*, 1980); these changes cause a higher operating temperature due to a reduction in the maximal rate of heat transfer from the body core to the skin. Combined with the lower maximal cardiac stroke volume due to the lower central blood volume, the $\dot{V}o_{2\,max}$ should be reduced and the ability to prolong exercise at a high intensity should be compromised.

The question of whether blood flow to the active skeletal muscles can be maintained at appropriate rates during prolonged exercise in the heat is, in my mind, still an open one. If muscle blood flow is compromised, the rate of delivery of fuels and oxygen may become inadequate to meet the muscle's requirements, and fatigue will occur. Brown *et al.* (1982) claimed, from measurements of the relative rates of blood lactate accumulation during intense exercise in cool and hot conditions, that muscle blood flow might be lower in the heat. This confirmed the observations by Bell *et al.* (1983) of a lower muscle blood flow in sheep exercising in the heat compared with responses in a cool condition. However, as noted above (Rowell *et al.*, 1965), hepatic blood flow becomes progressively reduced during exercise in the heat and this may account for a reduced clearance of lactate by the liver, explaining the more rapid rate of its accumulation. Recently, Savard *et al.* (1988) reported that muscle blood flow was not reduced during exercise in the heat. They induced a heat load by using a water-perfused suit to clamp skin temperature at an artificially high level. While it is not yet clear to what extent the decrease in cardiac output

during upright, submaximal exercise in the heat (Rowell *et al.*, 1966) is reflected in a reduction in muscle blood flow, it is clear that the onset of fatigue occurs earlier.

Exercise in the cold

Generally speaking, cold stress is not an issue in so far as exercise performance or fatigue is concerned. The rate of heat production during exercise is sufficiently great to cause the risk of hyperthermia to be considered a potential problem, not the risk of hypothermia. The latter risk occurs occasionally during prolonged exercise when fatigue develops, heat production becomes reduced with the decrease in muscular activity and the participant is either inadequately clothed or the clothing is wet (promoting excessive evaporative cooling when inappropriate to thermoregulation).

The one environment that presents a cold stress during exercise, and therefore a legitimate risk of hypothermia, is the water. Water has a specific heat which is about 4000 times that of air and a thermal conductivity which is about 25 times greater. Thus, the heat transfer characteristics of water are much greater than those of air. Even when the body's rate of heat production is elevated 10–15-fold above resting levels, as can be the case during prolonged swimming, if the water temperature is low and the body's insulation is also relatively low, internal body temperature will fall steadily until it reaches a level at which confusion and disorientation occur and muscular activity cannot continue. Indeed, Keatinge (1969) cited press reports that attributed the many deaths associated with the sinking of the Titanic in April 1912 to drowning despite the fact that the Carpathia reached the scene of the disaster in less than 2 h and there were more than an adequate number of flotation devices available.

Because of its thermal properties, water has a much greater heat transfer coefficient than air and provides practically no insulation at its interface with the skin surface. Thus, the heat that reaches the skin surface from the body core is transferred rapidly to the water and the skin temperature rapidly approaches water temperature upon immersion. Since, as in an air environment, the heat flux from the body surface is a function of both the heat transfer coefficient and the skin-to-environment temperature gradient, the actual rate of heat flow from the body core to the water can be minimized if the resistance to heat flow from the core to the skin surface is large, thereby minimizing the rate of heat transfer from the core to the skin. This can be accomplished in any individual by maximal constriction of the skin vasculature, an autonomic response to body cooling; protection is more effective in fat than in thin individuals, due to the fact that fat is a relatively underperfused tissue having a thermal conductivity around half of that of muscle and a third of that of blood. Thus, the relative thickness of the subcutaneous fat layer is the primary determinant of heat flow from the body to the water. Keatinge (1960) recognized this years ago and this fact has been confirmed in subsequent studies which involved submaximal swimming (Holmér & Bergh, 1974).

To evaluate the driving force for heat loss to the water and the difference in this drive between resting and exercising conditions, we made measurements of heat flow and skin temperature while immersed and during swimming (Nadel et al., 1974). The heat transfer coefficient from the skin to the water was elevated threefold during swimming (independent of the swimming speed, to our surprise). Absolute values were close to those predicted from theoretical analyses (Rapp, 1971) and copper manikin studies (Witherspoon et al., 1971). However, knowledge of the heat transfer coefficient does not allow the prediction of the rate of development of hypothermia. The latter is dependent on the product of the transfer coefficient (elevated during swimming) and the skin-to-water temperature gradient (narrowed during swimming), as well as the rate of heat production (elevated during swimming) and the core-to-skin heat conductance (also elevated

during swimming). It appears that the best defence against body cooling in cold water is fat. The thermoregulatory system is relatively inadequate in the water because of water's great heat transfer properties.

Hypothermia should be avoided if optimal performance is the goal. Bergh and Ekblom (1979) showed that a decline of accompanied peak aerobic power and performance body cooling in the water. A decrease in performance in hypothermic athletes is the consequence of several possible factors, including an increased viscosity of skeletal muscle, requiring greater forces to overcome, an increased resistance to maximal blood flow, reducing maximal oxygen delivery, and a reduced maximal nerve conduction velocity, limiting the ability to transmit signals for repeated contractions.

Conclusions

The environment places many limits on the ability to perform an endurance task. In this chapter the limits imposed by thermal characteristics have been described. Limits imposed by clothing were not discussed; clothing imposes a barrier for optimal convective and evaporative cooling in a warm environment and offers an insulation against excessive convective and evaporative cooling in a cold environment. The effects of hyperthermia and hypothermia on performance generally occur via their influence on the body's ability to transfer oxygen from the environment to the contracting skeletal muscles, as outlined in the introduction to this chapter. Excessive body heating during exercise reduces the effectiveness of the circulatory system by limiting the heart's ability to deliver blood flow at the required rates to skin and muscle. Excessive body cooling during exercise is much more unusual than excessive heating, but is a real risk during exercise in the water.

References

Bell, A.W., Hales, J.R.S., King, R.B. & Fawcett, A.A. (1983) Influence of heat stress on exercise-induced changes in regional blood flow in sheep. *J. Appl. Physiol.* **55**, 1916–1923.

Bergh, U. & Ekblom, B. (1979) Physical performance and peak aerobic power at different body temperatures. *J. Appl. Physiol.* **46**, 885–889.

Brengelmann, G.L., Johnson, J.M., Hermansen, L. & Rowell, L.B. (1977) Altered control of skin blood flow during exercise at high internal temperatures. *J. Appl. Physiol.* **43**, 790–794.

Brown, N.J., Stephenson, L.A., Lister, G.L. & Nadel, E.R. (1982) Relative anaerobiosis during heavy exercise in the heat. *Fed. Proc.* **41**, 1677.

Edwards, R.H.T. (1981) Human muscle function and fatigue. In: *Human Muscle Fatigue: Physiological Mechanisms*, Ciba Foundation Symposium No. 82, pp. 1–18. Pitman Medical, London.

Holmér, I. & Bergh, U. (1974) Metabolic and thermal response to swimming in water at varying temperatures. *J. Appl. Physiol.* **37**, 702–705.

Johnson, J.M., Rowell, L.B., Niederberger, M. & Eisman, M.M. (1974) Human splanchnic and forearm vasoconstrictor responses to reductions of right atrial and aortic pressures. *Circ. Res.* **34**, 515–524.

Keatinge, W.R. (1960) The effects of subcutaneous fat and of previous exposure to cold on the body temperature, peripheral blood flow and metabolic rate of men in cold water. *J. Physiol (Lond.)* **153**, 166–178.

Keatinge, W.R. (1969) *Survival in Cold Water*. Blackwell Scientific Publications, Oxford.

Mitchell, J.W., Nadel, E.R. & Stolwijk, J.A.J. (1972) Respiratory weight losses during exercise. *J. Appl. Physiol.* **32**, 474–476.

Nadel, E.R., Bullard, R.W. & Stolwijk, J.A.J. (1971) Importance of skin temperature in the regulation of sweating. *J. Appl. Physiol.* **31**, 80–87.

Nadel, E.R., Cafarelli, E., Roberts, M.F. & Wenger, C.B. (1979) Circulatory regulation during exercise in different ambient temperatures. *J. Appl. Physiol.* **46**, 430–437.

Nadel, E.R., Fortney, S.M. & Wenger, C.B. (1980) Effect of hydration state on circulatory and thermal regulations. *J. Appl. Physiol.* **49**, 715–721.

Nadel, E.R., Holmér, I., Bergh, U., Åstrand, P.-O. & Stolwijk, J.A.J. (1974) Energy exchanges of swimming man. *J. Appl. Physiol.* **36**, 465–471.

Nadel, E.R., Pandolf, K.B., Roberts, M.F., Wenger, C.B. & Stolwijk, J.A.J. (1974) Mechanisms of thermal adaptation to exercise and heat. *J. Appl. Physiol.* **37**, 515–520.

Nishi, Y. & Gagge, A.P. (1970) Direct evaluation of convective heat transfer coefficient by naphthalene sublimation. *J. Appl. Physiol.* **29**, 603–609.

Nose, H., Mack, G.W., Shi, X. & Nadel, E.R. (1988) Role of osmolality and plasma volume during rehydration in humans. *J. Appl. Physiol.* **65**, 325–331.

Rapp, G.M. (1971) Convection coefficients of man in a forensic area of thermal physiology. *J. Physiol. (Paris)* **63**, 392–396.

Rowell, L.B. (1983) Cardiovascular adjustments to thermal stress. In: Shepherd, J.M. & Abboud, F.M. (eds) *Handbook of Physiology: The Cardiovascular System III*, pp. 967–1023. The American Physiological Society, Bethesda, MD.

Rowell, L.B., Blackmon, J.R., Martin, R.H., Mazzarella, J.A. & Bruce, R.A. (1965) Hepatic clearances of indocyanine green in man under thermal and exercise stresses. *J. Appl. Physiol.* **20**, 384–394.

Rowell, L.B., Marks, H.J., Bruce, R.A., Conn, R.D. & Kusumi, F. (1966) Reductions in cardiac output, central blood volume and stroke volume with thermal stress in normal men during exercise. *J. Clin. Invest.* **43**, 1801–1816.

Saltin, B., Gagge, A.P. & Stolwijk, J.A.J. (1968) Muscle temperature during submaximal exercise in man. *J. Appl. Physiol.* **25**, 679–688.

Savard, G.K., Nielsen, B., Laszczynska, I., Larsen, B.E. & Saltin, B. (1988) Muscle blood flow is not reduced in humans during moderate exercise and heat stress. *J. Appl. Physiol.* **64**, 649–657.

Stitt, J.T. (1979) Fever versus hyperthermia. *Fed. Proc.* **38**, 39–43.

Tripathi, A., Mack, G.W. & Nadel, E.R. (1989) Peripheral vascular reflexes elicited during lower body negative pressure. *Aviat. Space Environ. Med.* **60**, 1187–1193.

Wenger, C.B., Roberts, M.F., Stolwijk, J.A.J. & Nadel, E.R. (1975) Forearm blood flow during body temperature transients produced by leg exercise. *J. Appl. Physiol.* **38**, 58–63.

Witherspoon, J.M., Goldman, R.F. & Breckenridge, J.R. (1971) Heat transfer coefficients of humans in cold water. *J. Physiol. (Paris)* **63**, 459–462.

Chapter 17

Economy of Movement and Endurance Performance

EDWARD C. FREDERICK

Efficiency versus economy

Most sports biomechanists think of efficiency as the ratio of power output to power input. In other words, efficiency expresses the proportion of metabolic power required to produce a given physical power output. If we look at the power produced, for example on a cycle ergometer, relative to the metabolic power expended we see that humans have a gross efficiency of about 15%. To generate 45 W of power on a cycle ergometer, we need to expend about 300 W of metabolic power (Stegemann, 1981).

The problem with such calculations is that they do not completely measure the mechanical power produced. When we pedal a cycle ergometer, work is being done to move the mass of the limbs and trunk, to perform a variety of non-productive counter movements, and to sustain isometric 'work'. If one simply sits on an ergometer and pedals with no load, for example, oxygen intake increases because physical work is being done although no *measurable work* is being performed. Much of this unmeasurable work is excluded from most calculations of efficiency. In addition, as Lafortune and Cavanagh (1983) have pointed out, significant work is being done on the cycle ergometer itself, in distorting the frame and bending components, and this work is not included in that measured by a conventional ergometer. Such examples underscore the diffi-

culties in assessing mechanical power and efficiency.

It turns out to be very difficult to measure or to calculate the precise mechanical power output of a moving human body, and so exact measurements of efficiency are not possible for sports movements. However, the concept is an interesting one and helpful in elucidating the influence of biomechanics on endurance performance, and so it is a topic worth exploring further with these limitations firmly in mind.

Let us start with the assumption that we are dealing with endurance sports where metabolic power is limiting. A given athlete trains physiological systems to the point where a certain level of metabolic power consumption can be sustained for a set amount of time and the limit then becomes the amount of mechanical power that can be developed, given the metabolic power available. A runner, for example, might be able to sustain 90% of maximal oxygen intake ($\dot{V}_{O_2 \, max}$) for 30 min. That corresponds to about 1500 W for a champion class runner. The total mechanical power requirement of running at a speed of 330 m·min^{-1} is roughly 800 W. In this example, the runner is then constrained only by the amount of physical work that can be performed with the available energy during the allotted time. The more efficiently the runner moves, the faster he or she can run.

Such an improvement in efficiency might be

179

affected by changing the pattern of movement to reduce mechanical power output that does not contribute to forward movement (e.g. by reducing unnecessary excursions of the centre of mass of the body). Or, as we have previously discussed, the runner might modify a number of extrinsic factors that are increasing the extraneous workload, for instance, reducing air resistance with a wind suit or wearing lighter shoes. If power requirements can be reduced to say 750 W by manipulating these factors then the athlete would be able to run about 6% faster with the same expenditure of metabolic power. This is a gross oversimplification of a complex topic but it underscores the influence of mechanical constraints and biomechanical adaptations upon endurance performance.

It becomes clear from Chapter 15 that a number of factors that influence endurance are closely linked to the moderation of extraneous mechanical work and an improved efficiency of movement. But, as mentioned, work and power output are difficult to determine for complex movements such as those used in sports. For this reason, physiologists and biomechanists usually retreat to the relative comfort of the term 'economy of movement'.

Economy of movement is defined as the relative metabolic power or energy required to perform a given task. The task might be, for example, to swim at a velocity of 100 m·min^{-1}, to run at 300 m·min^{-1}, or to dribble a soccer ball 100 m in 20 s. Metabolic power requirements are usually measured via oxygen intake. The notion here is that the less energy it takes to perform the task, the more economical the movement.

By inference, we might also be tempted to say that the movement is more efficient, but that may not be the case. In fact, in most cases of improved economy, the agent of change is more likely a reduction in the mechanical power requirement. In this case, efficiency may actually remain unchanged or even decrease.

Factors that affect economy of movement

Economy of movement is important in all endurance sports, but its role has been particularly well explored in distance running. A number of authors have shown a strong correlation between success in distance running and the economy of running (Costill & Fox, 1969; Costill & Winrow, 1970; Gregor & Kirkendall, 1978). So it is desirable to modify running style, and presumably the patterns of movement used in other endurance sports, in a way that improves the economy of movement. The contribution of biomechanics is to determine what kinetic and kinematic patterns are consistent with greater economy.

Factors that have been shown to influence the economy of movement can be divided into two principal categories: extrinsic and intrinsic. Tables 17.1 and 17.2 summarize a number of such factors.

Extrinsic factors include the effects of environment, surfaces and equipment. Intrinsic factors include biological rhythms, kinanthropometric, psychological and biomechanical variables. The tables include factors that have been shown by direct experimental evidence to affect economy as well as factors that have been shown to be statistically correlated with economy. Because factors with a statistical relationship may not have a direct effect on economy, those factors are indicated with an asterisk.

Under kinanthropometric constraints such as body weight and leg length, one should also include the distribution of body weight. As an example, consider the predicted effect of foot size on the economy of running. Extreme departures from the normal foot size at a given height can bring advantages or disadvantages to the endurance athlete. The relationship between foot size and the calculated energy required to transport the feet during running (Frederick, 1987) shows that people with bigger feet expend significantly more energy to main-

Table 17.1 Extrinsic factors known to influence the economy of movement. These factors can be positively or negatively associated with economical movement.

Extrinsic factor	Reference
Environmental factors	
Ambient temperature	Sato *et al.* (1983)
Wind	Pugh (1971)
Surface-related factors	
Grade	Pugh (1971)
Surface compliance	Passmore & Durnin (1955); Ralston (1981)
Surface resilience	Strydom *et al.* (1966)
Equipment-related factors	
Orthotics	Hayes *et al.* (1983)
Shoe sole hardness	Frederick *et al.* (1983)
Shoe weight	Frederick (1985c)
Weight on head or trunk	Soule & Goldman, (1969)

Table 17.2 Intrinsic factors known to influence the economy of movement. These factors can be positively or negatively associated with economical movement.

Intrinsic factor	Reference
Kinanthropometric factors	
Body weight	Cureton *et al.* (1978)
Leg length*	van der Walt & Wyndham (1973)
Psychological factors	
Relaxation	Benson *et al.* (1978)
Hypnotic suggestion	Morgan & Brown (1983)
Biological rhythms	
Circadian rhythms	Reilly & Brooks (1982)
Circannual rhythms	Zahorska-Markiewicz & Markiewicz (1984)
Kinetic and kinematic factors	
Centre of mass excursion*	Williams (1980)
Mechanical energy transfers	Pierrynowski *et al.* (1980); Shorten *et al.* (1981)
Net positive work rate*	Williams (1980)
Impact force*	Williams (1980)
Foot strike*	Williams (1980)
Foot contact time*	Williams (1980)
Extraneous arm motion*	Williams (1980)
Angle of trunk inclination*	Williams (1980)
Angle of shank inclination*	Williams (1980)
Lower knee flexion velocity in support	Frederick *et al.* (1983)
Plantar flexion at toe-off*	Williams (1980)
Stride length	Cavanagh & Williams (1982)

* Statistical association rather than direct experimental evidence.

tain a given running speed. At the extremes of foot size this effect is large enough to have a significant effect on endurance performance. One can imagine a host of other anatomically mediated biomechanical effects, but this is a poorly explored area.

Many of the factors listed in Tables 17.1 and 17.2, such as foot size, are immutable, or simply a consequence of the circumstances of the movement or the environment in which the movement is performed. Others, however, are changeable and beg to be explored as potential keys to economical movement. This is especially true of factors connected with the kinetics and kinematics of movement.

Improving economy biomechanically

A few central themes have the potential to unite these variables into a single mechanism or group of mechanisms that have broader implications for improved economy of movement. One such theme is the transfer of energy between and within body segments. Both Williams (1980) and Shorten et al. (1981) have shown a strong statistical association between segmental energy transfer and economical movement, and their mathematical models support that notion. Likewise, Norman et al. (1985) have shown that a major biomechanical factor related to success in cross-country skiing is the capacity to effect greater transfers of mechanical energy. And Pierrynowski et al. (1980) have elaborated on the role of energy transfer in walking efficiency.

However, there are problems with between segment energy transfer calculations, because the constraints are selected on an arbitrary basis, independently of the pattern of muscle activation. Within segment transfers do not suffer from these problems and so may yield more useful insights. In either case, several of the biomechanical variables correlated with economical movement may in fact be cross-correlated with the segmental transfer of energy. Such factors as the angle of the shank,

knee flexion velocity and net positive work rate (Williams, 1980) may be part of a multisegmental strategy to enhance segmental energy transfers.

These observations should be followed up in two ways. Firstly, a synthesis of improved mathematical models that incorporate electromyographic data and more precise anatomical measurements of the line of pull of muscles might help us to predict what kinematic adjustments in movement patterns might cause greater transfers of energy. Secondly, we need to test these ideas experimentally. A starting point might be to determine which kinematic patterns the models predict will enhance energy transfer and then to examine whether such energy transfers improve economy. It has been suggested that this might be done by using biofeedback techniques to modify subjects' kinematics and then to test this hypothesis (Frederick, 1985b). Sanderson and Cavanagh (1986) have recently demonstrated the feasibility of feedback training as a means of modifying the biomechanics of cycling. This approach shows great promise for future investigations of this subject.

Another possible mechanism for more economical movement is the excursion of the body's centre of mass, although this approach has its limitations. Point-mass models treat the body as if it were a single point mass located at its centre of mass. Such models have illuminated some of the factors underlying the work−energy relationship, but they suffer from the fundamental problem that kinetic energy is not a vector quantity. So, tracking the body centre of mass is not sufficient to estimate the total kinetic energy of the body. Shorten (1983) has shown that this method underestimates the total kinetic energy of the body even if the kinetic energy of the limbs relative to the centre of mass is factored in. Because of this inherent limitation, we do not have the support of good mechanical models to pursue this possibility experimentally.

In fact, there is an interesting paradox that

deals with the economy of running and the excursion of the centre of mass. It helps to elucidate some of the problems with point-mass models:

1 Peak vertical ground reaction forces appear to be proportional to body mass.

2 It is generally observed that as running speed increases the vertical excursion of the centre of gravity *decreases*.

3 When running speed increases, oxygen intake and force increase even though the centre of mass has a lesser excursion.

This paradox undermines the common assertion that reducing centre of mass excursion in running will improve running economy. It may, but there are other confounding factors.

Despite this limitation of mathemical modelling, there may still be a specific effect due to the excursion of the body's centre of mass. Although a direct association has never been proven, good sense suggests that a number of the intrinsic variables which correlate with economy are probably cross-correlated with centre of mass excursion. Such variables as leg length, stride length, and angle of the shank, knee flexion, plantar flexion at toe-off and angle inclination of the trunk may be linked with the excursion of the centre of mass. It would be interesting directly to test the role of these effects on economy by experimentally manipulating kinematics.

A third possibility is that the storage and return of strain energy in tendon and muscle is a major determinant of running economy. We might test the importance of this factor by training subjects to run with styles that our models (e.g. Pierrynowski *et al.* 1980; Williams, 1980; Shorten, 1983) predict should enhance or diminish elastic storage. Indeed, it may be that most of the kinetic and kinematic factors associated with an economical running style are subsets of a strategy to maximize the elastic storage of energy. Such factors as foot strike index, contact time, knee flexion, stride length, leg length, and so on may contribute to the storage of strain energy.

Even these three larger themes of energy transfer, centre of mass excursion and strain energy storage may be interconnected. Indeed, one sees very quickly how mechanically interdependent these factors are. We need a rational approach to dealing with a synthesis of these ideas and the link-segmental approach seems the best hope for leading us through this maze of seemingly linked ideas.

Strategies for optimization have been proposed by Hatze (1983) and Hay (1973). Optimization might be another interesting approach to improving economy of movement, even though the methods are not specifically suited to this problem. Despite this limitation it would seem that the optimization of repetitive movements used in endurance sports should lead to greater economy and enhanced endurance.

Summary

Biomechanical factors play a broad and varied role in the development of endurance. Mechanical constraints on endurance performance include gravity, mass, friction, centripetal force, and both aerodynamic and hydrodynamic lift and drag. Biomechanical factors influence endurance mainly through changes in the mechanical power requirements resulting from these constraints. Such changes in mechanical power are usually expressed as improvements in efficiency, or more commonly, the energetic economy of movement. A review of the intrinsic and extrinsic factors affecting the economy of movement points to several potential areas for future improvement in endurance performance via the manipulation of kinetic and kinematic factors. This is one of the areas of research on endurance performance that should lead to significant advances in the next decade. Further elaborations of mathematical models and the development of feedback techniques for testing theories about what makes movements economical should give us new insights into the role of biomechanics in endurance performance.

References

Benson, H., Dryer, T. & Hartley, L.H. (1978) Decreased oxygen consumption during exercise with elicitation of the relaxation response. *J. Hum. Stress* **4**, 38–42.

Cavanagh, P.R. & Williams, K.R. (1982) The effect of stride length variation on the oxygen uptake during distance running. *Med. Sci. Sports Exerc.* **17**, 30–35.

Costill, D.L. & Fox, E.L. (1969) Energetics of marathon running. *Med. Sci. Sports Exerc.* **1**, 81–86.

Costill, D.L. & Winrow, E. (1970) Maximal oxygen uptake among marathon runners. *Arch. Phys. Med. Rehab.* **51**, 317–320.

Cureton, K.J., Sparling, P.B., Evans, B.W., Johnson, S.M., Kong, U.D. & Purvis, J.W. (1978) Effect of experimental alterations in excess weight on aerobic capacity and distance running performance. *Med. Sci. Sports Exerc.* **10**, 194–199.

Frederick, E.C. (1985a) The energy cost of load carriage on the feet during running. In: Winter, D.A., Norman, R.W., Wells, R.P., Hayes, K.C. & Patla, A.E. (eds) *Biomechanics IX -B*, pp. 295–300. Human Kinetics, Champaign, Illinois.

Frederick, E.C. (1985b) Synthesis, experimentation and the biomechanics of economical movement. *Med. Sci. Sports Exerc.* **17**, 44–47.

Frederick, E.C. (1985c) The energy cost of load carriage on the feet during running. In: Winter, D.A., Norman, R.W., Wells, R.P., Hayes, K.C. & Patla, A.E. (eds) *Biomechanics IX -B*, pp. 295–300. Human Kinetics, Champaign, Illinois.

Frederick, E.C. (1987) Biomechanical aspects of endurance. In: MacLeod, D., Maughan, R., Nimmo, M., Reilly, T. & Williams, C. (eds) *Exercise — Benefits, Limits, and Adaptations*, pp. 205–219. E. & F.N. Spon, London.

Frederick, E.C., Clarke, T.E., Larsen, J.L. & Cooper, L.B. (1983) The effects of shoe cushioning on the oxygen demands of running. In: Nigg, B.M. & Kerr, B.A. (eds) *Biomechanical Aspects of Sport Shoes and Playing Surfaces*, pp. 107–114. University of Calgary, Calgary, Alberta.

Gregor, R.J. & Kirkendall, D. (1978) Performance efficiency of world class female marathon runners. In: Asmussen, E. & Jorgensen, K. (eds) *Biomechanics VI-B*, pp. 40–45. University Park Press, Baltimore, Maryland.

Hatze, H. (1983) Computerized optimization of sports motions: an overview of possibilities, methods and recent developments. *J. Sports Sci.* **1**, 3–12.

Hay, J.G. (1973) Some thoughts on the ultimate in high jumping technique. *Sixth Congress of the International Track and Field Association*, Madrid, 1973.

Hayes, J., Smith, L. & Santopietro, F. (1983) The effects of orthotics on the aerobic demands of running. *Med. Sci. Sports Exerc.* **15**, 169.

Lafortune, M.A. & Cavanagh, P.R. (1983) Effectiveness and efficiency in bicycle riding. In: Matsui, H. & Kobayashi, K. (eds) *Biomechanics VIII-B*, pp. 928–936. University Park Press, Baltimore, Maryland.

Morgan, W.P. & Brown, D.R. (1983) Hypnosis. In: Williams, M. (ed.) *Ergogenic Aids in Sport*, pp. 223–252. Human Kinetics, Champaign, Illinois.

Norman, R., Caldwell, G. & Komi, P. (1985) Differences in body segment energy utilization between world-class and recreational cross-country skiers. *Int. J. Sports Biomech.* **1**, 253–262.

Passmore, R. & Durnin, J.V.G.A. (1955) Human energy expenditure. *Physiol. Rev.* **35**, 801–836.

Pierrynowski, M.R., Winter, D.R. & Norman, R.W. (1980) Transfers of mechanical energy within the total body and mechanical efficiency during treadmill walking. *Ergonomics* **23**, 147–156.

Pugh, L.G.C.E. (1971) The influence of wind resistance in running and walking and the mechanical efficiency of work against gravity. *J. Physiol.* **213**, 255–276.

Ralston, H.J. (1981) Energy expenditure. In: Inman, V.T., Ralston, H.J. & Todd F. (eds) *Human Walking*, pp. 62–77. William & Wilkins, Baltimore, Maryland.

Reilly, T. & Brooks, G.A. (1982) Investigation of circadian rhythms in metabolic responses to exercise. *Ergonomics* **25**, 1093–1107.

Sanderson, D. & Cavanagh, P.R. (1986) An investigation of the use of augmented feedback to modify the application of forces to the pedals during cycling. *Med. Sci. Sports Exerc.* **18**(2), S63.

Sato, M., Yasutaka, S., Inuoue, K., Fukuba, Y., Fujiie, K. & Yoshioka, H. (1983) The effect of air temperature on maximal oxygen uptake. *J. Anthropol. Soc. Nippon* **91**, 377–388.

Shorten, M. (1983) Mechanical energy models and the efficiency of human movement. *Int. J. Model. Simul.* **3**, 15–19.

Shorten, M.R., Wooten, S.A. & Williams, C. (1981) Mechanical energy changes and the oxygen cost of running. *Eng. Med.* **10**, 213–217.

Strydom, N.B., Bredell, G.A.G., Benade, A.J.S., Morrison, J.F., Vigoen, H.J. & van Graan, C.H. (1986) The metabolic cost of marching at 3 mph over firm and sandy surfaces. *Eur. J. Appl. Physiol.* **23**, 166–170.

Soule, R.G. & Goldman, R.F. (1969) Energy cost of loads carried on the head, hands or feet. *J. Appl. Physiol.* **27**, 687–690.

Stegemann, J. (1981) *Exercise Physiology: Physiologic Bases of Work and Sport*. Yearbook Medical, Chicago, Illinois.

Williams, K.R. (1980) *A biomechanical and physiological*

evaluation of running efficiency. Unpublished doctoral dissertation. Pennsylvania State University.

van der Walt, W.H. & Wyndham, C.H. (1973) An equation for prediction of energy expenditure of walking and running. *J. Appl. Physiol.* **34**, 559–563.

Zahorska-Markiewicz, B. & Markiewicz, A. (1984) Circannual rhythm of exercise metabolic rate in humans. *Eur. J. Appl. Physiol.* **52**, 328–330.

PART 3

MEASUREMENTS OF ENDURANCE

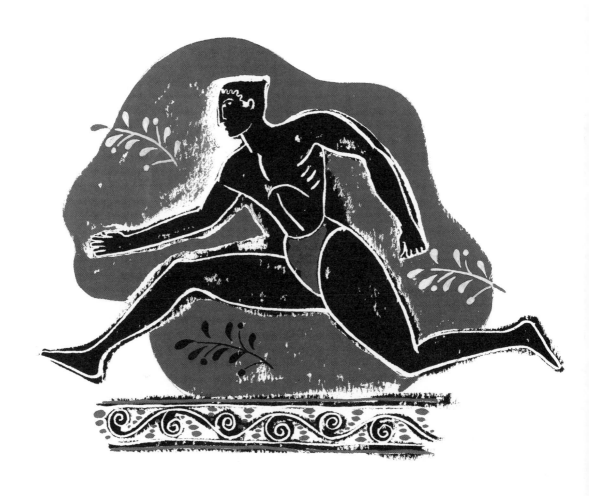

Chapter 18

Factors to be Measured

PER-OLOF ÅSTRAND

Athletic competition represents the classical test of physical fitness and performance. Under such conditions the performance may be measured objectively in metres and centimetres, and in time down to hundredths of seconds in some events. In sport shooting there is the point system. In gymnastics, figure skating and diving, the skill is judged subjectively. From a scientific point of view we have the inevitable question: why does one athlete in one particular competition perform better than the others? Figure 18.1 presents a simple effort to break down an analysis of physical performance into some basic components. If, without exception, élite athletes in one event

have a high maximal oxygen intake the event is apparently very demanding aerobically; that is the case in rowers, for whom oxygen intake in litres per minute is critical. In events such as middle- and long-distance running the aerobic power, expressed in $ml \cdot kg^{-1} \cdot min^{-1}$, must be high. In endurance events, aerobic processes dominate. Figure 18.2 is an effort to summarize the factors that should be considered when analysing the aerobic demands of various events and the individual's potential to perform well. There are precise methods to measure the aerobic power because for each litre of oxygen consumed in the cells about 20 kJ is yielded for the resynthesis of adenosine triphosphate (ATP) (range 19.7–21.2 kJ, depending on the proportions of carbohydrate and free fatty acids metabolized). Unfortunately we have no good methods to quantify anaerobic power accurately. However, this is not a dramatic handicap when endurance is being considered.

Most of the measurements related to physiological and behavioural aspects of sports are made under standardized conditions in laboratories. Under field conditions, measurements can be very difficult and sophisticated studies during important competitions are more or less impossible to carry out. Therefore, the question is to what extent can we extrapolate our knowledge from studies in laboratories to field conditions? Is there a risk that we generalize too much? There is a specificity in the human response to a particular exercise and in the effects of training. For example, two identical twins

Physical performance

Energy output
Aerobic processes
Anaerobic processes

Neuromuscular function
Strength
Technique

Psychological factors
Motivation
Tactics

Fig. 18.1 Basic factors influencing physical performance.

189

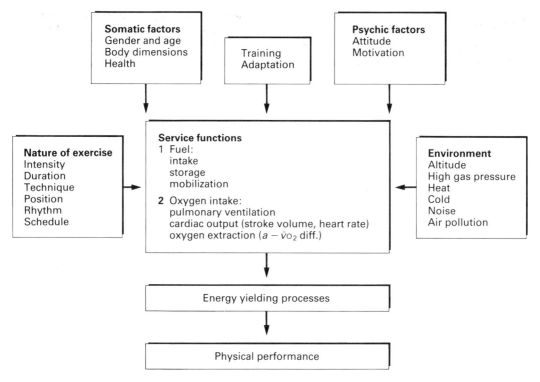

Fig. 18.2 Factors influencing the power and capacity for aerobic muscular activity. From Åstrand & Rodahl (1986), with permission.

were top swimmers but one of the sisters gave up training. Some years later their maximal oxygen intakes were measured both when they were running on a treadmill and when swimming in a flume. On that occasion they were students in physical education and were well trained. The sister who also under-took intensive swimming training attained the same maximal aerobic power when running as when swimming, 3.6 l·min^{-1}. Her sister, now not swim-trained, reached a similar maximum when running, 3.6 l·min^{-1} but achieved only 2.8 l·min^{-1} when swimming (Holmér & Åstrand, 1972). Unfortunately we cannot explain the nature of the specificity of training. We have access to telemetric systems to transmit signals triggered by heart rate, blood pressure and muscle activity which do not bother the subjects. There are efforts to construct lightweight equipment to follow pulmonary ventilation and oxygen intake under field conditions, but inevitably the subject becomes restricted. For analyses of blood and muscle specimens we must 'go under the skin', which sometimes worries athletes. Cycle ergometers and treadmills are supplemented with equipment for rowing, canoeing, swimming and skiing (see Chapter 20). Computerized methods are developed for the study of locomotion and body composition.

There is a danger with equipment that produces printed data because of the tendency to believe in all figures obtained from computers. For example, the sophisticated methods available to measure oxygen intake. Of key importance for reliability here is the calibration of the apparatus. Too many laboratory workers have forgotten how to analyse a gas chemically using Haldane or Scholander apparatus.

References

Åstrand, P.-O. & Rodahl, K. (1986) *Textbook of Work Physiology*. McGraw-Hill, New York.

Holmér, I. & Åstrand, P.-O. (1972) Swimming training and maximal oxygen uptake. *J. Appl. Physiol.* **33**, 510–513.

Chapter 19

Maximal Oxygen Intake

ROY J. SHEPHARD

Significance of maximal oxygen intake

Maximal oxygen intake measures the ability of the body to transport oxygen from ambient air to the working muscles, and it is one of the more important determinants of endurance performance. Indeed, if international performers in events such as cross-country skiing are compared with the general population (Table 19.1), their maximal oxygen intakes (with occasional male values as high as $85-90$ ml·kg^{-1}min^{-1}) lie as much as four to five standard deviations above the norm for a healthy young man (48 ± 8 ml·kg^{-1}min^{-1}). In events of 1-min duration, as much as 50% of the energy needs of the body may be satisfied by anaerobic metabolism, but if all-out activity is continued for 5 min, 80% of the required energy is derived from aerobic metabolism, and with 60 min of effort, 98% of metabolism is aerobic.

Criteria of maximal oxygen intake

The principle of measurement is simple. The intensity of large muscle effort is increased in either a stepwise progressive test or a series of several individual tests of suitably graded intensity until a 'plateau' of oxygen intake is reached (Fig. 19.1). The 'plateau' has been defined arbitrarily as an increase in oxygen consumption of less than 2 ml·kg^{-1}·min^{-1} with a further increase in the intensity of effort (for

example, a further 1% increase of treadmill grade at a consistent speed of running).

The demonstration of an oxygen consumption plateau is thought to imply that the individual who is being tested has reached a central limitation of effort — that is to say that under the particular conditions of measurement, the heart is unable to develop a larger maximal cardiac output, and is thus 'responsible' for the plateauing of oxygen transport. However, in practice, a proportion of subjects halt an intended maximal exercise test because of peripheral symptoms such as muscle weakness, pain or fatigue, despite the strong urgings of the investigator, and in many subjects a satisfactory oxygen consumption plateau cannot be demonstrated. There are then attempts to evaluate the 'quality' of the observed effort in terms of such subsidiary criteria of maximal performance as the peak heart rate (preferably at least 220 − the individual's age in years), the peak respiratory gas exchange ratio (carbon dioxide output : oxygen intake, a measure of metabolic acidosis, preferably higher than 1.10) and the peak blood lactate (preferably at least $10-12$ mmol·l^{-1} in young adults and around 8 mmol·l^{-1} in older individuals).

Demonstration of a centrally limited plateau of oxygen consumption depends upon the activation of a large muscle volume. Thus, plateaux are seen much less frequently during cycle ergometry (heavily dependent upon the quadriceps) than in uphill treadmill running (a task widely distributed over the major muscle

Table 19.1 Typical values of maximal oxygen intake in various sports. From Neumann (1988).

Type of event	Maximal oxygen intake ($ml \cdot kg^{-1} min^{-1}$)	
	Men	Women
Endurance sports		
Long-distance running	75–80	65–70
Cross-country skiing	75–78	65–70
Biathlon	75–78	—
Road cycling	70–75	60–65
Middle-distance running	70–75	65–68
Skating	65–72	55–60
Orienteering	65–72	60–65
Swimming	60–70	55–60
Rowing	65–69	60–64
Track racing	65–70	55–60
Canoeing	60–68	50–55
Walking	60–65	55–60
Games		
Football (soccer)	50–57	—
Handball	55–60	48–52
Ice hockey	55–60	—
Volleyball	55–60	48–52
Basketball	50–55	40–45
Tennis	48–52	40–45
Table tennis	40–45	38–42
Combative sports		
Boxing	60–65	—
Wrestling	60–65	—
Judo	55–60	50–55
Fencing	45–50	40–45
Power sports		
Sprint (200 m track)	55–60	45–50
Sprint track and field (100 m, 200 m)	48–52	43–47
Long jump	50–55	45–50
Competition consisting of several events (decathlon, septathlon)	60–65	50–55
Nordic combination (15 km ski walking and ski jumping)	60–65	—
Weightlifting	40–50	—
Discus throwing, shot-putting	40–45	35–40
Javelin throwing	45–50	42–47
Pole vaulting	45–50	—
Ski jumping	40–45	—
Technical-acrobatic sports		
Downhill skiing (Alpine disciplines)	60–65	48–53
Figure skating	50–55	45–50
Gymnastics	45–50	40–45
Rhythmic gymnastics	—	40–45
Sailing	50–55	45–50
Shooting	40–45	35–40

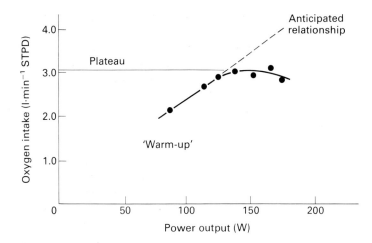

Fig. 19.1 Graph illustrating the principles of maximal oxygen intake measurement. After a 'warm-up', the power output on a sport-specific ergometer is increased progressively every 1–2 min until three successive increments augment the oxygen consumption by a total of less than 2 ml·kg^{-1}·min^{-1}. From Shephard (1982), with permission.

groups). Although the information on peak oxygen transport is more satisfying if a plateau has been reached, some authors maintain that peak values without a clear plateau are equally consistent and useful in the management of the athlete.

Preparations for a maximal effort test

The commonly recommended preparations for a maximal effort test include 24 h of rest, an overnight fast, and a room temperature of 22°C (Andersen et al., 1971; Shephard, 1977). It may be difficult to persuade a top athlete to accept 24 h of total rest, and indeed the state of the body would then be unrepresentative of normal conditions. However, the investigator should insist that the athlete take a lighter than average workout on the day preceding a maximal test. Some laboratories may also lack air conditioning; there is no evidence that a room temperature higher than 22°C has any direct influence on the results of a brief maximal oxygen intake test, although prolonged heat exposure, with resultant salt and mineral depletion, can have a negative effect upon test scores. If the room is hot, the comfort of the test subject can be improved by the use of a well placed fan. Often, the heat loss thus achieved is equivalent to a 2°C decrease in room temperature.

Test scores vary somewhat with the time of day. The largest values are observed in the morning (when central blood volume has been maximized by a night of recumbency). The time of testing should thus be noted carefully, and where possible it should be matched to the anticipated time of competition.

Choice of ergometer

In the general population, uphill treadmill running is regarded as the best method of eliciting a centrally limited maximal effort. However, such an approach gives an imprecise evaluation of aerobic potential in most types of endurance performer. One peculiarity of the endurance competitor is an ability to approach (or in some cases, even to exceed) the treadmill maximal oxygen consumption while performing their specific sport. A variety of special devices such as swimming flumes and kayaking ergometers have thus been devised to allow athletes to reach peak effort in a sport-specific manner (see below).

Irrespective of the choice of ergometer, there has been much discussion concerning the optimal type of test protocol. If the intent is simply to make an accurate measurement of maximal oxygen intake, the best recommendation seems to approximate the test plan for a normal healthy adult; exercise begins with a

3-min warm-up at 60–70% of the anticipated maximal oxygen intake. From the heart rate developed at this intensity of effort, it is possible to gauge and to move relatively precisely to a higher intensity of exercise that will demand 85–90% of aerobic power. After 2 min at 85–90% of aerobic power, further small increments of loading are made at 1–2 min intervals, with the intention of reaching both a plateau of oxygen consumption and subjective exhaustion over 9–11 min of heavy exercise (Andersen et al., 1971; Shephard, 1977; 1982).

If constraints of time require the concurrent estimation of ventilatory threshold, the warm-up is based upon 3 min of loadless operation of the ergometer. An attempt is then made to reach both an oxygen consumption plateau and subjective exhaustion, using from nine to 11 small and equal increments of effort, applied at 1-min intervals.

If a true central limitation of effort is reached, the athlete will commonly show a greying of the complexion and some loss of postural control. There may also be feelings of nausea, a confused response to questioning, and impending loss of consciousness. Depending on the circumstances of the test, the investigator must be prepared to offer support (particularly in treadmill testing, where unattended subjects have sometimes suffered unpleasant abrasions from falling against the moving parts of the machine).

A sudden cessation of effort can lead to collapse from a pooling of blood in the dilated vessels of the lower limbs, and it is advisable to allow a gentle cool-down of at least 1 min following exercise. This precaution is particularly important if the test is performed in a warm environment.

Use of ancillary equipment

If resources permit, it is desirable to use an automated system such as the Beckman Metabolic cart or the Jaeger ergostat to monitor oxygen consumption. These devices incorporate an infrared detector to measure carbon dioxide concentrations, a paramagnetic or electrochemical oxygen sensor, and a turbine or a screen flowmeter for the determination of respiratory minute volume. The data thus generated allow the online calculation of oxygen consumption at 20–30-s intervals. The investigator is thereby provided with an indication of progress towards an oxygen consumption plateau.

If a laboratory is less lavishly equipped, it is possible to obtain similar information by collecting expired gas samples in Douglas bags at 1-min intervals. The volume of expired gas is subsequently measured, using a carefully calibrated gasmeter or Tissot spirometer, and the expired gas concentrations are determined chemically, by Lloyd–Haldane or Scholander apparatus.

A continuous electrocardiogram provides a check on the safety of the test, and allows an accurate counting of heart rates. In sedentary individuals, it is customary to monitor at least three chest leads (CM-2, CM-4 and CM-6) during an exercise test (Fig. 19.2). The neutral lead is fixed to the back of the neck, one lead is secured to the manubrium sterni, and the exploring electrodes are placed in the V-2, V-4 and V-6 positions. However, in a young and healthy adult, a single (CM-5) lead is adequate for the purpose of most exercise tests. Some ingenuity in the placement of the electrodes may be needed in order to avoid electrical interference from muscle action potentials, particularly if the subject is operating a type of ergometer that requires arm movements, but a wandering baseline during exercise is an indication of poor electrode contact or inadequate preliminary abrasion of the skin. Abnormalities of heart rhythm may develop early in the recovery period, and it is thus wise to continue monitoring the electrocardiogram for at least 5 min after exercise has ceased.

The systemic blood pressure should be measured at 1-min intervals throughout a maximal exercise test. A standard sphygmomanometer cuff is adequate for this purpose. Systolic readings can be auscultated with

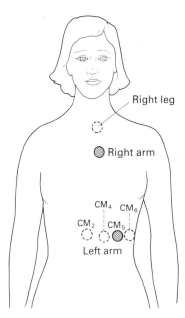

Fig. 19.2 Diagram illustrating the recommended placement of electrocardiography electrodes for an exercise test involving leg exercise. The lead marked 'right arm' is attached over the manubrium sterni, and the lead marked 'right leg' is attached to the nape of the neck. The lead labelled 'left arm' is attached 7–10 cm to the left of the midline, in the fifth interspace (CM-5 recording). From Shephard (1977), with permission.

reasonable confidence, and it can be assumed that the diastolic readings (which are hard to detect in vigorous exercise) remain relatively constant. Failure of the mean systemic blood pressure to rise with work rate implies a difficulty in sustaining cardiac stroke volume; this situation may be anticipated when maximal oxygen intake has been surpassed and the heart is starting to fail. A decline in systolic reading of more than 10 mmHg with a further increment of work rate is an urgent indication to halt an exercise test.

Safety precautions

The great majority of athletes who are tested will be extremely healthy individuals. Never-

theless, it is important to look for and observe both relative and absolute contraindications to testing (Tables 19.2 and 19.3), and to discontinue a test if any of the widely agreed warning signs or symptoms are noted (Table 19.4).

At all ages, there is a very slight risk that

Table 19.2 Relative contraindications to exercise testing, based on the recommendations of the American College of Sports Medicine. From American College of Sports Medicine (1986), with permission.

Resting diastolic blood pressure over 120 mmHg or resting systolic blood pressure over 200 mmHg
Moderate valvular heart disease
Digitalis or other drug effect
Electrolyte abnormalities
Fixed-rate artificial pacemaker
Frequent or complex ventricular irritability
Ventricular aneurysm
Cardiomyopathy including hypertrophic cardiomyopathy
Uncontrolled metabolic disease (such as diabetes, thyrotoxicosis, myxoedema)
Any serious systemic disorder (such as mononucleosis, hepatitis)
Neuromuscular, musculoskeletal or rheumatoid disorders that would make exercise difficult

Table 19.3 Absolute contraindications to maximal exercise testing, based on the recommendations of the American College of Sports Medicine. From American College of Sports Medicine (1986), with permission.

Recent acute myocardial infarction
Unstable angina
Uncontrolled ventricular dysrhythmia
Uncontrolled atrial dysrhythmia which compromises cardiac function
Congestive heart failure
Severe aortic stenosis
Suspected or known dissecting aneurysm
Active or suspected myocarditis
Thrombophlebitis or intracardiac thrombi
Recent systemic or pulmonary embolus
Acute infection
Third degree heart block
Significant emotional distress (psychosis)
A recent significant change in the resting electrocardiogram
Acute pericarditis

Table 19.4 Indications to halt a maximal exercise test, based on the recommendations of the American College of Sports Medicine. From American College of Sports Medicine (1986), with permission.

Subject requests to stop
Failure of the monitoring system
Progressive angina (stop at 3+ level or earlier on a scale of 1+ to 4+)
Two millimetres horizontal or downsloping ST-depression or elevation
Sustained supraventricular tachycardia
Ventricular tachycardia
Exercise-induced left or right bundle branch block
Any significant drop (10 mmHg) of systolic blood pressure, or failure of the systolic blood pressure to rise with an increase in exercise load after the initial adjustment period
Lightheadedness, confusion, ataxia, pallor, cyanosis, nausea or signs of severe peripheral circulatory insufficiency
Excessive blood pressure rise: systolic >250 mmHg; diastolic >120 mmHg
R on T premature ventricular complexes
Unexplained inappropriate bradycardia — pulse rate more than two standard deviations below age-adjusted normals
Onset of second or third degree heart block
Multifocal premature ventricular complexes
Increasing ventricular ectopy

maximal exercise may provoke ventricular fibrillation or cardiac arrest, and it is important that the investigator who is conducting the test should be familiar with the procedures for cardiac resuscitation. Emergency equipment should always be available to deal with such a contingency. There is no need for a physician to be present when testing a symptom-free athlete who is under the age of 35 years, but in older competitors medical coverage may be a wise precaution. The inherent risk of myocardial infarction is less for most types of endurance athlete than for the general population, but regular physical activity does not confer a total immunity from coronary vascular disease, and because athletes are high achievers, they may continue a test in the face of symptoms that would halt the effort of a sedentary person.

Possible use of submaximal tests

Partly because of fears that maximal tests have a greater tendency to provoke cardiac arrest, and partly because of a desire to eliminate the supposed discomfort of all-out effort, much research has been directed to possible submaximal indicators of aerobic potential.

The usual theoretical basis of submaximal test procedures has been the relationship between oxygen consumption (or the equivalent work rate) and heart rate. A roughly linear plot is obtained from 50% to near 100% of maximal oxygen intake. Unfortunately, because of some lability in the heart rate during submaximal exercise, slight departures from a linear heart rate : oxygen consumption relationship, and substantial interindividual variations in maximal heart rate, heart rate-based predictions of maximal oxygen intake show a coefficient of variation of 10−15% relative to directly measured values. Predicted values may have some application in determining the aerobic potential of large populations, and they may allow a rough assessment of changes in the condition of an individual from week to week; on the other hand, it is hardly useful to predict that the maximal oxygen intake of a cross-country skier is 80 ml·kg^{-1}·min^{-1} if the confidence intervals for this report extend from 60 to 100 ml·kg^{-1}·min^{-1}!

Other methods of predicting maximal oxygen intake have been based upon changes in the respiratory gas exchange ratio; this ratio increases progressively as maximum effort is approached. Such predictions seem no more precise than estimates based on the heart rate during submaximal activity.

Possible use of field tests

Given that a substantial part of the large maximal oxygen intake of the endurance competitor may be inherited rather than developed through rigorous training, one potential approach to national athletic success is to search extensively through the entire population in an attempt to discover unusually well endowed candidates. The number of individuals to be tested in such a search precludes the use of any sophisticated laboratory procedures, and the question thus arises as to whether a simple field test can provide an approximate measure of oxygen transport.

The most obvious solution is to measure the times achieved in a standardized athletic event. For example, runners can be compared in terms of the times that they take to cover a fixed distance, or the distance covered in a fixed time (Table 19.5). An immediate difficulty is that athletic selection is being made at ever younger ages, and the relationship between performance times and oxygen transport is not very close in young children. Much depends on the sport-specific skill of the individual and an appropriate choice of pace rather than upon peak oxygen transport; indeed, cynics have suggested that timed trials of running or swimming add little to information that could have been obtained from age, body mass and skinfold thicknesses.

If mass tests are contemplated, it is further quite difficult to standardize the precise conditions of measurement. Indoor running times, for example, may suffer from over-heated rooms or the need to made repeated turns in order to cover the required distance. Outdoor measurements are not only susceptible to differences of environmental temperature and humidity, but also face problems from wind, rain, and changing track or ground conditions.

Performance times thus provide an even less satisfactory measure of aerobic potential than laboratory submaximal exercise tests.

Interpretation of test results

In the general population, the reproducibility of maximal oxygen intake data depends very much upon the care adopted in calibrating the equipment, and the success of the observer in motivating subjects to an all-out, centrally limited maximal effort. But even with careful technique, there remains an unavoidable intra-individual test-to-test variation of 4–5%.

When testing endurance athletes, results are often no more precise. A competitor may be reluctant to give an all-out effort, fearing that this will impair performance in an upcoming contest, and in many cases maximal performance is hampered by differences in the pattern of exercise between normal competition and use of the test ergometer. For example, there are considerable functional differences between any of the normal swimming strokes and exercise on a swim-bench or a tethered swimming device. Likewise, a rowing machine provides only a limited simulation of experience in a racing shell. It is thus optimistic to assume that the accuracy of measurements in athletes will exceed the 4–5% cited for the general population.

Interindividual differences of mechanical efficiency also limit the match between a performer's competitive times and their maximal oxygen intake, and, given that most races are decided by margins much smaller than 4–5%, measurements of peak oxygen transport can allow only a very crude classification of competitors. If the treadmill maximal oxygen intake is substantially larger than the sport-specific measurement, this may indicate a need to concentrate athletic training upon local muscle development. If both treadmill and sport-specific values are low, then a general development of the cardiovascular system should be attempted, while if both treadmill and sport-specific values

Table 19.5 Some reported coefficients of correlation between the directly measured maximal oxygen intake and running speed. After data collected by Disch *et al.* (1975) and Shephard (1982). See Shephard (1982) for details of references.

Subjects	n	Authors	Coefficients of correlation with $V_{O_2 max}$
402 m			
College males	35	Wiley & Shaver (1972)	−0.22
College males	11	Ribisl & Kachadorian (1969)	−0.31
549 m			
Boys, 10 years	20	Larivière *et al.* (1974)	−0.58
Boys, 12−13 years	30	Metz & Alexander (1970)	−0.67
Boys, 14−15 years	30	Metz & Alexander (1970)	−0.27
Boys, grade 9	9	Doolittle & Bigbee (1968)	−0.62
Faculty and staff	87	Falls *et al.* (1966)	−0.64
Sedentary men	141	Drake *et al.* (1968)	−0.27
805 m			
Boys, 10 years	20	Larivière *et al.* (1974)	−0.37
College males	11	Ribisl & Kachadorian (1969)	−0.67
Physical education majors	10	Kearney & Byrnes (1974)	−0.30
College males	11	Byrnes & Kearney (1974)	−0.73
Physical education majors	11	Byrnes & Kearney (1974)	−0.04
Cross-country runners	11	Byrnes & Kearney (1974)	−0.42
1610 m			
College males	25	Wiley & Shaver (1972)	−0.29
College males	11	Ribisl & Kachadorian (1969)	−0.79
College males	11	Byrnes & Kearney (1974)	−0.72
Physical education majors	11	Byrnes & Kearney (1974)	−0.25
Cross-country runners	11	Byrnes & Kearney (1974)	−0.51
3220 m			
College males	11	Ribisl & Kachadorian (1969)	−0.85
College males	25	Wiley & Shaver (1972)	−0.47
Older males	24	Ribisl & Kachadorian (1969)	−0.86
4830 m			
College males	35	Wiley & Shaver (1972)	−0.43
8050 m			
Cross-country runners	17	Kearney & Byrnes (1974)	−0.38
9-min run			
Boys, 9−12 years	25	Coleman (1974)	0.82
Girls, 9−12 years	25	Coleman (1974)	0.71
12-min run			
Boys, 9−12 years	25	Coleman (1972)	0.82
Boys, 10 years	20	Larivière *et al.* (1974)	0.44
Boys, 11−14 years	17	Maksud & Coutts (1971)	0.65
Boys, grade 9	9	Doolittle & Bigbee (1968)	0.90
Girls, 9−12 years	25	Coleman (1974)	0.71
College males	7	Kearney & Byrnes (1974)	0.80
Physical education majors	10	Kearney & Byrnes (1974)	0.64
Cross-country runners	17	Kearney & Byrnes (1974)	0.28
Adult males	115	Cooper (1968a)	0.90
College females	30	Burris (1970)	0.74
College females	36	Katch *et al.* (1973)	0.67

are high but performance is poor, the implication is that the coach should concentrate upon improving technique.

In the general population, measured gains of maximal oxygen intake are sometimes used to encourage continued training. If an athlete shows substantial gains of oxygen transport, these can be used for a similar purpose. But as a peak of conditioning is approached, the gains are likely to be disappointingly small relative to the effort that has been expended, limiting the motivational value of such data for the high-performance athlete.

Overtraining may be associated with a decrease in maximal oxygen intake, but again the day-to-day margin of error in test data is sufficiently large that oxygen transport measurements cannot provide as sensitive an index of overtraining as measurements of performance times, serum enzyme levels and immune function.

The maximal oxygen intake has sometimes been used to monitor recovery of function following injury or illness. It also provides the denominator for such indices as ventilatory threshold. Finally, it may help in establishing an appropriate intensity of training sessions, and the grouped data for an entire team may be useful in evaluating the response to novel plans of training.

References

American College of Sports Medicine (1986) *Graded Exercise Testing and Exercise Prescription*. Lea & Febiger, Philadelphia.

Andersen, K.L., Shephard, R.J., Denolin, H., Varnauskas, E. & Masironi, R. (1971) *Fundamentals of Exercise Testing*. World Health Organization, Geneva.

Disch, J., Frankiewicz, R. & Jackson, A. (1975) Construct validation of distance run tests. *Res. Quart.* **46**, 169–176.

Neumann, G. (1988) Special performance capacity. In: Dirix, A., Knuttgen, H.G. & Tittel, K. (eds) *The Olympic Book of Sports Medicine*, Vol. 1, pp. 97–108. Blackwell Scientific Publications, Oxford.

Shephard, R.J. (1977) *Endurance Fitness*, 2nd edn. University of Toronto Press, Toronto.

Shephard, R.J. (1982) *Physiology and Biochemistry of Exercise*. Praeger Publishing, New York.

Chapter 20

Sport-Specific Ergometric Equipment

ANTONIO DAL MONTE, MARCELLO FAINA AND
CLAUDIO MENCHINELLI

The main objective of a modern functional evaluation of the athlete is to measure her or his
quality and efficiency in relation to the specific
discipline in question. Athletes are no longer
regarded as 'superstars', but as subjects who
must have, and increase, the psychological,
biomechanical and physiological qualities required by their sport. In other words, they
must have or develop qualities that conform to
the biophysiological, technical and psychological pattern deemed necessary for that sports
discipline.

Therefore it is clear that the functional evaluation of an athlete cannot be limited to the
application of 'generic' tests; methods of study
must be devised that stress the functional
characteristics shown by the various organs
and systems during the performance of each
competitive sport in order to supply reliable
and useful data and theories to researchers,
experts and athletes.

These concepts have influenced the investigations that have been carried out for 30 years
by the Department of Physiology and Biomechanics of the Institute of Sport Science of
the Italian National Olympic Committee of
Rome (CONI). The first prototypes of specific
ergometers were constructed about 30 years
ago. Some of these ergometers are unique
designs and are able to reproduce almost exactly
the typical movements of athletes during
competition.

Definition of specific ergometry

By sport-specific ergometry, we imply the
multidisciplinary science-based evaluation of
the athlete in conditions that simulate as closely
as possible a competition or phases of training
similar to competitions. In particular the following parameters must be considered:
1 The type of sport.
2 Spatial position.
3 Frequency of movement used during the
competition.
4 Power output.
5 Duration of test in order to simulate the
energy sources used by the athlete in her or his
performance.
6 The kinds of stress that the athlete will experience during competition.

From this definition we can deduce that
functional evaluation of the performances of
élite athletes has now become such a complex
field of study that multidisciplinary 'teams' of
researchers are needed. With regard to physiological and biomechanical evaluation, a distinction can be made between study in the
laboratory and in the field. Field methods are
generally used when it is not possible to reproduce or simulate in the laboratory all of the
conditions that may occur during competition.

Types of ergometers

Among the ergometers currently used in the

laboratory are the treadmill; the cycle ergo-meter; the kayak ergometer; ergometers for the Canadian canoe, and for the 'grinders' of sailing boats; specific ergometers for swimming; and ergometer pools for tests on aquatic sports (swimming, swimming with flippers, wind-surfing, canoeing and diving activities).

The treadmill is used to evaluate athletic disciplines connected with running or walking (500–10 000 m events, marathon runs, etc.). The cycle ergometer is used exclusively for evaluation of cyclists when the aim is to study the limits of strength, power and endurance shown by the cyclist in her or his typical move-ment pattern. The cycle ergometer has to have controls and characteristics that are not found on other ergometers; for this reason the ergo-meter used in our department has been specially designed and constructed.

The ergometer simulating kayak canoeing (Fig. 20.1) is made from two long cranks placed obliquely to simulate the continuity of the body of the paddle. The device is completed by a tripod bearing a canoe pedalling set, so that the athlete works from a position similar to that in the boat. A specific ergometer has been con-structed for the Canadian canoe (Fig. 20.2) so that the athlete maintains the same knee position as when paddling the canoe.

For rowing, two types of ergometers, are available. In the first, after Gjessing–Nilsen (Fig. 20.3), the bearing of the athlete (pedalling set and trolley) and the movement pattern reproduce the action of rowing, but the handle is fastened on to the edge of a sliding pole and can effect only a sagittal movement, whereas in reality the oar moves by rotating in corre-spondence with the rowlock. The resistance of the oar during its passage through the water is simulated by means of a brake equipped with a belt rolled up on a pulley. The second type of ergometer can reproduce the sport kinesiology, including passage through the water (Fig. 20.4). The system reproduces rowing and is made from a real oar installed on a boat-type rowlock; therefore, the rower is able to perform all the possible movements on the fulcrum constituted by the row-lock itself, just as in reality.

To improve the study of the above aquatic sport disciplines, and of other aquatic sports such as swimming, model-scale sailing, wind-surfing and diving, an ergometer pool was built in our Department (projected and designed by Dal Monte). Some of the characteristics of this flume are quite original (Fig. 20.5).

For cross-country skiing, a specific ergo-meter has also been constructed (Fig. 20.6). This device, installed on a treadmill, is made

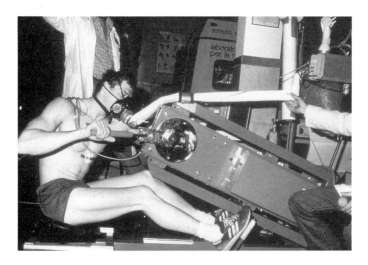

Fig. 20.1 Ergometer for kayak canoe, created and used at the Department of Physiology and Biomechanics of the Institute of Sport Science in Rome.

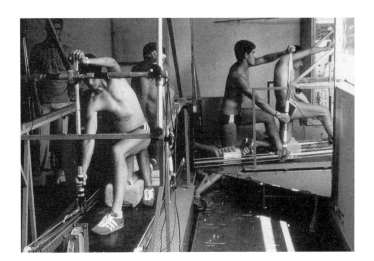

Fig. 20.2 Ergometer for laboratory reproduction of the technical kinetics of the Canadian canoe.

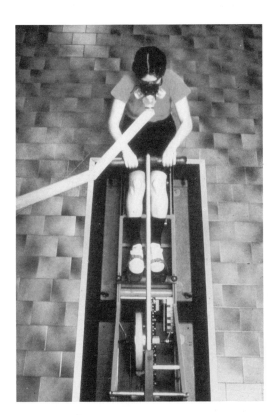

Fig. 20.3 Gjessing–Nilsen oar-ergometer for laboratory study of rowing.

from two tracks, one on each side, on which the ski poles are placed. The ski poles slide on the tracks, and a linear force-measuring transducer is located close to the hand-grip of the ski pole. During the pushing phase, resistance is provided by a mechanical brake with a belt rolled up on a pulley. Ski rollers are used with two tracks (2 m in length) to avoid side deviations during tests. The ski bindings are equipped with linear transducers for measuring the force on the skis. During the tests the subject is 'skiing' on the inclined treadmill at various speeds. By this method one can calculate the total work done by the subject to raise her or his body while skiing on the treadmill; the work done by the upper limbs; and the force applied by both the upper and lower limbs.

Recently, a new isokinetic ergometer has been constructed (Fig. 20.7). This device works in isokinetic conditions over 360° movements. It can be used to observe the lower limbs, upper limbs or both at the same time, in different spatial positions and at different speeds (0–240° r.p.m.). Aerobic and anaerobic metabolism can be studied according to the working protocol that is adopted. The device can also work at constant torque or at constant mechanical power.

Our institute also has a wind tunnel with a

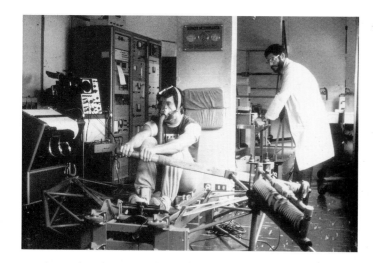

Fig. 20.4 Ergometer for reproducing the technical kinetics of rowing in the laboratory.

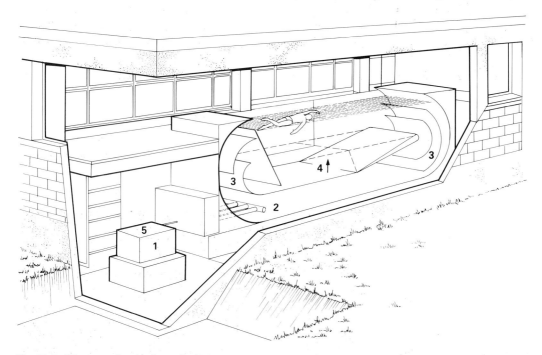

Fig. 20.5 Diagram of a test flume for diving sports used at the Institute of Sport Science. The flume is characterized by having a steady water flow throughout which can be varied over a wide range of velocities. The flume can be used for aquatic disciplines such as swimming, canoeing, windsurfing, model-scale sailing, diving activities, etc. This can be obtained by: (1) four parallel propellers; (2) a propulsion system; (3) a hydraulic system of alignment deflectors; (4) flow facility to reduce the chamber area by raising the floor, in order to generate a higher water flow; (5) cooling the engine by means of the flume water, which is consequently heated.

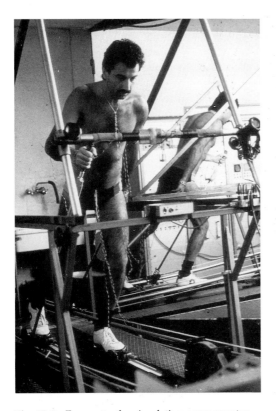

Fig. 20.6 Ergometer for simulating cross-country skiing. The apparatus allows the measurement of power and forces by each limb (arms and legs) using linear vertical displacement transducers applied on the 'ski rollers' and on the ski poles.

treadmill (Fig. 20.8). Its total dimensions are 9×18 m, and the test chamber is 5 m long, 3 m high and 3.2 m wide. This device permits the study of subjects, vehicles and equipment at full scale.

The treadmill belt, which moves at the same speed as the air, can reproduce the 'ground' effect and permit aerodynamic studies on moving, wheeled vehicles. In the wind tunnel, many endurance sports have been studied, particularly cycling (the testing of newly conceived wheels and frames and evaluation of the best position for the athlete) (Fig. 20.9). The results of these studies include the 'lenticular' wheels and the frame used by Francesco Moser in his 1-h record and by the Italian national team which won the team time-trial competition at the Olympic Games in Los Angeles.

In the wind tunnel, studies have also been carried out on race vehicles and equipment such as bob-sleighs, race motor-boats, go-karts, downhill skis, and crash helmets. The position of athletes when jumping from the ski-jumping board has also been studied.

Mobile ergometry

Some studies may be required at the competition site. For this reason our institute has

Fig. 20.7 The 'multifunctional isokinetic ergometer' makes it possible to test lower and upper limbs separately and simultaneously at constant speed, power and torque. Power and forces exerted during the test can be illustrated by power–velocity curves.

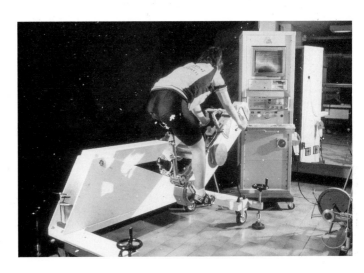

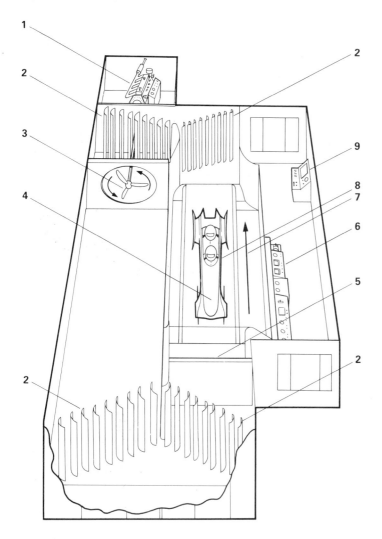

Fig. 20.8 View of a wind tunnel used at the Science Institute of Rome. 1 Engine; 2 corner vanes; 3 fan; 4 object under examination; 5 honeycomb screen; 6 control panel; 7 test section; 8 treadmill; 9 computer data system.

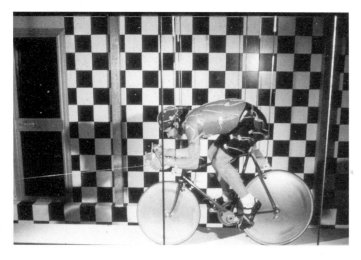

Fig. 20.9 The bicycle and the cyclist are subject to an aerodynamic evaluation. The wool threads, which permit visualization of the turbulence of the air, are visible.

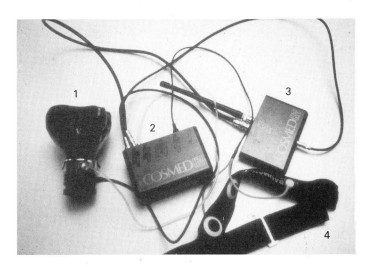

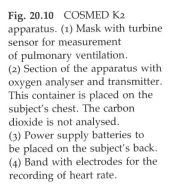

Fig. 20.10   COSMED K2 apparatus. (1) Mask with turbine sensor for measurement of pulmonary ventilation. (2) Section of the apparatus with oxygen analyser and transmitter. This container is placed on the subject's chest. The carbon dioxide is not analysed. (3) Power supply batteries to be placed on the subject's back. (4) Band with electrodes for the recording of heart rate.

prepared two mobile units that 'transfer' the laboratory directly to the field. In general, physiological and biomechanical data are transmitted via radio from miniaturized instruments worn by the athletes or installed on the 'athlete–vehicle' as a whole.

We have recently obtained the facility to record oxygen consumption ($\dot{V}o_2$) via radio-telemetry using a portable device which is small and light (weighing about 800 g) (Fig. 20.10). This is an integrated telemetric system which can be used to measure pulmonary ventilation, respiratory frequency, $\dot{V}o_2$ and heart rate. The instrument is called a COSMED K2, and was completely redesigned and tested in our department (Fig. 20.11).

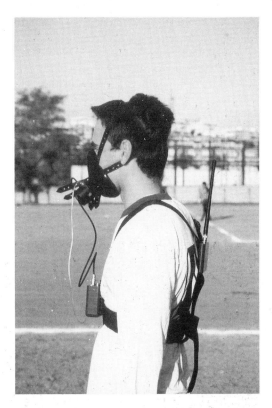

Fig. 20.11   Illustration of how the COSMED K2 equipment is applied to an athlete.

Chapter 21

Haemoglobin, Blood Volume and Endurance

NORMAN GLEDHILL

Determinants of endurance performance

Endurance performance is influenced by several factors, in particular maximal oxygen intake ($\dot{V}o_{2\,max}$), anaerobic threshold and running efficiency. However, since $\dot{V}o_{2\,max}$ can vary among individuals by as much as 200% (from $< 30\,ml\cdot kg^{-1}\cdot min^{-1}$ to $> 80\,ml\cdot kg^{-1}\cdot min^{-1}$), this factor must be regarded as the major determinant of endurance performance. By comparison, anaerobic threshold and running efficiency influence to only a modest degree the portion of an individual's $\dot{V}o_{2\,max}$ that is utilized during endurance performance (up to 20% and 5% of $\dot{V}o_{2\,max}$ respectively). $\dot{V}o_{2\,max}$, in turn, is determined by oxygen transport — the product of cardiac output and arterial oxygen content ($\dot{Q} \times Cao_2$). Further, since $\dot{Q}$ is influenced by blood volume (BV), and Cao_2 is determined almost entirely by the blood haemoglobin concentration ([Hb]), manipulation of BV and [Hb] can markedly affect the provision of oxygen to the working muscles, thereby having a significant influence on $\dot{V}o_{2\,max}$ and endurance performance.

Role of haemoglobin in oxygen transport

Oxygen is carried by blood both in physical solution and in combination with haemoglobin. The amount of dissolved oxygen is proportional to the partial pressure of oxygen (Po_2) in blood as follows: $Po_2 \times 0.003\,ml$ oxygen per 100 ml blood. Hence, under normal atmospheric conditions, dissolved oxygen contributes very little to the overall transport of oxygen in blood. In addition, oxygen undergoes an easily reversible chemical combination with haemoglobin, and this accounts for most of the blood's capacity to transport oxygen. Each gram of haemoglobin can combine with up to 1.39 ml of oxygen, so that variations in [Hb] can markedly affect oxygen transport.

Given the substantial influence of the oxygen-carrying capacity of blood upon endurance performance, a consideration of the relevant measurements is informative. Since haemoglobin is contained in red blood cells (RBCs), the total number of RBCs is of considerable importance to oxygen carriage. The RBC count is generally determined via automated counters, although measurements are possible using a standard light microscope and counting chambers. In normal healthy males the mean RBC count is $5.2 \times 10^6\cdot mm^{-3}$ (range $4.5{-}6.0 \times 10^6\cdot mm^{-3}$), and in normal healthy females it is $4.8 \times 10^6\cdot mm^{-3}$ (range $4.0{-}5.5 \times 10^6\cdot mm^{-3}$). Approximately 45% of the blood volume of a normal healthy male is RBCs (range 40–54%); this percentage is called the haematocrit. In normal healthy females the mean haematocrit is 41% (range 37–47%). The haematocrit can be determined via automated counters, or more simply by centrifugation to a packed cell volume. Most often, the reported haematocrit is not corrected for the effect of trapped plasma (factor = 0.96), or for the venous-to-whole body ratio (factor = 0.91). The concentration of haemoglobin in blood is generally determined via automated counters or by a spectrophotometric cyanmethaemoglobin assay technique. The mean [Hb] of normal healthy males is 15.5 g·100 ml^{-1} (range 14.0−18.0 g·100 ml^{-1}), and normal healthy females have a mean [Hb] of 13.8 g·100 ml^{-1} (range 12.0−16.0 g·100 ml^{-1}).

Anaemia and endurance performance

Severe clinical anaemia is associated with both a reduction in $\dot{V}O_{2\,max}$ and an impairment of endurance performance (Sproule et al., 1960). However, of greater relevance to the topic of endurance performance is the condition of sports anaemia − when the [Hb] of an athlete is below normal in the absence of any medical explanation (Clement & Sawchuk, 1984). Although the incidence of clinical anaemia is very low in well-nourished athletes, a suboptimal (low normal) [Hb] is frequently reported (Pate, 1983). In fact, [Hb] decreases as a function of intense endurance training (Frederickson et al., 1983), and small reductions in [Hb] are associated with reductions in $\dot{V}O_{2\,max}$ and endurance performance (Ekblom et al., 1972; Kanstrup & Ekblom, 1982). As an approximation of the relationship between anaemia and $\dot{V}O_{2\,max}$, a reduction in [Hb] of 0.3 g·100 ml^{-1} corresponds to a fall in $\dot{V}O_{2\,max}$ of 1%. Thus, if the [Hb] of an endurance athlete fell from 15.5 g·100 ml^{-1} to 14 g·100 ml^{-1}, it would be accompanied by a 5% decrease in $\dot{V}O_{2\,max}$ and a parallel impairment of endurance performance ability.

Given the important performance implications of haematological status, the ability to monitor this variable is receiving increasing attention. Haemoglobin is an iron-containing protein, and its synthesis thus depends on the presence of adequate amounts of iron in the bone marrow. Therefore, in addition to the customary measurements of [Hb], haematocrit and RBC count, current monitoring includes measurements of iron-related variables that can detect impending haematological problems before they are overtly manifested. Such indices include serum ferritin, serum iron, total iron binding capacity and saturation of transferrin. Individually, these indicators have limited value in monitoring iron deficiency, but when several are measured concurrently abnormalities are more easily and promptly detected. However, care must be taken in comparing values for the same athlete from samples measured using different assay kits or in different commercial laboratories. As well, the use of a single recommended value for each indicator to diagnose 'normal' vs. 'iron-deficient' values should be avoided in favour of kit-specific and laboratory-specific values (Ondracka & Gledhill, 1988).

Men and women normally lose approximately 1 mg of iron each day in sweat and stool, and women lose additional iron during menstruation. This loss must be balanced by the dietary intake of iron, and the recommended daily intake is 10 mg for males and 14 mg for females. Because only 10% of the ingested iron is absorbed, the daily intake normally matches the daily loss. Computer-processed nutritional intake analyses can be employed to monitor the adequacy of dietary iron intake and deficiencies can be corrected via a variety of tablet or liquid supplements (Clement & Sawchuk, 1984).

Erythrocythaemia and endurance performance

Blood doping, blood boosting and blood packing are terms used to describe the procedure of inducing erythrocythaemia − a [Hb] above the normal. Early investigators of blood doping employed a blood storage technique which resulted in considerable RBC loss, and they were therefore unable to achieve a significant increase in [Hb]. Consequently, it was commonly concluded from these studies that blood doping had no effect on $\dot{V}O_{2\,max}$ or endurance performance. However, given this major methodological shortcoming, the findings from such studies must be largely ignored. On the other hand, recent investigators of blood doping, who avoided this methodological problem and successfully induced a significant increase in [Hb], reported consequent increases in $\dot{V}_{O_2\,max}$ and endurance performance (Williams *et al.*, 1981; Robertson *et al.*, 1982; Celsing *et al.*, 1986; Spriet *et al.*, 1986; Brien & Simon, 1987). The $\dot{V}_{O_2\,max}$ increases by approximately 1% for each $0.3\,g\cdot100\,ml^{-1}$ increase in [Hb] (Gledhill, 1982; Celsing *et al.* 1986).

Improvements in endurance performance have been observed not only in laboratory experiments, but also under competitive conditions in cross-country skiing (Berglund & Hemmingson, 1987) and 10-km running (Brien & Simon, 1987). Moreover, the results of those members of the US cycling team who engaged in blood doping at the Los Angeles Olympics appear to substantiate the improvement of competitive performance (Pavelka, 1985). It should also be noted that inducing erythrocythaemia before exercising at altitude very effectively erased the adverse effect of aerohypoxia on $\dot{V}_{O_2\,max}$ and endurance performance (Robertson *et al.*, 1982).

It was long accepted that oxygen transport and haematocrit had an 'inverted U' relationship, such that increases in [Hb] above the optimal haematocrit (postulated to be 45%) would cause a decrease in oxygen transport. This was hypothesized to result from a decrease in $\dot{Q}$, due to increased blood viscosity and a consequent increase in peripheral resistance. However, the relationship was based on in vitro observations which do not accurately simulate in vivo conditions, especially during exercise. The effective in vivo viscosity, both at and above the optimal haematocrit, is considerably less than the corresponding in vitro viscosity, due to exercise-induced increases in temperature and blood vessel dimensions (Celsing *et al.*, 1986). Therefore, $\dot{Q}_{max}$, and hence oxygen transport, are not impaired up to a haematocrit of at least 52% (Thomson *et al.*, 1982; Spriet *et al.*, 1986).

Methodology of inducing erythrocythaemia

Erythrocythaemia can be induced by transfusing fresh blood from a matched donor (homologous transfusion), as was undertaken by some members of the US cycling team during the 1984 Los Angeles Olympics (Pavelka, 1985). Homologous transfusions are utilized routinely during the treatment of life-threatening medical conditions. However, even when strict clinical precautions are taken, such transfusions are associated with significant risks. For example, despite appropriate typing and matching of blood, there is a 3–4% incidence of minor transfusion reactions, consisting of fever, chills or malaise, and such delayed reactions can result in the destruction of transfused RBCs. Homologous transfusions also pose a risk of acquiring potentially fatal infections such as hepatitis B and AIDS (acquired immune deficiency syndrome).

Inducing erythrocythaemia via the removal, storage and subsequent reinfusion of a person's own blood (autologous infusion) avoids these dangers. The conventional clinical method of storing blood for autologous transfusion is to preserve the cells by refrigeration at 4°C. During refrigeration storage, the erythrocytes continue to age, and since the average lifespan of an RBC is 120 days, approximately 1% of any RBC population is lost each day. In the body, the byproducts of RBC breakdown are recycled, and the destruction of RBCs is matched by RBC synthesis through erythropoiesis. However, when blood is refrigeration-stored, there is a progressive build-up of cellular aggregates, and health authorities in North America have imposed a 3-week maximum refrigeration storage time on blood banks. (In some countries the allowable storage time is extended to 4–5 weeks.) At the end of a 3-week period of refrigeration, the number of stored RBCs has declined by approximately 15–20% (Valeri, 1976). Additional erythrocytes are lost during processing because they adhere to the storage containers and transfer tubing. As well, some erythrocytes become so fragile during storage that they break up shortly after they are infused (Valeri, 1976). The net result is that when blood is refrigeration-stored for the maximum allowable 3-week period, only 60% (approximately) of the RBCs that were removed are viable after infusion.

The glycerol cell-freezing technique of blood storage is utilized by blood banks to maintain a supply of rare blood types. Freeze-preservation requires laboratory personnel with considerable expertise and the use of sophisticated equipment. Unlike refrigeration, when blood is stored as frozen cells the ageing process of the RBCs is interrupted and the fragility of the stored cells is normal after reinfusion. Loss due to RBC handling is similar to that in the refrigeration process and amounts to approximately 15%, whether the storage time is 2 days or 2 years. Consequently, a major difference in the two storage techniques is that freeze-preserved cells can be safely stored for an indefinite period of time (Valeri, 1976). Therefore, by employing freeze-preservation it is possible not only to maximize the recovery of the stored RBCs (approximately 85%) but also to delay reinfusion of the cells as long as is necessary to ensure that the normal RBC count has been re-established in the donor.

Before blood is freeze-preserved, it is centrifuged, and the separated RBCs are combined with glycerol at a haematocrit of approximately 90%. At the conclusion of storage, the RBCs are carefully thawed, deglycerolysed via a series of washings, and reconstituted with physiological saline to a haematocrit of approximately 50%. Since the reconstituted 'blood' has essentially the same haematocrit as normal blood, the blood volume of the recipient is transiently increased, and there is no immediate increase in haematocrit. The acute hypervolaemia disappears over the next 24 h as the excess fluid is lost, and this haemoconcentration produces the final elevated haematocrit and [Hb] that is termed erythrocythaemia.

Time-course of RBC changes following blood removal and infusion

Following blood removal, the donor's [Hb] drops by approximately $1-1.5\%$ ($0.1-0.15$) g·100 ml^{-1}) for each 100 ml blood that has been removed. Thereafter, the [Hb] remains low for $1-2$ weeks before increasing rapidly toward the control level (Gledhill, 1982). The time required to re-establish the control [Hb] depends on: (i) the volume of blood removed (450 ml requires $3-4$ weeks recovery following phlebotomy, and 900 ml requires $4-5$ weeks recovery following phlebotomy); and (ii) the activity level of the donor following phlebotomy (after a 900 ml phlebotomy, up to 10 weeks' recovery is required for donors who continue endurance training). Consequently, 3 weeks after a 900 ml phlebotomy, the blood has regained only half of its $10-12\%$ reduction in [Hb]. After refrigeration storage, infusion of the 60% of the removed RBCs that are still viable cannot achieve a significant increase in [Hb]. Not surprisingly, therefore, studies of blood doping in which the refrigeration storage technique was employed did not achieve a significant increase in [Hb], and hence, the authors should not have expected to observe an increase in $\dot{V}o_{2\,max}$ and endurance performance. However, when RBCs are freeze-preserved, it is possible to wait until the control [Hb] has been re-established before infusing the 85% of the removed RBCs that are still viable after storage, thereby achieving a significant increase in [Hb].

After reinfusion of 900 ml freeze-preserved blood, the [Hb] increases to approximately 10% above control; it then progressively declines toward the control level over the next 120 days: a condition of erythrocythaemia is present for an extended period of time while the RBC count is gradually decreasing to the control level (Gledhill, 1982).

Detection of blood doping

The practice of blood doping to improve athletic performance was banned by the International

Olympic Committee in 1987, but there exists no reliable method to detect its use. Currently, athletes selected for doping control must provide a urine sample. However, the provision of a blood sample could also be required, so that the presence of a high [Hb], haematocrit and RBC count could easily be determined. The problem in detecting the use of blood doping is that of determining unequivocally that there is an *abnormally* high [Hb]. In all of the studies of induced erythrocythaemia to date, the [Hb] was within the range found in the general population, and a high normal [Hb] could be due to genetic endowment or altitude acclimatization. In fact, some athletes (who were not suspected of blood doping) competed in the 1976 Montreal Olympics with a [Hb] as high as 18 g·100 ml^{-1} (Clement *et al.*, 1977).

Investigators are currently endeavouring to develop an effective technique for detecting blood doping, and Berglund *et al.* (1987; 1989) have proposed that it might be possible to detect blood doping from analysis of a blood sample and an algorithm incorporating [Hb], erythropoietin, serum iron and bilirubin. As an indication of the effectiveness of this potential detection technique, if 20 athletes were tested for blood doping, and 10 had actually employed this manipulation, the detection technique would catch five of the 10 guilty athletes and would not falsely detect any of the 10 who had not employed blood doping. However, five guilty athletes would still not be detected, and because the technique is equivocal it is not commonly employed. Therefore, at present the only deterrents to the use of blood doping to improve performance are concern over the associated health risks and the integrity of the athletes and coaches involved.

A new form of blood doping

Erythropoietin is a hormone produced by the kidneys in response to either low levels of circulating haemoglobin or a low arterial Po_2. Recently, a synthetic version of erythropoietin was approved in North America for the treat-

ment of anaemia (Cowart, 1989). Unfortunately, erythropoietin could also be employed to improve endurance performance in the same manner as blood doping — by enhancing [Hb] and thereby oxygen transport. In this case, though, the increase would be accomplished simply by a series of injections. Evidence to substantiate this possibility has not yet been reported, but the theory is sound. However, the dose–response relationship between erythropoietin and increases in [Hb] is not presently known, and it is quite possible that erythropoietin injections could increase a normal haematocrit to the point that viscosity impairs $\dot{Q}_{max}$ and thereby $\dot{V}o_{2\,max}$ and endurance performance. It is also possible that the considerable accompanying increase in viscosity could lead to heart failure and death. Unfortunately, there is presently no effective technique to detect the use of synthetic erythropoietin, because it is indistinguishable from its endogenous counterpart. Therefore, we must once again rely on the integrity of the athletes and coaches and refrain from utilizing this unfair advantage.

Role of blood volume in oxygen transport and endurance performance

Changes in blood volume affect oxygen transport by altering stroke volume and thereby $\dot{Q}$ through changes in ventricular preload and the Frank–Starling mechanism. Resultant changes in $\dot{Q}_{max}$ in turn affect oxygen transport capacity and consequently $\dot{V}o_{2\,max}$. Hence, alterations in blood volume can influence endurance performance ability.

Blood volume can be estimated from body mass (77.5 ml blood per kg body mass) or measured with dilution techniques using radioactive labelled RBCs or Evan's blue dye (current supplier: New World Trading Corporation, Longwood, Florida, USA). In addition, changes in blood volume subsequent to the infusion of blood can be determined from knowledge of both the [Hb] and volume of infused blood (generally by weighing it, then converting it to a volume, using an assumed density of 1.037). The blood volume following infusion can then be calculated, based on the principle of mass balance, assuming 100% erythrocyte survival in vivo. (With freeze-preserved cells, it is not unreasonable to assume 100% in vivo survival following infusion, but with refrigeration storage some erythrocytes become fragile and break up shortly after they are infused.) The blood volume (BV) following infusion is determined via the equation:

$$(BV\ post \times [Hb]\ post) = (BV\ pre \times [Hb]\ pre) \\ + (BV\ infused \times \\ [Hb]\ infused)$$

Because alterations in blood volume are inter-related to changes in [Hb], when examining the effect of changes in blood volume on $\dot{V}o_{2\,max}$ and endurance performance it is necessary to specify the [Hb] that accompanies the hypervolaemia or hypovolaemia. For example, in the hours immediately following the infusion of RBCs for blood doping, there exists a transient hypervolaemia with no change in [Hb]. Within 1 day, or at the most 2 days, the excess fluid is excreted to re-establish normovolaemia, with an elevated [Hb] (actually a very slight hypervolaemia persists due to the increased oncotic pressure) (Spriet et al., 1986).

Hypervolaemia, accompanied by an above normal [Hb], increases both $\dot{V}o_{2\,max}$ and endurance performance (Kanstrup & Ekblom, 1984), but when hypervolaemia is accompanied by a subnormal [Hb], there is no change in $\dot{V}o_{2\,max}$ and possibly a decrease in endurance performance (Kanstrup & Ekblom, 1982; 1984; Green et al., 1987). When a greater reduction in [Hb] accompanies hypervolaemia, both $\dot{V}o_{2\,max}$ and endurance performance are impaired (Kanstrup & Ekblom, 1984).

Acute decreases in blood volume and a consequent elevation in [Hb] are compensated for in several hours by an expansion of the blood volume back to normovolaemia. However, the acute hypovolaemia and increased [Hb] are accompanied by a decrease in both $\dot{V}o_{2\,max}$ (Danzinger & Cumming, 1964) and endurance

performance (Saltin, 1964). When a subnormal [Hb] is accompanied by hypovolaemia, both $\dot{V}o_{2\,max}$ and endurance performance are considerably impaired (Kanstrup & Ekblom, 1982).

In summary, if [Hb] remains unchanged, an accompanying decrease in blood volume will generally lead to decreases in $\dot{V}o_{2\,max}$ and endurance performance. However, an increase in blood volume with no change in [Hb] will have no effect on $\dot{V}o_{2\,max}$ or endurance performance. Also, if blood volume remains unchanged, an accompanying decrease in [Hb] will lead to decreases in $\dot{V}o_{2\,max}$ and endurance performance, while an increase in [Hb] with no change in blood volume will produce increases in $\dot{V}o_{2\,max}$ and endurance performance. It can be concluded, therefore, that [Hb] (through alterations in total body haemoglobin) plays the dominant role in the influence of blood volume and [Hb] on $\dot{V}o_{2\,max}$ and endurance performance.

References

Berglund, B., Birgegard, G., Wide, L. & Philstedt, P. (1989) Effects of blood transfusions on some hematological variables in endurance athletes. *Med. Sci. Sports Exerc.* 21, 637–642.

Berglund, B. & Hemmingson, P. (1987) Effect of re-infusion of autologous blood on exercise performance in cross-country skiers. *Int. J. Sports Med.* 8, 231–233.

Berglund, B., Hemmingson, P. & Birgegard, G. (1987) Detection of autologous blood transfusions in cross-country skiers. *Int. J. Sports Med.* 8, 66–70.

Brien, A.J. & Simon, T.L. (1987) The effects of red blood cell infusion on 10-km race time. *J.A.M.A.* 257, 2761–2765.

Celsing, F., Svedenhag, J., Philstedt, P. & Ekblom, B. (1986) Effects of anaemia and stepwise induced polycythemia on maximal aerobic power in individuals with high and low hemoglobin concentrations. *Acta Physiol. Scand.* 129, 47–54.

Clement, D.B., Asmundson, R.C. & Medhurst, C.W. (1977) Hemoglobin values: comparative survey of the 1976 Canadian Olympic team. *J. Can. Med. Assoc.* 117, 614–616.

Clement, D.B. & Sawchuk, L.L. (1984) Iron status and sports performance. *Sports Med.* 1, 65–74.

Cowart, V.S. (1989) Erythropoietin: a dangerous new

form of blood doping? *Phys. Sportsmed.* **17**, 115–118.

Danzinger, R.G. & Cumming, G.R. (1964) Effects of chlorothiazide on working capacity of normal subjects. *J. Appl. Physiol.* **19**, 636–638.

Ekblom, B., Goldbarg, A.N. & Gullbring, B. (1972) Response to exercise after blood loss and reinfusion. *J. Appl. Physiol.* **33**, 175–180.

Frederickson, L.A., Puhl, J.L. & Runyan, W.S. (1983) Effects of training on indicies of iron status in young female cross-country runners. *Med. Sci. Sports Exerc.* **15**, 271–276.

Gledhill, N. (1982) Blood doping and related issues: a brief review. *Med. Sci. Sports Exerc.* **14**, 183–189.

Green, H.J., Jones, L.L., Hughson, R.L., Painter, D.C. & Farrance, B.W. (1987) Training-induced hypervolemia: lack of an effect on oxygen utilization during exercise. *Med. Sci. Sports Exerc.* **19**, 202–206.

Kanstrup, I.-L. & Ekblom, B. (1982) Acute hypervolemia, cardiac performance and aerobic power during exercise. *J. Appl. Physiol.* **52**, 1186–1191.

Kanstrup, I.-L. & Ekblom, B. (1984) Blood volume and hemoglobin concentration as determinants of maximal aerobic power. *Med. Sci. Sports Exerc.* **16**, 256–262.

Ondracka, S. & Gledhill, N. (1988) Evaluation of serum ferritin analysis techniques. *Can. J. Sports Sci.* **13**(3), 73–74.

Pate, R.R. (1983) Sports anemia: a review of the current research literature. *Phys. Sportsmed.* **11**, 115–127.

Pavelka, E. (1985) Olympic blood boosting. *Bicyling* April, 32–39.

Robertson, R.J., Gilcher, R., Metz, K. *et al.* (1982) Effect of induced erythrocythemia on hypoxia tolerance during physical exercise. *J. Appl. Physiol.* **53**(2), 490–495.

Saltin, B. (1964) Circulatory response to submaximal and maximal exercise after thermal dehydration. *J. Appl. Physiol.* **19**, 1125–1132.

Spriet, L., Gledhill, N., Froese, A.B. & Wilkes, D.L. (1986) Effect of graded erythrocythemia on cardiovascular and metabolic responses to exercise. *J. Appl. Physiol.* **61**, 1942–1948.

Sproule, B.J., Mitchell, J.H. & Miller, W.F. (1960) Cardiopulmonary physiological responses to heavy exercise in patients with anemia. *J. Clin. Invest.* **39**, 378–388.

Thomson, J., Stone, J.A., Ginsburg, A.D. & Hamilton, P. (1982) O_2 transport during exercise following blood reinfusion. *J. Appl. Physiol.* **53**, 1213–1219.

Valeri, C.R. (1976) *Blood Banking and The Use of Frozen Blood Products.* CRS Press, Cleveland.

Williams, M.H., Wesseldine, S., Somma, T. & Schuster, R. (1981) The effect of induced erythrocythemia upon 5-mile treadmill run time. *Med. Sci. Sports Exerc.* **13**, 169–175.

Chapter 22

Muscular Endurance and Blood Lactate

ROY J. SHEPHARD

Introduction

Muscular endurance and the accumulation of lactate in both the exercising muscles and blood stream, with ensuing problems in the regulation of acid−base balance, make a substantial contribution to an individual's overall performance in endurance competition.

The classical view of physical performance was that subjects pursued activity in a purely aerobic mode until their maximal oxygen intake was reached (Margaria *et al.*, 1963), only drawing upon anaerobic effort during occasional jockeying for position and the final sprint to the finish line. Four primary arguments suggested that a competitor might be wise to adopt such tactics. First, anaerobic activity is extremely inefficient metabolically; whereas each molecule of glucose phosphate can generate 39 molecules of adenosine triphosphate (ATP) during aerobic metabolism, only three molecules of ATP can be generated by the incomplete breakdown of the carbohydrate to lactate (Shephard, 1982). Second, any anaerobic component of activity is necessarily dependent upon the metabolism of carbohydrate, and thus depletes the limited body reserves of glycogen. Third, the accumulation of lactate causes local weakness and pain in the working muscles. Finally, the build-up of hydrogen ions stimulates a vigorous hyperventilation that is distressing for the subject and diverts a substantial fraction of the available cardiac output from the limbs to the chest muscles.

On the other hand, if endurance effort is extended beyond 30 min, there is increasing evidence that maximal oxygen intake is not the sole criterion of performance. Indeed, results are often correlated more closely with blood lactate measurements than with maximal oxygen intake (Table 22.1; Jacobs, 1986; Iwaoka *et al.*, 1988). Likewise, an evaluation of training may show that long-term endurance is improving despite a stagnation of gains in oxygen transport, this change reflecting the development of anaerobic mechanisms (Williams *et al.*, 1967; Heck *et al.*, 1985; Henritze *et al.*, 1985). It has also been argued that lactate measurements provide a simple method of evaluating a number of important characteristics of the active musculature, including the proportion of slow-twitch muscle fibres (Farrell *et al.*, 1979; Tesch *et al.*, 1981), capillary density (Tesch *et al.*, 1981; Jacobs *et al.*, 1983) and enzyme activity (Sjödin *et al.*, 1982). Moreover, several authors have argued that lactate levels should be the primary guide to the intensity of endurance training (Jacobs, 1986; Stegmann & Kindermann, 1982).

Muscular endurance

Muscular endurance is normally examined as the ratio of the peak force that can be generated by a muscle at any given time, relative to the peak force that was possible during a single brief initial effort. It is possible to consider muscular endurance with respect to a prolonged isometric contraction, a series of rhythmically

215

Table 22.1 Coefficients of correlation of maximal oxygen intake and blood lactate variables with endurance performance. From Jacobs (1986), with permission (see original paper for details of references).

Type of performance	Coefficient of correlation		Reference
	Maximal oxygen intake	Lactate	
42.2-km run	0.91	0.98	Farrell *et al.*, 1979
19.3-km run	0.91	0.97	
15.0-km run	0.89	0.97	
9.7-km run	0.86	0.96	
3.2-km run	0.83	0.91	
90-km run	n.s.	0.93	Jooste *et al.*, 1981
10-km run	0.75	0.84	Kumagi *et al.*, 1982
6.2-km run	0.49	0.84	
5-km run	0.46	0.95	
Race walking	0.62	0.94	Hagberg & Coyle, 1983
30-km run	0.71	0.76	Lehmann *et al.*, 1983
21.1-km run	0.81	0.88	Williams & Nute, 1983
10-km run	Lower	>0.89	Allen *et al.*, 1985

n.s., not significant.

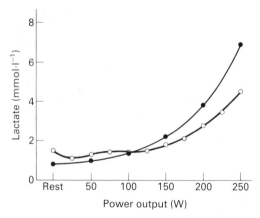

Fig. 22.1 Influence of ramp function on the relationship between power output and blood lactate readings. A comparison of two cycle ergometer tests with load increments of 25 and 50 W·min^{-1}, respectively. From Jacobs (1986), with permission.

repeated dynamic contractions, or a series of rhythmic contractions on an isotinetic dynamometer. In each of these cases, the decrement of force with time probably reflects a local accumulation of lactate, with an inhibition of glycolysis and a failure of ATP regeneration in the active muscle fibres (Tesch & Wright, 1983). The overall loss of muscle force thus depends on the proportion of muscle fibres in which lactate concentration has exceeded the limiting value for continued contractile function.

In very prolonged activities, muscle endurance may be limited by other factors, particularly a depletion of intramuscular glycogen reserves (Hultman, 1971). Muscle biopsy makes plain a progressive depletion of glycogen stores in individual fibres. In activities that last longer than 1 h, reliance is placed mainly upon the function of slow-twitch muscle fibres. As muscle glycogen reserves are depleted, a continuation of activity depends increasingly on the output of growth hormone and cortisol (Shephard & Sidney, 1975), with mobilization of alternative fuels (liver glycogen, proteolysis and lipolysis; Shephard, 1983). The decrease of blood glucose concentration over a very prolonged contest can be sufficient to cause a clinically significant hypoglycaemia, with a negative impact upon cerebral function (Noakes *et al.*, 1985). Other metabolites (glucose and fatty acids) are carried to the exercising muscle by the blood stream, but the rate of transfer is not enough to sustain the peak force of contraction observed at the beginning of exercise (Lloyd, 1966). Particular difficulty is encountered at points in the competition when anaerobic effort is required (for example, the cyclist who must climb a hill), since any anaerobic exercise has become dependent on an adequate supply of carbohydrate.

The training of muscular endurance can influence performance positively in several ways. First, as muscles become stronger, they contract at a smaller fraction of their maximum voluntary force. Perfusion thus occurs more readily, and a given effort can be sustained without recourse to the anaerobic activity that would cause an accumulation of lactate and a decrease of muscle force. Because the increase of bulk in the active muscle offers a larger peripheral vascular conductance (see Chapter 8), there is usually quite a close correlation between lean body mass and maximal oxygen intake (Davies & van Haaren, 1973), although in most endurance sports muscle hypertrophy also has the practical disadvantage of increasing total body mass and thus the load that must be transported (Shephard, 1982). Moreover, endurance training increases the local activity of aerobic enzymes (Holloszy, 1973); this change facilitates a continuation of aerobic metabolism at low partial pressures of oxygen, encouraging the metabolism of fat, with a resultant sparing of intramuscular glycogen. Finally, the size of intramuscular glycogen stores tends to be greater in well-trained individuals than in those who are not accustomed to endurance activity.

Blood lactate

While the critical variable limiting endurance performance is the intramuscular lactate concentration, the need for biopsy specimens limits the possibility of evaluating intracellular changes on a repeated basis. In contrast, a combination of peripheral venous catheterization and modern enzymatic techniques (Maughan, 1982; Karlsson et al., 1983) allows a fairly rapid and frequent measurement of blood lactate concentrations if desired (although Jacobs et al. (1985) have argued that much of the necessary information for management of an endurance athlete can be obtained from a single measurement of blood lactate during submaximal exercise).

When a small number of blood samples are needed, it is usual to take arterial or arterialized capillary blood specimens. The latter are collected by application of a chemical vasodilator or hot water to the ear lobe or the fingertip, followed by a sharp needle puncture. It is important to cleanse the skin of lactate secreted by the sweat glands, and to avoid squeezing the finger or ear (which could dilute the blood with extracellular fluid). If multiple readings are planned, a venous catheter is introduced, usually into the antecubital vein. Venous sampling has the important disadvantage of imposing a substantial time lag between release of lactate from the exercising muscles and its appearance in the blood specimens (Yoshida et al., 1982; Yeh et al., 1983). Moreover, if exercise is being performed on a cycle ergometer, but blood is being collected from the antecubital vein, the lactate formed in the quadriceps muscle has traversed the capillary beds of both the lungs and the forearm, with a potential for a substantial decrease of lactate concentrations en route (Yoshida et al., 1982; Orok et al., 1989).

Measurements of blood lactate concentrations can serve several purposes. They can help to define an optimal level of endurance training that lies just below an intensity at which substantial amounts of lactate accumulate in the blood stream (Sjödin et al., 1982; Stegmann et al., 1982). Measurements may also help to identify those who are well suited to long-distance competition in terms of fibre type, local capillary supply and muscle enzyme characteristics; current evidence suggests that those who have the characteristics allowing a good performance in events such as marathon races can operate very close to their peak aerobic power before significant accumulations of lactate occur (Costill, 1972; Neumann, 1983). Lactate data may further contribute to the design of an interval training plan, the length of recovery intervals being adjusted to assure no more than a modest accumulation of lactic acid in the working muscles or the circulating blood (Tesch & Wright, 1983; Yates et al., 1983). Operation at a blood lactate concentration of $3-5$ mmol·l^{-1} seems optimal in terms of developing a good anaerobic threshold (Sjödin et al., 1982; Hurley et al., 1984).

The original hypothesis of a sudden transition from aerobic to anaerobic activity was built around a very limited database, obtained during brief bouts of treadmill exercise (Margaria et al., 1963). More precise and more extensive measurements have since established that lactate can begin to accumulate in the arterial blood at efforts ranging from 50% to 70% of maximal oxygen intake, depending on the nature of the exercise that is being performed and the proportion of the skeletal musculature that has been activated (Shephard et al., 1968; 1989). Some authors have coined the term 'anaerobic threshold' for this phenomenon (Wasserman et al., 1973), although there does not seem to be any very clearcut threshold. The intensity of effort at which blood lactate first begins to increase depends on the ramp function (Hughson & Green, 1982; Campbell et al., 1989) and the type of exercise that is being undertaken, and is highly individualized. If steady state effort is pursued at $60-70\%$ of maximal oxygen intake, it is common for the blood lactate to rise at first, but subsequently to return toward resting values if the effort is continued (Kay & Shephard, 1969). At a somewhat larger fraction of maximal oxygen intake (80–90%), the blood lactate concentration rises progressively until a level is reached where the subject is exhausted. Recovery following exercise is also slowed as the duration of exercise is extended (Freund et al., 1990).

The increase of blood lactate concentration observed during exercise is a complex phenomenon (Brooks, 1985; 1987; Davis, 1985), depending upon the various factors that influence the input and egress of lactic acid from the muscles (Zouloumian & Freund, 1981) and the circulation (Eldridge, 1975; Jacobs, 1986). Under well-controlled laboratory conditions, intramuscular concentrations of lactate are influenced by both the overall rate of pyruvate metabolism (an influence independent of local oxygen partial pressures; Huckabee, 1958; Jobsis & Stainsby, 1968; Connett et al., 1984) and the extent of any local hypoxia in the muscle fibres. Because of a varying perfusion of the local capillary supply and differences in local intramuscular enzyme concentrations, one type of fibre within a given muscle may be functioning aerobically while another must resort to anaerobic metabolism. Lactate can thus diffuse from the anaerobically contracting fibres and be metabolized by fibres that are still operating aerobically. Moreover, the nature of the physical activity undertaken may be such that one muscle group is operating at a larger fraction of its maximal force, and therefore lacks adequate perfusion, while a second muscle group that is contracting less vigorously is not only able to function aerobically, but can also metabolize lactate originating from the first muscle group (Mazzeo et al., 1982).

The blood concentration of lactate depends firstly on the rate of diffusion from the muscle fibre into the blood stream. This is a relatively slow process; at normal temperatures, peak blood concentrations are reached $1-2$ min after a brief maximal effort such as a standard maximal oxygen intake test, but the time lag may be even longer in a cold environment (Bergh & Ekblom, 1979; Blomstrand et al., 1984). During a typical large muscle endurance activity, the function of key glycolytic enzymes is inhibited when the local lactate concentration reaches $30-40$ mmol·l^{-1}; the corresponding peak blood concentration does not usually exceed $10-12$ mmol·l^{-1}, although it can occasionally rise to 30 mmol·l^{-1} with a suitably designed interval training programme (Hermansen & Stensvold, 1972). The ratio of intramuscular to blood lactate concentration is influenced by the total volume of muscle that is functioning anaerobically, and by the total circulating blood volume (Shephard et al., 1989). Other influences are the proportion of carbohydrate in the diet and thus the extent of glycogen reserves (Jansson, 1980; Maughan & Poole, 1981; Greenhaff et al., 1988), the extent of tissue buffering and the rate of diffusion of hydrions from the muscles into the blood stream (Hughson & Green, 1982), the rate of metabolism of lactate (locally, in better oxygenated muscle fibres, in other muscles that are contracting less vigorously, and in the liver; Shephard, 1983), the blood flow carrying lactate away from the active muscles (particularly during recovery; Boileau et al., 1983), and the rate of excretion of lactic acid by the kidneys and the sweat glands (Lamont, 1987).

Under competitive conditions, the rate of lactate formation may vary over the course of an event. For instance, a distance cyclist may have to exert a much greater force on the pedals when ascending a rise than when covering level ground or a downhill gradient. Lactate thus accumulates during the climb, to be metabolized during the subsequent descent. While there are many potential situations where the accumulation of lactic acid can influence physical performance, the maximal potential accumulation of lactate is relatively small. There are practical difficulties in translating lactate into an equivalent quantity of oxygen delivery (Rieu et al., 1988), but if data are expressed in such terms DiPrampero et al. (1971) have suggested that the average person can generate the equivalent of 70 ml·kg^{-1} of oxygen by anaerobic metabolism. During the first minute of sustained activity, this would satisfy some 50% of requirements in an endurance athlete with a maximal oxygen intake of 70 ml·kg^{-1}·min^{-1}. However, if the activity were to be extended over a 1-h event, the maximal potential anaerobic contribution would drop to less than 1%.

Anaerobic threshold

There has been much controversy over the past 10 years as to both the existence and the definition of an anaerobic threshold (Brooks, 1985; 1987; Davis, 1985). The basic concept, originally described by Jervell (1929) and Owles (1930), and popularized by Wasserman et al. (1973), is straightforward enough. If a person engages in a task of progressively increasing intensity, a point is reached where effort can no longer be sustained by aerobic means. Thus, anaerobic metabolism supervenes. The blood lactate concentration rises, and if respiratory variables are being plotted against the increasing work rate, a disproportionate increase of ventilation is seen. Identification of the threshold can sometimes be facilitated by plotting the data in logarithmic form (Beaver et al., 1985).

The literature is unfortunately rather confusing, different authors using, among other terms, anaerobic threshold, the aerobic/anaerobic threshold, the onset of blood lactate accumulation (OBLA), the onset of plasma lactate accumulation, the lactate threshold, the lactate turning point, the maximal steady state, the individual anaerobic threshold, excess lactate and aerobic capacity (Jacobs, 1986) to describe similar but not necessarily identical phenomena. At the classical anaerobic threshold of Wasserman et al. (1973), the ventilatory equivalent for oxygen (which to this point in a continuous, ramp function exercise test has been decreasing) begins to increase again. The respiratory gas exchange ratio also begins to increase rapidly, although the ratio of ventilation to carbon dioxide output continues to fall. The turning point of the ventilatory equivalent for oxygen is the easiest method of identifying the anaerobic threshold (Davies et al., 1986; Reinhard et al., 1979), although the exercise test must begin at a low enough initial power output to accommodate the occasional individual with a turnpoint as low as 35–40% of maximal oxygen intake (McLellan, 1987). If the search is concentrated on finding a disproportionate increase in ventilation relative to work rate or carbon dioxide output, the breakpoint tends to be set at a higher power output (Beaver et al., 1986), corresponding to a second breakpoint that has been identified by other observers who make a more detailed analysis of the ventilatory record (McLellan, 1987). Irrespective of the specific criterion that is sought, the various breakpoints can be seen fairly readily during a large muscle task such as cycling or treadmill running, but it becomes much harder to identify any clear breakpoint when the activity involves a small group of muscles and the rise of blood lactate concentration is proportionately smaller (Shephard et al., 1989).

If effort is concentrated on identifying a single breakpoint, findings for an activity that involves most of the body musculature seem quite reproducible, not only in athletes but also in sedentary patients with a low aerobic power. Readings are consistent from one day's test to another and from one observer to another (Kavanagh et al., 1990). Further, in debilitated subjects, a measurement of the absolute ventilatory threshold may provide a better method of assessing fitness than attempts to carry a maximal effort test through to voluntary exhaustion. Authors who identify two breakpoints in the ventilation curve argue that the first reflects an increase of ventilation in proportion to oxygen consumption, sometimes calling this the ventilatory threshold or the aerobic threshold (Ribeiro et al., 1985). It may indicate a local intramuscular accumulation of lactate, without any substantial increase of blood lactate concentration (Systrom et al., 1990). A further possible factor is an increasing recruitment of fast-twitch fibres as the intensity of work is increased (Helal et al., 1987). There have been claims that such a ventilatory threshold corresponds to a blood lactate concentration of 2 $mmol\cdot l^{-1}$, although other authors have objected that the correspondence to this hypothetical value is poor (Davis et al., 1983; Aunola & Rusko, 1984), and that any relationship between ventilatory threshold and blood lactate concentrations is coincidental rather than causal (Hagberg, 1984; Neary et al., 1985; Gaesser & Poole, 1986).

If two thresholds are identified, then the

second is termed 'anaerobic'; at this point, the blood lactate concentration rises more steeply, ventilation becomes disproportionate to carbon dioxide output, and arterial Pco_2 falls (Ribeiro et al., 1985). With the usual ramp function test, the second breakpoint is said to correspond to a blood lactate concentration of about 4 $mmol\cdot l^{-1}$, although it is unclear whether blood lactate or a peripheral neurogenic drive is responsible for the hyperventilation (Hagberg et al., 1982; Dempsey et al., 1985).

Critics of the double breakpoint concept have noted that the identification of even a single threshold can be quite subjective, and they reason that the accuracy of the ventilation curve rarely warrants the fitting of two breakpoints. Further, they maintain that the particular shape of curve that is observed in any given experimental or athletic situation depends substantially upon the ratio of active muscle mass to blood volume, and is also influenced by the intensity/time curve for the exercise under consideration (Hughson & Green, 1982; Campbell et al., 1989).

When investigating anaerobic function, the measurement of ventilation plainly has attractions as a less invasive approach than the collection of blood samples. Investigators have thus persisted in their attempts to identify both ventilatory and anaerobic thresholds, using these values in the regulation of training prescriptions for athletes and sedentary patients alike (Stegmann & Kindermann, 1982; Jacobs, 1986). There remains the inconvenience of breathing through a tightly fitting facemask or mouthpiece as the breakpoints are determined, and interest has thus been aroused by suggestions that an analogous breakpoint can be detected in a plot of heart rate against power output or oxygen consumption (Conconi et al., 1982; Droghetti et al., 1985). It is easy to envisage how the increasing hydrion concentration can lead to the onset of a disproportionate hyperventilation as lactate accumulates in the blood stream. However, the theoretical basis of the Conconi heart-rate test is less certain. The heart rate/power output relationship is also influenced by changes of stroke volume, arterio-venous oxygen difference, core temperature and catecholamine secretion as the intensity of exercise is increased. Nevertheless, there could possibly be an added respiratory pumping of blood, an irradiation of impulses from the respiratory to the vasomotor centres and some stimulation of vasomotor centres from periph-eral muscular chemoreceptors as anaerobic effort supervenes. In an apparent direct contra-diction of the hypothesis of Conconi and associ-ates, other observers (for instance, Åstrand, 1960) have suggested that there is a linear relationship between heart rate and power output over the range between 50% and 100% of maximal oxygen intake. Thus the concept of a disproportionate tachycardia at the anaerobic threshold has not to date gained wide credence (Ribeiro *et al.*, 1985; Kuipers *et al.*, 1988; Francis *et al.*, 1989).

Acid−base balance

Acid−base status is commonly evaluated using the micro-Åstrup apparatus, a specialized de-vice that can equilibrate blood with known concentrations of carbon dioxide in oxygen and measure the resultant pH. The data yield estimates of pH, $P\text{CO}_2$, HCO_3', base excess, and standard bicarbonate reserve (Comroe, 1974). Under normal resting conditions, the blood pH is in the range 7.35−7.45. During long-distance running events, there is commonly a decrease to 7.15−7.25 (a somewhat smaller change than is observed in sprint competitions). The more rapidly the normal resting values are restored after exercise, the less the residual fatigue that the competitor experiences.

The total buffer base of whole blood is the sum of buffer anions (bicarbonate in plasma and red cells, haemoglobin, plasma protein, and the phosphate content of plasma and red cells). The base excess relative to standard nor-mal values can be computed using the Siggard−Andersen nomogram; the estimate is based on two of total plasma CO_2, pH, and $P\text{CO}_2$ (Comroe, 1974). For example, with a pH of 7.4

and a $P\text{CO}_2$ of 5.3 kPa (40 mmHg), the base excess is zero. However, if a lactate-related bicarbonate loss has brought about a lower pH at this carbon dioxide pressure, a negative base excess is calculated. The resultant base excess values show a high correlation with blood lac-tate, and Keul *et al.* (1969) have suggested that the blood lactate concentration (mmol·l^{-1}) can be estimated as (0.54 − base excess/1.25). The decrease of base excess that is incurred over the course of an athletic event represents an overall deficit of 'alkaline radicals' associated with the accumulation of not only lactic acid, but also pyruvic acid, ketoacids and fatty acids in the circulation. A good performer on a standard cycle ergometer test shows only about half the decrease in base excess seen in a bad performer.

The standard bicarbonate, or alkaline reserve, provides a second measure of any metabolic acidosis. It may be defined as the bicarbonate concentration observed at a standard tempera-ture of 37°C and a standard CO_2 pressure of 5.3 kPa (40 mmHg). Normal resting values range from 22 to 26 mmol·l^{-1}, but values can drop as low as 15 mmol·l^{-1} following exhausting ex-ercise (Shephard, 1983). Some 95% of the de-crease induced by all-out exercise is attributable to an accumulation of lactic acid and pyruvic acid, with the remaining 5% of change being caused by an accumulation of free fatty acids. There are some problems of interpretation of both base excess and standard bicarbonate levels during athletic competition, since the measurements assume a fixed core temperature of 37°C. During prolonged exercise, there may be substantial departures from the assumed temperature due to either hyperthemia or hypothermia.

The impact of lactate accumulation upon per-formance depends essentially upon the related change of hydrion concentration. The critical intramuscular pH for an inhibition of glycolysis is around 7.0. Likewise, the impact of a rising blood lactate concentration upon ventilatory function depends on the arterial acid−base balance.

Buffering capacity can increase during adaptation to carbon dioxide retention (a compensated respiratory acidosis). This has traditionally been described in submariners (Schaefer *et al.*, 1971), but it can also arise through repeated underwater exploration using self-contained underwater breathing apparatus. In contrast, the hyperventilation associated with exploration of high altitudes leads to a progressive loss of carbon dioxide, with a compensating adjustment of buffering by the kidneys; a normal resting pH is restored, but the person concerned has a poor tolerance of anaerobic activity because the loss of bicarbonate buffering is not fully compensated by the increased haemoglobin level (Shephard, 1982). At altitude, attempts have been made to treat the acute symptoms of respiratory alkalosis by the administration of acetazolamide, a carbonic anhydrase inhibitor (see Chapter 43). The athlete who prepares for endurance competition by altitude training will normally develop the hyperventilation-related handicap of a reduced serum bicarbonate concentration (see Chapter 43). Banister and Woo (1976) suggested the possibility of simulating altitude training by having teams rebreathe through long tubes during their practices. Such 'tube breathing' has the advantage that subjects are presented simultaneously with a combination of hypoxia and hypercarbia. In theory, haemoglobin formation is then stimulated without the disadvantage of reducing bicarbonate reserves. However, in practice the technique is rather clumsy, and experience to date has not shown any great gains in performance from tube rebreathing, possibly because the tubes can be used for only a brief period each day. A further potential option is to modify the acid−base balance by the deliberate ingestion of bicarbonate preparations. This plainly is a form of doping, although because of the prevalence of bicarbonate in the human body it would be extremely difficult to detect such an abuse. Observations have shown that such an approach can increase the speed of a short-distance run by a substantial 3%, although the dosage and the timing of bicarbonate ingestion

are critical to success (Wilkes *et al.*, 1983). To the author's knowledge, there have been no studies of the impact of bicarbonate doping upon endurance performance. If a sufficient dose of a bicarbonate preparation (at least 0.3 $g \cdot kg^{-1}$ body mass) were given at an appropriate point before or during a race, it might serve to counter some of the adverse effects of lactate accumulation, although it would also have the adverse effect of causing gastric discomfort (Horswill *et al.*, 1988).

References

Åstrand, I. (1960) Aerobic work capacity in men and women with special reference to age. *Acta Physiol. Scand.* **49** (Suppl. 169), 1−92.

Aunola, S. & Rusko, H. (1984) Reproducibility of aerobic and anaerobic thresholds in 20−50 year old men. *Eur. J. Appl. Physiol.* **53**, 260−266.

Banister, E.W. & Woo, W. (1976) Effects of simulated altitude training on aerobic and anaerobic power. *Eur. J. Appl. Physiol.* **38**, 55−69.

Beaver, W.L., Wasserman, K. & Whipp, B.J. (1985) Improved detection of lactate threshold during exercise using a log-log transformation. *J. Appl. Physiol.* **59**, 1936−1940.

Beaver, W.L., Wasserman, K. & Whipp, B.J. (1986) A new method for detecting anaerobic threshold by gas exchange. *J. Appl. Physiol.* **60**, 2020−2027.

Bergh, U. & Ekblom, B. (1979) Physical performance and peak aerobic power at different body temperatures. *J. Appl. Physiol.* **46**, 885−889.

Blomstrand, E., Bergh, U., Essén-Gustavsson, B. & Ekblom, B. (1984) Influence of low muscle temperature on muscle metabolism during intense dynamic exercise. *Acta Physiol. Scand.* **120**, 229−236.

Boileau, R.A., Misner, J.E., Dykstra, G.L. & Spitzer, T.A. (1983) Blood lactic acid removal during treadmill and bicycle exercise at various intensities. *J. Sports Med.* **23**, 159−167.

Brooks, G.A. (1985) Anaerobic threshold: review of the concept and directions for future research. *Med. Sci. Sports Exerc.* **17**, 22−31.

Brooks, G.A. (1987) Lactate production during exercise: oxidizable substrate versus fatigue agent. In: Macleod, D., Maughan, R., Nimmo, M., Reilly, T. & Williams, C. (eds) *Exercise — Benefits, Limits, and Adaptations.* E. & F.N. Spon, London.

Campbell, M.E., Hughson, R. & Green, H.J. (1989) Continuous increase in blood lactate concentration during different ramp exercise protocols. *J. Appl. Physiol.* **66**, 1104−1107.

Comroe, J.H., (1974) *Physiology of Respiration*, 2nd edn. Year Book Publishers, Chicago.

Conconi, F., Ferrari, M., Ziglio, P.G., Droghetti, P. & Codeca, L. (1982) Determination of the anaerobic threshold by a non-invasive field test in runners. *J. Appl. Physiol.* **52**, 869–873.

Connett, R.J., Gayeski, T.E. & Honig, C.R. (1984) Lactate accumulation in fully aerobic, working dog gracilis muscle. *Am. J. Physiol.* **246**, H120–H128.

Costill, D.L. (1972) Physiology of marathon running. *J.A.M.A.* **221**, 1024–1029.

Davies, C.T.M. & van Haaren, J.P.M. (1973) Maximum aerobic power and body composition in healthy East African older male and female subjects. *Am. J. Phys. Anthrop.* **39**, 395–401.

Davies, S.F., Iber, C., Keene, S.A., McArthur, C.D. & Path, M.J. (1986) Effect of respiratory alkalosis during exercise on blood lactate. *J. Appl. Physiol.* **61**, 948–952.

Davis, J.A. (1985) Anaerobic threshold: review of the concept and directions for future research. *Med. Sci. Sports Exerc.* **17**, 6–18.

Davis, J.A., Caiozoo, V.J., Lamarra, N. & Ellis, J.F. (1983) Does the gas exchange anaerobic threshold occur at a fixed blood lactate concentration of 2 or 4 mM? *Int. J. Sports Med.* **4**, 89–93.

Dempsey, J.A., Vidruk, E.H. & Mitchell, G.S. (1985) Pulmonary control systems in exercise: update. *Fed. Proc.* **44**, 2260–2270.

DiPrampero, P.E. (1971) Anaerobic capacity and power. In: Shephard, R.J. (ed.) *Frontiers of Fitness* pp. 155–173. C.C. Thomas, Springfield, Illinois.

Droghetti, P., Borsetto, C., Casoni, I. *et al.* (1985) Noninvasive determination of the anaerobic threshold in canoeing, cross-country skiing, cycling, roller, and ice skating, rowing and walking. *Eur. J. Appl. Physiol.* **53**, 299–303.

Eldridge, F.L. (1975) Relationship between turnover and blood concentration in exercising dogs. *J. Appl. Physiol.* **39**, 231–234.

Farrell, P.A., Wilmore, J.H., Coyle, E.F., Billing, J.E. & Costill, D.L. (1979) Plasma lactate accumulation and distance running performance. *Med. Sci. Sports Exerc.* **11**, 338–344.

Francis, K.T., McClatchen, P.R., Sumsion, J.R. & Hansen, D.E. (1989) The relationship between anaerobic threshold and heart rate linearity during cycle ergometry. *Eur. J. Appl. Physiol.* **59**, 273–277.

Freund, H., Oyono-Enguéllé, S., Heitz, A. *et al.* (1990) Comparative lactate kinetics after short and prolonged submaximal exercise. *Int. J. Sports Med.* **11**, 284–288.

Gaesser, G.A. & Poole, D.C. (1986) Lactate and ventilatory thresholds: disparity in time course of adaptations to training. *J. Appl. Physiol.* **61**, 999–1004.

Greenhaff, P.L., Gleeson, M. & Maughan, R.J. (1988) Diet-induced metabolic acidosis and the performance of high intensity exercise in man. *Eur. J. Appl. Physiol.* **57**, 254–259.

Hagberg, J.M. (1984) Physiological implications of the lactate threshold. *Int. J. Sports Med.* **5**, 106–109.

Hagberg, J.M., Coyle, E.F., Carroll, J.E., Miller, J.M., Martin, W.H. & Brooke, M.H. (1982) Exercise hyperventilation in patients with McArdle's disease. *J. Appl. Physiol.* **52**, 991–994.

Heck, H., Mader, A., Hess, G., Mücke, S., Müller, R. & Hollman, W. (1985) Justification of the 4 mmol/l lactate threshold. *Int. J. Sports Med.* **6**, 117–130.

Helal, J.N., Guezennec, C.Y. & Goubel, F. (1987) The aerobic–anaerobic transition: reexamination of the threshold concept including an electromyographic approach. *Eur. J. Appl. Physiol.* **56**, 643–649.

Henritze, J., Weltman, A., Schurrer, R.L. & Barlow, K. (1985) Effects of training at and above the lactate threshold on the lactate threshold and maximal oxygen intake. *Eur. J. Appl. Physiol.* **54**, 84–88.

Hermansen, L. & Stensvold, I. (1972) Production and removal of lactic acid during exercise in man. *Acta Physiol. Scand.* **86**, 191–201.

Holloszy, J.O. (1973) Biochemical adaptations to exercise: aerobic metabolism. *Exerc. Sport Sci. Rev.* **1**, 45–71.

Horswill, C.A., Costill D.L., Fink, W.J. *et al.* (1988) Influence of sodium bicarbonate on sprint performance: relationship to dosage. *Med. Sci. Sports Exerc.* **20**, 566–569.

Huckabee, W.E. (1958) Relationships of pyruvate and lactate during anaerobic metabolism. II. Exercise and formation of O_2 debt. *J. Clin. Invest.* **37**, 255–271.

Hughson, R.L. & Green, H. (1982) Blood acid–base and lactate relationships studied by ramp work tests. *Med. Sci. Sports* **14**, 297–302.

Hultman, E. (1971) Muscle glycogen stores and prolonged exercise. In: Shephard, R.J. (ed.) *Frontiers of Fitness.* C.C. Thomas, Springfield, Illinois.

Hurley, B.F., Hagberg, J.M., Allen, W.K. *et al.* (1984) Effect of training on blood lactate levels during submaximal exercise. *J. Appl. Physiol.* **56**, 1260–1264.

Iwaoka, K., Hatta, H., Atomi, Y. & Miyashita, M. (1988) Lactate, respiratory compensation thresholds, and distance running performance in runners of both sexes. *Int. J. Sports Med.* **9**, 306–309.

Jacobs, I. (1986) Blood lactate: implications for training and sports performance. *Sports Med.* **3**, 10–25.

Jacobs, I., Schéle, R. & Sjodin, B. (1983) A single blood lactate determination as an indicator of cycle ergometer endurance capacity. *Eur. J. Appl. Physiol.* **50**, 355–364.

Jacobs, I., Schéle, R. & Sjodin, B. (1985) Blood lactate

vs exhaustive exercise to evaluate aerobic fitness. *Eur. J. Appl. Physiol.* **54**, 151–155.

Jansson, E. (1980) Diet and muscle metabolism in man. *Acta Physiol. Scand.* (Suppl.) **487**, 1–24.

Jervell, O. (1929) Milchsäureuntersuchungen im Blot bei Nephritidien. *Acta Med. Scand.* **72**, 262–273.

Jobsis, F. & Stainsby, W. (1968) Oxidation of NADH during contractions of circulated skeletal muscle. *Resp. Physiol.* **4**, 292–300.

Karlsson, J., Jacobs, I., Sjodin, B. *et al.* (1983) Semi-automatic blood lactate assay: experiences from an exercise laboratory. *Int. J. Sports. Med.* **4**, 52–55.

Kavanagh, T.J., Mertens, D.J., Myers, M.G., Baigrie, T. & Shephard, R.J. (1990) Assessment of patients with congestive failure: ventilatory threshold or aerobic power determination. *Proc. Int. Congr. Cardiol.*, Manila, C1656.

Kay, C. & Shephard, R.J. (1969) On muscle strength and the threshold of anaerobic work. *Int. Z. Angew. Physiol.* **27**, 311–328.

Keul, J., Doll, E. & Keppler, D. (1969) *Muskelstoffwechsel.* J.A. Barth, Munich.

Kuipers, H., Keizer, H.A., deVries, T., van Rijthoven, P. & Wijts, M. (1988) Comparison of heart rate as a non-invasive determinant of anaerobic threshold with the lactate threshold when cycling. *Eur. J. Appl. Physiol.* **58**, 303–306.

Lamont, L.S. (1987) Sweat lactate secretion during exercise in relation to women's aerobic capacity. *J. Appl. Physiol.* **62**, 194–198.

Lloyd, B.B. (1966) Presidential Address, Section 1 (Physiology and Biochemistry). In: *Advancement of Sciences*, pp. 515–530. British Association for Advancement of Science, London.

McLellan, T.M. (1987) The anaerobic threshold: concept and controversy. *Aust. J. Sci. Med. Sport* **19**, 3–8.

Margaria, R., Cerretelli, P., DiPrampero, P.E., Massari, C. & Torelli, G. (1963) Kinetics and mechanisms of oxygen debt contraction in man. *J. Appl. Physiol.* **18**, 371–377.

Maughan, R.J. (1982) A simple, rapid method for the determination of glucose, lactate, pyruvate, alanine, 3-hydroxybutyrate and acetoacetate on a single 20 μl blood sample. *Clin. Chim. Acta* **122**, 231–240.

Maughan, R.J. & Poole, D.C. (1981) The effects of glycogen loading regimen on the capacity to perform anaerobic exercise. *Eur. J. Appl. Physiol.* **46**, 211–219.

Mazzeo, R.S., Brooks, G.A., Budinger, T.F. & Schoeller, D.A. (1982) Pulse injection, ^{13}C tracer studies of lactate metabolism in humans during rest and two levels of exercise. *Biomed. Mass Spectrom.* **9**, 310–314.

Neary, P.J., MacDougall, J.D., Bachus, R. & Wenger, H.A. (1985) The relationship between lactate and ventilatory thresholds: coincidental or cause and effect? *Eur. J. Appl. Physiol.* **54**, 104–108.

Neumann, G. (1983) Metabole Regulation bei Langzeitausdauerleistungen. *Med. Sport* **23**, 169.

Noakes, T.D., Nathan, M., Irving, R.A. *et al.* (1985) Physiological and biochemical measurements during a 4-day surf-ski marathon. *S. Afr. Med. J.* **67**, 212–216.

Orok, C.J., Hughson, R.L., Green, H.J. & Thomson, J.A. (1989) Blood lactate responses in incremental exercise as predictors of constant load performance. *Eur. J. Appl. Physiol.* **59**, 262–267.

Owles, W.H. (1930) Alterations in the lactic acid content of the blood as a result of light exercise and associated changes in the CO_2 combining power of the blood and in the alveolar CO_2 pressure. *J. Physiol.* **69**, 214–237.

Reinhard, U., Müller, P.H. & Schmülling, R.M. (1979) Determination of anaerobic threshold by the ventilation equivalent in normal individuals. *Respiration* **38**, 36–42.

Ribeiro, J.P., Fielding, R.A., Hughes, V., Black, A., Bochese, M.A. & Knuttgen, H.G. (1985) Heart rate break point may coincide with the anaerobic and not the aerobic threshold. *Int. J. Sports Med.* **6**, 220–224.

Rieu, M., Duvallet, A., Scharapan, L., Thieulart, L. & Ferry, A. (1988) Blood lactate accumulation in intermittent supramaximal exercise. *Eur. J. Appl. Physiol.* **57**, 235–242.

Schaefer, K.E., Bond, G.F., Mazzone, W.F., Carey, C.R. & Dougherty, J.H. (1971) Carbon dioxide retention and metabolic changes during prolonged exposure to high pressure environment. *Aerospace Med.* **39**, 1206–1215.

Shephard, R.J. (1982) *Physiology and Biochemistry of Exercise.* Praeger Publishing, New York.

Shephard, R.J. (1983) *Biochemistry of Physical Activity.* C.C. Thomas, Springfield, Illinois.

Shephard, R.J., Allen, C., Benade, A.J.S. *et al.* (1968) Standardization of submaximal exercise tests. *Bull. W.H.O.* **38**, 765–776.

Shephard, R.J., Bouhlel, E., Vandewalle, H. & Monod, H. (1989) Anaerobic threshold, muscle volume and hypoxia. *Eur. J. Appl. Physiol.* **58**, 826–832.

Shephard, R.J. & Sidney, K.H. (1975) Effects of physical exercise on plasma growth hormone and cortisol levels in human subjects. *Exerc. Sport Sci. Rev.* **3**, 1–30.

Sjödin, B., Schéle, R., Karlsson, J., Linnarsson, D. & Willensten, R. (1982) The physiological background of onset of blood lactate accumulation (OBLA). In: Komi, P.V. (ed.) *Exercise and Sport Biology*, pp. 43–56. Human Kinetics, Champaign, Illinois.

Stegmann, H. & Kindermann, W. (1982) Comparison of prolonged exercise tests at the individual anaerobic threshold and the fixed anaerobic threshold of 4 mmol/l. *Int. J. Sports Med.* **3**, 105−110.

Systrom, D.M., Kanarck, D.J., Kohler, S.J. & Kazemi, H. (1990) ^{31}P nuclear magnetic resonance spectroscopy study of the anaerobic threshold in humans. *J. Appl. Physiol.* **68**, 2060−2066.

Tesch, P.A., Sharp, D.S. & Daniels, W.L. (1981) Influence of fiber type composition and capillary density on onset of blood lactate accumulation. *Int. J. Sports Med.* **2**, 252−255.

Tesch, P.A. & Wright, J.E. (1983) Recovery from short term intense exercise: its relation to capillary blood supply and blood lactate concentration. *Eur. J. Appl. Physiol.* **52**, 98−103.

Wasserman, K., Whipp, B.J., Koyal, S.N. & Beaver, W.L. (1973) The anaerobic threshold and respiratory gas exchange during exercise. *J. Appl. Physiol.* **35**, 236−243.

Wilkes, D., Gledhill, N. & Smyth, R. (1983) Effect of acute induced metabolic alkalosis on 800-m racing times. *Med. Sci. Sports Exerc.* **15**, 277−280.

Williams, C.G., Wyndham, C.H., Kok, R. & von Rahden, M.J. (1967) Effect of training on maximum oxygen intake and anaerobic metabolism in man. *Int. Z. Angew. Physiol.* **24**, 18−23.

Yates, J.W., Gladden, L.B. & Cresanta, M.K. (1983) Effects of prior dynamic leg exercise on static effort of the elbow flexors. *J. Appl. Physiol.* **55**, 891−896.

Yeh, M.P., Gardner, R.M., Adams, T.D., Yanowitz, F.G. & Crapo, R.O. (1983) 'Anaerobic threshold': problems of determination and validation. *J. Appl. Physiol.* **55**, 1178−1186.

Yoshida, T., Takeuchi, N. & Suda, Y. (1982) Arterial versus venous blood lactate increase in the forearm during incremental bicycle exercise. *Eur. J. Appl. Physiol.* **50**, 87−93.

Zouloumian, P. & Freund, H. (1981) Lactate after exercise in man. III. Properties of the compartment model. *Eur. J. Appl. Physiol.* **46**, 135−147.

Chapter 23

Metabolism in the Contracting Skeletal Muscle

JAN HENRIKSSON

Major metabolic pathways of the muscle cell: an overview

Introduction

Ultimately, endurance performance is dependent on metabolism in the contracting muscles. Muscle metabolism is a broad concept, including all the chemical reactions that take place in the muscle cell. An important part of muscle metabolism is the uptake of fuels from the blood and their subsequent degradation to yield energy in a form that can be used by the muscle cell, e.g. to perform contractile work or to build new cellular material in a continuous cycle of degradation and synthesis. Muscle metabolism further includes: (i) the hepatic mobilization of glucose from glycogen; and (ii) the mobilization of fatty acids from triglycerides in the adipose tissue and the transport of these compounds to the muscle. The metabolic processes are regulated via a complicated chemical interaction of the body's different organs.

The muscle cell is unique in the sense that its metabolic rate can vary over a very wide range, increasing more than 200 times from rest to maximal exercise. The major portion of this increase is due to processes related to the production of chemical energy for the contracting filaments. The most important principles of energy metabolism in skeletal muscle also apply to the majority of other tissues in the body.

For most chemical compounds in the body, the net turnover is zero, i.e. their degradation over a given period of time equals their resynthesis. Therefore, only a limited number of compounds constitute quantitatively important reactants and products in the net metabolic equation. The total body metabolism can thus be simplified as consisting of a rather small number of biochemical pathways that have a significant impact on the cellular metabolic equilibrium. These include: (1) the complete oxidation of carbohydrates, fats (and proteins); (2) the net transformation of carbohydrates into fats and of proteins into carbohydrates (gluconeogenesis) and fats; (3) the net formation of ketoacids (acetoacetic acid and β-hydroxybutyric acid) from fatty acids (liver only); (4) the net formation of lactic acid from carbohydrates (glycogen), the pathway known as anaerobic glycolysis; and (5) the oxidation of alcohol, during times of alcohol intake, which may make up a significant portion of the body's metabolism and partly replace the oxidation of carbohydrates and fats.

The degradation of glycogen is correctly termed glycogenolysis. In the present chapter, however, in order to avoid confusion, the term glycogenolysis is avoided and instead glycolysis is used to mean both glycolysis from glucose and glycolysis from glycogen.

The initial steps in the oxidation of alcohol occur almost exclusively in the liver. This is likely to explain why the maximal turnover of alcohol is not increased by physical exercise, despite the fact that its hepatic degradation product, acetic acid, is transported to skeletal muscle and other organs for final oxidation.

For contracting muscle only (1), (4) and gluconeogenesis are of quantitative importance. These biochemical pathways, as well as the energy exchange between adenosine triphosphate (ATP) and phosphocreatine, are discussed below.

Muscle metabolism: general principles

The muscle cell obtains its energy by degrading carbohydrates and fats to smaller molecules. As a result of this degradation, part of the energy stored in the carbohydrate and fat molecules is released and used by the cell to cover its energy demands. Proteins, the third large group of organic compounds, are not normally used as a fuel by skeletal muscles. This makes sense physiologically, since proteins constitute the building blocks of the cells in the body. This is especially true of skeletal muscle cells, due to their high content of the contractile proteins (myosin and actin). However, in situations where the body's energy supply is compromised, such as in long-term starvation, proteins (including those derived from muscle tissue) will also be used as a fuel in the energy metabolism of muscle.

All energy originates from the sun. The chlorophyll of green plants trap solar energy in the photosynthetic process, where carbon dioxide is combined with water to yield carbohydrate (starch and sucrose) (see Fig. 23.1). Carbohydrates and proteins contain approximately 17 kJ of energy per gram, while fats contain more than twice as much: 39 kJ$\cdot$g^{-1} (corresponding to 29 kJ$\cdot$g^{-1} of adipose tissue). From an energy point of view, fat is thus by far the best storage fuel (Fig. 23.2). One drawback, however, is that once transformed to fat for storage, carbohydrates and proteins cannot be reformed. The carbon skeleton of five of the 20 amino acids, from which proteins are formed, can theoretically be synthesized from fatty acids, but human cells can synthesize only one

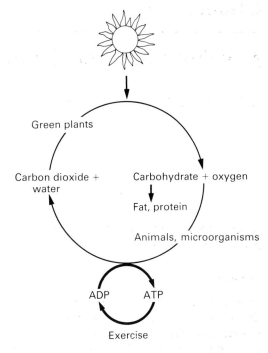

Fig. 23.1 Schematic view of the cycle of carbon compounds in nature. The chlorophyll of green plants trap solar energy in the photosynthetic process. In this process, carbon dioxide is combined with water to yield carbohydrate (starch and sucrose), with the formation of oxygen. Solar energy is thus incorporated into these carbohydrates, and is 'transferred' to fats and proteins when part of the carbohydrates is used to synthesize these compounds in plants or animals. In cells of animals and microorganisms, oxygen is utilized in the combustion of carbohydrates, fats (and proteins), whereby carbon dioxide and water are reformed. The energy thus released permits the synthesis of adenosine triphosphate (ATP), the cell-specific energy source. ADP, adenosine diphosphate.

of these. The remaining four belong to the group of 'essential' amino acids, which must be taken in via the diet.

Another product of photosynthesis is oxygen. The circle is closed when, in muscle and other cells, oxygen is utilized in the combustion of carbohydrates, fats (and proteins), whereby carbon dioxide and water are reformed (see Fig. 23.1). For further studies, the reader is

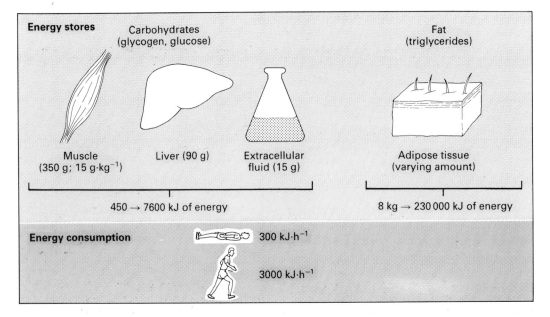

Fig. 23.2 The approximate magnitude of the largest body stores of carbohydrates and fat. The energy content of these compounds is compared with energy consumption at rest and during relatively intense exercise ($\dot{V}o_2 = 2.5$ l·min^{-1}).

referred to standard textbooks of biochemistry and physiology. Three which, in the present context, have been found to be of particular value are those by McMurray (1983), Newsholme and Leech (1983) and Åstrand and Rodahl (1986).

Enzyme-catalysed reactions

In cellular energy metabolism, fats and carbohydrates are degraded successively in small steps. Each step (reaction) is made possible (catalysed) by one enzyme. Enzymes are small proteins, one specific enzyme existing for each of the thousands of chemical reactions that occur in the body. Without these biological catalysts, all chemical reactions would proceed very slowly at body temperature. Different chemical processes each involve a characteristic number of steps. For example, the degradation of glucose to lactate requires a sequence of 10 enzyme reactions (Fig. 23.3). The ultimate goal of the energy metabolism in muscle is to release the energy bound in the carbohydrate and fat molecules. Therefore, it is to be expected that most of the reactions occur with a loss of energy, the energy content of the product being less than that of the substrate. Such reactions are termed exergonic. There are also several reactions (Fig. 23.3), where energy must be added in order for the reaction to occur (endergonic reactions, e.g. A→B, C→D) and other reactions with little or no energy exchange (e.g. B→C, J→Z). The cell can make use of the energy released in reactions only where there is a large energy loss (in Fig. 23.3, steps F→G and I→J). In other reactions involving an energy loss, the liberated energy cannot be used by the cell and is released as heat instead in Fig. 23.3, steps D→E, E→F, G→H). The generated heat, although a byproduct, contributes to the maintenance of normal body temperature in homoiothermal species.

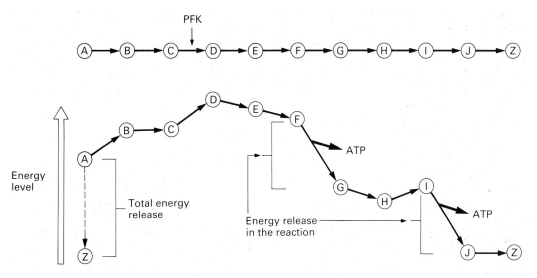

Fig. 23.3 Schematic illustration of the chemical reactions involved in the glycolytic pathway. A symbolizes glucose, J pyruvate and Z lactate. Each arrow symbolizes one chemical reaction and one enzyme step. The letters B–I represent metabolic intermediates between glucose and pyruvate. 6-Phosphofructokinase (PFK), the rate-limiting enzyme of glycolysis, catalyses the reaction C→D. The energy contents of the different compounds are indicated at the bottom of the figure. In reactions where there is a large energy loss, the released energy is utilized in the resynthesis of adenosine triphosphate (ATP). From McMurray (1983), modified with permission.

How cells make use of the liberated energy

In reaction steps with a sufficiently large energy release, the liberated energy is used to synthesize a cell-specific, energy-rich compound, ATP. ATP is of paramount importance since it is the only form of energy the cell can use directly. The structure of the ATP molecule is illustrated in Fig. 23.4.

The three phosphate groups are an important feature of this molecule. These are bound with high-energy chemical bonds. This means that their formation involves the utilization of a large amount of energy, but also that much energy is liberated when the bond is broken (hydrolysed). In order to bind a phosphate group to ADP, adenosine diphosphate, to give rise to ATP, approximately 70 joules per gram of ADP or 5×10^{-20} joules per molecule of ADP are required. If less energy than this is liberated in a specific reaction, no ATP can be produced

at this step, and all of the liberated energy is released as heat. When the muscle is activated, the outermost phosphate group of the ATP molecule is cleaved off enzymatically, liberating energy for the contracting filaments (see Fig. 23.1). ATP is stored in each muscle cell, but in an amount sufficient for only a few seconds of intense contraction. Thus, for the muscle to continue contracting, it is essential that ATP should be continuously resynthesized from ADP, at a very high rate. Over 24 h, the total weight of the ATP produced and consumed in the human body generally exceeds the body weight.

Major metabolic pathways of the muscle cell: an overview

The cell utilizes four major metabolic pathways to degrade and obtain energy from fats and carbohydrates. These are glycogenolysis/

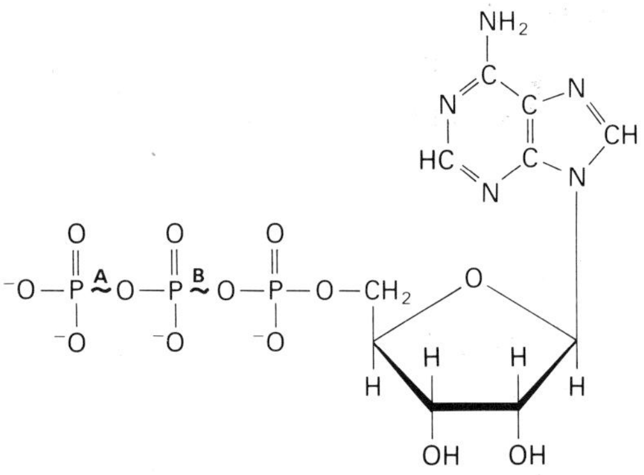

Adenosine triphosphate (ATP)

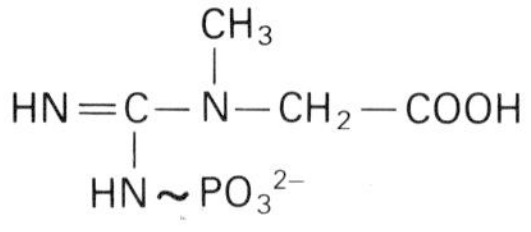

Phosphocreatine

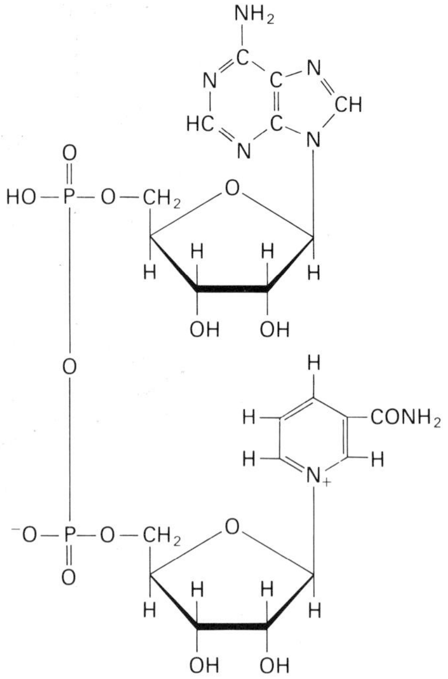

Nicotinamide adenine dinucleotide (NAD$^+$)

Fig. 23.4 Three key substances in cellular energy metabolism: ATP, NAD$^+$ and phosphocreatine. ATP contains two phosphate groups bound by high-energy bonds (**A** and **B**). (The bond of the innermost phosphate group contains less energy.) The energy released when these bonds are hydrolysed is the only form of energy that can be used directly by the cell. When bond **A** is hydrolysed, ATP is converted to adenosine diphosphate (ADP). The cleaving of the next phosphate group (bond **B**) converts ADP to adenosine monophosphate (AMP). ATP is subsequently resynthesized from ADP (or AMP) via the energy that is released in the cellular degradation of carbohydrates and fats. ATP may also be resynthesized from ADP using energy liberated by cleavage of the high-energy phosphate group of phosphocreatine (PO$_3{}^{2-}$). The function of NAD$^+$ is to take up electrons (and hydrogen), which are released at several points in the cellular degradation of carbohydrates and fats (and proteins). These are incorporated in the NAD$^+$ molecule in the lower nitrogen-containing ring and result in the conversion (reduction) of NAD$^+$ to NADH. NADH subsequently donates its electrons to the mitochondrial respiratory chain. The electron flow in the respiratory chain represents the body's most important energy source in producing ATP (three molecules of ATP per molecule of NADH). Note the similarity between the configuration of the ATP and NAD$^+$ molecules; both are termed nucleotides. $\sim$ symbolizes a high-energy bond.

glycolysis, the fatty acid degradation system (β-oxidation), the citric acid cycle and the respiratory chain (Fig. 23.5). A metabolic pathway, or enzyme system, is a group of enzymes which catalyse a consecutive chain of reactions. One such enzyme system, anaerobic glycolysis, is illustrated in Fig. 23.3.

The enzymes of a specific metabolic pathway

are often located close to each other in the same cellular compartment. Each cell in the body is delineated by a cell membrane, inside which are many different organelles such as the nucleus, the mitochondria and the sarcoplasmic reticulum. In skeletal muscle cells, the most abundant structures in the cytoplasm are the contractile filaments, myosin and actin,

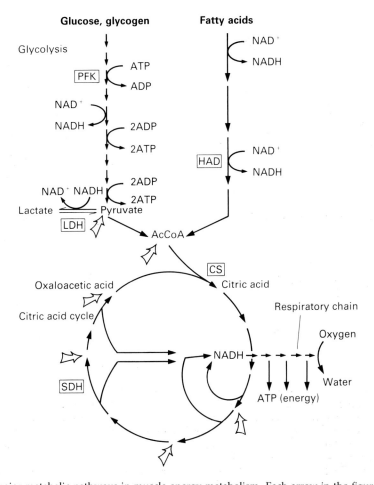

Fig. 23.5 The major metabolic pathways in muscle energy metabolism. Each arrow in the figure designates a chemical reaction, i.e. one enzyme step; the metabolic intermediates are illustrated only as the empty space between arrows. Enzymes, the levels of which are commonly used as a measure of the capacity of their respective metabolic pathways, are indicated: 6-phosphofructokinase (PFK) and lactate dehydrogenase (LDH) of glycolysis; 3-hydroxyacyl CoA dehydrogenase (HAD) of the fatty acid β-oxidation pathway; and citrate synthase (CS) and succinate dehydrogenase (SDH) of the citric acid cycle. The proteins enter this system when their building blocks, the amino acids, are degraded to different metabolic intermediates in glycolysis and the citric acid cycle or to AcCoA (acetyl coenzyme A) (see the open arrows). The figure indicates that in each of two steps of glycolysis, two molecules of ATP are formed. This is explained by the fact that the glucose molecule (which contains six carbon atoms) is split to yield two three-carbon units in the step following the PFK reaction. It should be noted that there is a cost of one additional ATP molecule to phosphorylate glucose. To increase clarity, the two molecules of carbon dioxide and the GTP (guanosine triphosphate) molecule, which is formed in the citric acid cycle, have been omitted from the figure. ⇗, entry of amino acids.

which in concert with several other proteins execute the contractile activity. The glycolytic enzymes are located in the cytoplasm, close to the contractile filaments. Thus, the ATP pro-

duced via the glycolytic pathway is formed near the site of its use. Part of the muscle store of ATP and phosphocreatine is likewise in close proximity to the contractile filaments. The other three major metabolic pathways in muscle energy metabolism (fatty acid β-oxidation, the citric acid cycle and the respiratory chain) are, unlike glycolysis, strictly aerobic. Most of the enzymes of aerobic metabolism are localized in one specific cellular organelle, the mito-chondrion. The fatty acid β-oxidation enzymes are arranged in the inner space of the mito-chondria (the matrix), whereas many enzymes of the citric acid cycle and components of the respiratory chain are situated on the inner mito-chondrial wall. Thus, the substrates for the aerobic pathways, such as fatty acids and pyruvate, must be transported into the mito-chondria from the cytoplasm and, conversely, the ATP produced in aerobic processes must be transported from mitochondria to the cyto-plasmic site of use. This is one reason why the maximal power is lower in the aerobic pathways than in anaerobic glycolysis.

Oxidation–reduction

Oxidation and reduction reactions have a cen-tral position in cellular metabolism. Oxidation is chemically defined as a release of electrons. Reduction is its counterpart, i.e. an electron uptake. The reactant that receives electrons in a specific chemical reaction will be reduced and, conversely, the reactant that donates the elec-trons will be oxidized. In many oxidation–reduction (redox) reactions, the electrons are released or incorporated via hydrogen atoms (a proton with an associated electron) or hy-dride ions (a proton with an associated pair of electrons). The term dehydrogenation is there-fore used synonymously with oxidation. The major substrates of energy metabolism, e.g. glucose and fatty acids, are generally more reduced than their degradation products, such as carbon dioxide and water. They therefore have a greater tendency to release electrons (and hydrogen). The entire degradation of carbohydrates and fats to carbon dioxide and water is therefore often termed oxidation. The central cellular substance in redox reactions is the compound NAD^+, nicotinamide adenine dinucleotide (see Fig. 23.4). NAD^+ functions as an electron carrier. This means that it can easily take up or release electrons and hydrogen. At several points in the cellular degradation of carbohydrates and fats, hydride ions are re-leased from the metabolic intermediates and taken up by NAD^+, and a proton is liberated into the medium (Fig. 23.5). In this process NAD^+ is reduced to NADH. NADH sub-sequently donates its electrons to the mito-chondrial respiratory chain. The electron flow through the respiratory chain represents the body's most important energy source in pro-ducing ATP (three ATP molecules per molecule of NADH).

ATP production from phosphocreatine

Phosphocreatine also has a high-energy phos-phate bond (see Fig. 23.4) with a similar energy content to that of the corresponding bond in the ATP molecule. When this bond is enzy-matically cleaved, the released energy can be used to resynthesize one molecule of ATP from ADP. This is the fastest way available for ATP resynthesis in the cell, because it occurs without activation of the carbohydrate and fat degra-dation systems. The cellular store of phospho-creatine is three times that of ATP; if used up completely, these two compounds would yield sufficient energy for 5–10 s of intense muscle activity. There is no cellular system that can directly utilize the energy derived from phos-phocreatine. Its function is that of a 'buffer substance' which can rapidly resynthesize ATP during muscle contraction.

In muscular exercise of longer duration than 5–10 s, other ATP-regenerating systems must come into play. None of the remaining systems has, however, the same maximal power as the phosphocreatine reaction (McGilvery, 1975). The exercise intensity must therefore be re-duced accordingly. Below, these other ATP-regenerating systems (anaerobic glycolysis, carbohydrate oxidation and fat oxidation), are described in order of decreasing maximal power.

ATP production from glycolysis

GENERAL BACKGROUND

In glycolysis, glucose or glycogen molecules are broken down to pyruvate (or lactate) (Fig. 23.5). If glucose is the starting substance of glycolysis, the net gain is two ATP molecules per molecule of glucose consumed. If the starting substance is glycogen, the gain per molecule of glucose is three molecules of ATP. In one of the glycolytic reactions hydride ions are released to NAD$^+$ (Fig. 23.5), which is transformed into NADH. The cellular content of NAD$^+$ is sufficient for only a few seconds of maximal glycolytic activation. Therefore, a prerequisite glycolytic energy production is that NADH continuously releases its electrons and hydrogen in order to reform NAD$^+$. This release may occur in two different ways. The most advantageous is the release of electrons and protons to the mitochondrial respiratory chain, with the subsequent formation of three molecules of ATP per molecule of NADH. This demands in turn an adequate cellular supply of oxygen, since the respiratory chain is strictly aerobic. In this situation, the glycolytically formed pyruvate is transported from the cytoplasm into the mitochondrion to be converted to acetyl coenzyme A (acetyl CoA) and further degraded in the citric acid cycle (Fig. 23.5).

When the oxygen supply is inadequate, for instance during intense exercise, or when the glycolytic rate is high, part of the NAD$^+$ is reformed via an alternative mechanism. This involves the transfer of electrons and hydrogen from NADH to pyruvate ($C_3H_4O_3$), which is then transformed into lactate ($C_3H_6O_3$). No ATP is regenerated in this reaction, but NAD$^+$ is reformed, thus enabling continued ATP production via the glycolytic pathway. The formation of lactate and protons as a consequence of an insufficient oxygen supply can be readily understood, but why does a high glycolytic rate also lead to an increased production of lactate? The probable reason is that, in this situation, the cytoplasmic NADH con-

centration must be set at a higher level in order to establish a sufficiently high driving pressure for the transport of cytoplasmic NADH into the mitochondrial respiratory chain. This is necessary because a high glycolytic rate results in more NADH having to be transported into the mitochondrion. An increased cytoplasmic NADH content automatically leads to more pyruvate being converted to lactate (Fig. 23.5). The two causes of lactate formation are closely linked, since a relative lack of oxygen automatically leads to a high glycolytic rate in the muscle cell. The drawbacks of lactate formation are: (i) that the possibility of obtaining ATP from NADH in the respiratory chain is not utilized; and (ii) that the pH is gradually reduced, leading to impaired muscle function.

Part of the lactate formed in muscles during intense exercise is released to the blood stream and is subsequently taken up by the liver or by other muscles. A large part, however, remains in the muscle, where one portion follows the opposite route, i.e. it is utilized to resynthesize glucose and glycogen. A large portion is subsequently reconverted to pyruvate and further degraded in the citric acid cycle. The energy yield for the resynthesis of ATP is the same, whether the degradation of glycogen goes directly via pyruvate into the mitochondrion or makes a 'detour' to lactate first. The importance of this route is illustrated by the fact that following a bout of intense exercise, lactate disappearance occurs markedly faster when a subject continues to exercise at a lower intensity than during complete rest. The exercise intensity most suitable for this purpose has been found to be one demanding approximately 40% of the person's $\dot{V}o_{2\,max}$ (Åstrand & Rodahl, 1986).

ANAEROBIC GLYCOLYSIS

In this pathway (Figs 23.3 & 23.5), where glycogen is gradually converted to lactate without the participation of oxygen, ATP is regenerated from ADP, at a rate of about one third to one half of that of the phosphocreatine reaction (McGilvery, 1975). The high rate of ATP regeneration in anaerobic glycolysis is due to the fact that the mitochondrial oxidative processes need not be activated. The price for such independence is lactate, or more correctly H^+, accumulation, which gradually fatigues the muscle. The starting point of this pathway is glycogen. Glycogen, essentially a branched chain of glucose molecules, is stored in skeletal muscle in varying amounts, normally between 15 and 25 $g \cdot kg^{-1}$ muscle (see Fig. 23.2; see also Chapter 12). In glycolysis, about 1 kJ of energy is released per gram of glycogen degraded. Roughly half of this amount is used to re-synthesize ATP; the remaining half is released as heat.

AEROBIC GLYCOLYSIS (CARBOHYDRATE OXIDATION)

Anaerobic glycolysis constitutes the main source of energy in intense exercise of short duration (under 2 min). Longer exercise periods require that the main energy delivery occurs through aerobic processes. Carbohydrate oxidation occurs without the accumulation of lactate and accompanying protons and is therefore tolerated longer by the muscle cell. In addition, a much larger portion of the stored energy is utilized for ATP formation. The power of aerobic glycolysis is about half of that in anaerobic glycolysis. In a given muscle, these processes may occur simultaneously; in one fraction of the muscle aerobic metabolism may dominate, while other muscle cells, due to their enzyme characteristics and blood supply, may derive a large part of their energy supply from anaerobic metabolism. The lower the exercise intensity, the more aerobic metabolism predominates.

The aerobic degradation of carbohydrates is limited by the cellular supply of glycogen. It has been shown that 10–20 km of running is sufficient to deplete the muscle store of glycogen (Saltin & Karlsson, 1971). The capacity to exercise 70–80% of maximal oxygen intake is thus largely dependent on the pre-exercise store of muscle glycogen (Bergström *et al.*, 1967). The

muscle glycogen content varies; it can be markedly increased by a diet rich in carbohydrates and is decreased following fasting and muscular exercise (Bergström *et al.*, 1967; Saltin & Hermansen, 1967; see Chapter 12).

HYPOGLYCAEMIA AS A CAUSE OF FATIGUE

Which factor is likely to limit endurance at exercise intensities lower than those at which the muscle stores of glycogen are the major limiting factor? Paradoxically, fatigue may then be related to a lack of blood glucose. Although the predominant energy supply, for instance during moderate running, may be derived from fat combustion, there is always also some increase in the rate of muscle glucose oxidation. The carbohydrate needed for this purpose is derived from muscle glycogen as well as from an increased uptake of glucose from the blood. Blood glucose is regulated by the liver, which releases glucose in an amount that should balance the amount used by the different tissues of the body. The liver normally possesses a glycogen store of about 90 g, plus some capacity for *de novo* glucose synthesis (gluconeogenesis).

The increased glucose uptake by the exercising muscles may, if continued for several hours, result in a depletion of the liver's glycogen stores, and the rate of gluconeogenesis may not be sufficient to avert hypoglycaemia. This rapidly affects the brain and nervous system, since these organs are normally restricted to blood glucose as their energy substrate. Due to a feeling of weakness and dizziness, the individual is forced to stop the exercise, or may continue only after ingesting glucose (Pruett, 1971; see also Chapter 30).

If the rate of exercise is sufficiently low, the point where liver glucose production becomes limiting is never reached. Possible causes of fatigue under these conditions include changes in the membrane potential of the muscle cell, leading to impaired excitability (Sjögaard, 1990; see also Chapters 9 & 10).

ATP production from fatty acid degradation

Free fatty acids, originating from the adipose tissue and taken up by muscle cells, or originating from the stores of triglycerides which exist inside the muscle cells, are transported into the mitochondria for further degradation. The transport across the mitochondrial wall requires that the fatty acids are bound to carnitine. Inside the mitochondria, the fatty acids are degraded stepwise to acetyl CoA, as in aerobic glycolysis (Fig. 23.5).

The most abundant fatty acids give rise to eight or nine molecules of acetyl CoA. The degradation, termed β-oxidation, requires four enzymes. No ATP is directly formed in this pathway; large amounts of NADH are generated instead. Continued operation of the β-oxidation pathway requires the regeneration of NAD^+ from NADH by the respiratory chain. However, there is no anaerobic alternative available, as is the case for glycolysis. β-oxidation is therefore strictly oxygen dependent, and all ATP regeneration occurs in the respiratory chain. Acetyl CoA constitutes the common degradation product of carbohydrates, fats and, to some extent, proteins (Fig. 23.5). This explains why an overconsumption of carbohydrates and proteins is stored as fat in the body. It is noteworthy that a *net* transformation of fatty acids to carbohydrates cannot occur in the cells of the body. The reason is that the reaction pyruvate→acetyl CoA is unidirectional.

In spite of the body's large supply of adipose tissue, fatty acid combustion is not always an appropriate fuel for contracting skeletal muscle. The reason is that the energy released per unit time is only about half of that of aerobic glycolysis (McGilvery, 1975). This may be explained by the comparatively low enzymatic capacity of the free fatty acid transport and oxidation pathways. The practical consequence of this is that when the carbohydrate stores are depleted, it is not possible to continue at the same pace. To avoid or delay a slowing of pace, the pre-exercise carbohydrate stores may be increased by consuming a diet rich in carbohydrates. The maximal pace that it is possible to maintain with predominantly fat oxidation varies with the muscle enzymatic capacity for fat combustion as well as the muscle capillarization. The effect of training on these systems is described in Chapter 5.

Citric acid cycle and the respiratory chain

The citric acid cycle and respiratory chain are central pathways in the metabolism of muscle and other cells (Fig. 23.5). The starting point is acetyl CoA, which reacts with oxaloacetic acid, the final product of the citric acid cycle, to give rise to citric acid. Then follows a circle of eight enzymatic reactions, the last one ending with a regeneration of oxaloacetic acid. Two carbon atoms, equivalent to the carbon content of acetyl CoA, have by then disappeared as carbon dioxide in the expired air. In addition, one molecule of ATP and four molecules of NADH have been formed. The latter molecules are oxidized in the respiratory chain, which results in the generation of three molecules of ATP per molecule of NADH. The respiratory chain consists of iron-containing proteins, the so-called cytochromes. The first cytochrome of the chain is reduced by NADH, regenerating NAD^+. This cytochrome reduces the following cytochrome, and so on. The last cytochrome in the chain (cytochrome a) finally reduces oxygen brought to the muscle cell via the blood. Thus, in this step, oxygen combines with the electrons and hydrogen contained in the hydride ion originally incorporated in NADH, plus the proton released to the medium when NADH was formed. The product of this reaction is water. The flow of electrons along the respiratory chain represents an energy source, which is utilized at three locations along the chain to regenerate ATP from ADP and inorganic phosphate.

The final degradation of acetyl CoA in the citric acid cycle and the ensuing reactions in the respiratory chain are by far the cell's largest energy source. By way of comparison, anaerobic glycolysis (glycogen→lactate) yields less than

10% of the amount of energy released when pyruvate, instead of being converted to lactate, is converted to acetyl CoA and subsequently metabolized in the citric acid cycle and the respiratory chain.

How to determine the metabolic capacity of skeletal muscle

The capacity of a metabolic pathway is mainly decided by the amount of pathway enzymes contained in the cell. Some enzymes are in this context more important than others: these have been termed rate-limiting or flux-generating enzymes. Such an enzyme has a low activity and constitutes a bottleneck in a pathway. Generally, however, as was discussed in Chapter 5, it is possible to obtain a good estimation of the cellular capacity of a specific metabolic pathway by measuring the maximal activity of any one of its enzymes. Enzymes commonly used as a measure of the capacity of their respective metabolic pathway are indicated in Fig. 23.5.

The study of muscle metabolism during exercise in humans

Due to its large mass and high exercise energy expenditure, skeletal muscle dominates metabolism in the exercising body. Muscle metabolism can therefore be studied indirectly via analyses of blood samples or expired air. Lavoisier, in 1789, was the first to use oxygen ('*air vital*') intake measurements in an attempt to quantify the aerobic combustion of food-stuffs in muscle induced by exercise (Séguin & Lavoisier, 1862). Lavoisier, who might be called the first exercise physiologist, was active in Paris during the latter part of the eighteenth century, just before the French Revolution.

In the latter part of the nineteenth century, improved techniques allowed a more accurate determination of oxygen intake and carbon dioxide production. In concert with the development of ergometers, such as the cycle ergo-meter, these techniques made possible more precise quantification of the relationship between exercise intensity and aerobic metabolism. During that period several groups used the respiratory quotient, RQ, to estimate the relative extent to which carbohydrates and fats contributed to exercise metabolism. RQ is the ratio between the body's carbon dioxide production and its oxygen consumption. Proteins had been excluded as an important fuel for the exercising muscle by Pettenkofer and Voit (1866), who estimated protein combustion by measuring the urinary nitrogen output. The pitfalls of determining the true RQ, lactate (H^+) formation and hypo- or hyperventilation, were already known at that time and could be avoided. The question as to whether carbohydrate alone, or fat and carbohydrate combined, delivered the energy for muscular exercise was, however, left unanswered for many decades. The matter was first resolved in the groundbreaking experiments of Benedict and Cathcart (1913), Krogh and Lindhard (1920), and Hohwü Christensen and Hansen (1939). RQ-determination of expired air or over the exercising muscles (arteriovenous differences of oxygen and carbon dioxide) is still one of the most widely used methods in muscle metabolic research.

Biochemical determinations in muscle

At the beginning of the twentieth century a new line of research was introduced, that of muscle biopsy analysis. On the basis of biochemical determinations, Fletcher and Hopkins (1907), using an improved technique for extracting substances from isolated muscle, were able to show that lactic acid is formed from glycogen stored in the muscle. In the years before and after the Second World War, new methods were developed with a sensitivity and precision not previously seen. As early as 1935, a method was described for the determination of glucose-6-phosphate dehydrogenase, based on absorption in the near-ultraviolet wavelength range, as the pyridine nucleotide

NADPH was produced (Negelein & Haas, 1935). This represented a new analytical approach, that of enzymatic analysis. Greengard (1956) was the first to describe fluorometric pyridine nucleotide methods, which now allow the measurement of almost every substance and enzyme of biological interest (Lowry & Passonneau, 1972).

During the past decade, high performance liquid chromatography (HPLC) has largely replaced the enzymatic techniques for metabolite analyses of muscle homogenates. In addition, many other techniques have been introduced; examples are bioluminiscence assays (see Campbell & Simpson, 1979), capillary electrophoresis (CE; see Kennedy et al., 1989) and radioimmunoassays (RIA). Several of these techniques have advantages over the pyridine nucleotide methods, in that they allow the determination of many metabolites in each assay (e.g. HPLC, CE) or are faster (e.g bioluminiscence) or more sensitive (e.g. RIA, and generally also the bioluminiscent methods). Enzymatic techniques are likely to remain an essential tool, however, due to their high degree of flexibility and precision, and the fact that their sensitivity can be substantially improved by enzymatic cycling (Fig. 23.6). The enzymatic analytical technique based on pyridine nucleotides is still the method of choice for the determination of the maximal activity of muscle enzymes (Chapter 5). Concurrently with the development of new analytical methods, new techniques have become available for the study of single muscle cells (Fig. 23.7; Fig. 5.3) (Lowry & Passonneau, 1972; Essén et al., 1975), as well as for the subcellular fractionation of muscle and the measuring of transport phenomena across the muscle cell membrane.

Catheterization and radioactive techniques

The described methodological advances made possible a tremendous increase in the understanding of the metabolic processes involved in cellular energy metabolism. Up to the 1950s, however, all detailed studies of these processes in skeletal muscle had to be restricted to experimental animals or in vitro systems. A methodological development of decisive importance for the extension of these studies to humans was the introduction of the catheterizaton technique (Seldinger, 1953). With this technique, small catheters could be introduced subcutaneously and directed via the circulatory system to almost any organ in the body, e.g. Fig. 23.8. The technique has enabled researchers to study the relative importance of substrates stored in the muscle cells vs. that of substrates brought to the muscle cells by the blood stream. Measurements of arteriovenous differences of substances such as glucose, free fatty acids, lactate and pyruvate in resting and exercising muscles, as well as in the liver and other organs, have been very important in elucidating the fate of such metabolites (see Pernow & Saltin, 1971). Quantitative data on the flux of various substances across different muscle beds has required the development of methods for the determination of local blood flow. The product of blood flow and the arteriovenous difference of a compound represents the uptake or release of that compound over unit time. The dye dilution technique has been found to be a reliable method for the determination of blood flow in the liver (Bradley et al., 1945) and the extremities (Wahren, 1966; Jorfeldt & Wahren, 1971). An alternative method, used to estimate blood flow in exercising muscle, is thermodilution (Jorfeldt et al., 1978; Andersen & Saltin, 1985).

Another very important technique has been the use of labelled compounds, notably ^{14}C or ^{3}H compounds. Tracer techniques have been used to investigate the metabolism of free fatty acids and glucose in human muscle at rest and during exercise (see Hagenfeldt, 1975; Searle, 1976; and references in Pernow & Saltin, 1971). With this technique, a small amount of radioactive isotope, for instance ^{14}C-or ^{3}H-labelled glucose, equivalent to a few weeks of normal background cosmic radiation, is infused intravenously. From determinations of the specific activity of the compound in the blood, its total

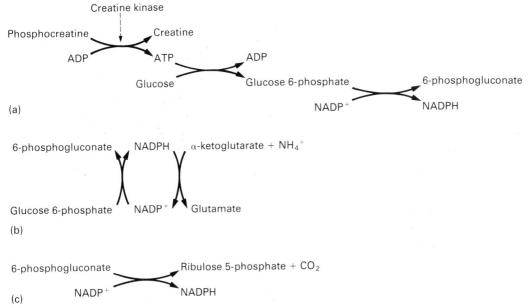

Fig. 23.6 Example of a fluorometric pyridine nucleotide method for measuring enzymes or metabolites in muscle samples or fragments of muscle fibres. It is applicable to any substance that can be made to oxidize or reduce NAD^+ or $NADP^+$, directly or indirectly. In the example shown, phosphocreatine or creatine kinase is measured by the NADPH formed in (a). In the case of creatine kinase, enough NADPH is produced to be measured by means of its own fluorescence. However, for phosphocreatine, considerable amplification may be necessary because the phosphocreatine present in 20 ng dry muscle fibre is only about 2 pmol, whereas the creatine kinase in the same amount of muscle can break down 2000 times this amount of phosphocreatine in 1 h. Fortunately, the amplification is easy: the excess $NADP^+$ is destroyed with NaOH and heat, and the sample is added to a reagent with components to carry out the rapidly repeating enzymatic cycle shown in (b). After a sufficient number of cycles, the enzymes are killed with heat or alkali and the 6-phosphogluconate is measured by the fluorescence of the NADPH formed from extra $NADP^+$ in the final enzymatic step (c). The amplification that can be achieved in this way is rather impressive. Cycling rates of up to 30 000 per hour can be obtained by using high levels of the two enzymes (in this case glutamic and glucose-6-phosphate dehydrogenase). By incubating for long periods, an overall amplification of 400 000 times may be achieved (Lowry & Passonneau, 1972; Chi *et al.*, 1978).

turnover in the body can be determined. It is furthermore possible to study the different degradation pathways of a compound by measuring the specific activity of its metabolites. The usefulness of radioactive methods to quantitate the flux through different metabolic pathways is hampered, however, by the inevitable exchange of isotopes that occurs in the tissues (Landau, 1986; Sahlin, 1987).

Muscle biopsy technique

The use of a needle technique to obtain muscle biopsy specimens was described more than 100 years ago by Charrière and Duchenne (1865). The reintroduction of the technique by Bergström (1962) opened a new field of research in human physiology. Together with the catheterization technique described above, the biopsy method has been extensively used over the past three decades and has led to an in-

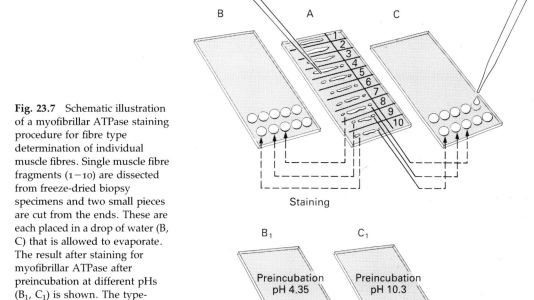

Fig. 23.7 Schematic illustration of a myofibrillar ATPase staining procedure for fibre type determination of individual muscle fibres. Single muscle fibre fragments (1−10) are dissected from freeze-dried biopsy specimens and two small pieces are cut from the ends. These are each placed in a drop of water (B, C) that is allowed to evaporate. The result after staining for myofibrillar ATPase after preincubation at different pHs (B_1, C_1) is shown. The type-identified fibre fragment (A) is subsequently used for biochemical analysis. From Essén *et al.* (1975), modified with permission.

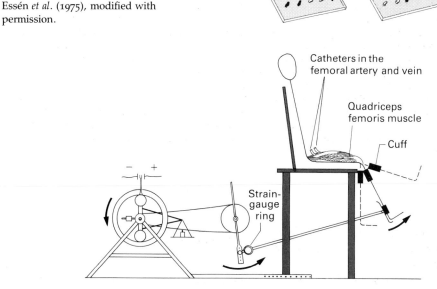

Fig. 23.8 A one-leg model for the study of metabolic regulation in skeletal muscle. One of the subject's legs is attached to a cycle ergometer in such a way that, during exercise, only the quadriceps femoris muscle is activated. Exercise is performed by pulling a rod attached to the ankle of the subject and to the crank of a modified Krogh cycle ergometer. The flywheel momentum returns the relaxed leg. Detailed studies of metabolic processes are made possible by arterial and venous catheterization and muscle biopsy analysis. Quantitative data on the flux of various substances are obtained by blood flow determinations, using thermodilution or dye dilution techniques. To minimize blood sampling from tissues other than active muscles, the circulation to the lower leg is occluded with a pressure cuff. From Andersen & Saltin (1985).

depth understanding of the metabolic processes occurring in exercised muscle.

The Bergström needle (Fig. 23.9) is 3–5 mm in diameter, the outer cylinder having a small window close to the tip of the needle. After anaesthetizing the skin and the tissue immediately above the muscle fascia (e.g. with 1 ml 1% lidocaine), a small incision (approximately 5 mm) is made, extending through the muscle fascia. When the needle is inserted into the muscle, tissue bulges into the needle window and can be cut with the sharp edge of the inner cylinder. The obtained piece of muscle generally weighs 20–100 mg. Larger samples may be obtained by means of a suction device attached to the needle (Edwards *et al.*, 1983) or by replacing the needle with a Weil–Blakesley conchotome (Fig. 23.9, Henriksson, 1979). The latter is an alligator forceps, which is as easy to use as the biopsy needle and therefore has replaced it in many laboratories. Apart from the Bergström needle, several other biopsy needles are in current use (Nichols *et al.*, 1968; Siperstein *et al.*, 1968; Young *et al.*, 1978).

The needle or conchotome technique is important because, unlike the surgical muscle biopsy procedure, it allows repeated sampling from the same muscle. In addition, subjects need not restrict their activity after a biopsy has been performed. The lateral aspect of the thigh muscle has been the most common biopsy site for physiological and clinical studies, but biopsies have been performed in many other muscles as well. These include the deltoid, biceps and triceps brachii, gastrocnemius, soleus and tibialis anterior muscles. For a more detailed description of the biopsy procedure, the reader is referred to the review by Edwards *et al.* (1980) and, for methods applied to and results obtained by the biopsy technique, to the review by Saltin and Gollnick (1983).

Recent techniques for the study of muscle metabolism

During the past decade, nuclear magnetic resonance (NMR) spectroscopy has become available at many university centres. It is a completely atraumatic technique for studying muscle metabolism continuously (see Shulman, 1983). The method is based on the fact that atomic nuclei with an odd number of nucleons (protons and neutrons) have an intrinsic magnetism that makes each such nucleus a magnetic dipole. Such nuclei include the proton (H-1), the carbon-13 nucleus (C-13, 1.1% of all carbon atoms) and the phosphorus-31 nucleus (P-31). Metabolites containing these nuclei can be

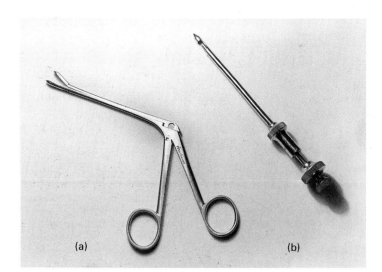

(a)   (b)

Fig. 23.9 The Weil–Blakesley conchotome (a) and the Bergström biopsy needle (b). The length of the needle is 14 cm.

measured after two fields have been applied to the tissue. One is a strong magnetic field, which causes the nuclear dipoles to align either with the field (less energy stored) or against it. The other field consists of electromagnetic radiation in the radiofrequency portion of the spectrum; at a given magnetic field strength, each nucleus will 'flip' over in the magnetic field, absorbing radiophotons (resonating) when the field has a certain frequency. The precise frequency of resonance, however, differs for a given nucleus depending on which other chemical groups are bound to it. Different compounds can be localized and quantified on the basis of the 'chemical shift' of the resonance frequency. To date, most NMR studies of human muscle metabolism have been conducted with P-31 (see Wilkie *et al.*, 1984), but for the future, because of the ubiquitous presence of carbon, C-13 NMR looks particularly promising.

Other new and important techniques in muscle metabolic research include positron emission tomography (PET) and microdialysis. With PET, extremely short-lived isotopes may be injected into the blood stream and their behaviour in specific tissues (uptake, release, metabolism, receptor binding) may be studied with an external camera (see Phelps *et al.*, 1986). The microdialysis technique (Delgado *et al.*, 1972; Ungerstedt & Pycock, 1974) utilizes a hollow probe continuously perfused with physiological fluid. The microdialysis probe constitutes an 'artificial blood vessel' inserted into the tissue, where diffusion of chemical substances will occur in the direction of the lowest concentration. Constituents of the muscle extracellular space can be collected for analysis, and foreign compounds may be added to the extracellular space via the dialysis probe so that their effect on the muscle cell may be monitored (Henriksson *et al.*, 1990).

Acknowledgements

The author wishes to express his appreciation to Ms Ulla Siltberg for her help in the preparation of the manuscript.

References

Andersen, P. & Saltin, B. (1985) Maximal perfusion of skeletal muscle in man. *J. Physiol.* **366**, 233–249.

Åstrand, P.-O. & Rodahl, K. (1986) *Textbook of Work Physiology*, 3rd edn. McGraw-Hill Book Company, New York.

Benedict, F.G. & Cathcart, E.P. (1913) *Muscular Work. Carnegie Institute of Washington.* Publication No. 187.

Bergström, J. (1962) Muscle electrolytes in man. *Scand. J. Clin. Lab. Invest.* **14** (Suppl. 68), 1–110.

Bergström, J., Hermansen, L., Hultman, E. & Saltin, B. (1967) Diet, muscle glycogen and physical performance. *Acta Physiol. Scand.* **71**, 140–150.

Bradley, S.E., Ingelfinger, F.J., Bradley, G.P. & Curry, J.J. (1945) The estimation of hepatic blood flow in man. *J. Clin. Invest.* **24**, 890–897.

Campbell, A.K. & Simpson, J.S.A. (1979) Chemi- and bio-luminescence as an analytical tool in biology. In: Kornberg, H.L., Metcalfe, J.C., Northcote, D.H., Pogson, C.I. & Tipton, K.F. (eds) *Techniques in the Life Sciences, Biochemistry — Vol. B2/II. Techniques in Metabolic Research, Part II, B 213*, pp. 1–56. Elsevier/North-Holland Scientific Publishers, Ireland.

Charrière, M. & Duchenne, G.B. (1865) Emporte pièce histologique. *Bull. Acad. Med.* **30**, 1050–1051.

Chi, M.M.-Y., Lowry, C.V. & Lowry, O.H. (1978) An improved enzymatic cycle for nicotinamide-adenine dinucleotide phosphate. *Anal. Biochem.* **89**, 119–129.

Delgado, J.M.R., Defeudis, F.V., Roth, R.H., Ryugo, D.K. & Mitruka, B.K. (1972) Dialytrode for long term intracerebral perfusion in awake monkeys. *Arch. Int. Pharmacodyn. Ther.* **198**, 9–21.

Edwards, R.H.T., Round, J.M. & Jones, D.A. (1983) Needle biopsy of skeletal muscle: a review of 10 years experience. *Muscle Nerve* **6**, 676–683.

Edwards, R.H.T., Young, A. & Wiles, M. (1980) Needle biopsy of skeletal muscle in the diagnosis of myopathy and the clinical study of muscle function and repair. *N. Engl. J. Med.* **302**, 261–271.

Essén, B., Jansson, E., Henriksson, J., Taylor, A.W. & Saltin, B. (1975) Metabolic characteristics of fibre types in human skeletal muscle. *Acta Physiol. Scand.* **95**, 153–165.

Fletcher, W.M. & Hopkins, F.G. (1907) Lactic acid in amphibian muscle. *J. Physiol.* **35**, 247–309.

Greengard, P. (1956) Determination of intermediary metabolites by enzymic fluorimetry. *Nature (Lond.)* **178**, 632–634.

Hagenfeldt, L. (1975) Turnover of individual free fatty acids in man. *Fed. Proc.* **34**, 2246–2249.

Henriksson, J., Fuchi, T., Oshida, Y. & Ungerstedt, U. (1990) Microdialysis for in vivo studies of skeletal muscle glucose metabolism. *Acta Physiol. Scand.* **140**(1), 9A.

Henriksson, K.G. (1979) 'Semi-open' muscle biopsy technique. A simple outpatient procedure. *Acta Neurol. Scand.* **59**, 317–323.

Hohwü Christensen, E. & Hansen, O. (1939) I. Zur Methodik der Respiratorischen Quotient-Bestimmungen in Ruhe und bei der Arbeit. II. Untersuchungen über die Verbrennungsvorgänge bei langdauernder, schwerer Muskelarbeit. III. Arbeitsfähigkeit und Ernährung. *Skand. Arch. Physiol.* **81**, 137–171.

Jorfeldt, L., Juhlin-Dannfelt, A., Pernow, B. & Wassén, E. (1978) Determination of human leg blood flow: a thermodilution technique based on femoral venous bolus injection. *Clin. Sci.* **54**, 517–523.

Jorfeldt, L. & Wahren, J. (1971) Leg blood flow during exercise in man. *Clin. Sci.* **41**, 459–473.

Kennedy, R.T., Oates, M.D., Cooper, B.R., Nickerson, B. & Jorgenson, J.W. (1989) Microcolumn separations and the analysis of single cells. *Science* **246**, 57–63.

Krogh, A. & Lindhard, J. (1920) The relative value of fat and carbohydrate as source of muscular energy. *Biochem. J.* **14**, 290–363.

Landau, B.R. (1986) A potential pitfall in the use of isotopes to measure ketone body production. *Metabolism* **35**, 94.

Lowry, O.H. & Passonneau, J.V. (1972) *A Flexible System of Enzymatic Analysis.* Academic Press, New York.

McGilvery, R.W. (1975) The use of fuels for muscular work. In: Howald, H. & Poortmans, J.R. (eds) *Metabolic Adaptation to Prolonged Physical Exercise*, pp. 12–30. Birkhäuser Verlag, Basel.

McMurray, W.C. (1983) *Essentials of Human Metabolism*, 2nd edn. Lippincott, Philadelphia.

Negelein, E. & Haas, E. (1935) Über die Wirkungsweise des Zwischenferments. *Biochem. Z.* **282**, 206–220.

Newsholme, E.A. & Leech, A.R. (1983) *Biochemistry for the Medical Sciences.* John Wiley & Sons, Chichester.

Nichols, B.L., Hazlewood, C.F. & Barnes, D.J. (1968) Percutaneous needle biopsy of quadriceps muscle: potassium analysis in normal children. *J. Pediatr.* **72**, 840–852.

Pernow, B. & Saltin, B. (1971) *Muscle Metabolism During Exercise.* Proceedings of a Karolinska Institutet Symposium held in Stockholm, Sweden, September 6–9, 1970. Plenum Press, New York.

Pettenkofer, M. & Voit, C. (1866) Untersuchungen über den Stoffverbrauch des normalen Menschen. *Zeitschr. F. Biol.* **2**, 537.

Phelps, M., Mazzeota, J. & Schelbert, H. (eds) (1986) *Positron Emission Tomography. Principles and Application for the Brain and Heart.* Raven Press, New York.

Pruett, E.D.R. (1971) *Fat and carbohydrate metabolism in exercise and recovery, and its dependence upon work load severity.* Institute of Work Physiology, Oslo.

Sahlin, K. (1987) Lactate production cannot be measured with tracer tehniques. *Am. J. Physiol.* **252**, E439–E440.

Saltin, B. & Gollnick, P.D. (1983) Skeletal muscle adaptability: significance for metabolism and performance. In: Peachey, L.D., Adrian, P.H. & Geiger, S.R. (eds) *Handbook of Physiology. Skeletal Muscle,* 1983, Section 10, pp. 555–631. American Physiological Society, Bethesda, Maryland.

Saltin, B. & Hermansen, L. (1967) Glycogen stores and prolonged severe exercise. In: Blix, G. (ed.) *Nutrition and Physical Activity*, p. 32., Almqvist & Wiksell, Uppsala.

Saltin, B. & Karlsson, J. (1971) Muscle glycogen utilization during work of different intensities. In: Pernow, B. & Saltin, B. (eds) *Muscle Metabolism During Exercise*, pp. 289–299. Plenum Press, New York.

Searle, G.L. (1976) The use of isotope turnover techniques in the study of carbohydrate metabolism in man. In: Besser, G.M., Bierich, J.R., Bondy, P.K., Daughaday, W.H., Franchimont, P. & Hall, R. (eds) *Clinics in Endocrinology and Metabolism. Vol. 5, No. 3. Disorders of Carbohydrate Metabolism Excluding Diabetes*, pp. 783–804. W.B. Saunders, London.

Séguin, A. & Lavoisier, A.L. (1862) *Oeuvres de Lavoisier,* Vol. II. p. 688 (*Mémoires de l'Academie des Sciences 1789*, p. 185). Academie des Sciences, Paris.

Seldinger, S.I. (1953) Catheter replacement of the needle in percutaneous arteriography. A new technique. *Acta Radiol. (Stockholm)* **39**, 368–376.

Shulman, R.G. (1983) NMR spectroscopy of living cells. *Sci. Am.* **248**, 86–93.

Siperstein, M.D., Unger, R.H. & Madison, L.L. (1968) Studies of muscle capillary basement membranes in normal subjects, diabetic, and prediabetic patients. *J. Clin. Invest.* **47**, 1973–1999.

Sjögaard, G. (1990) Exercise-induced muscle fatigue: the significance of potassium. *Acta Physiol. Scand.* **140** (Suppl.), 593.

Ungerstedt, U. & Pycock, C. (1974) Functional correlates of dopamine neurotransmission. *Bull. Schweiz Akad. Med. Wiss.* **1278**, 1–13.

Wahren, J. (1966) Quantitative aspects of blood flow and oxygen uptake in the human forearm during rhythmic exercise. *Acta Physiol. Scand.* **67** (Suppl.), 269.

Wilkie, D.R., Dawson, M.J., Edwards, R.H.T., Gordon, R.E. & Shaw, D. (1984) ^{31}P NMR studies of resting

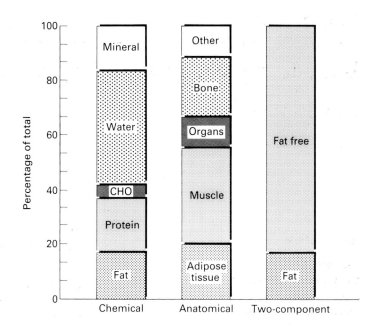

Fig. 24.1 Illustration of the chemical, anatomical and two-component models of body composition. CHO, carbohydrate.

While the concept of lean body mass is sound, it is problematic from an assessment point of view. How can you differentiate essential from non-essential lipid? Thus, it is now recommended that all investigators adopt the concept of fat-free mass, defined as the mass of all body tissues minus that of extractable fat (Lohman, 1986). As techniques are advanced to allow the assessment of other elements of body composition, the simple two-component model will be expanded to include these other measurable components.

Measurement of body composition

There are a number of procedures to assess body composition. In the laboratory, the densitometric technique has been regarded as the 'gold standard' or criterion technique. The density of the human body can be determined accurately by measuring the total mass of the body and its volume, since density = mass/volume. The volume of the body can be measured directly as the volume of water displaced by a subject when immersed in water,

or by the body's loss of weight when weighed underwater, since:

$$V_B = \frac{W_A - W_{H_2O}}{D_{H_2O}}$$

where V_B = body volume, W_A = body weight in air, W_{H_2O} = body weight in water and D_{H_2O} = density of water, corrected for water temperature. The measured body volume must be corrected for any air trapped within the body at the time of the weighing, such as gas in the gastrointestinal tract or the volume of air remaining in the lungs at the time of weighing. The volume of gastrointestinal tract gas is generally small, and is either ignored or a constant correction of 100 ml is used. The volume of air in the lung must be measured, because it is sizeable and can greatly influence the accuracy of the resulting calculations. The final equation for computing body density is:

$$D_B = \frac{W_A}{\left(\dfrac{W_A - W_{H_2O}}{D_{H_2O}}\right) - RLV}$$

where D_B = body density, RLV = residual lung volume and the remaining abbreviations are as above. Assuming that the body weight, underwater weight and lung volume are each obtained correctly, the resulting body density value will be accurate. The main problem with the densitometric technique is in the translation of body density to relative body fat. With the two-component model, it is critical to have an accurate estimate of the densities of the fat-free and fat tissue. There is little disagreement as to the density of the fat tissue, because this value is consistent among different sites in the same individual as well as between individuals. A value of 0.9007 g·cm^{-3} is generally assumed. There is, however, considerable interindividual variation in the density of the fat-free body mass. To define a density for the fat-free mass, one must assume that the densities of the component tissues are known and constant. Further, it is necessary to assume that each accounts for a constant proportion of the fat-free mass (for example, that muscle always represents 50% of the fat-free mass). Violations of any of these assumptions will lead to error when translating body density into relative body fat. The density of the fat-free mass is generally assumed to be 1.100 g·cm^{-3} for a chemically mature individual, but evidence now supports the use of lower values in children, females and the elderly (Lohman, 1981) and higher values in black people (Schutte et al., 1984). Population-specific equations are now available for translating body density into relative body fat values. An excellent review by Lohman (1986) discusses this issue relative to children and youth.

Additional procedures proposed for assessing body composition can be classified as either field or laboratory methods. The field methods use anthropometric measurements (girths, diameters and skinfolds) to estimate body density, fat-free body mass, and absolute and relative body fat. These methods are discussed below. The laboratory methods (Table 24.1) are now discussed briefly, borrowing from the reviews of Behnke and Wilmore (1974), Lohman (1984), Wilmore (1984) and Brodie (1988).

Hydrometry, or the assessment of total body water, involves isotopic dilution, using tracers such as deuterium oxide or tritium oxide. Ethanol and antipyrine are also potential tracers. Water is assumed to account for 73.2% of fat-free tissue. Thus, fat-free mass = (total body water)/0.732.

Spectrometry requires the use of a whole body counter to measure the γ-radiation from ^{40}K, a radioactive isotope which is naturally present in small quantities in the human body. The body's ^{40}K content is directly proportional to the total body potassium which, in turn, constitutes a relatively stable proportion of the fat-free body mass. A liquid scintillation counter is usually used to assess ^{40}K. The subject is placed horizontally in the well of the counter, which is surrounded by a layer of liquid scintillatory solution. This solution converts the photon energies of the γ-rays into

Table 24.1 Techniques for the measurement of fat, fat-free mass, muscle and bone. From Lohman (1984).

Fat and fat-free body	Muscle	Bone
Densitometry	Spectrometry (^{40}K)	Photon absorptiometry
Hydrometry	Ultrasonics	Radiographics
Spectrometry (^{40}K)	Radiographics	Neutron activation
Ultrasonics	Neutron activation	NMR
Radiographics	NMR	Computed tomography
Electrical conductivity	Computed tomography	
Neutron activation	Creatinine excretion	
NMR	Serum creatinine	
Computed tomography	Urinary 3-methylhistidine	

light impulses or scintillations. The impulses are detected by photomultiplier tubes mounted around the outer wall of the chamber, and the signals are then amplified and converted into proportional voltages.

Ultrasonics utilizes high-frequency sound waves to differentiate between tissue types. Sound waves pass into the tissue, and when a change in density is encountered, a portion of these waves generated by a special transducer is reflected, sensed and converted to electrical impulses; these impulses are then simplified and recorded. The thickness and density of the tissue through which the ultrasonic waves pass determine the characteristics of the reflected sound wave.

Radiographic analysis of body composition uses soft tissue X-rays to differentiate between the various layers of skin, fat, muscle and bone. This technique has been confined largely to the upper arm, but the tissue proportions for this region have been reported to be highly correlated with total body composition.

Measurement of the *electrical conductivity* of the body has been proposed as a method of estimating fat-free body mass, due to the difference in electrical conductivity between fat-free and fat tissue. During the early 1980s, two instruments were introduced to assess the body's electrical conductivity; TOBEC (total body electrical conductivity) and a bioelectrical impedance device. With TOBEC (Fig. 24.2), the individual is placed inside a large polaroidal coil and a small radiofrequency current is passed through the body. The procedure takes less than 1 min per assessment, with minimal risk and no subject discomfort. Initial studies have indicated excellent agreement of TOBEC data with the results of densitometry and spectrometry. With the bioelectric impedance device, four skin electrodes are attached — two on the arm and two on the foot — and a radio-

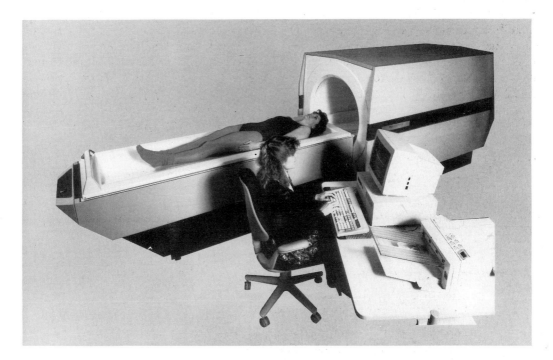

Fig. 24.2 The TOBEC device for measuring body composition. (Courtesy of EM-SCAN Inc., Springfield, Illinois.)

frequency signal is introduced into the deep tissues of the body (800 μA at 50 kHz). Whole body impedance (Fig. 24.3) is supposedly closely related to total body water. Considerable research has tested its validity in the assessment of total body composition. While the standard error of measurement is acceptable for normal adults, Graves *et al.* (1987) have reported relatively large errors of measurement in élite female distance runners.

Neutron activation analysis is a fairly new technique, whereby fast neutrons are captured by specific elements in the body and unstable isotopes are produced which revert to a stable condition following the emission of one or more γ-rays. The body thus becomes temporarily radioactive, and the emissions are recorded in a whole body counter. Both total body nitrogen and total body potassium can be estimated. At this time, neutron activation analysis remains an experimental technique, but it has considerable promise for the future.

Nuclear magnetic resonance (NMR) imagery is clearly a future technique for determining regional and total body composition. In this method, the body is exposed to a static magnetic field that affects the rotation of the nucleus of atoms with an odd number of protons or neutrons. The body is then exposed to an alternating magnetic field of the same frequency. After removing the attenuating magnetic field, measurement of one or more parameters of these nuclei enables the formation of body images. This method, while very expensive, has considerable promise for detailed body composition analyses.

Computed tomography is an X-ray scanning technique which provides cross-sectional images. It has been used to assess the composition of the trunk and the limbs, at the level of the mid-thigh, mid upper arm, and the entire forearm. However, the relationship between local scans and total body composition has yet to be determined.

Photon absorptiometry has been used to measure the mineral content of a cross-section of bone. A beam of photons from a ^{125}I source is directed at the extremity; the amount that passes through the limb is inversely proportional to the mineral content of the underlying bone. Dual-photon absorptiometry (^{153}Gd), a more recent development, has been found to provide an excellent estimate of total body composition.

Creatinine excretion, total plasma creatinine, and 3-methylhistidine have been proposed as indices of muscle mass. While these markers appear to be accurate indices of total body

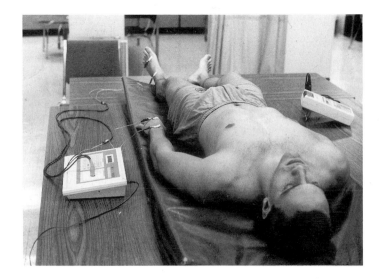

Fig. 24.3 The bioelectric impedance device for measuring body composition.

muscle, it is less clear how applicable these techniques would be in the determination of total body composition.

Field methods for estimating body density, fat-free body weight, and absolute and relative body fat use girths, bony diameters and skinfolds. Body composition was first estimated from skinfolds in 1951. In the 1960s and 1970s, many investigators developed linear multiple regression equations to estimate body composition from anthropometric variables. Typically, a number of anthropometric variables was measured on a selected population such as college-age males, college-age females or wrestlers, and then, using the hydrostatic weighing technique as the criterion, multiple regression equations were derived, using stepwise, linear regression procedures. These equations were later found to be population-specific, that is they yielded accurate fat predictions only when used on populations similar to the population from which the equation had been derived (Wilmore, 1983). This created considerable confusion, because clinicians and practitioners were faced with the necessity of selecting an equation appropriate to the population they were evaluating. In addition, recognition that many of the previously established equations were population-specific led to a further proliferation of new equations for specific populations.

It is now recognized that the relationship between the sum of skinfolds and total body density is curvilinear, and not linear as was assumed in most of the original multiple regression equations (Pollock & Jackson, 1984). This has led to the development of quadratic equations which are generalizable, rather than specific to a given population. Coefficients of correlation with hydrostatically determined body density are similar for linear and for generalized, quadratic equations, but the standard errors of estimate (s.e.e.) for the quadratic equations are generally much lower (Pollock & Jackson, 1984). In particular, the quadratic equations minimize large prediction errors that would occur with linear equations at the ex-

tremes of the body density distribution, as, for example, in endurance-trained athletes.

Pollock and Jackson (1984) state that the sum of several skinfolds provides the most representative estimate of subcutaneous body fat; this value is more highly correlated with body density than are readings from individual sites. The correlations with individual skinfold sites are generally ≥ 0.90, and the correlations with various combinations of summed skinfold sites are typically > 0.97. Consequently, they recommended that the sum of three or more skinfold sites be used to estimate body density.

For the clinician and practitioner, the use of skinfold calipers will provide a simple and inexpensive, yet accurate, estimate of the endurance athlete's body composition. The Jackson and Pollock equations for males, and the Jackson, Pollock and Ward equations for females, are considered by this author to be the best generalized equations available. Coefficients normally range from $r = 0.85$ to 0.95 (with a s.e.e. of about 3%) when these equations are correlated with body density determined hydrostatically in various populations of males and females, athletes and non-athletes alike. Refer to Pollock and Wilmore (1990) for more specific details on these equations, descriptions of the specific sites used, procedures and equipment selection.

Practical application of body composition and body energy stores data

This last section discusses the practical application of the above information to the selection and training of athletes, including a more detailed discussion of how body composition and body energy stores affect endurance performance. Endurance athletes attempt to minimize their fat stores, because excess weight negatively affects endurance performance. Cureton and Sparling (1980) subjected male and female runners to submaximal and maximal treadmill runs, and to an all out 12-min run. Each male completed all testing under normal conditions and also while carrying external weight added to the trunk to simulate the relative body fat of the female to which he had been matched. With the added weights, the cost of submaximal exercise was increased and the maximal oxygen intake per unit of body mass was reduced (Fig. 24.4). Pate *et al.* (1985) matched men and women runners on the basis of their times to complete a 24.2-km (15-mile)

road race. In this matched population, no difference in relative body fat was found between the women and men (17.8% vs. 16.3% respectively). Normally, male runners are much leaner than female runners, and this is postulated as an important cause of differences in running performance between élite men and women distance runners (Wilmore *et al.*, 1977).

Since body composition can greatly affect

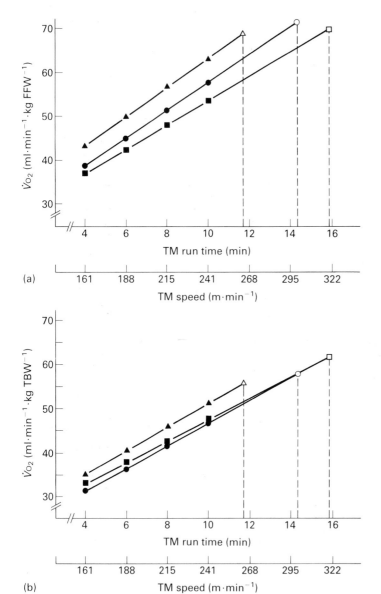

(a)

(b)

Fig. 24.4 Mean submaximal and maximal oxygen intake expressed relative to both (a) fat-free weight (FFW); and (b) total body weight (TBW) in men and women distance runners. The men completed the submaximal and maximal tests twice, once under normal conditions and once with weights attached to the trunk. TM, treadmill; ■, male, no weights; ●, male, with weights ▲, female. Open symbols refer to maximal oxygen intake values. From Cureton & Sparling (1980).

Table 24.2   Relative body fat values for male and female athletes (mainly élite competitors). From Wilmore & Costill (1988); see for details of references.

Athletic group or sport	Sex	Age (years)	Height (cm)	Body mass (kg)	Relative fat (%)	Reference
Baseball	Male	20.8	182.7	83.3	14.2	Novak
	Male	—	—	—	11.8	Forsyth
	Male	26.0	185.4	87.5	16.2	Gurry
	Male	27.3	185.8	86.4	12.6	Coleman
	Male	27.4	183.1	88.0	12.6	Wilmore
Pitchers	Male	26.7	188.1	89.8	14.7	Coleman
Infielders	Male	27.4	183.1	83.2	12.0	Coleman
Outfielders	Male	28.3	185.9	85.6	9.9	Coleman
Basketball	Female	19.1	169.1	62.6	20.8	Sinning
	Female	19.4	173.0	68.3	20.8	Vaccaro
	Female	19.4	167.0	63.9	26.9	Conger
Centres	Male	27.7	214.0	109.2	7.1	Parr
Forwards	Male	25.3	200.6	96.9	9.0	Parr
Guards	Male	25.2	188.0	83.6	10.6	Parr
Bicycling	Male	—	180.3	67.1	8.8	Burke
	Female	—	167.7	61.3	15.4	Burke
Canoeing/paddlers	Male	23.7	182.0	79.6	12.4	Rusko
	Male	20.1	179.9	76.3	10.4	Vaccaro
Dancing						
Ballet	Female	15.0	161.1	48.4	16.4	Clarkson
General	Female	21.2	162.7	51.2	20.5	Novak
Fencers	Male	20.4	174.9	68.0	12.2	Vander
Football (US)	Male	19.3	186.8	93.1	13.7	Smith
	Male	20.3	184.9	96.4	13.8	Novak
	Male	—	—	—	13.9	Forsyth
Defensive	Male	17–23	178.3	77.3	11.5	Wickkiser
Backs	Male	24.5	182.5	84.8	9.6	Wilmore
Offensive	Male	17–23	179.7	79.8	12.4	Wickkiser
Backs	Male	24.7	183.8	90.7	9.4	Wilmore
Linebackers	Male	17–23	180.1	87.2	13.4	Wickkiser
	Male	24.2	188.6	102.2	14.0	Wilmore
Offensive	Male	17–23	186.0	99.2	19.1	Wickkiser
Linemen	Male	24.7	193.0	112.6	15.6	Wilmore
Defensive	Male	17–23	186.6	97.8	18.5	Wickkiser
Linemen	Male	25.7	192.4	117.1	18.2	Wilmore
Quarterbacks Kickers	Male	24.1	185.0	90.1	14.4	Wilmore
Golf	Female	33.3	168.9	61.8	24.0	Crews
Gymnastics	Male	20.3	178.5	69.2	4.6	Novak
	Female	14.0	—	—	17.0	Pařízková
	Female	15.2	161.1	50.4	13.1	Moffatt
	Female	19.4	163.0	57.9	23.8	Conger
	Female	20.0	158.5	51.5	15.5	Sinning
	Female	23.0	—	—	11.0	Pařízková
	Female	23.0	—	—	9.6	Pařízková
Ice hockey	Male	22.5	179.0	77.3	13.0	Rusko
	Male	26.3	180.3	86.7	15.1	Wilmore
Jockeys	Male	30.9	158.2	50.3	14.1	Wilmore

Continued overleaf

Table 24.2 (*Continued*)

Athletic group or sport	Sex	Age (years)	Height (cm)	Body mass (kg)	Relative fat (%)	Reference
Orienteering	Male	31.2	—	72.2	16.3	Knowlton
	Female	29.0	—	58.1	18.7	Knowlton
Pentathlon	Female	21.5	175.4	65.4	11.0	Krahenbuhl
Racketball	Male	25.0	181.7	80.3	8.1	Pipes
Lightweight	Male	21.0	186.0	71.0	8.5	Hagerman
	Female	23.0	173.0	68.0	14.0	Hagerman
Rowing	Male	25.6	192.0	93.0	6.5	Secher
Rugby	Male	28.1	181.6	86.3	9.1	Maud
Skiing	Male	25.9	176.6	74.8	7.4	Sprynarová
Alpine	Male	16.5	173.1	65.5	11.0	Song
	Male	21.0	178.0	78.0	9.9	Veicsteinas
	Male	21.2	176.0	70.1	14.1	Rusko
	Male	21.8	177.8	75.5	10.2	Haymes
	Female	19.5	165.1	58.8	20.6	Haymes
Cross-country	Male	21.2	176.0	66.6	12.5	Niinimaa
	Male	22.7	176.2	73.2	7.9	Haymes
	Male	25.6	174.0	69.3	10.2	Rusko
	Female	20.2	163.4	55.9	15.7	Haymes
	Female	24.3	163.0	59.1	21.8	Rusko
Nordic	Male	21.7	181.7	70.4	8.9	Haymes
Combination	Male	22.9	176.0	70.4	11.2	Rusko
Skijumping	Male	22.2	174.0	69.9	14.3	Rusko
Soccer	Male	26.0	176.0	75.5	9.6	Raven
US Junior	Male	17.5	178.3	72.3	9.4	Kirkendahl
US Olympic	Male	20.6	179.3	72.5	9.1	Kirkendahl
US Collegiate	Male	20.0	175.3	72.4	10.9	Kirkendahl
US National	Male	22.5	178.6	76.2	9.9	Kirkendahl
MISL	Male	26.9	177.3	74.5	10.5	Kirkendahl
Skating	Male	21.0	181.0	76.5	11.4	Kusko
Speed	Male	—	181.0	73.6	9.0	Vanlugen
Figure	Male	21.3	166.9	59.6	9.1	Niinimaa
	Female	16.5	158.8	48.6	12.5	Niinimaa
Swimming	Male	15.1	166.8	59.1	10.8	Vaccaro
	Male	20.6	182.9	78.9	5.0	Novak
	Male	21.8	182.3	79.1	8.5	Sprynarová
	Female	19.4	168.0	63.8	26.3	Conger
Sprint	Female	—	165.1	57.1	14.6	Wilmore
Middle distance	Female	—	166.6	66.8	24.1	Wilmore
Distance	Female	—	166.3	60.9	17.1	Wilmore
Synchronized swimming	Female	20.1	166.2	55.8	24.0	Roby
Tennis	Male	—	—	—	15.2	Forsyth
	Male	42.0	179.6	77.1	16.3	Vodak
	Female	39.0	163.3	55.7	20.3	Vodak
Track and field	Male	21.3	180.6	71.6	3.7	Novak
	Male	—	—	—	8.8	Forsyth
Runners						
Distance	Male	22.5	177.4	64.5	6.3	Sprynarová
	Male	26.1	175.7	64.2	7.5	Costill
	Male	26.2	177.0	66.2	8.4	Rusko
	Male	26.2	177.1	63.1	4.7	Pollock

Table 24.2 (*Continued*)

Athletic group or sport	Sex	Age (years)	Height (cm)	Body mass (kg)	Relative fat (%)	Reference
	Male	40–49	180.7	71.6	11.2	Pollock
	Male	47.2	176.5	70.7	13.2	Lewis
	Male	55.3	174.5	63.4	18.0	Barnard
	Male	50–59	174.7	67.2	10.9	Pollock
	Male	60–69	175.7	67.1	11.3	Pollock
	Male	70–75	175.6	66.8	13.6	Pollock
	Female	19.9	161.3	52.9	19.2	Malina
	Female	32.4	169.4	57.2	15.2	Wilmore
	Female	37.8	165.1	54.1	15.5	Upton
	Female	43.8	161.5	53.8	18.3	Vaccaro
Middle distance	Male	20.1	178.1	71.9	6.9	Wilmore
	Male	24.6	179.0	72.3	12.4	Rusko
Sprint	Female	20.1	164.9	56.7	19.3	Malina
	Male	20.1	178.2	72.8	5.4	Wilmore
	Male	46.5	177.0	74.1	16.5	Barnard
Cross-country	Female	15.6	164.2	51.1	15.3	Butts
	Female	15.6	163.3	50.9	15.4	Butts
Race walking	Male	26.7	178.7	68.5	7.8	Franklin
Discus	Male	26.4	190.8	110.5	16.3	Wilmore
	Male	28.3	186.1	104.7	16.4	Fahey
	Female	21.1	168.1	71.0	25.0	Malina
Jumpers and hurdlers	Female	20.3	165.9	59.0	20.7	Malina
Shot put	Male	22.0	191.6	126.2	19.6	Behnke
	Male	27.0	188.2	112.5	16.5	Fahey
	Female	21.5	167.6	78.1	28.0	Malina
Triathlon	Male	—	—	—	7.1	Holly
	Female	—	—	—	12.6	Holly
Volleyball	Male	26.1	192.7	85.5	12.0	Puhl
	Female	19.4	166.0	59.8	25.3	Conger
	Female	19.9	172.2	64.1	21.3	Kovaleski
	Female	21.6	178.3	70.5	17.9	Puhl
Weight lifting						
Power	Male	24.9	166.4	77.2	9.8	Sprynarová
	Male	25.5	173.6	89.4	19.9	Hakkinen
	Male	26.3	176.1	92.0	15.6	Fahey
Olympic	Male	25.3	177.1	88.2	12.2	Fahey
Body builders	Male	25.6	176.9	87.6	13.4	Hakkinen
	Male	27.6	178.8	88.1	8.3	Pipes
	Male	29.0	172.4	83.1	8.4	Fahey
	Female	27.0	160.8	53.8	13.2	Freedson
Wrestling	Male	11.3	141.2	34.2	12.7	Sady
	Male	15–18	172.3	66.3	6.9	Katch
	Male	19.6	174.6	74.8	8.8	Sinning
	Male	20.6	174.8	67.3	4.0	Stine
	Male	22.0	—	—	5.0	Pařízková
	Male	23.0	—	79.3	14.3	Taylor
	Male	24.0	173.3	77.5	12.7	Hakkinen
	Male	26.0	177.8	81.8	9.8	Fahey
	Male	27.0	176.0	75.7	10.7	Gale

endurance performance, what is the recommended body composition for an élite endurance athlete? There must be an optimal value, above or below which the athlete's performance is negatively affected. This is an important question, but there is, as yet, no easy answer. First, there are substantial errors inherent in existing techniques for measuring body composition. Even the better laboratory techniques have a 1—3% error rate in the measurement of body density (Lohman, 1984). Further, the optimal value is greatly influenced by individual variability (Wilmore, 1983). Not every male endurance athlete will achieve his best performance at 8% body fat. Some will reach lower values and still improve performance, while others will find it impossible to get down to 8% fat and will have to compete at higher values. Wilmore (1983) has thus suggested that a range of values should be set for male and female competitors in a given sport, recognizing individual variability and methodological error (Table 24.2).

While body composition assessment can be used to select individuals with potential for endurance sports, diet and exercise can effectively reduce the body fat stores of athletes who might initially be considered to lie outside the range of values appropriate for a given sport (Wilmore & Costill, 1988). However, a word of caution must be given at this point. Endurance athletes can get down to weights that are below their personal optimal levels. Weight and eating disorders, particularly anorexia nervosa and bulimia nervosa, are becoming a major concern in both male and female endurance athletes who are attempting to get down to the lowest weight possible to gain a competitive edge. This problem must be kept in mind when prescribing weights, or relative body fats, for the élite endurance athlete.

Finally, it is important to come back to the topic of body energy stores. Muscle and liver glycogen are the most important energy stores for endurance athletes. As the intensity of activity increases, there is a greater reliance on carbohydrate as the energy source (Costill, 1988), but stores of carbohydrate are very limited compared with the energy stored in fat. Fat is thus a valuable energy source. However, at the extremely high intensities of effort experienced during actual competition, carbohydrate is the preferred energy substrate, and the endurance athlete's performance is greatly affected if the carbohydrate substrate is no longer available (Costill, 1988). At one time it was hypothesized that women would be better endurance athletes then men because they had larger energy stores of fat and were supposed to be better burners of fat. Subsequent research has proven this to be wrong (Wilmore & Costill, 1988). Protein can provide energy for physical activity, but is a minor source during endurance activities. It serves as a precursor for gluconeogenesis, but humans are unable to generate a significant amount of glycogen through this pathway (Costill, 1988). Thus, the endurance athlete must concentrate on measures that will increase the glycogen-storing capacity of the muscles and liver, and will attenuate the use of glycogen during intense competitive activity.

References

Behnke, A.R. & Wilmore, J.H. (1974) *Evaluation and Regulation of Body Build and Composition.* Prentice-Hall, Englewood Cliffs, New Jersey.

Brodie, D.A. (1988) Techniques for measurement of body composition, Part I and II. *Sports Med.* **5,** 11—40, 74—98.

Costill, D.L. (1988) Carbohydrates for exercise: dietary demands for optimal performance. *Int. J. Sports Med.* **9,** 1—18.

Cureton, K.J. & Sparling, P.B. (1980) Distance running performance and metabolic responses to running in men and women with excess weight experimentally equated. *Med. Sci. Sports Exerc.* **12,** 288—294.

Graves, J.E., Pollock, M.L. & Sparling, P.B. (1987) Body composition of elite female distance runners. *Int. J. Sports Med.* **8,** 96—102.

Lohman, T.G. (1981) Skinfolds and body density and their relation to body fatness: a review. *Hum. Biol.* **53,** 181—225.

Lohman, T.G. (1984) Research progress in validation of laboratory methods of assessing body composition. *Med. Sci. Sports Exerc.* **16,** 596—603.

Lohman, T.G. (1986) Applicability of body composition techniques and constants for children and youths. *Exerc. Sport Sci. Rev.* **14**, 325−357.

Pate, R.R., Barnes, C. & Miller, W. (1985) A physiological comparison of performance-matched female and male distance runners. *Res. Q. Exerc. Sport* **56**, 245−250.

Pollock, M.L. & Jackson, A.S. (1984) Research progress in validation of clinical methods of assessing body composition. *Med. Sci. Sports Exerc.* **16**, 606−613.

Pollock, M.L. & Wilmore, J.H. (1990) *Exercise in Health and Disease: Evaluation and Prescription for Prevention and Rehabilitation*, 2nd edn. W.B. Saunders, Philadelphia.

Schutte, J.E., Townsend, E.J., Hugg, J., Shoup, R.F., Malina, R.M. & Blomqvist, C.G. (1984) Density of lean body mass is greater in Blacks than Whites. *J. Appl. Physiol.* **56**, 1647−1649.

Wilmore, J.H. (1983) Body composition in sport and exercise: directions for future research. *Med. Sci. Sports Exerc.* **15**, 21−31.

Wilmore, J.H. (1984) *Design issues and alternatives in assessing physical fitness among apparently healthy adults in a health examination survey of the general population*. Paper prepared for NHANES III, Department of Health and Human Services, Washington, D.C.

Wilmore, J.H., Brown, C.H. & Davis, J.A. (1977) Body physique and composition of the female distance runner. *Ann. N. Y. Acad. Sci.* **301**, 764−776.

Wilmore, J.H. & Costill, D.L. (1988) *Training for Sport and Activity: The Physiological Basis of the Conditioning Process*, 3rd edn. William C. Brown, Dubuque, Iowa.

Chapter 25

Personality and Endurance Performance: the State–Trait Controversy

LARRY M. LEITH

Introduction

Athletes and coaches are realizing that success in high-level sports competition is 10–20% physiological and 80–90% psychological (Kozar & Lord, 1983). The past two decades have witnessed a proliferation of research aimed at developing a science of superior athletic performance. It has become obvious that the physiology, biomechanics and psychology of an élite athlete differ markedly from these of individuals who have not reached world-class status. Of concern to this chapter are those psychological constructs that have the potential to distinguish between athletes of differing abilities. More specifically, attention will be focused on personality factors and their possible role in endurance sports performance.

In the present context, personality will be defined as the individual's unique psychological make-up or, more formally, 'the underlying, relatively stable, psychological structures and processes that organize human experience and shape a person's actions and reactions to the environment' (Lazarus & Monat, 1979, p. 1). The study of personality and the role it may play in a successful athletic performance have interested sport psychologists for decades. Perhaps this is because the topic has potential for more than mere academic interest. Consider the practical value of finding answers to the following important questions: (a) Do athletes possess relatively enduring personality characteristics? (b) Can these characteristics be measured? (c) Do winners possess personality profiles that differ from losers? (d) Is there a personality prototype for the endurance athlete? (e) Can personality testing be used as a screening device? (f) Can coaches and sport psychologists intervene to change these characteristics, or are they relatively resistant to change? The desire to answer such questions has resulted in a deluge of personality studies in the sport environment. Fisher (1984) has indicated that 'over 1000 studies were conducted in this so-called heyday of sport personality research' (p. 70). In spite of the tremendous volume of research, the unfortunate conclusion remains that limited knowledge has resulted with specific value for either the coach or the sport psychologist. This leaves two inescapable interpretations: (a) either personality characteristics are not very important as determinants of performance; or (b) the current experimental methodology is inadequate. Which explanation is correct? To answer this question, it is important to examine the history of personality assessment in sport, and to trace its evolution to the present day. This will be accomplished by reviewing the state–trait controversy, and suggesting future avenues of research with potential to aid the practitioner who is working with endurance athletes.

Trait theories of personality

Trait theories have generated a tremendous

amount of personality research, including most sport personality studies. The trait paradigm's key assumption is that traits, being relatively stable characteristics, can predict an athlete's behaviour in a wide variety of circumstances. Practitioners searching for personality profiles in athletes or athletic groups are implicitly adopting a trait perspective. By administering standard personality tests, for example, Cattell's 16 Personality Factor (16PF), the California Psychological Inventory (CPI), the Minnesota Multiphasic Personality Inventory (MMPI) and the Edward's Personal Preference Schedule (EPPS), to athletes, researchers have looked for common personality denominators. Their next step was to make cross-sectional comparisons between athletes and non-athletes or between élite and less talented performers. Using this approach, Alderman (1974) and Morgan (1980) have proposed the following personality traits to be characteristic of superior athletes: (a) outgoing and socially confident; (b) dominant; (c) self-assertive and self-assured; (d) tough-minded; (e) hard-driving; (f) competitively aggressive; (g) extroverted; (h) self-confident; (i) emotionally stable; and (j) highly achievement oriented. Of special interest to the practitioner working with endurance athletes would be the traits of being tough-minded, hard-driving, competitively aggressive, and highly achievement oriented.

Morgan and Pollock (1977) have indicated that such a relationship exists between personality characteristics and athletic performance in élite distance runners. In reality, however, the research consensus maintains that traits are notoriously poor predictors of behaviour. Fisher (1984) has reported that personality traits explain no more than 10% of behavioural variability in any given situation. This finding is very damaging to the trait model of behaviour. The glaring inability of traits to predict behaviour and thus to identify successful athletes has led researchers to explore different research paradigms.

Trait versus state theories of personality

According to Anastasi (1988, p. 555), 'a long-standing controversy regarding the generalizability of personality traits versus the situational specificity of behaviour reached a peak in the late 1960s and the 1970s'. Researchers started to focus their attention on narrowly defined behaviours of specific contextual interest, rather than measuring broadly defined traits. Perhaps the best example of this differentiation is witnessed in the State–Trait Anxiety Inventory (STAI). When this instrument was constructed, state anxiety (A-State) was defined as a transitory emotional condition characterized by subjective feelings of tension and apprehension. Such states were believed to vary in intensity over time. Trait anxiety (A-Trait), on the other hand, was seen as a relatively stable measure of the individual's anxiety-proneness. The differentiation between state and trait accents the notion that situational factors are important in personality assessment. For example, a distance runner may score relatively low on trait anxiety, but much higher on state anxiety. This would be a likely scenario on a race day, when the athlete was highly activated and nervous about his or her forth-coming performance. The idea of considering both trait and state in conjunction with the situation has led to an interactional perspective upon personality assessment. The following section reviews this position, and examines research with particular relevance to endurance athletes.

An interactional theory of personality assessment

The interactional paradigm of personality assessment has evolved from social learning theory. It attempts to integrate the influence of both the person and the situation on overt behaviour. Bandura (1977, pp. 11–12) expresses this social learning viewpoint ·as follows: 'psychological functioning is explained in terms of a continuous reciprocal interaction of personal and environmental determinants'. In recent years, both sport psychology and general personality theory have moved away from trait theories and closer to social learning theories. According to Gill (1986, p. 28), 'most personality psychologists do not accept traits as primary determinants of behaviour, but most do acknowledge the existence of some consistent individual differences'. As a result, various sport psychologists have now applied the interactional perspective to their research efforts.

One of the first efforts in this regard involved the Sport Competition Anxiety Test (SCAT); this instrument was designed to detect situational variables in competition that may be anxiety provoking. The test differs from the conventional questionnaires that have been used in sport psychological studies in two important respects. First, the instrument is sport specific. All questions are sport related. This feature provides more meaningful direction for the sport practitioner. Second, it takes the specific situation into consideration, rather than making assumptions based solely upon underlying traits. This consideration of the person as well as the situation is characteristic of interactional personality research. Another widely used test within this paradigm is the Profile of Mood States (POMS). This instrument was designed to measure mood at specific times such as 'the last 7 days' or 'right now'. As a result, the interaction of the individual and the specific situation is evaluated at a particular moment. An excellent review of POMS-related sport research is provided by LeUnes & Hayward (1988). They identified 56 sport-related research papers that had used the POMS since its introduction to sport psychology in 1975. The afore-mentioned research article analysed POMS research by sport category. Several research papers dealt exclusively with endurance sports events. While a summary of the results is beyond the scope of this chapter, the reader is encouraged to review individual studies directly related to his or her endurance sport. As a general summary, however, the results remain varied and somewhat inconsistent.

An interactionist approach avoids making simple, absolute predictions concerning the relationship between personality and behaviour. According to Gill (1986, p. 28), it further suggests that 'considerable research is needed to identify personality characteristics that influence specific behaviours in varying situations and to determine how those personality characteristics interact with varying situational factors'.

The current status of sport personality

The initial section of this chapter painted a rather bleak picture of personality research in the sport environment. A cursory review of the sport sciences literature reveals that personality research studies dwindled drastically during the late 1970s and early 1980s. Since that time, however, there has been a re-emergence of interest in sport personality. Several factors have been responsible for this resurrection. First, the state–trait controversy has served an heuristic function. It has revitalized the study of personality and led to the emergence of the interactional paradigm. Second, this combined interest in the person and the situation has created optimism concerning the potential of personality research to aid the practitioner. Finally, the adapting of psychological tests to specific sport situations holds much promise for future research efforts. Personality is still far from a perfect predictor of human behaviour and sport performance. It is entirely possible, however, that it can become one more tool in the practitioner's arsenal of screening and intervention tools. The next section provides specific suggestions concerning the use of sport personality research for endurance athletes.

Sport personality and endurance sports: implications for practitioners

What implications and recommendations can

be gleaned from sport personality research? The following suggestions provide the practitioner with specific directions for use in endurance sports.

1 The use of an 'average personality profile' appears inappropriate. All too often, researchers have taken psychological measures and averaged them across a number of individuals to produce a mean or average personality score. The problem with this approach is that the resultant scores do not represent any single athlete. Average values are often affected by extreme scores, leaving a mean value with little real or practical significance. Fisher (1984) concurs with this analysis, suggesting that data analysis must be ipsative, not normative. In other words, individual data must be analysable to keep individual differences alive. Although it is easier and less time consuming to collapse athletes' personality data into mean scores, in so doing we lose the idiosyncratic nature of an individual athlete's behavioural response. One-on-one personality testing with endurance athletes is a necessary prerequisite of the interactional approach. It also provides data that are qualitatively more meaningful.

2 Trait personality assessment is fraught with methodological problems. In spite of this fact, it still seems intuitively obvious that certain personality characteristics lend themselves to augmented endurance performance. Earlier in the chapter, it was shown that Alderman (1974) and Morgan (1980) have linked certain personality traits with athletic performance. If we look specifically at endurance sports, personality characteristics such as tough-minded, hard-driving, competitively aggressive, and highly achievement oriented can only be advantageous to performance outcome. More ipsative research is needed to establish the specific value of these personality traits to endurance athletes. Similarly, other specific tests would appear to be of value to the practitioner working with endurance athletes. For example, the Test of Attentional and Interpersonal Style (TAIS) has potential to identify the mental preparation strategies that are used by those competing in

endurance events. Athletes scoring high on narrow internal focus would benefit most from the use of mental imagery while training or competing. They would also profit most from techniques to monitor individual fatigue and avoid 'hitting the wall' of exhaustion before completing an event. Research of this nature should have practical significance for the coach of endurance athletes. To date, no studies have apparently addressed this phenomenon.

3 Finally, the interactional paradigm can be of special value if new tests are developed or existing tests are adapted to be sport and situation specific. For example, the Sport Competition Anxiety Test (SCAT) could be of value in identifying athletes who experience excessive anxiety. This is a particular problem for endurance athletes, because excessive worry uses valuable nervous energy. By targeting susceptible athletes, the coach is able to implement appropriate therapeutic techniques such as progressive muscular relaxation. This in turn will lower the athlete's anxiety level and conserve valuable psychic energy for the upcoming competition. Another example of a sport and situation specific test is the Causal Dimension Scale (CDS). This test measures an athlete's attribution of causality to a performance outcome. A marathoner who attributes failure in a race to external, unstable causes such as the weather or faulty time-splits is not usually addressing the specific problem at hand (for instance, lack of proper conditioning). By identifying faulty outcome attribution, the coach can help the athlete rectify the true causes of poor performance. If used properly, personality testing can thus be a valuable tool for the sport practitioner.

References

Alderman, R.B. (1974) *Psychological Behavior in Sport.* Saunders, Philadelphia.

Anastasi, A. (1988) *Psychological Testing,* 6th edn. Collier Macmillan, London.

Bandura, A. (197*1*) *Social Learning Theory.* Prentice-Hall, Englewood Cliffs, New Jersey.

Fisher, A.C. (1984) New directions in sport personality research. In: Silva, J. & Weinberg, R. (eds) *Psychological Foundations of Sport*, pp. 70–80. Human Kinetics, Champaign, Illinois.

Gill, D.L. (1986) *Psychological Dynamics of Sport*. Human Kinetics, Champaign, Illinois.

Kozar, B. & Lord, R. (1983) Psychological considerations for training the elite athlete. In: Hall, E.R. & McIntyre, M. (eds) *Olympism: A Movement of the People. Proceedings of the United States Olympic Academy VII*, pp. 78–96. Texas Tech University, Lubbock, Texas.

Lazarus, R.S. & Monat, A. (1979) *Personality*, 3rd edn.

Prentice-Hall, Englewood Cliffs, New Jersey.

LeUnes, A. & Hayward, S. (1988) Annotated bibliography on the profile on mood states in sport, 1975–1988. *J. Sport Behav.* **11**, 213–239.

Morgan, W.P. (1980) Personality dynamics and sport. In: Suinn, R.M. (ed.) *Psychology in Sports: Methods and Applications*, pp. 145–155. Burgess, Minneapolis.

Morgan, W.P. & Pollock, M.L. (1977) Psychological characteristics of the elite distance runner. *Ann. N. Y. Acad. Sci.* **301**, 382–403.

Chapter 26

Sensory Processes and Endurance Performance

ENZO CAFARELLI

Introduction

According to Mountcastle (1975), 'Sensations are set by the encoding functions of sensory nerve endings and by the integrated neural mechanics of the central nervous system'. The sensations that occur during prolonged exercise are caused by the electrical expressions of physiological change brought about by disturbances in homoeostasis. The perception of these simple signals, however, is a function of memories and associations acquired over repetitions of similar experiences. This chapter focuses on simple, conscious sensation; we will leave to others the task of explaining the relationship between simple sensation and complex human thought. The overall objectives are to discuss: (i) the characteristics of the internal environment that influence sensory processes during prolonged exercise; and (ii) the role that sensory processes play in performance. Because this area of inquiry has received little direct investigation, much of what follows will be inferred from related work. The following specific questions will be discussed:

1 Is there a distinct neuromuscular sensory system, with a control strategy common to all humans?

2 What sensations occur during exercise and how are they measured?

3 What physiological factors influence the response characteristics of this system?

4 Can sensation alter performance?

Neuromuscular mechanisms for sensory processes during exercise

Much of the early work in this area was not rigorously mechanistic, but it has provided some valuable observations on sensory processes and exercise (Borg & Noble, 1974; Pandolf, 1983). For the most part, these early studies used Borg's category scale of perceived exertion during numerous different exercise protocols, making inferences about the underlying mechanism. Several authors suggested that the overall level of sensory intensity, as expressed in the category judgements, was an integration of signals from muscles and joints as well as cardiorespiratory inputs (Borg & Noble, 1974; Cafarelli, 1982; Robertson, 1982; Pandolf, 1983). Most authors have been circumspect about the specific receptors that may have served this process and there have been very few attempts to synthesize relevant data in some way that is meaningful, given our understanding of sensory physiology.

Receptors

To some extent, the nature of the peripheral sensory receptors determines the ensemble of parameters that reach consciousness. During exercise of any form, the numerous and sophisticated receptors of the neuromuscular system make major input to the central nervous system (CNS). During locomotor exercise, an enormous amount of sensory information reaches the CNS from the active limbs. The sources of this afferent activity are the muscle spindles and Golgi tendon organs in muscle, receptors embedded in the joint capsule and skin receptors (Shepherd, 1983; Martin, 1985). In addition, small, unmyelinated, polymodal 'c' fibres, whose free endings are liberally distributed throughout deep tissue, respond to mechanical, thermal and chemical energies (Kniffki *et al.*, 1978). The parameters derived from these receptors are: muscle length, tension and position, mechanical pressure, temperature, and the concentration of some ions — the most likely being H^+ (Kniffki *et al.*, 1978). Figure 26.1 shows the approximate location of these receptors in the knee joint (Shepherd, 1983). The cortical projection of this afferent activity, in so far as it can be localized, is probably areas 1, 3a and 5 of the somatosensory cortex (Shepherd, 1983). It is highly unlikely that sensory input about cardiac frequency is part of the ensemble, because appropriate receptors have not been demonstrated.

Second only to the active limbs is the sensory input from the respiratory apparatus. Receptors in the diaphragm and in the chest wall convey information relative to the work of these muscles in achieving the required ventilation (Killian & Campbell, 1983). Undoubtedly, other receptors in the airway are sensitive to specific

energies in that area and transmit such data to the CNS. The resulting dyspnoeic sensations may be distinct from the exercise intensity (Cafarelli & Noble, 1976) or they may be proportional to the energy expenditure (Robertson, 1982; Killian & Campbell, 1983).

In addition to these inputs, there is a contribution of corollary discharge or central feedforward (McCloskey, 1981) that irradiates from the motor centres of the cortex to various other control centres. For example, feedforward may play a role in controlling the cardiovascular and respiratory systems during exercise (Dempsey *et al.*, 1979; Rowell, 1980; Hobbs, 1982). Numerous experiments have shown that the sensations of force (Cafarelli, 1988), velocity and position (McCloskey, 1978; 1981) are partially driven by the outflow from the motor cortex to the somatosensory cortex and thence into consciousness. This feedforward component is responsible for the increase in force sensation that occurs when the same force is developed over a period of time (Cafarelli, 1988). Some argue that there is a 'sense of effort' that is a reflection of how hard one must try in order to achieve a desired motor outcome (McCloskey, 1978; Killian & Campbell, 1983). According to McCloskey (1981) it is the change in motor outflow that is responsible for the increased sense of effort that accompanies repeated muscular contractions.

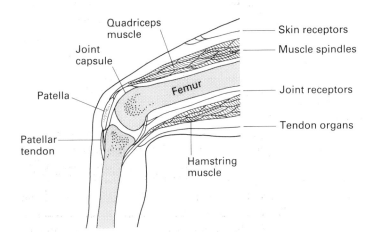

Fig. 26.1 Location of peripheral receptors that probably contribute to conscious muscle sensation. Group IV afferents are not shown. From Shepherd (1983), with permission.

What information reaches the brain?

Given that any sensory process requires specific receptors, and that only a limited number of receptors is available for muscle sensation during exercise, what information is actually transmitted to the brain? Muscle tissue is rich in sophisticated mechanoreceptors. Muscle spindles, for example, are surpassed only by the eye as sensory receptors. It is not surprising, therefore, that sensations during any form of exercise are derived from the basic information of length and tension that is transmitted from muscle. Although joint receptors exist, these appear to be active only at the extremes of the range of motion (Shepherd, 1983). Thus the basic information is in response to muscle length and tension, and these are signalled by the spindle afferents and the Golgi tendon organs. From this information the parameters of force, position and velocity are derived (McCloskey, 1978; Shepherd, 1983). Figure 26.2 shows schematically how peripheral information may be integrated in the CNS. Note that muscle contains the contractile apparatus, the metabolic machinery to provide adenosine triphosphate (ATP) for contraction, and the receptors to regu-

late contraction and monitor the internal environment. Mechanoreceptors are somewhat more involved in the process, because they provide information to the somatosensory cortex and because they also modulate the outflow along the final common pathway. Moreover, muscle spindles can adjust their sensitivity through the γ motor system (not shown in Fig. 26.2).

Thermal energy and the products of metabolism during exercise alter the internal environment of the muscle, thus affecting the very processes that produced them. As a consequence, there are both local and central effects of changing the internal environment. For example, the accumulation of H^+ has direct inhibitory effects on metabolism and the contractile proteins, and additional recruitment of muscle fibres would be required to maintain a constant motor output. In addition, decreased pH stimulates small, 'c' fibres (Kniffki et al., 1978); this information is transmitted directly to the somatosensory cortex and is probably responsible for the 'burning sensation' that accompanies intense, fatiguing contractions.

The optimal temperature for enzymatic function in muscle is about 41°C, which is 5−6°

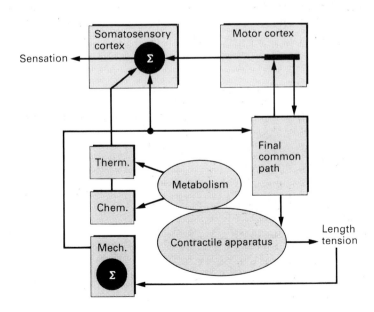

Fig. 26.2 Schematic representation of how the neuromuscular system may produce and modulate conscious sensation during muscular contraction. See text for explanation. Modified from Cafarelli (1988).

higher than the usual muscle temperature at rest. Immediately after the onset of exercise, the accumulation of heat actually helps muscle function. At some point, temperature-sensitive fibres in the muscle may be stimulated to provide conscious thermal sensations. On the other hand, it is well known that cutaneous thermal receptors are active during exercise, but that these sensations are easily discerned from those arising from muscular activity; it is possible to exercise at a very low intensity and still feel quite hot (Pandolf *et al.*, 1972).

During prolonged exercise, it appears a simple matter to distinguish between numerous different sensations. For example, the sensations of force, velocity and position are probably derived from the comparison of the corollary discharge of the motor command to the somatosensory cortex and feedback from the peripheral mechanoreceptors (McCloskey, 1978; Cafarelli, 1982). These sensations are then modulated by additional feedback from other peripheral receptors. Moreover, reflex spindle feedback to the anterior horn helps modulate output along the final common pathway (Fig. 26.2). The greater the error between the desired motor outcome and the actual muscle length and tension, the greater the γ motor activity. Since γ motor drive is known to project to the cortex as well as on to the motor neuron pool of the homonymous muscle, it will also tend to increase the output of the motor cortex (Matthews, 1982).

Dyspnoea

Respiratory contributions to the ensemble of sensory processes that occur during exercise are largely a function of the work of breathing (Killian & Campbell, 1983). As the metabolic requirement for any level of exercise increases, so does the respiratory minute volume, and these respiratory sensations are clearly distinguished from other muscular sensations (Robertson, 1982). Whether they actually play a role in limiting exercise may depend on the extent of the dyspnoea. Respiratory sensations

seem of little consequence until the metabolic requirement for exercise exceeds 60–70% of $\dot{V}_{O_2 max}$ (Cafarelli & Noble, 1976; Robertson, 1982). In any case, the mechanism for transducing respiratory sensations is essentially the same as for other muscle sensations (Killian & Campbell, 1983) and probably operates as shown in Fig. 26.2.

Fatigue of the respiratory muscles could indeed limit exercise, but this is liable to occur only in respiratory disorders, when any level of exercise requires a large fraction of the maximum voluntary ventilation (Killian & Jones, 1984). Because minute ventilation during maximal exercise is normally considerably less than the maximal voluntary ventilation, it is unlikely that dyspnoea is a major consideration when highly trained athletes perform endurance exercise.

Measurement of sensory processes

The nature of prolonged exercise limits the techniques that may be used to measure sensory processes in humans. Although standard psychophysical methods have been used to observe the relation between sensory stimulus and response, only a few have been applied during prolonged exercise. The most prevalent method is the category rating scale of Borg (Borg & Noble, 1974; Pandolf, 1983) (Figs 26.3 and 26.4). This is an interval scale, where alternate intervals have a descriptive phrase. While this type of measurement has been extremely useful in describing the general behaviour of the sensory system during exercise, it suffers from two major short-comings when studying long-term activity. The first is that an interval scale has no ratio properties; that is, '10' does not indicate a sensory intensity twice as great as '5'. One of the most revealing aspects of any system is the rate at which the output changes in response to each stimulus increment (Marks, 1974). This information cannot be gained from interval (category) scales. A more recent version of this instrument has been constructed so that it does have ratio properties, but the revised

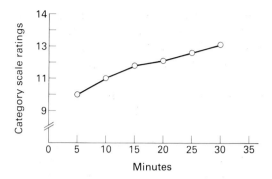

Fig. 26.3 Category scale ratings during 30 min of cycling at 100 W. Note that there is only a slight increase in sensation at this low intensity of exercise but that no apparent sensory steady state is achieved. Modified from Morgan (1973).

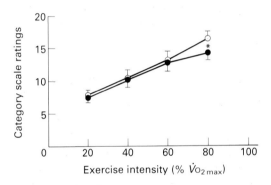

Fig. 26.4 Category scale ratings as a function of exercise intensity during cycling. Control data show an almost perfectly linear relation, which is how the scale was intended to behave. When body fluid buffering capacity is enhanced by ingesting $NaHCO_3$, sensory intensity is significantly reduced at the load where greatest H^+ accumulation would be expected. This suggests that H^+ accumulation contributes to conscious muscle sensation. *, $p < 0.05$; ○, control; ●, HCO_3. Modified from Robertson *et al.* (1986).

format has seen limited use (Borg, 1982). A second shortcoming of interval scales that is particularly egregious with respect to prolonged exercise is that when the upper limit of the scale is known to the subject, the selection of all other intervals is biased. For example, in determining the time-course of a sensation

as it changes during prolonged exercise, the subject tends to conserve intervals (Gescheider, 1976). Experiments designed to study differences between more than one condition are thus biased, because the subjects must choose the same terminal interval category.

The method of magnitude estimation has been used to measure sensory processes during exercise, although not nearly so often as category scales. With this technique, the subject expresses the magnitude of a sensation as a number; an infinite set of numbers is thus available (Fig. 26.5). The major drawback of magnitude estimation is that it is not particularly well suited to interindividual comparisons, or to the study of absolute sensory intensities (Marks, 1974). However, in most sensory experiments the question of interest is the way in which sensory intensity varies with some attribute of the stimulus intensity. Be-

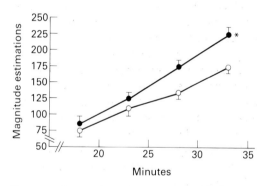

Fig. 26.5 Sensory intensity measured with the method of magnitude estimation during cycling at 80% of $\dot{V}_{O_2\,max}$. This is the last 20 min of a continuous 35-min ride; the load was only 40% of $\dot{V}_{O_2\,max}$ in the first half. Because this is a ratio scale, it follows that sensory intensity was 2.4 times greater at the end of the control condition than it was at the 17th minute, and that the terminal sensory intensity in the experimental condition was 28% higher than in the control condition. In this case ingesting NH_4Cl was intended to decrease body fluid pH. Like the data in Fig. 26.4, this suggests that H^+ accumulation contributes to conscious muscle sensation, probably via excitation of group IV afferents. The asterisk (*) indicates that there was a significant interaction between the two conditions at $p < 0.05$. ○, Control; ●, NH_4Cl. Modified from Kostka & Cafarelli (1982).

cause magnitude estimation is a direct scaling technique, it is possible to calculate the gain of the sensory system under any set of conditions for each subject. Magnitude estimation presents problems in data analysis, especially when individual subjects choose numbers that differ by an order of magnitude. Nevertheless, because it is a direct technique, and because it gives unbiased estimates of the way in which sensory intensity grows with stimulus intensity, it is eminently suited for measuring sensory processes during prolonged exercise. A complete description of a magnitude estimation experiment may be found in Marks (1974).

Nature of sensory processes during prolonged locomotor exercise

Having considered the neuromuscular sensory system in general and the methods of measurement that may reveal its behaviour, it is now time to consider sensory processes during prolonged exercise. Very few direct experiments have been conducted. Therefore, the discussion below is speculative.

Increases in sensory intensity indicate some change in either the internal environment *or* in the way in which the CNS integrates peripheral afferent activity. If we assume that fatigue, which is defined here as the loss of force-producing capacity, is the reciprocal of increased force sensation (Cafarelli, 1988), then any causes of fatigue will also influence sensation. Although an extensive literature on fatigue processes has not answered all questions in this area, it has been suggested that the causative agents are those that either accumulate in and around muscle or exert an influence by their absence (MacLaren et al., 1989). It is beyond the scope of this chapter to consider all possible causes of fatigue, but it may be of some benefit to discuss how the sensory system may operate when faced with an accumulation and/or a depletion of fatigue-related substances during prolonged exercise.

Generally speaking, substances that accumu-

late within the cell and in the extracellular fluid are the products of accelerated metabolism and heightened membrane activity. For example, hydrogen ions (H^+) dissociated from lactate during glycolysis have a deleterious effect on both the contractile proteins and enzymatic function (MacLaren et al., 1989). More recently, an extracellular accumulation of potassium (K^+), the major intracellular cation, has been implicated in fatigue (MacLaren et al., 1989). Electrical phenomena in muscle and nerve depend on the appropriate distribution of inorganic ions across the membrane. Thus, when this distribution is upset, excitation may be impaired (MacLaren et al., 1989). The concentrations of glycogen in muscle and liver, and blood glucose levels, have been studied on numerous occasions to determine how the availability and depletion of these substrates may limit performance (Conlee, 1987). Conlee (1987) concluded that fatigue is associated with muscle glycogen depletion. However, glycogen depletion need not be total in order for endurance performance to abate (Fig. 26.6).

Using Fig. 26.2 as a guide, it is possible to speculate on how the neuromuscular system operates to provide conscious sensation during prolonged exercise. Four assumptions must be made. First, this scenario is speculative; very few data are available, although the model generally accommodates what is known about physiological changes during endurance exercise. Second, only known receptors are used; non-specific receptors are not postulated. Third, central feedforward contributes to conscious sensation; there are numerous indirect data that attest to its participation in various physiological processes (McClosk' y, 1978; 1981; Cafarelli, 1988). Fourth, the example focuses on locomotor muscle, but extends to the muscles of respiration and thus it can account for exercise-dependent respiratory sensations. These assumptions apply to moderately intense (60–70% of $\dot{V}o_{2\,max}$) steady-state locomotor exercise.

At the very outset of exercise, all sensations derive from the force of contraction (Cafarelli, 1982). These are mediated through mechano-

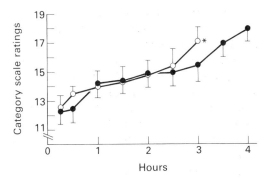

Fig. 26.6 Category scale ratings during cycling at 70–74% of $\dot{V}O_{2\,max}$ for up to 4 h. During the experimental condition, subjects were given a glucose solution in order to maintain blood glucose. The ride was terminated when the subjects could no longer maintain the required power output. These data suggest that there is some relationship between substrate availability and conscious muscle sensation. Compare these category scale data with those in Fig. 26.3. Note that during the first hour of exercise at 80% of $\dot{V}O_{2\,max}$ (this figure) the judgements increase by 1.5 points and that at 100 W (Fig. 26.3) the judgements increase by 1.5 points after only 15 min. Moreover, even after 3–4 h of cycling, when subjects were incapable of maintaining the required power output, they did not choose the maximal rating. This illustrates how category scales can be biased when a subject knows the duration of the experiment and tries to 'conserve' categories. ○, Control; ●, subjects given glucose. * indicates a significant difference from the control. Modified from Coyle et al. (1986).

receptors in muscle, primarily the spindle Ia afferents, as well as the so-called group IV 'ergoceptive afferents' (Kniffki et al., 1978), and are compared with a copy of the motor outflow. This phase is characterized by a rapid increase in the intensity of sensation, which then slows markedly as a metabolic steady state is attained (Fig. 26.7). The level of dynamic force sensation is set by the intensity of the repetitive contractions required to achieve locomotion. The sensations of velocity, effort and position are all discernible by themselves (McCloskey, 1978). Pain, temperature and chemoreception are probably of little consequence during the first few minutes of exercise.

Once a metabolic steady state has been achieved, sensory intensity changes slowly, unless there are mitigating circumstances. Experimentally manipulating P_{O_2} haemoglobin concentration [Hb] (Robertson, 1982), pH (Kostka & Cafarelli, 1982; Robertson, 1982), plasma volume (E.R. Nadel, personal communication) and feeding carbohydrate (Coyle et al., 1986) all affect sensory intensity. Thus, alterations in the internal environment caused by repetitive contractions help modulate the sensory intensity originally set by the mechanoreceptors. For example, as the small, oxidative motor units begin to fatigue, they lose their force generating capacity and additional units must be recruited in order to maintain a given power output. This leads to an increase in drive from the motor cortex, a copy of which is fed forward to the somatosensory cortex and compared with afferent information. The sensations of force and effort both increase under these conditions (McCloskey, 1981; Gandevia, 1987; Cafarelli, 1988).

In the final stages of prolonged exercise, the 'basic' afferent feedback from peripheral mechanoreceptors and the feedforward of motor outflow are modulated by feedback from the ubiquitous 'c' fibres which are excited by H^+ (Kniffki et al., 1978), thermal energy (Shepherd, 1983) and muscle activation (Kniffki et al., 1978). The depletion of glycogen somehow hampers the rate of ATP synthesis (Conlee, 1987) and forces the recruitment of additional motor units, which themselves tend to rely more heavily on glycolysis and produce more lactate and H^+. Central and peripheral afferent signals increase under these conditions, as does conscious sensation. Ultimately, the intensity of force, effort and perhaps pain sensation outweigh the conscious drive to continue exercise (Brück & Olschewski, 1987), and the power output must be reduced.

In summary, sensory processes that occur during prolonged, steady-state exercise arise from peripheral mechanoreceptors *and* from a copy of the motor output. These two separate signals are compared in the somatosensory

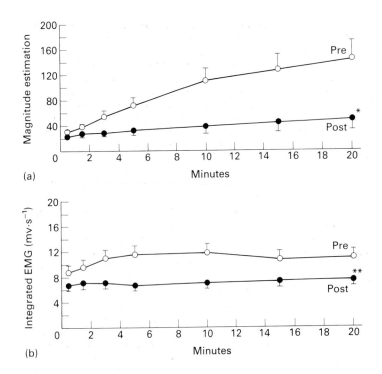

Fig. 26.7 Magnitude estimates of dynamic force and vastus lateralis electromyogram (EMG) during single-leg cycling at 70% of $\dot{V}O_2$ peak before and after endurance training. The reduction in sensory intensity before and after training shown in (a) occurs at the same time as a reduction in neural drive (EMG) (b) required to produce the same power output. Control subjects showed no changes in either sensory intensity or neural drive. These findings suggest that the sensation of dynamic force during cycling is related not only to the changes normally seen in trained muscle but also to the reduction in neural drive. A single asterisk (*) indicates a significant interaction and two (**) indicate a significant main effect ($p < 0.05$) (E. Cafarelli, J. Liebesman & J. Kroon, unpublished data).

cortex, and the *difference* between them drives conscious sensation. As the consequences of sustained muscular activity alter the internal environment, this information is transmitted from the periphery and modulates the basic signal. When sensory intensity exceeds the drive to continue, power output must be reduced.

Acknowledgements

The author's work is supported by the Natural Science and Engineering Research Council of Canada. The assistance of Monica B. Hamilton in preparing this manuscript is gratefully acknowledged.

References

Borg, G. (1982) A category scale with ratio properties for intermodal and interindividual comparisons. In: Geissler, H. & Petzold, P. (eds) *Psychophysical Judgement and the Process of Perception*, pp. 25–34. VEB Deutscher Verlag der Wissenschaften, Berlin.

Borg, G. & Noble, B. (1974) Perceived Exertion. In Wilmore, J. (ed.) *Exercise and Sports Sciences Reviews*, pp. 131–153. Academic Press, New York.

Brück, K. & Olschewski, H. (1987) Body temperature and related factors diminishing the drive to exercise. *Can. J. Physiol. Pharmacol.* **65**, 1274–1280.

Cafarelli, E. (1982) Peripheral contributions to the perception of effort. *Med. Sci. Sports* **14**, 382–389.

Cafarelli, E. (1988) Force sensation in fresh and fatigued human skeletal muscle. In: Pandolf, K. (ed.) *Exercise and Sports Sciences Reviews*, pp. 139–168. MacMillan Publishing, New York.

Cafarelli, E. & Noble, B. (1976) The effect of inspired carbon dioxide on subjective estimates of exertion during exercise. *Ergonomics* **19**, 581–589.

Conlee, R. (1987) Muscle glycogen and exercise endurance: a twenty-year perspective. In: Pandolf, K. (ed.) *Exercise and Sports Sciences Reviews*, pp. 1–28. MacMillan Publishing, New York.

Coyle, E., Coggan, A., Hemmert, M. & Ivy, J. (1986) Muscle glycogen utilization during prolonged strenuous exercise when fed carbohydrates. *J. Appl. Physiol.* **61**, 165–172.

Dempsey, J., Pellegrino, D., Aggarwal, D. & Olson, E. (1979) The brain's role in exercise hyperpnea. *Med. Sci. Sports* **11**, 213–220.

Gandevia, S. (1987) Roles for perceived voluntary motor commands in motor control. *Trends Neurosci.*

10, 81–85.

Gescheider, G. (1976) *Psychophysics: Method and Theory*. Lawrence Earlbaum Associates, Hillsdale, New Jersey.

Hobbs, S. (1982) Central command during exercise: parallel activation of the cardiovascular and motor system by descending command signals. In: Smith, O., Calosy, R. & Weiss, S. (eds) *Circulation, Neurobiology and Behavior*, pp. 217–231. Elsevier, New York.

Killian, K. & Campbell, E.J.M. (1983) Dyspnea and exercise. *Annu. Rev. Physiol.* **45**, 465–479.

Killian, K. & Jones, N. (1984) The use of exercise testing and other methods in the investigation of dyspnea. *Clin. Chest Med.* **5**, 99–108.

Kniffki, K., Mense, S. & Schmidt, R. (1978) Responses of group IV afferent units from skeletal muscle to stretch, contraction, and chemical stimulation. *Exp. Brain Res.* **31**, 511–522.

Kostka, C. & Cafarelli, E. (1982) Effect of pH on sensation and vastus lateralis electromyogram during cycling exercise. *J. Appl. Physiol.* **52**, 1181–1185.

McCloskey, D.I. (1978) Kinesthetic sensibility. *Physiol. Rev.* **58**, 763–792.

McCloskey, D.I. (1981) Corollary discharges: motor commands and perception. In: Brooks, V. (ed.) *Handbook of Physiology, Section I: The Nervous System, Vol. II, Motor Control, Part II*, pp. 1415–1447. American Physiology Society, Bethesda, Maryland.

MacLaren, D., Gibson, H., Parry-Billings, M. & Edwards, R.H.T. (1989) A review of metabolic and physiological factors in fatigue. In: Pandolf, K. (ed.) *Exercise and Sports Sciences Reviews*, pp. 29–66. Williams and Wilkins, Baltimore.

Marks, L. (1974) *Sensory Processes: The New Psychophysics*. Academic Press, New York.

Martin, J.H. (1985) Receptor physiology and submodality coding in the somatic sensory system. In: Kandel, E. & Schwartz, J. (eds) *Principles of Neural Science*, 2nd edn, pp. 285–300. Elsevier, New York.

Matthews, P.B.C. (1982) Where does Sherrington's 'muscular sense' originate? Muscles, joints, corollary discharges? *Annu. Rev. Neurosci.* **5**, 189–218.

Morgan, W. (1973) Psychological factors influencing perceived exertion. *Med. Sci. Sports* **5**, 97–103.

Mountcastle, V.B. (1975) The view from within: pathways to the study of perception. *Johns Hopkins Med. J.* **136**, 109.

Pandolf, K.B. (1983) Advances in the study and application of perceived exertion. In: Terjung, R. (ed.) *Exercise and Sports Sciences Reviews*, pp. 118–153. Franklin Institute Press, Philadelphia.

Pandolf, K.B., Cafarelli, E., Noble, B. & Metz, K. (1972) Perceptual responses during prolonged work. *Percept. Mot. Skills* **35**, 975–980.

Robertson, R. (1982) Central signals of perceived exertion during dynamic exercise. *Med. Sci. Sports* **14**, 390–396.

Robertson, R., Falkel, J., Drash, A. *et al.* (1986) Effect of blood pH on peripheral and central signals of perceived exertion. *Med. Sci. Sports Exerc.* **18**, 114–122.

Rowell, L. (1980) What signals govern the cardiovascular responses to exercise? *Med. Sci. Sports* **12**, 307–315.

Shepherd, G. (1983) *Neurobiology*. Oxford University Press, New York.

Chapter 27

Environmental Extremes and Endurance Performance

KENT B. PANDOLF AND ANDREW J. YOUNG

Introduction

The environmental extremes of heat, cold, high terrestrial altitude and air quality each pose a threat to the endurance performance of competitive athletes. This chapter, which primarily concerns the environmental extremes of heat and cold, describes how to assess a particular environment, when competition should be modified and, if appropriate, when competition should be curtailed. In addition, strategies are presented for each of the environmental extremes which should help to optimize individual performance.

Environmental heat stress

Assessment of the thermal environment

Proper assessment of the thermal environment should consider ambient temperature, humidity, wind velocity and radiant heat in order to characterize the level of environmental heat stress imposed on the competitor. One index of environmental heat stress that may have application for competitive athletic endurance performance is the wet bulb globe temperature (WBGT). For outdoor environments with solar load, $WBGT = 0.7\ T_{wb(n)} + 0.2\ T_g + 0.1\ T_{db}$, where $T_{wb(n)}$ is the naturally convected wet bulb temperature which incorporates a wetted sensor exposed to natural air movement, T_g is the temperature of a black globe thermometer 15 cm in diameter, and T_{db} is the dry bulb

temperature. Portable WBGT meters are available commercially, and are simple to operate while offering a digital display of the WBGT index. While WBGT is an easily understood and measured index, it is empirically based rather than rationally derived from heat transfer theory. Examples of rationally derived environmental indices, which may be more appropriate for quantifying human heat strain and endurance performance, are the heat stress index (HSI) and the new effective temperature (ET). The various environmental heat stress indices are discussed in detail elsewhere (Gonzalez, 1988; Santee & Gonzalez, 1988).

The American College of Sports Medicine (ACSM) has published a position stand on the prevention of thermal injuries during distance running, based in part on the WBGT index (ACSM, 1987). For instance, when the WBGT is greater than 28°C (82°F), ACSM suggests that athletic competition should be curtailed or rescheduled until a lower WBGT is prevalent. When the WBGT is at or below 28°C, ACSM proposes the use of colour-coded flags to alert athletic participants and officials to the risk of thermal stress. A red flag denotes high risk and is associated with a WBGT of 23–28°C (73–82°F), while an amber flag represents moderate risk when WBGT is 18–20°C (65–73°F), and a green flag represents low risk when WBGT is below 18°C (65°F). These WBGT values are applicable to athletes dressed in running shorts, shoes and a T-shirt, while different clothing systems and differing durations of activity would necessitate further adjustments in the WBGT values associated with each level of risk. Finally, ACSM recommends that in regions where environmental heat stress is prevalent, athletic competition should begin in the early morning (before 08.00 h), or in the evening (after 18.00 h) in order to lessen the effects of solar load.

Competitive strategies

During endurance exercise in the heat, human thermoregulation is known to be primarily influenced by exercise–heat acclimatization state (Wenger, 1988), level of aerobic fitness (Armstrong & Pandolf, 1988), hydration level (Sawka & Pandolf, 1990) and clothing worn (Gonzalez, 1987). In addition, competitors with a previous history of heat illness such as heat stroke will generally display greater exercise–heat intolerance than those not so predisposed. A discussion of heat illnesses and their influence on human endurance performance is beyond the scope of this section, but has been previously reviewed in detail (Hubbard & Armstrong, 1988; see also Chapter 42).

Exercise–heat acclimatization: The classical physiological adjustments during exercise–heat acclimatization are a potentiated sweating response, reduced heart rate, and lowered skin and rectal temperatures, while exercise–heat tolerance is greatly improved as illustrated in Fig. 27.1. Figure 27.1 depicts the improvement in exercise–heat tolerance for 24 males who attempted 100 min of exercise (1.56 m·s^{-1}) at 49°C and 20% relative humidity on each of 7 days. No subject completed the 100-min walk on day 1, 40% were successful by day 3, 80% by day 5, and all but one subject were successful by the seventh acclimatization day. Complete exercise–heat acclimatization occurs after 10–14 days of exposure; however, about 75% of the physiological acclimatization responses are developed by the end of the first week. Regular heavy exercise in the heat is the most effective method for developing heat acclimatization (Wenger, 1988). Daily 100-min

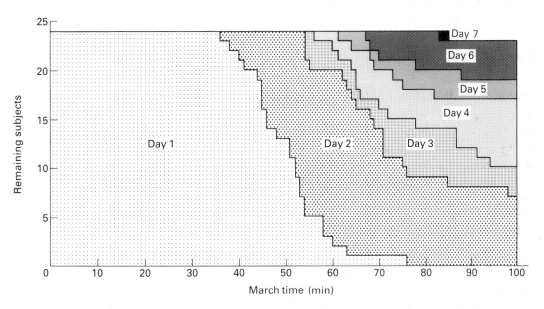

Fig. 27.1 Relationship between improvement in exercise–heat tolerance (march time) and the number of remaining subjects (24 male volunteers) attempting 100 min of exercise (1.56 m·s^{-1}) at 49°C and 20% relative humidity over 7 days of repeated testing. (US Army Research Institute of Environmental Medicine, unpublished data.)

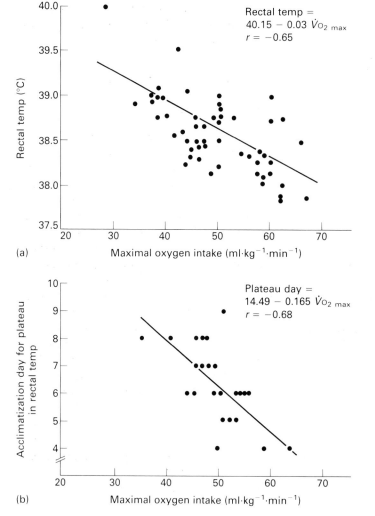

(a)

(b)

Fig. 27.2 Relationship between $\dot{V}_{O_2 \, max}$ and (a) rectal temperature in a hot–humid environment or (b) the acclimatization day for a plateau in rectal temperature during dry-heat exposure. From Armstrong & Pandolf (1988).

exercise bouts seem optimal to induce the heat-acclimatization process. Competitive athletes who expect to participate in an event involving environmental heat stress should train in the hot environment for at least 1 week before participation in order to help maximize their endurance performance.

Aerobic fitness: Researchers generally agree that high aerobic fitness achieved through endurance training reduces the physiological strain during exercise in the heat (Armstrong & Pandolf, 1988). Figure 27.2 presents obser-

vations from different hot climates (hot–humid, Fig. 27.2a; hot–dry, Fig. 27.2b) and shows that maximal oxygen intake accounts for between 42% and 46% of the variability in core temperature after 3 h of exercise in the heat, or the heat acclimatization day for a plateauing of core temperature. However, the improvement of aerobic fitness by endurance training must be associated with significant elevations in core temperature during the training process in order to improve exercise–heat tolerance (Armstrong & Pandolf, 1988). It has also been hypothesized that high aerobic fitness is a major factor in the small decay of acclimatization and the rapid reacclimatization of individuals after they have stopped exercising in the heat. Endurance athletes should be at peak levels of aerobic fitness in order to maximize the potential benefits associated with improved exercise—heat tolerance.

Hydration level: In general, dehydration degrades endurance exercise performance, and there is no evidence that dehydration can benefit endurance (Sawka & Pandolf, 1990). In addition, humans do not appear to adapt to chronic dehydration. Table 27.1 presents a summary of research studies investigating the influence of dehydration on maximal aerobic power ($\dot{V}o_{2\,max}$) and physical work capacity. Physical performance is clearly diminished even at marginal levels of dehydration (1% decrease of body mass), with alterations in $\dot{V}o_{2\,max}$ requiring at least a 2% decrease due to water loss. Greater body water deficits are associated with progressively larger reductions in physical work capacity. Furthermore, dehydration results in a much larger reduction in physical work capacity in a hot compared with a thermally neutral temperature. Prolonged endurance exercise that places large demands on aerobic metabolism is more likely to be affected adversely by dehydration than is short-term exercise. Therefore, endurance athletes should be encouraged to avoid becoming dehydrated during events in hot environments and should target their loss of body water to 2% or less of body mass.

Clothing: Proper clothing helps to optimize performance of the competitive endurance athlete in the heat (Gonzalez, 1987; 1988). For hot environments, the proper clothing ensemble must allow evaporative heat transfer, but it should be lightweight and afford solar protection. Light-coloured clothing is preferred during endurance exercise in the heat. In general, synthetic materials have most of the thermal advantages of materials made of natural fibres such as cotton, and most synthetic fabrics are not affected by microorganisms. Endurance athletes should select their clothing for performance in hot environments with great care.

Environmental cold stress

Physiological effects of cold

Humans rely primarily on behavioural techniques (for example, clothing and shelter) to gain cold protection, but such avoidance strategies are of limited use when endurance athletes are competing outdoors in cold weather. Peripheral vasoconstriction, which limits body heat loss, and muscular shivering, which increases metabolic heat production, are the major physiological responses to cold. However, as exercise intensity increases, the demand for blood flow to the active muscles overrides cold-induced vasoconstriction (Toner & McArdle, 1988) and shivering is suppressed (Horvath, 1981; Young, 1990). Despite inhibition of shivering and compromised insulation from skin and active muscle, metabolic heat production during high-intensity endurance exercise in cold air is generally sufficient to maintain thermal balance and body temperature (Toner & McArdle, 1988). In contrast, some athletes may not defend body temperatures during high-intensity exercise in cold water, despite a high rate of metabolic heat production (Toner & McArdle, 1988).

Cold-associated injuries are reviewed in detail elsewhere (see Chapter 42; Hamlet, 1988). Cold injuries can be localized (periphery) or generalized (whole body). The localized injuries most likely to be experienced during acute exposure to cold air temperatures are frostnip and the more serious condition of frostbite. Both result from tissue freezing, limited to superficial skin layers with frostnip, but extending through the skin and even subcutaneous tissue with frostbite (Hamlet, 1988). Skin freezes at tissue temperatures below $-2°C$. Whole body cooling occurs when the rate of metabolic heat production due to exercise and/or shivering is less than the rates of conductive

Table 27.1 Summary of studies investigating the influence of hypohydration on maximal aerobic power ($\dot{V}o_{2max}$) and peak power output. From Sawka & Pandolf (1990).

Study	n	Dehydration procedure	Weight Δ (%)	Test environment	Exercise mode	Maximal aerobic power	Peak power output
Armstrong et al. (1985)	8	Diuretics	−1	Neutral	TM	NC	→ (6%)
Caldwell et al. (1984)	16	Exercise	−2	Neutral	CY	NC	→ (7 W)
	15	Diuretics	−3	Neutral	CY	→ (8%)	→ (21 W)
	16	Sauna	−4	Neutral	CY	→ (4%)	→ (23 W)
Saltin (1964)	10	Sauna, exercise, heat, diuretics	−4	Neutral	CY	NC	→ (?)
Craig & Cummings (1966)	9	Heat	−2	Hot	TM	→ (10%)	→ (22%)
			−4	Hot	TM	→ (27%)	→ (48%)
Buskirk et al. (1958)	13	Exercise, heat	−5	Neutral	TM	→ (−0.22 l·min⁻¹)	—
Webster et al. (1988)	7	Exercise in heat, sauna	−5	Neutral	TM	→ (7%)	→ (12%)
Herbert & Ribisl (1971)	8	?	−5	Neutral	CY	—	→ (17%)
Houston et al. (1981)	4	Fluid restriction	−8	Neutral	TM	NC	—

* CY, cycle ergometer; NC, no change; TM, treadmill.

and evaporative heat loss at the skin and via the respiratory tract. An individual is considered hypothermic when the core temperature (T_C) falls below 35°C.

Assessment of the thermal environment

Cold air and wind chill: Air temperature, wind speed, solar radiation and humidity are all determinants of environmental stress experienced during outdoor sporting events in winter. No single cold stress index integrates the effect of these factors on the potential for body heat loss. Wind chill formulae allow cooling power for combinations of air temperature and wind speed to be expressed as the still air temperature which would result in the same heat flow through bare skin (Santee & Gonzalez, 1988). Table 27.2 depicts the equivalent chill temperature for different wind speeds and air temperatures (Gonzalez, 1986).

Although widely reported, wind chill temperatures really only estimate the danger of cooling the exposed flesh of *sedentary* persons, and windproof clothing greatly reduces wind chill effects (Kaufman & Bothe, 1986; Santee & Gonzalez, 1988). Thus, the danger zones indicated in Table 27.2 probably apply to competitors in endurance sports only before the start of the event or during recovery, and events in which participants maintain high metabolic rates need not be cancelled due to wind chill alone. Safety surveillance of competitors should be increased when conditions reach the dangerous zones indicated in Table 27.2, because injured or fatigued athletes may be unable to sustain the high metabolic rates and high skin temperatures (T_{sk}) which would protect them from wind chill. In contrast to heat stress, wind chill effects pose a greater danger to non-exercising spectators and competition officials than to competitors.

With an air temperature of 5°C, heat loss in

Table 27.2 Cooling power of wind on exposed flesh expressed as an equivalent temperature under calm conditions. The actual thermometer reading (°C) and wind speed (m·s^{-1}) are used to calculate an equivalent chill temperature. From Gonzalez (1986).

Wind speed (m·s^{-1})	Actual thermometer reading (°C)												
	10	5	0	−5	−10	−15	−20	−25	−30	−35	−40	−45	−50
	Equivalent chill temperature (°C)												
Calm	10	5	0	−5	−10	−15	−20	−25	−30	−35	−40	−45	−50
2	9	4	−1	−6	−11	−16	−21	−26	−32	−37	−42	−47	−52
4	5	−1	−7	−13	−19	−25	−31	−37	−43	−49	−55	−61	−67
6	3	−4	−10	−17	−23	−30	−37	−43	−50	−56	−63	−69	−76
8	1	−6	−13	−20	−27	−34	−41	−48	−55	−62	−69	−76	−83
10	0	−8	−15	−22	−30	−37	−44	−51	−59	−66	−73	−81	−88
12	−2	−9	−17	−24	−32	−39	−47	−54	−62	−69	−77	−84	−92
14	−2	−10	−18	−25	−33	−41	−48	−56	−64	−72	−79	−87	−95
16	−3	−11	−19	−26	−34	−42	−50	−58	−65	−73	−81	−89	−97
18	−3	−11	−19	−27	−35	−43	−51	−59	−67	−75	−83	−90	−98
20*	−4	−12	−20	−28	−36	−44	−52	−60	−68	−76	−84	−91	−99

Little danger	Increasing danger	Great danger
In events of less than 5 h with dry skin; maximum danger from false sense of security (WCI < 1400)	Danger from freezing of exposed flesh within 1 min (WCI 1400–2000)	Flesh may freeze within 30 s (WCI > 2000)

* Wind speeds > 20 m·s^{-1} have little additional effect. WCI, wind chill index.

wet clothes may be double that under dry conditions (Kaufman & Bothe, 1986). Water has a much higher thermal capacity than air; therefore, heat conduction away from the skin is more rapid when clothing is wet than when it is dry (Gonzalez, 1988). However, it can be estimated (Stolwijk & Hardy, 1977) that with an air temperature of 5°C and continuous rain, an individual capable of sustaining high intensity endurance exercise (600 W) would maintain T_c above 35°C for 7 h. In this situation, fatigue rather than body cooling would limit performance.

Cold water: During exercise at a given metabolic rate, skin heat conductance can be 70 times greater in water than in air at the same temperature (Gonzalez, 1988). Thus, marathon swimmers and triathletes can experience considerable body heat loss even in relatively mild water temperatures. However, there is con-

siderable variability between individuals in the water temperature below which heat loss cannot be balanced by the heat produced through exercise and shivering (Toner & McArdle, 1988). Whether or not an individual experiences a decline in T_c during exercise in water will be influenced by anthropomorphic factors, metabolic rate, sustained aerobic capacity and water temperature, all of which interact in a complex manner to determine thermal responses in water. Studies of survival time following accidental immersion and body cooling rates during experimental cold water immersion enable prediction of safe, marginally safe and lethal immersion durations as a function of water temperature. As shown in Fig. 27.3, such predictions have been based on resting or moderately active persons. The estimates are of times of death from hypothermia or drowning from an inability to maintain consciousness or sustain useful physical ac-

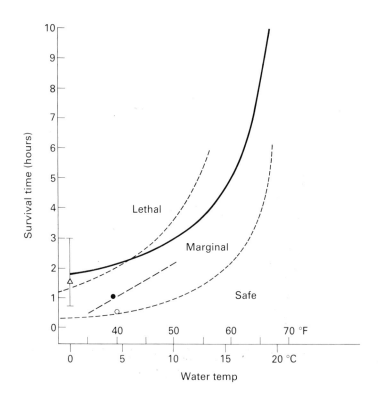

Fig. 27.3 Estimated survival time during immersion in water of varying temperature. From Toner & McArdle (1988).

tivity (Toner & McArdle, 1988). While these predictions may not be completely applicable to athletes exercising intensely, it seems prudent to limit endurance competitions so that expected immersion durations do not exceed the predicted safe zone for a given water temperature. Whenever water temperatures are colder than generally considered comfortable, competitors should be closely monitored during the start of an event, since sudden plunging into cold water can produce ventricular arrhythmias as well as gasping and hyperventilation; both of the latter could result in water aspiration and drowning (Hamlet, 1988).

Performance factors

Anthropomorphic factors: Body size and shape, as well as the amount and distribution of body fat, influence heat loss. Individuals with a small surface area relative to body mass and a thick layer of subcutaneous fat are best able to resist body cooling (Toner & McArdle, 1988; Young, 1990). Figure 27.4 shows how fat thickness influences critical temperature (the ambient temperature below which shivering ensues and the effects of peripheral vasoconstriction are degraded). Fat individuals tolerate low temperatures without shivering better than lean persons; however, the effect is more pronounced in cold water than in cold air (Toner & McArdle, 1988). Thus, on land, any thermoregulatory advantage of extra body fat and a low surface area to mass ratio would probably be overshadowed by the increased cardiovascular and biomechanical stress of carrying excess weight. In contrast, moderate amounts of subcutaneous fat provide both buoyancy and substantial insulation in cold water (Toner & McArdle, 1988). Long-distance swimmers with a body fat content of 9% or less may be at a distinct thermoregulatory disadvantage in cool water compared to those with 12% or more (Young, 1990).

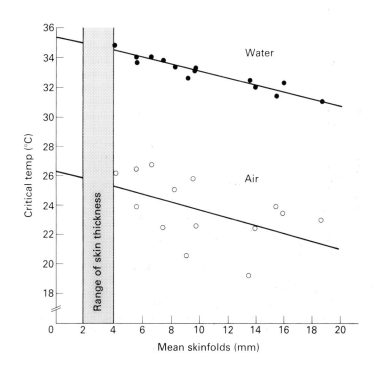

Fig. 27.4 Comparison of critical temperatures in water and air in relation to subcutaneous body fat. From Smith & Hanna (1975).

Aerobic fitness: High aerobic fitness may enable better maintenance of body temperatures in the cold. This might reflect a larger muscle mass available for shivering in fit individuals (Toner & McArdle, 1988), together with some insulation from the muscle bulk. The primary benefit of aerobic fitness during endurance competition in the cold is that it allows a higher sustained exercise intensity and a greater metabolic heat production.

Hydration level: As in the heat, athletes competing in cold environments should avoid fluid deficits greater than 2% body mass. Although sweating is less marked, ventilatory fluid losses during exercise in the cold can be more pronounced than in warm air. In addition, cold-induced diuresis contributes to body water loss (Toner & McArdle, 1988), and thermal inputs to thirst may be diminished (Sawka & Pandolf, 1990).

Clothing: There is a wide variety of clothing available to provide protection during exercise in both cold air and water. The biophysics of cold-weather athletic clothing has been considered in detail elsewhere (Gonzalez, 1987). Heat production during high-intensity exercise can be sufficient to prevent a fall in deep body temperature without the need for heavy clothing even when the air temperature is extremely low. However, the skin of the fingers, nose and ears may be susceptible to freezing injuries and should be protected when wind chill conditions are extreme. Athletes dressed for optimal performance during events may be inadequately protected from cold before starting, or when exercise ceases due to fatigue, injury or completion of the event.

Cold acclimatization: Humans develop physiological adaptations to chronic cold exposure. However, there is no evidence that cold acclimatization influences thermoregulatory responses during exercise (Young, 1990).

High terrestrial altitude

Assessment of the environment

Assessing high altitude stress is relatively simple. As altitude increases, the barometric pressure decreases, resulting in a reduction in the partial pressure of oxygen in inspired air. Although barometric pressure and inspired oxygen pressure are easily measured, this is normally unnecessary. Most endurance competitions take place at elevations below 3000 m, where variations in barometric pressure due to local weather patterns and gravitational effects have little physiological significance. Furthermore, investigators have usually reported altitude effects as a function of the elevation above sea level as obtained from a map.

Physiological effects of high altitude

Physiological responses to exercise at altitude are reviewed elsewhere (Chapter 43; Grover *et al.*, 1986; Young & Young, 1988; Young, 1990). The reduction in $\dot{V}o_{2\,max}$ is the principal factor influencing the endurance performance of athletes at high altitude. Figure 27.5 shows the decrement in $\dot{V}o_{2\,max}$ at high altitude. There is no measurable decrement below 1000 m and a small and variable decrement between 1000 and 2000 m, but above 2000 m the $\dot{V}o_{2\,max}$ decreases by about 10% for each additional 1000 m ascended (Grover *et al.*, 1986). The influence of the altitude-induced reduction in $\dot{V}o_{2\,max}$ on submaximal endurance exercise is illustrated in Fig. 27.6. Neglecting the effects of reduced air density (which may be significant for cyclists), running or cycling at a given velocity at high altitude elicits the same oxygen intake, but this represents a higher percentage of $\dot{V}o_{2\,max}$ at high altitude than at sea level. Therefore, muscle glycogen use and lactate accumulation will be accelerated (Young, 1990), the perception of exertion will be greater, and the endurance will be curtailed at altitude (Young & Young, 1988). Altitude acclimatization leads to an improvement in endurance,

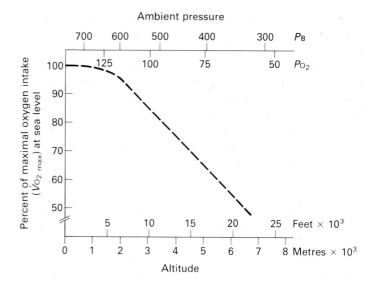

Fig. 27.5 Effects of reduced partial pressure of oxygen at high altitude on maximal oxygen intake ($\dot{V}_{O_2\,max}$) when expressed as a percentage of $\dot{V}_{O_2\,max}$ at sea level. Modified from Grover *et al.* (1986).

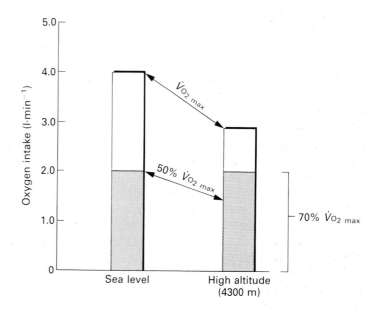

Fig. 27.6 Effects of high altitude on the relationship between a fixed absolute power output of cycle ergometer exercise, oxygen intake ($\dot{V}_{O_2}$) and the relative exercise intensity (%$\dot{V}_{O_2\,max}$). From Young & Young (1988). □, Steady-state $\dot{V}_{O_2}$ for cycle exercise at power output of 100 W.

but sea-level capacity is not restored (Young & Young, 1988).

Competitive strategies

Acclimatization: Endurance is impaired by the occurrence of high altitude illnesses in addition to the direct physiological effects of acute hypoxia. The illnesses, which are reviewed else-where (Malconian & Rock, 1988), not only impair endurance performance, but can also be life threatening. Rapid ascent and early intense exercise may increase susceptibility or exacerbate symptoms of high altitude illnesses, and young adult males may be at particular risk of high altitude pulmonary oedema (Malconian & Rock, 1988). The occurrence and severity of altitude illnesses diminish with acclimatization, especially when combined with staging (stops at intermediate altitude). Athletes ascending to high altitude should stop for 24 h upon reaching 2500 m, and a further 24-h stop should be allowed for every additional 600 m ascended (Malconian & Rock, 1988). Acute mountain sickness, the most common altitude illness at moderate elevations (< 5000 m), resolves in 3–7 days in most persons (Malconian & Rock, 1988). Cardiovascular adaptations are apparent after about 8 days at moderate altitude (Grover et al., 1986), but metabolic adaptations contributing to improved endurance may require up to 3 weeks of acclimatization (Young & Young, 1988; Young, 1990).

Training: Similarities between altitude acclimatization and physical training have led to the suggestion that altitude training is advantageous for sea-level competition. However, no scientific evidence supports this contention. Athletes will be unable to sustain the same intensity of exercise during training at altitude as at sea level. In addition, individuals who develop their racing pace at high altitude will find that pace too slow at sea level. Physical training at sea level does not lessen the decrement in $\dot{V}o_{2\,max}$ at altitude (Grover et al., 1986). For lowlanders competing at high altitude, the principal concern is how to maintain their fitness while acclimatizing. Increased emphasis on high intensity 'interval' type training may offset reductions in endurance training and allow muscle power to be maintained (Young & Young, 1988).

Air quality

In addition to the environmental extremes of heat, cold and high altitude, poor air quality or air pollution is another environmental stressor which can affect human endurance performance adversely (Pandolf, 1988; see also Chapter 44). Air pollutants have been categorized as primary or secondary. Primary pollutants include carbon monoxide, sulphur and nitrogen oxide, and primary particulates. Secondary

pollutants result from interactions of primary pollutants and include ozone, peroxyacetyl nitrate and certain aerosols.

Primary pollutants

Carbon monoxide does not appear to impair submaximal exercise performance; however, breathing carbon monoxide significantly reduces maximal exercise performance when the carboxyhaemoglobin exceeds 4.3%. The threshold level of sulphur dioxide that affects submaximal exercise performance is between 1.0 and 3.0 p.p.m.; however, no research has been reported concerning the effects of this pollutant upon maximal exercise performance. No research has been reported to evaluate maximal exercise performance after nitrogen dioxide exposure, but such exposure does not seem to affect submaximal exercise performance adversely. The physiological effects of primary particulate exposure have not been studied during exercise in humans.

Secondary pollutants

While ozone exposure does not appear to alter submaximal exercise performance at light to moderate exercise intensities, exposure to ozone during heavy exercise can limit performance, due primarily to severe respiratory discomfort and alterations in pulmonary function. Submaximal and maximal exercise performance are not altered dramatically during peroxyacetyl nitrate exposure. The sulphate aerosols, sulphuric acid and the nitrate aerosols produce minimal adverse effects during exercise.

Environmental stressor interactions

Human performance of submaximal or maximal exercise can be expected to suffer under the combined stressors of excessive heat, humidity and poor air quality. The interactive effects of breathing cold polluted air may increase the degree of exercise-induced bronchospasm and adversely affect exercise performance in susceptible individuals. The adverse effects of certain pollutants such as carbon monoxide may be enhanced at high altitude, due to a greater degree of hypoxaemia.

Air quality assessment

The rate and severity of air pollution episodes are known to be influenced by environmental and meteorological factors, as well as the time of day (Pandolf, 1988). Primary pollutants such as carbon monoxide and also the nitrogen oxides display daily peaks clearly associated with peak traffic conditions, and have their highest levels in midwinter. Secondary pollutants such as ozone have a distinctive pattern related to sunlight, with peak daily values in the afternoon and peak seasonal values in the summer or early autumn. In addition to sunlight, other meteorological factors known to influence air quality are wind speed and vertical temperature gradient.

Historical air pollution episodes have led to development of public guidelines to help assess potential health problems associated with poor air quality (Pandolf, 1988). In turn, certain nations such as the USA have developed national average air quality standards relative to many pollutants (such as carbon monoxide, ozone, sulphur dioxide and total suspended particulates). When poor air quality is expected, officials associated with athletic endurance events should contact sources analogous to the US Environmental Protection Agency for information about pending air quality to aid in decisions concerning the curtailment or delay of competition.

Disclaimer and distribution statements

The views, opinions and/or findings in this report are those of the authors, and should not be construed as an official Department of the Army position, policy or decision, unless so designated by other official documentation.

Approved for public release; distribution is unlimited.

References

American College of Sports Medicine (1987) The prevention of thermal injuries during distance running. *Med. Sci. Sports Exerc.* **19**, 529–533.

Amstrong, L.E., Costill, D.L. & Fink, W.J. (1985) Influence of diuretic-induced dehydration on competitive running performance. *Med. Sci. Sports Exerc.* **17**, 456–461.

Armstrong, L.E. & Pandolf, K.B. (1988) Physical training, cardiorespiratory physical fitness and exercise-heat tolerance. In: Pandolf, K.B., Sawka, M.N. & Gonzalez, R.R. (eds) *Human Performance Physiology and Environmental Medicine at Terrestrial Extremes,* pp. 199–226. Benchmark Press, Indianapolis.

Buskirk, E.R., Iampietro, P.F. & Bass, D.E. (1958) Work performance after dehydration: effects of physical conditioning and heat acclimation. *J. Appl. Physiol.* **12**, 189–194.

Caldwell, J.E., Ahonen, E. & Nousiainen, U. (1984) Differential effects of sauna-, diuretic-, and exercise-induced hypohydration. *J. Appl. Physiol.* **57**, 1018–1023.

Craig, F.N. & Cummings, E.G. (1966) Dehydration and muscular work. *J. Appl. Physiol.* **21**, 670–674.

Gonzalez, R.R. (1986) Work in the north: physiological aspects. *Arctic Med. Res.* **44**, 7–17.

Gonzalez, R.R. (1987) Biophysical and physiological integration of proper clothing for exercise. In: Pandolf, K.B. (ed.) *Exercise and Sport Sciences Reviews,* pp. 261–295. Macmillan, New York.

Gonzalez, R.R. (1988) Biophysics of heat transfer and clothing considerations. In: Pandolf, K.B., Sawka, M.N. & Gonzalez, R.R. (eds) *Human Performance Physiology and Environmental Medicine at Terrestrial Extremes,* pp. 45–95. Benchmark Press, Indianapolis.

Grover, R.F., Weil, J.V. & Reeves, J.T. (1986) Cardiovascular adaptation to exercise at high altitude. In: Pandolf, K.B. (ed.) *Exercise and Sport Sciences Reviews,* pp. 269–302. Macmillan, New York.

Hamlet, M.P. (1988) Human cold injuries. In: Pandolf, K.B., Sawka, M.N. & Gonzales, R.R. (eds) *Human Performance Physiology and Environmental Medicine at Terrestrial Extremes,* pp. 435–466. Benchmark Press, Indianapolis.

Herbert, W.G. & Ribisl, P.M. (1971) Effects of dehydration upon physical working capacity of wrestlers under competitive conditions. *Res. Quart.* **43**, 416–423.

Horvath, S.M. (1981) Exercise in a cold environment. In: Miller, D.I. (ed.) *Exercise and Sport Sciences Reviews,* pp. 221–263. Franklin Institute Press, Philadelphia.

Houston, M.E., Marrin, D.A., Green, H.J. & Thomson, J.A. (1981) The effect of rapid weight loss on physiological functions in wrestlers. *Physician Sportsmed.* **9**, 73–78.

Hubbard, R.W. & Armstrong, L.E. (1988) The heat illnesses: biochemical, ultrastructural and fluid-electrolyte considerations. In: Pandolf, K.B., Sawka, M.N. & Gonzalez, R.R. (eds) *Human Performance Physiology and Environmental Medicine at Terrestrial Extremes*, pp. 305–359. Benchmark Press, Indianapolis.

Kaufman, W.C. & Bothe, D.J. (1986) Wind chill reconsidered, Siple revisited. *Aviat. Space Environ. Med.* **57**, 23–26.

Malconian, M.K. & Rock, P.B. (1988) Medical problems related to altitude. In: Pandolf, K.B., Sawka, M.N. & Gonzalez, R.R. (eds) *Human Performance Physiology and Environmental Medicine at Terrestrial Extremes*, pp. 545–563. Benchmark Press, Indianapolis.

Pandolf, K.B. (1988) Air quality and human performance. In: Pandolf, K.B., Sawka, M.N. & Gonzalez, R.R. (eds) *Human Performance Physiology and Environmental Medicine at Terrestrial Extremes*, pp. 591–629. Benchmark Press, Indianapolis.

Saltin, B. (1964) Aerobic and anaerobic work capacity after dehydration. *J. Appl. Physiol.* **19**, 1114–1118.

Santee, W.R. & Gonzalez, R.R. (1988) Characteristics of the thermal environment. In: Pandolf, K.B., Sawka, M.N. & Gonzalez, R.R. (eds) *Human Performance Physiology and Environmental Medicine at Terrestrial Extremes*, pp. 1–43. Benchmark Press, Indianapolis.

Sawka, M.N. & Pandolf, K.B. (1990) Effects of body water loss on exercise performance and physiological functions. In: Gisolfi, C.V. & Lamb, D.R. (eds) *Perspectives in Exercise Science and Sports Medicine: Fluid Homeostasis During Exercise*, Vol. 3,

pp. 1–38. Benchmark Press, Indianapolis.

Smith, R.M. & Hanna, J.M. (1975) Skinfolds and resting heat loss in cold air and water: temperature equivalence. *J. Appl. Physiol.* **39**, 93–102.

Stolwijk, J.A.J. & Hardy, J.D. (1977) Control of body temperature. In: Lee, D.H.K., Falk, H.L., Murphy, S.D. & Geiger, S.R. (eds) *Handbook of Physiology, Section 9: Reactions to Environmental Agents*, pp. 45–68. American Physiological Society, Bethesda, Maryland.

Toner, M.N. & McArdle, W.D. (1988) Physiological adjustments of man to the cold. In: Pandolf, K.B., Sawka, M.N. & Gonzalez, R.R. (eds) *Human Performance Physiology and Environmental Medicine at Terrestrial Extremes*, pp. 361–399. Benchmark Press, Indianapolis.

Webster, S.F., Rutt, R.A. & Weltman, A. (1988) Effects of typical dehydration practices on performance. *Med. Sci. Sports Exerc.* **20**, S20 (abstract).

Wenger, C.B. (1988) Human heat acclimatization. In: Pandolf, K.B., Sawka, M.N. & Gonzalez, R.R. (eds) *Human Performance Physiology and Environmental Medicine at Terrestrial Extremes*, pp. 153–197. Benchmark Press, Indianapolis.

Young, A.J. (1990) Energy substrate utilization during exercise in extreme environments. In: Pandolf K.B. & Hollozsy, J.O. (eds) *Exercise and Sport Sciences Reviews*, pp. 66–117. Williams & Wilkins, Baltimore.

Young, A.J. & Young, P.M. (1988) Human acclimatization to high terrestrial altitude. In: Pandolf, K.B., Sawka, M.N. & Gonzalez, R.R. (eds) *Human Performance Physiology and Environmental Medicine at Terrestrial Extremes*, pp. 497–543. Benchmark Press, Indianapolis.

PART 4

PRINCIPLES OF
ENDURANCE PREPARATION

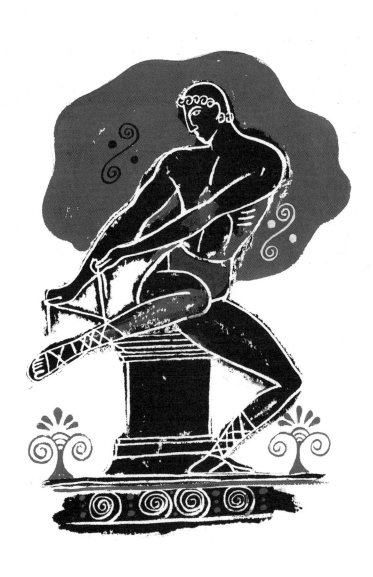

Chapter 28

Influences of Biological Age and Selection

PER-OLOF ÅSTRAND

Chronological versus biological age

Chronological age is a good reference point for the analysis of biological data, particularly in the case of children and teenagers. However, in physical activity programmes young people are nearly always teamed against each other by chronological age.

It is an inevitable evolutionary consequence that individuals within a species are different in many ways. Tanner has established the general framework of biological age (Tanner, 1989). The most reliable criterion for assessing biological age is skeletal or bone age. However, the method of establishing bone age is quite complicated: it needs special apparatus (X-ray) and is time consuming. More readily applicable methods are measurements of physical characteristics such as body height and mass at least twice a year, and observations on the development of secondary sex characteristics, such as breasts, pubic hair development and time of first menstruation in girls, and genital and pubic hair in boys. Figure 28.1 gives an example of the growth of height in one boy.

During the first years of life the child grows rapidly, followed by a slower growth rate for about a 10-year period. Then comes a second spurt, when the increase in height is, on average, about 8 cm per year for girls, and about 10 cm for boys (northern Europe and North America). A girl's first menstruation normally occurs shortly after this accelerated growth period, with a time lag of about 1 year. The

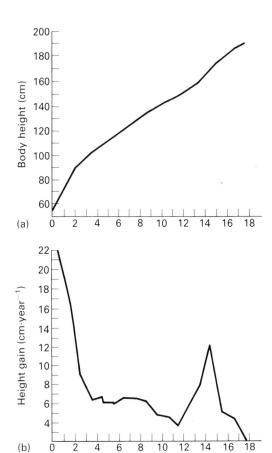

Fig. 28.1 The growth in height of a French boy recorded by his father De Montbeillard, 1759–1777. (a) shows the gradual gain during the 18-year period; (b) shows the height gain each year. Note the accelerated growth at about the age of 14–15 years ('peak height velocity'). From Tanner (1962), with permission.

285

development of the sex characteristics for both girls and boys is also related to this adolescent growth spurt, which is referred to as the age at peak height velocity (PHV−age). A peak body mass velocity is usually observed some months later. Results from a Swedish longitudinal study are presented in Fig. 28.2 (Lindgren, 1978). The PHV−age occurred as early as 9.5 years for one girl, but was delayed until the age of 15 years for another. In the boys' group, one had his adolescent growth spurt at the age of 11 years, another boy had his as late as 17 years. The PHV−age was, on average, at age 12 for girls and 2 years later for boys. At the age of about 13 years, the majority of the girls were already 'young women', while the boys were still children. In this study the PHV−ages varied around five chronological years within each gender and the total variation was at least seven chronological years (Fig. 28.2). The greatest

interindividual variation in biological age was between the chronological ages 12−14 years. Table 28.1 illustrates the quite dramatic interindividual difference in body size and maximal aerobic power in 13-year-old girls and boys.

The characterization of an individual on the basis of an age scale may be practical, but it is biologically unsound. However, an alternative basis for classification is not easy to find. At any rate, it is important to be aware of the problem. Because the adolescent growth spurt has a profound effect on physical performance, it is not only unfair, but may also possibly be harmful, to group children athletically according to age. An individual who has developed early may be at the top of his or her class athletically for a period of time, causing the parents and coach to overestimate his or her athletic talent. In time, his or her classmates may catch up, only to show that the early success was not due to talent but was simply a matter of early maturation. For a relatively long period, the early maturer may achieve success and be held in high esteem by her or his peers. In contrast, the late maturer is left behind in relation to athletic success in events where body size is important. It may be traumatic to find one is a champion one minute but only an average athlete the next; the interest in sports may be lost.

As an individual ages, the genetic code may have more of an effect on the function of systems of key importance for physical performance than environment and lifestyle. However, a change in lifestyle can definitely modify the 'biological age', either upward or downward, at almost any chronological age.

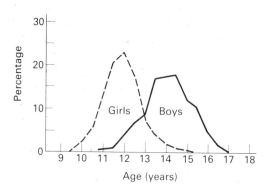

Fig. 28.2 Distribution of age at peak height velocity for girls ($n = 358$) and boys ($n = 373$). Modified from Lindgren (1978).

Table 28.1 Range of scores (R) in height, body mass and $\dot{V}o_{2\,max}$ for boys and girls aged 13 years in the Growth and Fitness Study in Sydney 1972−1973. From Russo *et al.* (1975).

	Range of scores at the age of 13 years	
Characteristic	Boys	Girls
Height (cm)	134−181 (R = 47)	141−170 (R = 29)
Body mass (kg)	29−84 (R = 55)	28−79 (R = 51)
$\dot{V}o_{2\,max}$ (ml·kg^{-1}·min^{-1})	31−77 (R = 46)	18−74 (R = 56)

Early specialization in sports

The early maturer who eventually becomes a 'retired athlete' might have specialized in one or two events but had real talent for another event which she or he never tried. There are anecdotal reports of intense, successful coaching in high jumping or basketball with prepubertal girls and boys. If height gain after PHV−age stops at 160 and 170 cm respectively, then the wrong sports were chosen. Again, perhaps these individuals had talents for sports where body height was not a basic prerequisite for success. Therefore, children and teenagers should be stimulated to be physically active and to try many different sports − a 'smörgåsbord'. It is a special challenge for parents, teachers, coaches and administrators to promote activities that maintain the late maturer's interest and adherence.

In a study of Swedish élite tennis players it was reported that five male players who were very highly placed in the international ranking list had participated in all-round sports activities up to the age of about 14 years. They then discovered that they were most successful in tennis, and so specialized 100% in tennis. Another five players, who were as good or even better according to prize lists at the age of 10−11 years, specialized much earlier, at about the age of 11 years. Apparently they were early maturers, but they did not have enough talent for tennis to reach the world's élite standard.

Training can improve muscular strength, aerobic and anaerobic power in children (Zanner et al., 1989). However, athletic training should be under the guidance and supervision of experienced coaches. Parents, teachers and coaches must have a good knowledge of the distinction between chronological and biological age.

Maffulli (1990) points out that 'during the growth spurt a dissociation between bone matrix formation and bone mineralisation occurs, thus leaving the child with the risks of chronic moderate-to-high overloading, sudden great overload, and diminished bone strength'.

Also, epiphyseal plate ('growth plate') injuries can have disastrous consequences. An early specialization with frequent, repetitive, monotonous activities may induce overload on the young athlete's musculoskeletal system. (Certainly the adult athlete also takes risks; see Chapter 35.) Endurance running is a typical stress factor, and each step can contribute to a cumulative microtrauma. The marathon should be prohibited for children and young teenagers. In Sweden the minimum age for participation is 17 years, which is quite logical because, according to Fig. 28.2, all individuals have by then passed their PHV−age.

Talent identification and development

At the 1988 Seoul Olympic Scientific Congress two sessions were devoted to this theme. No doubt it is the ambition of sports associations and coaches to find young presumptive champions and keep them in a 'nursery' with efficient training facilities. In my opinion that is a doubtful strategy. As pointed out, children and teenagers should be stimulated and helped to try a wide variety of sports. Sports for young people should not be too serious: they should be fun and games. During growth it is hard to decide who will develop the best physical structure for a particular sport discipline. At one stage it was believed that muscle biopsy might reveal whether a person had a fibre type that was optimal for a specific sport activity. However, with the exception of long-distance runners and skiers, top athletes in other sports, e.g. players in ball games, exhibit a wide variety of fibre types. Success in a sport is highly genotype dependent. The person who wants to become a champion must be very careful when selecting her or his parents! Figure 28.3 gives an example of two sedentary males who started an intensive training programme comparable to those of top athletes. They made impressive progress, with an increase in maximal oxygen intake from 40−45 ml·kg^{-1}·min^{-1} to about 60 ml·kg^{-1}·min^{-1}, but that was the definite ceiling: it is far from the 80 ml·kg^{-1}·min that

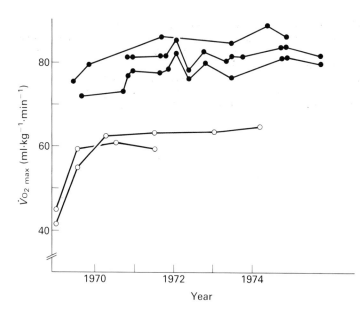

Fig. 28.3 Maximal oxygen intake in three internationally successful cross-country skiers (●) and in two 'normal' subjects (○) who started an intensive physical training of aerobic power in 1969. (Courtesy of U. Bergh & B. Ekblom.)

Table 28.2 Number of medals won by the East German national swimming team in the European Championship (EC) and the World Championship (WC) out of the total possible to win.

	Women		Men	
	Gold	Silver	Gold	Silver
EC in Rome 1983	15/15	12/12	1/15	6/15
EC in Sofia 1985	14/15	10/12	2/15	6/15
WC in Madrid 1986	13/16	8/13	1/16	4/15

characterizes élite cross-country skiers and middle-distance runners. Bouchard *et al.* (1988) reported that 77% of the variance in maximal aerobic power training response seemed to be genotype dependent. The subjects were monozygotic twins. About 5% of a sedentary population improved less than 5% with a given training programme. Another 5% of the population improved the maximal aerobic power by 60% or more. The authors pointed out that at present there are no genetic markers that can be used to type an individual for sensitivity to training.

At the Seoul Congress there was a discussion of East German successes in talent identifi-cation and development. East German female swimmers have been extremely successful in European and World Championships (Table 28.2). However, the male swimmers have definitely not been so outstanding. Apparently the problem in other countries has been to identify, develop and stimulate women with a talent for swimming.

References

Bouchard, C., Boulay, M.R., Simoneau, J.-A., Lortie, G. & Pérusse, L. (1988) Heredity and trainability of aerobic and anaerobic performances. *Sports Med.* **5**, 69–73.

Lindgren, G. (1978) Growth of schoolchildren with early, average and late ages of peak height velocity. *Ann. Hum. Biol.* **5**, 253–267.

Maffulli, N. (1990) Intensive training in young athletes: the orthopaedic surgeon's viewpoint. *Sports Med.* **9**, 229–243.

Tanner, J.M. (1962) *Growth of Adolescence*, 2nd edn.

Blackwell Scientific Publications, Oxford.

Tanner, J.M. (1989) *Foetus into Man. Physical Growth from Conception to Maturity*, 2nd edn. Castlemead Publications, Ware.

Zanner, C.W., Maksud, M.G. & Melichna, J. (1989) Physiological considerations in training young athletes. *Sports Med.* **8**, 15–31.

Chapter 29

Endurance Conditioning

JAN SVEDENHAG

Introduction

The increased interest during the past two decades in endurance training, and especially in long-distance running, has created unique opportunities for more thorough studies on the physiology of endurance conditioning and racing performance. This has led to a better understanding of the factors determining endurance capacity. However, some of the basic training principles and physiological changes associated with endurance conditioning have been known for half a century or more.

In this chapter, general training considerations and specific training factors are discussed. First, however, the basic physiological factors determining success in endurance events will be reviewed. Because most of the applied research carried out by the present author has dealt with male middle- and long-distance runners (of various abilities), and since running is one of the oldest and most widespread sports around the globe, the runner will form the basis of these discussions.

Physiological factors related to endurance performance and their interrelations

Maximal oxygen intake

Since the 1930s it has been known that the maximal oxygen intake ($\dot{V}o_{2\,max}$) is exceptionally high in élite endurance event athletes.

These high values are thought to be due to a combination of training effort and natural endowment. Early studies of élite runners (Robinson *et al.*, 1937; Åstrand, 1955) measured values of up to 81.5 ml·kg^{-1}·min^{-1} in champion athletes. This is comparable to the $\dot{V}o_{2\,max}$ observed in élite runners of today (highest value ever obtained by us in a runner, 87.7 ml·kg^{-1}·min^{-1}; mean for a 5000–10000 m group, 78.7 ml·kg^{-1}·min^{-1}). Thus, improvements in competitive results for middle and long distances seen over the last 50 years cannot be ascribed to a higher $\dot{V}o_{2\,max}$ of today's élite runners. Although evidently important, the maximal oxygen intake is only one of the factors that determines success in middle- and long-distance events. This is illustrated by the large variation in performance between marathon runners of equal $\dot{V}o_{2\,max}$ and vice versa (see Sjödin & Svedenhag, 1985).

Oxygen cost of movement

During the 1970s and 1980s, there has been growing interest in how best to utilize the maximal aerobic capacity in endurance events. During running, the submaximal oxygen intake is directly related to the running velocity. However, at a given running speed, the submaximal oxygen requirement (in ml·kg^{-1}·min^{-1}) may vary considerably between subjects (Costill *et al.*, 1973; Svedenhag & Sjödin, 1984). In contrast, differences may be small or non-existent when groups of élite runners from different distances are compared (Svedenhag & Sjödin, 1984). In élite distance runners with a relatively narrow range in $\dot{V}O_{2\,max}$, the running economy at different speeds has been found to be significantly correlated ($r = 0.79-0.83$) with performance in a 10-km race (Conley & Krahenbuhl, 1980). There is also a surprisingly wide (about 20%) variation in the oxygen cost of running at a given speed between marathon runners of similar performance capacities (Sjödin & Svedenhag, 1985). A low oxygen cost of running (i.e. good running economy) is truly beneficial. As was the case for $\dot{V}O_{2\,max}$, however, there is a relatively poor correlation between the oxygen cost of running and performance (e.g. $r = -0.55$ in a marathon with a large variation in performance; Sjödin & Svedenhag, 1985).

Because the oxygen cost of running has been thoroughly studied for only two decades, any long-term trend for élite runners cannot be assessed. However, except for obvious improvements in long-distance racing shoes, and in track and spikes, the improved results of the past 50 years (especially in long-distance running) are likely to be explained by improvements in running economy and/or in the ability to exercise at a high percentage of $\dot{V}O_{2\,max}$ for long periods of time (implying an increase of lactate threshold).

Total aerobic capacity

A given performance in an endurance event, such as running, can be attained in different ways. Two kinds of élite runners with different physiological characteristics can be distinguished. One category of runners is characterized by a high $\dot{V}O_{2\,max}$ but a relatively poor running economy. The second category, of runners has an excellent running economy, but a relatively low $\dot{V}O_{2\,max}$. In many cases the overall result of these differences is a fairly even performance level. Both the accomplished training and various natural abilities ought to explain these differences in the oxygen cost of running and in $\dot{V}O_{2\,max}$. Only the outstanding

runner has excellent values in both regards.

To help account for these individual differences in relation to performance, the fractional utilization of $\dot{V}O_{2\,max}$ when running at a specific speed (e.g. 15 km·h^{-1} or 20 km·h^{-1}) can be calculated. The %$\dot{V}O_{2\,max}$ value calculated in this way has been found to be significantly correlated with performance over various long distances. This value can be regarded as the total aerobic running capacity of the runner. For instance, in a heterogeneous group of runners marathon (Sjödin & Svedenhag, 1985), the relationship between fractional utilization of $\dot{V}O_{2\,max}$ at a submaximal speed of 15 km·h^{-1} and performance was as good as $r = -0.94$ ($n = 35$). This is because the %$\dot{V}O_{2\,max}$ value expresses the effects of $\dot{V}O_{2\,max}$ and of running economy, both of which may be separately related to performance.

In recent years, another way of expressing the combined effect of running economy and $\dot{V}O_{2\,max}$ has won some popularity; that is, to extrapolate the running economy line of an individual up to her or his $\dot{V}O_{2\,max}$ value and use the running velocity at which this occurs. Especially for middle-distance runners with high racing velocities, this may be the preferred mode of expression.

Depending on the treadmill test results, some training advice can be given. A runner with poor running economy should place emphasis on training to improve running economy (such as technique intervals with relatively long rest periods, hill training, general strength and stretching). On the other hand, a runner who needs an increase in $\dot{V}O_{2\,max}$ (and is judged to have the capacity to do it) may accordingly adjust her or his training programme (e.g. more 'fartlek' in a hilly terrain, long intense intervals and lactate threshold training).

Lactate threshold

The 'anaerobic threshold' concept is reviewed in earlier chapters of this book. This chapter has used the 4 mmol·l^{-1} blood lactate concentration as the highest steady-state level of lactate that can be sustained during running (expressed as the corresponding running velocity of each subject, $V_{La\,4}$). From a practical and experimental viewpoint I have found this $V_{La\,4}$ to be an excellent marker of training status and form. In several studies (e.g. Farrell *et al.*, 1979), a clear relationship between lactate threshold and performance in long distances has been shown. A correlation of $r = 0.97$ was found between $V_{La\,4}$ and competitive marathon speed (Sjödin & Svedenhag, 1985) (over marathon times ranging from 2 : 12 to 3 : 52 h). The lactate threshold is also the best single predictor in long-distance running, from 5 km to marathon distances.

High correlations are found between the lactate threshold and long-distance running speed because the lactate threshold is dependent on several variables which are all related to performance. The 4 mmol·l^{-1} lactate threshold (expressed as a velocity) is thus a function of $\dot{V}_{O_2\,max}$, the oxygen cost of running and $\%\dot{V}_{O_2\,max}$ at $V_{La\,4}$ (Fig. 29.1). An improvement in one of these factors (e.g. the oxygen cost of running), with the other factors unchanged, will result in an analogous improvement in the lactate threshold. However, an unbalanced training programme, which over-emphasizes one or a few training elements, may lead to opposite changes in these factors with, at best, an unchanged lactate threshold as the overall result.

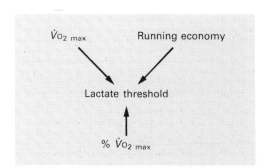

Fig. 29.1 Interrelationship between different physiological variables of importance for performance in middle- and especially long-distance running.

With physical endurance training, the lactate curve is known to be shifted to the right relative to $\dot{V}_{O_2\,max}$, resulting in lower lactate levels at the same $\%\dot{V}_{O_2\,max}$ and a higher $\%\dot{V}_{O_2\,max}$ at the lactate threshold (as $V_{La\,4}$). In our marathon study (Sjödin & Svedenhag, 1985), $\%\dot{V}_{O_2\,max}$ at $V_{La\,4}$ was similar (88%) in two sub 3-h groups but was slightly lower (85%) in the slow runners. However, this value was not significantly different between élite marathon runners and élite runners in the 400 m and 800-m events (88%, 84% and 83%, respectively) (Svedenhag & Sjödin, 1984). Furthermore, if trained long-distance runners have a slightly lower lactate threshold than untrained or less endurance-trained subjects (as suggested by Stegmann *et al.*, 1981), the $\%\dot{V}_{O_2\,max}$ value at the individual lactate thresholds could be completely equal in the above comparisons. In all, this may indicate that the rightward shift of the lactate threshold relative to $\dot{V}_{O_2\,max}$ may occur largely as an early response to training. The excessive amounts of training done by some endurance athletes thus appears to have little or no effect in shifting the lactate curve (as $\%\dot{V}_{O_2\,max}$) further to the right.

Training at the speed corresponding to the 'anaerobic threshold' is widely used as a means of improving performance in marathon running. As for the early rightward shift of the lactate curve, such a training effort would appear to be rather fruitless for a previously trained individual. An improvement in the anaeroic threshold velocity after threshold training in previously well-trained runners may be due mostly to effects on the running economy and the $\dot{V}_{O_2\,max}$ (Sjödin *et al.*, 1982; see below). Evidently, there may be an intricate interplay between training and the different physiological variables that determine running performance.

Endurance factor

Another aspect of performance is the question of the closeness to $\dot{V}_{O_2\,max}$ that can be attained during competition. Obviously, this value is dependent on the distance as well as on environmental factors. The $\%\dot{V}o_{2\,max}$ at the race pace ($\%\dot{V}o_{2\,Ma}\cdot\dot{V}o_{2\,max}^{-1}$, determined on the treadmill; Ma, marathon speed) has been found in the literature to range between 60% in slow to 86% in élite marathon runners. In our marathon study (Sjödin & Svedenhag, 1985), the $\%\dot{V}o_{2\,Ma}\cdot\dot{V}o_{2\,max}^{-1}$ was the same, on average 80%, in both élite runners (mean time 2:21) and good runners (2:37) but was significantly lower (71%) in the slow runners (3:24). Likewise, the percentage of lactate threshold velocity ($\%V_{La\,4}$) performed during a marathon was significantly lower in slow runners (85%) than in good or élite runners (92−93%). These findings suggest that the $\%\dot{V}o_{2\,max}$ that can be maintained during a marathon race differs with performance capacity. These differences would be even greater if the effect of wind resistance (proportional to the third power of velocity) was accounted for. In experienced runners who prepare for the event with adequate endurance training (such as our sub 3-h marathon runners) the $\%\dot{V}o_{2\,Ma}\cdot\dot{V}o_{2\,max}^{-1}$ may be similar. The lower $\%\dot{V}o_{2\,max}$ in the slowest runners may be due not only to a lack of adequate endurance training (with a lower capacity to metabolize fat and save glycogen) but also to the longer period of exertion and/or to inadequate running and racing experience.

General training considerations

Even though there may be several ways of reaching the goal, for each individual there ought to be an optimal training programme that provides the easiest, fastest and/or least hazardous way of achieving a given endurance performance. A complete adjustment of the training programme to the individual athlete is rather utopian. With a good training log, 'Fingerspitzgefühl', and recurrent physiological and medical tests, the athlete and the coach, together with their physiological/medical advisers, may be well on their way. To get even further, however, more knowledge regarding the normal responses to different types of training is needed.

The more you train, the less additive training effect can be expected. However, relatively little is known about the physiological changes that accompany the small but important improvements in performance in already well-trained athletes. For the completely untrained, the precise training elements do not seem so important; the subject will most certainly improve anyway. For example, several studies of previously untrained subjects have not found any difference in physiological effects or performance improvements between continuous and interval running training programmes (even though training intensity has been found to be positively related to $\dot{V}o_{2\,max}$ increases; Wenger & Bell, 1986). For the well trained, on the other hand, the composition and rate of progression of the different training elements (with quantity and quality clearly specified), together with the timing and lengths of the recovery periods, may be decisive.

Less training may be needed to preserve a raised physiological capacity or performance level than to attain it in the first place. This seems, however, to be applicable mostly to 'slow-responding' variables such as $\dot{V}o_{2\,max}$, while endurance or skeletal muscle mitochondrial capacity need almost continuous stimulation (i.e. training) to maintain the capacity.

Physiological effects of specific training

Effects on maximal oxygen intake

Ten well-trained élite runners (belonging to the Swedish national team) with judged capacity for improvement were followed with regular treadmill tests for a year (from January to January) (Svedenhag & Sjödin, 1985). Of these, five were middle-distance runners (mean age 21.2 years) and five were long-distance runners (22.6 years). From the competitive season before to the one following this test year, the average 1500-m time improved from 3:45.0 to 3:40.8 min, but the 800-m time was essentially unchanged (1:50) (middle-distance runners), and the 5000-m time improved from 14:11 to 13:43 min (long-distance runners).

The $\dot{V}O_{2\,max}$ (ml·kg^{-1}·min^{-1}) rose significantly from winter to the competitive summer season (from 74.2 to 77.4; +4.5%) (Fig. 29.2). In some part (+1.3%) this was due to a slightly lower body mass during the competitive season. By the following winter, the $\dot{V}O_{2\,max}$ was almost back to the starting level. The increase in $\dot{V}O_{2\,max}$ may seem small, but is probably of great importance in a race with runners of similar performance level. The increase in $\dot{V}O_{2\,max}$ from winter to summer is probably related to the increase in the number of weekly high-intensive workouts, which tripled between January to May and the competitive summer season for these runners (Svedenhag & Sjödin, 1985). The blood lactate concentration, measured 30 s after the $\dot{V}O_{2\,max}$ test, rose significantly during the same period. This relation-

ship between training intensity and $\dot{V}O_{2\,max}$ is compatible with the findings of Wenger and Bell (1986) (see above).

Effects on oxygen cost of running

In our study of 10 élite middle- and long-distance runners (Svedenhag & Sjödin, 1985), the oxygen costs of running at 15 and 20 km·h^{-1} were determined. The training response differed from that for $\dot{V}O_{2\,max}$. The oxygen cost of running (ml·kg^{-1}·min^{-1}) improved successively during the test year and was 3–4% lower at the last test than on the first test occasion (specified running velocities). For $\dot{V}O_2$ at 20 km·h^{-1} ($\dot{V}O_{2\,20}$), this improvement in oxygen cost of running was significant (Fig. 29.3). There was no change in body mass on a year-to-year basis. Furthermore, in a larger group of élite runners who were followed for 22 months, progressive and significant improvements in both $\dot{V}O_{2\,15}$ and $\dot{V}O_{2\,20}$ were found (Svedenhag & Sjödin, 1985). All runners had been familiarized with and tested on the treadmill at least once before commencing the study. Thus, our data suggest a slow but progressive improvement in running economy in élite runners. At the same time, the $\dot{V}O_{2\,max}$ was unchanged from year to year (comparisons for the same month). This indicates that it may take longer to improve running economy than it takes to reach an individual's maximum obtainable level of $\dot{V}O_{2\,max}$ (which in itself may take several years of hard rational training). This could at least partly explain improved performance levels seen in runners who already have been training for several years.

In a study on 11 marathon runners, the effect of hill training on different physiological characteristics was investigated (B. Sjödin & J. Svedenhag, unpublished observations). Besides their normal training routine, a programme of hill training with 'bounce' running in an almost 400-m long, firm and even uphill slope was added. The hill training was performed with periodically varying intensity over a 12-week period. After the training period

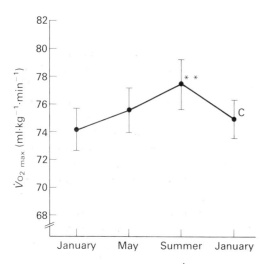

Fig. 29.2 Maximal oxygen intake ($\dot{V}O_{2\,max}$) of 10 élite runners on four occasions during the course of a year. Analysis of variance (ANOVA) with subsequent calculation of the least significant difference was applied. The symbol ** denotes a significant difference ($p<0.01$) from the first January value. The letter C denotes a significant difference ($p<0.05$) from the summer value. Values are means ± standard errors. From Svedenhag & Sjödin (1985), with permission.

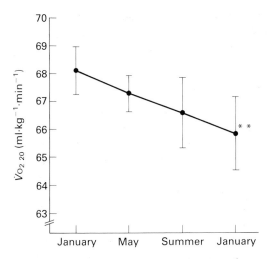

Fig. 29.3 Oxygen cost of running at 20 km·h^{-1} ($\dot{V}_{O_2\,20}$) of 10 élite runners tested on four occasions during the course of a year. Analysis of variance (ANOVA) with subsequent calculation of the least significant difference was applied. The symbol ** denotes a significant difference ($p<0.01$) from the first January value. Values are means ± standard errors. From Svedenhag & Sjödin (1985).

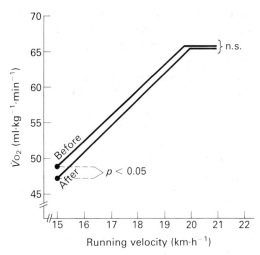

Fig. 29.4 Oxygen cost of running in 11 marathon runners before and after 12 weeks of additional hill training. At 15 km·h^{-1} there was a significant improvement in running economy ($p<0.05$). $\dot{V}_{O_2\,max}$ was unchanged. (B. Sjödin & J. Svedenhag, unpublished observations.)

the oxygen cost of running was significantly lowered (Fig. 29.4). This improvement was greatest at relatively low running velocities (3% at 15 km·h^{-1}). This effect may, theoretically, be related to development of the elastic components in the musculature engaged in running.

Effects on the lactate threshold

The effect of specific training on the lactate threshold was studied in a group of middle- and long-distance runners consisting of two 800-m and six 1500–5000-m runners. In addition to their normal training routine, the subjects ran a fast distance workout on a treadmill once a week, 20 min per workout, for 14 weeks. The speed was set at each individual's 4 mmol·l^{-1} lactate threshold. Blood lactate concentrations were controlled at each workout. As a result of this threshold training, the speed at lactate threshold ($V_{La\,4}$) increased signifi-

cantly (Sjödin *et al.*, 1982) (Fig. 29.5). Normal training before and after the lactate threshold training period did not affect the threshold velocity (Fig. 29.5). The runners who were closest to their individual lactate threshold (i.e. who showed the smallest accumulation of blood lactate during the fast distance training) showed the greatest improvements. The enhancement of the lactate threshold velocity was related to a decrease in the oxygen cost of running ($\dot{V}_{O_2\,15}$, from 50.6 to 49.2 ml·kg^{-1}·min^{-1}, $p<0.05$). For the 1500–5000-m runners the $\dot{V}_{O_2\,max}$ also increased significantly (from 68.7 to 71.0 ml·kg^{-1}·min^{-1}, $p<0.01$).

Lactate threshold training thus had a good overall effect on two of the factors that determine lactate threshold (see above). The fast distance training seems especially suitable for runners of 10000 m to marathon distances, while the threshold velocity in these cases is at or near the actual racing velocity, thereby simultaneously providing good (optimal?) training

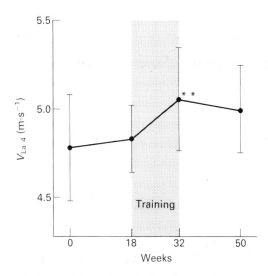

Fig. 29.5 The running velocity corresponding to a blood lactate concentration of 4 mmol·l^{-1} ($V_{La\ 4}$) in seven well-trained runners was measured twice before and twice after 14 weeks of additional '$V_{La\ 4}$' training. ** indicates a significant difference ($p < 0.01$) from the previously measured value. Values are means ± standard deviations. From Sjödin *et al.* (1982).

in running technique. For shorter distances, more planned running economy training is needed, and is indeed recommended (e.g. technique intervals at racing speed).

References

Åstrand, P.-O. (1955) New records in human power. *Nature* **176**, 922–923.

Conley, D.L. & Krahenbuhl, G.S. (1980) Running economy and distance running performance of highly trained athletes. *Med. Sci. Sports Exerc.* **12**, 357–360.

Costill, D.L., Thomason, H. & Roberts, E. (1973) Fractional utilization of the aerobic capacity during distance running. *Med. Sci. Sports* **5**, 248–252.

Farrell, P.A., Wilmore, J.H., Coyle, E.F., Billing, J.E. & Costill, D.L. (1979) Plasma lactate accumulation and distance running performance. *Med Sci. Sports* **11**, 338–344.

Robinson, S., Edwards, H.T. & Dill, D.B. (1937) New records in human power. *Science* **83**, 409–410.

Sjödin, B., Jacobs, I. & Svedenhag, J. (1982) Changes in onset of blood lactate accumulation (OBLA) and muscle enzymes after training at OBLA. *Eur. J. Appl. Physiol.* **49**, 45–57.

Sjödin, B. & Svedenhag, J. (1985) Applied physiology of marathon running. *Sports Med.* **2**, 83–99.

Stegmann, H., Kindermann, W. & Schnabel, A. (1981) Lactate kinetics and individual anaerobic threshold. *Int. J. Sports Med.* **2**, 160–165.

Svedenhag, J. & Sjödin, B. (1984) Maximal and submaximal oxygen uptakes and blood lactate levels in elite male middle- and long-distance runners. *Int. J. Sports Med.* **5**, 255–261.

Svedenhag, J. & Sjödin, B. (1985) Physiological characteristics of elite male runners in and off-season. *Can. J. Appl. Sport Sci.* **10**, 127–133.

Wenger, H.A. & Bell, G.J. (1986) The interactions of intensity, frequency and duration of exercise training in altering cardiorespiratory fitness. *Sports Med.* **3**, 346–356.

Chapter 30

Diet, Vitamins and Fluids: Intake Before and After Prolonged Exercise

BODIL NIELSEN

Introduction

The food we consume must ultimately assure an energy balance, and water must also be drunk to balance the losses. While lack of food can be tolerated for several weeks — due to the large energy stores in adipose tissue and tissue proteins — water deprivation leads to severe problems after only a few days. However, for optimal function, and especially before an endurance event, both the energy stores and the water compartments of the body must be filled. Further, it is necessary to supply the 'essential elements of nutrition', namely specific amino acids, minerals and vitamins, needed for building and maintaining the different cells in the body and their products. Deficiencies in these substances take longer to show up — several months — and can therefore be difficult to demonstrate.

Diet and energy balance

All cells in the body use energy for their general activity — the 'cost of living' at rest. To this basal metabolic rate (about $100\,kJ\cdot kg^{-1}$ body mass$\cdot day^{-1}$) is added the energy needed for 'activity'. This total energy demand should be balanced by the energy intake in the food. An excess energy intake is stored as fat, resulting in overweight and obesity, while in the case of a negative balance, the energy stores of the body will be used, resulting in weight loss;

in the long term, reduced performance capacity will occur.

The carbohydrates, fats and proteins in the diet supply practically all of the energy required by the body. From the energetic point of view, it makes no difference whether the energy is delivered by oxidation of 1 g protein (1 g yields about 17 kJ), 1 g carbohydrate (1 g yields about 17 kJ) or 0.44 g fat (1 g yields about 39 kJ). After digestion and absorption in the gastrointestinal canal, these dietary constituents appear in the blood in the form of hexoses (mostly glucose, maltose and fructose from carbohydrate), triacylglycerols (from fats) and amino acids (from protein). Most of the ingested food is oxidized in the cells. The rest is stored for the time being in the energy depots of the body. These include the *carbohydrate stores* of glycogen in the liver and in muscle tissue, and the much larger *fat stores* in adipose tissue (beneath the skin, around the organs of the abdomen, and also in the muscle tissues). After absorption, amino acids may be oxidized, split and rebuilt to protein in the liver (transaminated); converted to more specific proteins in the tissues; or converted and stored as either glycogen or fat (after deamination). There are no specific *protein stores*.

Energy for muscular activity

The fuel that is used during muscle activity depends on the intensity and duration of the work. A more detailed discussion is presented in Chapters 12 & 33. The direct energy source for muscle contractions is adenosine triphosphate (ATP). However, the stores of ATP can supply energy for only a few seconds of maximal exercise, which may require more than 200 kJ·min^{-1}. Phosphocreatine can restore ATP and supply energy for a few more seconds. But for physical activity of longer duration additional ATP energy must be supplied, either from glycogenolysis/glycolysis (anaerobic breakdown of glycogen/glucose) or by oxidative phosphorylation (aerobic energy liberation) of glycogen or free fatty acids (Table 30.1).

The energy stores of the body are the backup for the ATP supply during prolonged muscular activity, and their size will determine the possible duration of the activity. Thus, the task in preparation for endurance activity is to achieve an optimal build-up of stores (see Chapter 12) and during activity the successful endurance competitor protracts their degradation.

Exercise and substrates

The rate at which the energy stores are utilized depends on the individual's maximal aerobic power and, as indicated above, on the type, intensity and duration of the exercise. Before the circulation and oxygen delivery have been adjusted to the sudden increase in demand at the onset of exercise, the main fuel is glycogen, broken down anaerobically. In the 'steady state' of continued light exercise the energy is derived from a mixture of carbohydrate and fat, in nearly the same proportions as that used at rest immediately before exercise. At rest this is determined by the composition of diet and its proportions of fat and carbohydrate. Protein provides, at most, only 5–10% of the total energy requirement.

At exercise intensities higher than about 50–60% of $\dot{V}_{O_2 max}$, the relative importance of carbohydrate is increased. It seems that substrate utilization is determined by local conditions in the muscle, involving the oxygen availability.

During prolonged moderate exercise there is a gradual change in substrate utilization, from predominantly carbohydrate towards more and more fat. This change seems to be induced by the gradual depletion of the glycogen depots in the muscles and liver, and the consequent fall in blood glucose.

When the *muscle glycogen stores* have been depleted, the exercise can no longer be continued at the previous rate. In accordance with this finding, endurance time is proportional to the glycogen content of the muscles (Bergström

Table 30.1 Approximate energy stores of a 'normal' rested well-fed man (75 kg, 20 kg active muscles).

Substance	Concentration (mmol·kg^{-1})	Total amount (g)	Energy content (kJ)
High-energy phosphates			
Adenosine triphosphate (muscle)	5.5	Trace	5
Phosphocreatine (muscle)	17	Trace	15
Carbohydrate			
Glycogen (muscle)	80–>200	270–>400	4500–6500
Glycogen (liver)	300–500	80–100	1500–2500
Glucose (blood)	5	3.5	60
Fat			
Triacylglycerols (adipose tissue)	—	>7000	>275 000
Triacylglycerols (muscle)	10–15	50–80	2000–3000
Fatty acids (blood)	0.3–0.6	Trace	

et al., 1967). The ability to perform anaerobic exercise also decreases with the availability of glycogen, as reflected by the lowering of the peak blood lactate concentration after repeated bouts of exhausting exercise.

The smaller *glycogen store* in the *liver* (about 100 g) is especially important for the maintenance of an adequate blood glucose concentration. The central nervous system depends almost exclusively on blood glucose as its energy substrate. During prolonged exercise the exercising muscles extract increasing amounts of glucose from the blood as the muscle glycogen becomes depleted. This may cause a hypoglycaemia, which depresses the brain's function, with a feeling of general fatigue. A supply of glucose, for example taken as a drink in solution, will, within minutes, restore the blood-sugar concentration and so the ability to exercise (Fig. 30.1) (Christensen & Hansen, 1939).

The *fat stores* in the body are found mainly in subcutaneous tissue, the subcutis, and in the mesentery between the intestines. These stores amount to from 6% to more than 30% of body mass, a total of from 4 to over 15–20 kg, and they contain a high energy content per unit mass.

The contribution of fat (free fatty acids) to metabolism is important for exercise of longer duration. The rate of utilization of free fatty acids is controlled partly by their concentration in plasma. This is increased by mobilization of free fatty acids from adipose tissue as a result of exercise stimulation of the sympathetic system and by a gradual fall in blood glucose concentration during prolonged exercise. The capacity for fat oxidation in the muscles is increased following longlasting endurance training. However, oxidation of fat demands that a certain amount of carbohydrate oxidation takes place at the same time (free fatty acids combine with acetyl coenzyme A, an intermediate in carbohydrate breakdown, before they can enter the Krebs cycle). Therefore, when the carbohydrate stores are completely empty, the fat stores are available only to the extent that glucose can be provided by hepatic gluconeogenesis.

Although it has long been believed that proteins play no significant role as an energy source in exercise, it now appears that they can supply intermediates necessary to the Krebs cycle in situations where these have been depleted (e.g. oxaloacetic acid). Proteins may also contribute to the provision of glucose during prolonged exercise through gluconeogenesis in the liver using alanine formed in skeletal muscle. Finally amino acids themselves are oxidized during prolonged exercise. The contribution of amino acids to the substrate supply represents only a small percentage (5–10%) (Felig & Wahren, 1971; Rennie *et al.*, 1981).

Only during prolonged starvation are cellu-

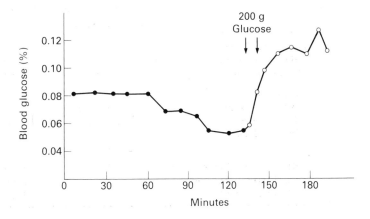

Fig. 30.1 Effect of prolonged exercise on blood glucose concentration after a fat diet. At 120 min the subject was unable to continue exercising, but 200 g glucose in solution (drunk in interval between arrows) restored the blood glucose and exercise performance. From Christensen & Hansen (1939).

lar proteins, for example from liver and muscle tissue, degraded on a larger scale to glucose (gluconeogenesis) and oxidized, thereby promoting the fat oxidation described above.

Food intake before exercise

The energy requirements of athletes are higher than those of 'ordinary active persons' (about $10-12$ MJ·day^{-1}). But for athletes in general all that is necessary is to eat a varied, well-balanced diet in sufficient amounts. With the increased food intake, the necessary proteins, vitamins and minerals will automatically be supplied.

However, in many sports the performance level is so high, and the training effort so intense, that the daily energy intake, more than double that of a normal person, can become a problem. Long-distance runners, cyclists and rowers have been recorded to have energy intakes of about 20 MJ.

Tour de France cyclists have been followed over several successive days (Poty et al., 1982; Brouns, 1988) and their average intake was found to be between 22 and 25 MJ. In some extreme conditions, for example the 'Wasa lopp', 86 km of cross-country skiing in Sweden, and bicycling in Norway from Trondheim to Oslo (the 'greatest endurance test', 560 km in one stretch), the performances require about 38 MJ and 55 MJ respectively (Costill & Kardel, 1980).

In such conditions, and also during the intense training the endurance athlete goes through before a competition, it can be difficult to eat enough, due to both lack of time and the reduced appetite associated with such strenuous exercise. It becomes a problem to eat sufficiently and to take in enough carbohydrate to refill the glycogen stores after daily training (Kirsch & Ameln, 1981; Kirwan et al., 1988). It is therefore important that the food offered is of high energy content. Further, the large volume that must be consumed should be spread over several meals in order to avoid discomfort from distension of the stomach. Supplementation with carbohydrate-rich drinks is recommended in addition to normal meals.

A diet which is 65–70% carbohydrate has been found beneficial for maintenance of muscle glycogen content in swimmers and rowers during periods of everyday training. This is much higher than the 40–45% carbohydrate intake found in the diet of the average person in Denmark (Kiens et al., 1990).

The recommended 'everyday diet' for an athlete does not differ much from that for everyone else: it should be varied, 'well balanced' and sufficient. In preparation for an endurance event, on the other hand, manipulation of the diet may be used to 'supercompensate' the glycogen stores in the muscles and in this way to secure an optimal build-up of reserves (Chapter 12).

On the day of the competition (in view of the discomfort of a full stomach during strenuous exercise), it is generally advised not to eat later than 2.5–3 h before an effort. Solid food has been found to remain in the gastrointestinal canal for 4–6 h after a meal, while a liquid meal may pass through the stomach and be completely absorbed 4 h after intake. Intake of liquid carbohydrate, rapidly absorbable mono- and di-hexoses, 1–2 h before competition would 'optimize' replenishment of the liver glycogen store up to the start. However, until recently this has been considered to be detrimental to performance, because (in subjects who fasted overnight) it produced a fall in blood glucose concentration at the onset of exercise (Bøje, 1940). Further, it could perhaps inhibit fat utilization and thus decrease endurance. However, several studies have now shown that in non-fasting persons, ingestion of carbohydrate-containing fluids during warming up some hours after a meal does not lower the blood glucose level during exercise.

Diet and restoration of food stores after exercise

Restoration of muscle glycogen stores after complete depletion takes more than 20 h. The rate of restoration depends on the diet (Ivy

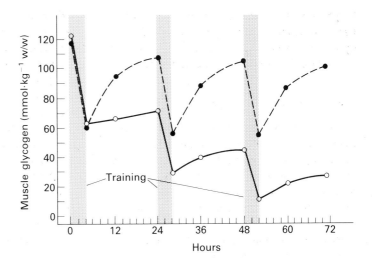

Fig. 30.2 Training of 2 h per day for 3 days on a 'normal' diet (40–60% carbohydrate) (○) or on a carbohydrate-rich diet (70% carbohydrate) (●). Only on the carbohydrate-rich diet were runners able to maintain muscle glycogen. From Costill & Miller (1980), with permission.

et al., 1988; Kirwan *et al.*, 1988): carbohydrate-rich diets result in a more effective replenishment than a mixed diet (see Fig. 30.2). Comparisons of glycogen resynthesis with glucose, fructose and sucrose feeding have been made. Glucose and sucrose appear to be similar, while a slower rate of resynthesis is seen with fructose. The muscle glycogen build-up also seems to be faster with mono- and di-hexoses and with easily digested and metabolized polysaccharides than with the larger starch molecules and the more slowly digested and absorbed polysaccharides found in beans, pasta, corn, etc. (Kiens *et al.*, 1990). The rate of glucose uptake in muscle is faster immediately after exercise as a result of a contraction-induced increase in insulin sensitivity (Bergström & Hultman, 1966; Richter *et al.*, 1989). It can therefore be recommended that sugar-containing fluids be drunk and that sweets be eaten in the restitution period immediately after exercise, when a fast muscle glycogen restoration is needed (Fig. 30.3).

On the other hand, fructose has been found to induce the largest glycogen restoration in the liver (Nilsson & Hultman, 1974; Conlee *et al.*, 1987).

Proteins and exercise

Although the daily recommended protein intake of 1 $g \cdot kg^{-1}$ body mass is easily met by a normal balanced diet, some studies have demonstrated a negative nitrogen balance in individuals who are training (Gontzea *et al.*, 1974; Brouns, 1988; Meredith *et al.*, 1989), especially in physically active athletes with a high energy intake. Thus a doubling of the recommended intake may assure nitrogen balance even in heavy-weight training athletes. At present more studies are needed to determine conclusively whether or not chronic physical training alters the daily requirements for protein and/or individual amino acids. However, it must also be borne in mind that protein-rich diets have been linked with cancer (Grobstein, 1982) and with renal problems, including glomerular sclerosis (Meyer *et al.*, 1983).

Vitamins

If something is good for you then more will be even better! That is the reasoning behind the widespread intake of vitamins, both in the general population and among performers of sport. Vitamins are a group of chemically un-

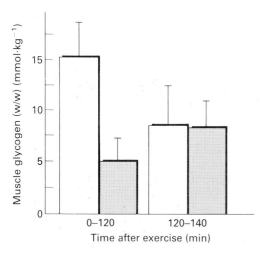

Fig. 30.3 Change in muscle glycogen content in exercised muscles after 2 and 4 h rest. The build-up was fastest when carbohydrate was taken immediately after exercise. Carbohydrate intake: □, immediately; ▨, after 2 h. From Ivy *et al.* (1988), with permission.

related substances that are essential in small amounts for the maintenance of normal metabolic functions. Because they cannot be synthesized within the body they must be obtained from exogenous sources (see Table 30.2). Vitamins can be divided into water-soluble and fat-soluble types. Water-soluble vitamins (vitamin C and the B group) cannot be stored in the body, and must be supplied constantly in the diet. If taken in excess they are excreted in the urine. The fat-soluble vitamins (A, D, E and K) are stored, primarily in the liver, but also in fat tissue. This means that they can be accumulated to levels that have toxic effects. Many of the B group vitamins serve as enzymes and coenzymes for fat and carbohydrate metabolism (e.g. B_1, B_2, B_6, pantothenic acid) while the full biochemical function of others (e.g. vitamins C, A and E) are still to be elucidated.

Vitamins and performance

There are indications that the capacity for physical performance deteriorates with vitamin deficiencies. The effects of deficiencies of water-soluble vitamins include poor coordination and muscular weakness. Diets poor in vitamin B_1 (thiamine) also induce symptoms of fatigue and leg pain during exercise. Few studies on deficiencies of the B complex vitamins (B_6, pantothenic acid, folic acid) and vitamin B_{12} have been made with respect to physical performance. No effects on physical performance were observed (Manore *et al.*, 1988). Of the fat-soluble vitamins only vitamin A has been studied in relation to performance. A period of 6 months on a deficient diet has no effect (van der Beek, 1985).

In well-nourished populations on a mixed diet, and even more in athletes with a large dietary intake, vitamin deficiencies are not likely to be a problem. However, many athletes, especially women, do not have a large energy intake and they may have a vitamin-deficient diet (Belko *et al.*, 1983; Guilland *et al.*, 1989). The question then is whether vitamin supplementation would improve performance, as many people believe. Recent well-controlled (double-blind) studies have not been able to demonstrate positive effects on performance by vitamin supplementation, from either the water- or the fat-soluble group. Excess intake of water-soluble vitamins may not be harmful, the excess simply being excreted in the urine, although large doses of vitamin C have been claimed to cause urinary stone formation and impaired copper absorption. Excessive intake of fat-soluble vitamins, on the other hand, is known to have toxic effects.

In conclusion, a vitamin pill per day may cause no harm, and may perhaps be beneficial for endurance athletes taking a very carbohydrate-rich diet including much refined sugar, which does not contain vitamins. But excessive intake of vitamins would at best be wasteful and may have harmful effects on health.

The demand for 'essential nutrients' has not been found to increase in proportion to energy output and physical performance. Therefore a diet of varied composition, covering the energy expenditure, will secure an adequate intake of

Table 30.2 Vitamins that are essential or probably essential to humans.

Group	Vitamin	Action	Source	Recommended daily intake
Water soluble	Thiamine (vitamin B_1)	Cofactor in pyruvic acid and α-ketoglutaric acid decarboxylation	Liver, unrefined cereal grains	1.5 mg ♂ 1.0 mg ♀
	Riboflavin (vitamin B_2)	Constituent of flavoproteins	Liver, milk	1.6 mg ♂ 1.3 mg ♀
	Niacin	Constituent of NAD^+, $NADP^+$	Yeast, lean meat, liver	18 mg ♂ 14 mg ♀
	Pyridoxine (vitamin B_6)	Coenzymes for certain decarboxylases and transaminases; converted in body into pyridoxal phosphate and pyridoxamine phosphate	Yeast, wheat, corn, liver	3 mg ♂ 2 mg ♀
	Pantothenic acid	Constituent of coenzyme A	Eggs, liver, yeast	4–7 mg
	Biotin	Catalyses carbon dioxide 'fixation' (in fatty acid synthesis, etc.)	Egg yolk, liver, tomatoes	160–200 µg
	Folates (folic acid) and related compounds	Coenzymes for 'one-carbon' transfer	Leafy green vegetables	400 µg
	Cyanocobalamin (vitamin B_{12})	Coenzyme in amino acid metabolism? Stimulates erythropoiesis	Liver, meat, eggs, milk	3 µg
	C (ascorbic acid)	Necessary for hydroxylation of lysine in collagen synthesis	Citrus fruits, leafy green vegetables	45 mg
Fat soluble	A (A_1, A_2)	Constituents of visual pigments; maintain epithelium	Yellow vegetables, fruit and liver	750 µg ♂ 500 µg ♀
	D group	Increases intestinal absorption of calcium and phosphate	Fish, liver	5 µg
	E group	Antioxidant, protects against oxidation of cell membrane	Milk, eggs, meat, leafy vegetables	10 mg ♂ 8 mg ♀
	K group	Catalyses synthesis of prothrombin and several other clotting factors in the liver	Leafy green vegetables	70–140 µg

these substances in most athletes, with the exception of those with excessively high energy requirements.

Fluid balance

In prolonged exercise, especially in hot environments, water and electrolytes are lost through sweating. Following sweat loss, the heart rate and body temperature increase to higher than normal levels. The ability to perform physical work is reduced and the tolerance to heat stress is reduced after a sweat loss inducing dehydration. A loss corresponding to only 1% of body mass has negative consequences (Adolph et al., 1947).

Sweat contains water and the same electrolytes as plasma and tissue fluids. However, due to the secretory processes in the sweat glands, the composition of sweat differs from that of plasma. The main electrolytes are Na^+ and Cl^-, but their concentrations in sweat are only about half of those in plasma (Table 30.3). This means that, while water and electrolytes are lost with sweating, electrolyte concentrations (osmolality) of the remaining body fluids are increased.

Both the volume change, through a reduced vascular filling, and the osmolality change have unfavourable effects on circulatory and thermoregulatory functions. The loss of volume results in a reduced filling of the vascular system and of the heart; the reduced stroke volume is compensated for by an increased heart rate for a given exercise intensity (Saltin, 1964).

The changed osmolality affects the sweating capacity. The sensitivity of the sweating mechanism to the stimulus of increased body temperature is decreased, so that the core temperature increases to a higher level than normal before sufficient sweat production occurs to achieve thermal equilibrium in a given environment (Nielsen, 1974).

The adverse effects of sweat loss can be reduced by fluid intake during exercise. A large number of studies have been conducted to find the ideal replacement fluid, which should supply water, electrolytes and energy (carbohydrate) (see review by Lamb & Brodowicz, 1986). One major obstacle is the speed with which the stomach can deliver the ingested drink to the intestine where the uptake (absorption) takes place. The rate of gastric emptying increases to a maximum at a gastric volume of about 600 ml and may decrease at higher volumes due to painful distension of the stomach (Costill & Saltin, 1974). This limits fluid absorption to about $1-1.2$ $l\cdot h^{-1}$, which can be considerably less than the rate of fluid loss in the sweat when exercise is performed in warm environmental conditions (Fig. 30.4).

The composition of the drink is also important. Fluids with high osmotic concentrations

Table 30.3 Electrolyte concentrations in blood plasma and in sweat. From Velar (1969).

Electrolytes and other constituents	Plasma concentration		Sweat concentration	
	mmol	$g\cdot l^{-1}$	mmol	$g\cdot l^{-1}$
Sodium	145	3.5	9-65	0.2-1.5
Potassium	4	0.15	4	0.15
Calcium	2.5	0.1	—	Small amount
Magnesium	1.5	0.04	—	Small amount
Chloride	103	3.5	6-43	0.2-1.5
Bicarbonate	24	1.5	—	Small amount
Proteins	2.5	70	—	0
Fats, glucose, small ions	—	15-20	—	Small amount

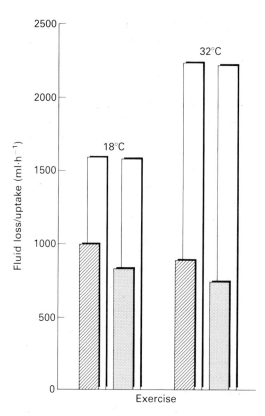

Fig. 30.4 Sweat loss compared with the maximal fluid uptake during running at 18°C and 32°C in seven élite marathon runners, running for 1 h at 95% of their marathon speed (80%$\dot{V}$O$_{2\,max}$). □, Sweat loss; ▨, water uptake; □ glucose polymer solution uptake. From Nielsen & Krog (1989).

Energy supplements in drinks

The reason for taking drinks with a higher osmolality than water is that carbohydrate intake during prolonged exercise is found to increase endurance and performance. In sports events lasting for less than 1−1.5 h, the available stored energy is generally ample to cover the expenditure. But for events of lasting 2 h or more, sugar solutions can supply energy and maintain the blood glucose level. For a measurable effect on muscle glycogen utilization, however, the rate of supply must be more than 40−60 g·h^{-1} (Hargreaves *et al.*, 1984).

In spite of the reduction in the rate of *fluid transfer* from the stomach with increasing concentration (osmolality) of glucose, the total *amount of glucose* passed on for uptake in the intestine increases with the concentration of the drink (Table 30.4).

In cold environments, cross-country skiers may ingest up to 1 litre of 30−40% flavoured sugar solutions in portions of 150−200 ml, providing up to 400 g glucose (50-km races). They do not have a large sweat loss and fluid requirement.

But problems arise during prolonged exercise in hot environments, where both fluid and carbohydrate are needed. Solutions of glucose polymers (chains of 10−20 glucose units) contain more energy per mole, due to the larger molecules, than an equal concentration of glucose. Recent studies have confirmed that glucose polymer solutions pass through the stomach more quickly than glucose solutions and, after being split to glucose, uptake in the intestine is rapid, while the rate of water absorption is reduced only slightly (Neufer *et al.*, 1986; Fig. 30.5). The rate of stomach emptying with an 8.8% glucose polymer solution (isosmotic) was not significantly reduced compared with water (Nielsen & Krog, 1989). With this solution the rate of glucose transfer to the gut was 85 and 65 g·h^{-1} in bicyclists exercising at 60%$\dot{V}$O$_{2\,max}$ and marathon runners at 80%$\dot{V}$O$_{2\,max}$, respectively. The first of these rates corresponds with the possible glucose uptake

are delayed in the stomach (Hunt & Pathak, 1960). This causes problems if 'energy substances', e.g. glucose, are added to the fluid. Fluids with more than 2.5% glucose (139 mmol·l^{-1}) have a lower rate of passage (Costill & Saltin, 1974) (Table 30.4).

Water is absorbed the quickest. The higher the osmolality, the slower the rate of emptying and the greater the secretion of fluid into the stomach and water transfer to the duodenum. By using hyperosmotic drinks the net gain of water is further delayed, because water is removed from the blood into the stomach and duodenum.

Table 30.4 Amount of fluid and glucose that passes through the stomach to the gut after 1 h when 200 ml solutions of various glucose concentrations are drunk every 12th minute.

	Glucose concentration (%)					
	0	2.5	5	10	20	40
Intake (ml)	1000	1000	1000	1000	1000	1000
Rate of emptying (ml·h^{-1})	1000	1000	800	600	350	200
Amount passed (g)	0	25	40	60	70	80

from a 40% glucose solution (see Table 30.4).

For the endurance athlete in warm environmental conditions ($> 30-35°C$), however, fluid balance is the most severe problem. It is therefore advisable to drink water (300 ml every 15 min) from the start of exercise. Intake of a 3–7% carbohydrate polymer solution towards the end of a $> 1-2.5$ h (marathon) performance, may help to maintain blood sugar, when the liver glycogen stores tend to be exhausted. In relation to the total energy cost of the run (about 10 MJ), the utilization of the exogenous (supplied) carbohydrate ($20-30$ g·h^{-1}) during a simulated marathon run as calculated from the respiratory exchange ratio, R was small (Nielsen & Krog, 1989). However, even with the maximal possible water intake, i.e. 300 ml every 15 min, a reduced performance due to dehydration must be expected in warm conditions.

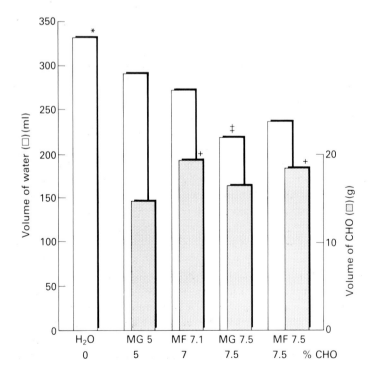

Fig. 30.5 Volume of water (□) and carbohydrate (▨) delivered from the stomach during 15 min of running after ingestion of 400 ml water or various carbohydrate solutions: MG 5, 3% maltin, 2% glucose; MF 7.1, 4.5% maltin, 2.6% fructose; MG 7.5, 5.5% maltin, 2% glucose; MF 7.5, 5.5% maltin, 2% fructose.
*, Significantly different from all other solutions; +, significantly different from MG 5;
‡, significantly different from H$_2$O, MG 5, MF 7.1. From Neufer et al. (1986), with permission.

Minerals in replacement fluids?

Even though electrolytes are lost in sweat, the water loss is relatively greater. Thus, in relation to the cell's environment, there is an excess of electrolytes after sweat loss. This means that the need to replace extracellular water is greater than the immediate need for electrolytes if there has been prolonged exercise with severe sweating.

Because it is difficult to replace the water loss, the addition of electrolytes such as sodium chloride tends to increase the body fluid osmolality and is thus harmful. After exercise the electrolytes have to be replaced; this is most readily and easily done by dietary intake, provided a sufficient amount of food and drink is consumed (a little extra salt may be added). In this way, with normal balanced feeding, the electrolyte loss is quickly restored.

Preparation in warm environments

If repeated training sessions involve high sweat losses, it is important that the fluid balance be maintained. A problem arises because the thirst sensation is inadequate: a 'voluntary dehydration' is apt to occur due to lack of thirst (Fig. 30.6). This is a particular problem in warm environments. Athletes must therefore be encouraged to drink more than they want, preferably in connection with meals, which should also normally supply sufficient sodium chloride to cover losses in sweat.

A reasonable way to control the fluid balance is for the athlete to check body weight every morning (at the same time and condition), trying to maintain a constant body mass. However, a change in body mass does not necessarily reflect the degree of dehydration. Water is chemically bound to glycogen and is liberated when glycogen is oxidized (about 3 $g \cdot g^{-1}$ glycogen). Changes in mass of up to about 1 kg may occur, depending on the glycogen content of the body. This water, together with the water liberated in the oxidative metabolism of carbohydrate and free fatty

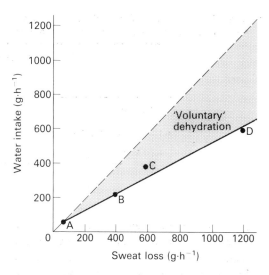

Fig. 30.6 Mean water intake vs. mean sweat loss during 4 h of resting or exercising in cool or hot conditions in four subjects initially in water balance. A, resting at 24°C; B, resting at 49°C; C, exercising at 24°C; D, exercising at 49°C. From Greenleaf & Sargent (1965), modified with permission.

acids, provides an 'internal water supply' to the body's water compartments during exercise. The body mass also shows changes from morning to morning due to biological variations in water content; for example in women up to $1-2$ kg water may by retained during the premenstrual phase of the menstrual cycle.

In preparation for competition in a warm environment, the athlete should fill the body water compartments by drinking about 1 litre of water (as milk or juice) in the evening before going to bed and a further $300-400$ ml before the warm-up. During the activity, $200-300$ ml should be consumed every 15 min, if possible, depending on the expected sweat loss (see Tables 30.5 & 30.6). Towards the end of the activity, glucose polymer solution ($4-8\%$) should be drunk instead of water.

The ability to perform in warm environments can be improved considerably by *acclimatization*. Repeated exposure to heat, preferably exercise in warm environments, improves the performance and endurance time. The main

Table 30.5 Predicted sweat loss per hour for runners of differing masses and running speeds at different temperatures.

Speed (km·h^{-1})	Body mass (kg)	Sweat loss in 1 h (ml)					
		10°C	15°C	20°C	25°C	30°C	35°C
15	50	610	610	750	895	1035	1085
15	60	770	770	930	1095	1260	1315
15	65	840	840	1015	1190	1365	1425
15	70	945	945	1120	1295	1470	1530
18	50	820	820	970	1120	1275	1330
18	60	1020	1020	1195	1370	1545	1605
18	65	1115	1115	1300	1485	1675	1740
18	70	1250	1250	1440	1625	1815	1880

Table 30.6 Recommended fluid intake: the maximal rate of passage of water and glucose from the stomach in cool and warm conditions is shown, with intake of water and 5% and 10% glucose solutions.

Drink	Maximal intake in cool environment*		Maximal intake in warm environment	
	Water (ml·h^{-1})	Glucose (g·h^{-1})	Water (ml·h^{-1})	Glucose (g·h^{-1})
Water	(4 × 300 ml) = 1200	0	(4 × 250 ml) = 1000	0
5% glucose	(4 × 250 ml) = 1000	50	(4 × 210 ml) = 840	40
10% glucose	(4 × 175 ml) = 700	70	(4 × 175 ml) = 700	70

Athletes are told to drink the fluid volume closest to the expected sweat loss (Table 30.5) with the highest possible glucose concentration. They should drink a portion of the chosen fluid every 15 min, but not more than the optimal quantity shown in Table 30.6.
* 'Cool environment' corresponds to a predicted sweat loss < 1200 ml·h^{-1} and exercise duration > 90 min (see Table 30.5).

changes are increased sweat production and a reduction in core temperature and heart rate for a given exercise intensity in a given set of environmental conditions (Eichna et al., 1950). These changes develop during 5–10 days of residence in the warm climate.

Inhabitants from a cool environment may benefit from artificial acclimatization, exercising in a climatic chamber or perhaps in a sauna, for about 1 h·day^{-1} for 8–10 days. In that way the athlete can become acclimatized to heat, while still being able to maintain a 'normal' training schedule in the familiar outdoor climate. It is a problem for athletes to train sufficiently before a competition when they also have to acclimatize by spending a prolonged time in a stressful environment before the event. This is true whether it is heat or high altitude they have to adjust to.

References

Adolph, E.F., Crown, A.H., Goddard, D.R. et al. (1947) Physiology of Man in the Desert. Interscience, New York.

Beek, van der E.J. (1985) Vitamins and endurance training. Food for running or faddish claims? Sports Med. 2, 175–197.

Belko, A.Z., Obarzanck E., Kalkwarf, H.J. et al. (1983) Effects of exercise on riboflavin requirements of young women. Am. J. Clin. Nutr. 37, 509–517.

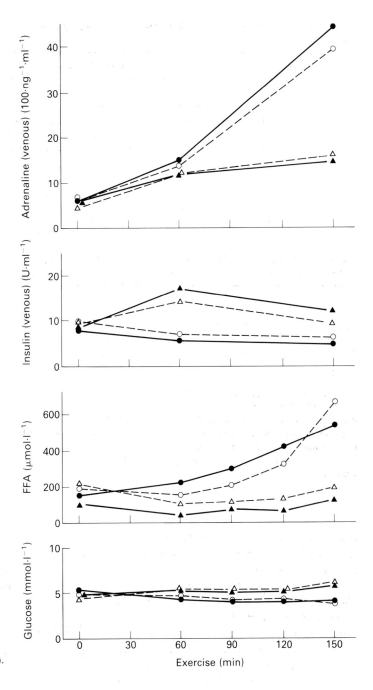

Fig. 30.7 Effect of intake of water and glucose polymer solution during 2.5 h of cycling. Blood glucose was maintained with glucose polymer, but decreased with water intake; free fatty acid (FFA) mobilization was produced by the increase in adrenaline. ●, Water at 18°C; ○, water at 32°C; ▲, glucose polymer solution at 18°C; △, glucose polymer solution at 32°C. From Nielsen & Krog (1989).

Bergström, J., Hermansen, L., Hultman, E. & Saltin, B. (1967) Diet, muscle glycogen and physical performance. *Acta Physiol. Scand.* **71**, 140–150.

Bergström, J. & Hultman, E. (1966) Muscle glycogen synthesis after exercise: an enhancing factor local-ized to the muscle cells in man. *Nature* **210**, 309–310.

Bøje, O. (1940) Arbeitshypoglykämie nach Gluco-seeingabe. *Scand. Archiv Physiol.* **83**, 308–312.

Brouns, F. (1988) *Food and fluid related aspects in highly trained athletes.* (Sportwetenschappelijke onderzoekingen, 15). De Vrieseborch, Haarlem, the Netherlands.

Christensen, E.H. & Hansen, O. (1939) Hypoglykämie, Arbeitsfähigkeit und Ermüdung. *Scand. Archiv Physiol.* **81**, 171−179.

Conlee, R.K., Lawler, R.M. & Ross, P.E. (1987) Effect of glucose or fructose feeding on glycogen repletion in muscle and liver after exercise or fasting. *Ann. Nutr. Metab.* **31**, 126−132.

Costill, D.L. & Kardel, K. (1980) *Energy for the long ride* (preliminary report). Muskelfysiologisk Institut, Oslo.

Costill, D.L. & Miller, J.M. (1980) Nutrition for endurance sport: carbohydrate and fluid balance. *Int. J. Sports Med.* **1**, 2−14.

Costill, D.L. & Saltin, B. (1974) Factors limiting gastric emptying during rest and exercise. *J. Appl. Physiol.* **37**, 679−683.

Eichna, L.W., Park, C.R., Nelson, N., Horwarth, S.M. & Palmes, E.D. (1950) Thermal regulation during acclimatization to hot dry environments. *Am. J. Physiol.* **163**, 585−597.

Felig, P. & Wahren, J. (1971) Amino acid metabolism in exercising man. *J. Clin. Invest.* **50**, 2703−2714.

Gontzea, I., Sutsescu, P. & Dimitrache, S. (1974) The influence of muscular activity on nitrogen balance and the need of man for proteins. *Nutr. Rev.* **10**, 35−43.

Greenleaf, J.E. & Sargent, F. II. (1965) Voluntary dehydration in man. *J. Appl. Physiol.* **20**, 719−724.

Grobstein, C. (1982) Protein. In: *Commission on Diet, Nutrition and Cancer*, pp. 106−122. National Research Council & National Academy Press, Washington, D.C.

Guilland, J.C., Penarando, T., Gallet, C., Boggio, V., Fuchs, F. & Klepping, J. (1989) Vitamin status of young athletes including the effects of supplementation. *Med. Sci. Sports Exerc.* **21**, 441−449.

Hargreaves, M., Costill, D.L., Coggang, A., Fink, W.J. & Nishibata, I. (1984) Effect of carbohydrate feedings on muscle glycogen utilization and exercise performance. *Med. Sci. Sports Exerc.* **16**, 219−222.

Hunt, J.N. & Pathak, J.D. (1960) The osmotic effects of some simple molecules and ions on gastric emptying. *J. Physiol. (Lond.)* **154**, 254−269.

Ivy, J.L., Katz, A.L., Cutler, C.L., Sherman, W.M. & Coyle, E.F. (1988) Muscle glycogen synthesis after exercise: effect of time of carbohydrate ingestion. *J. Appl. Physiol.* **64**, 1480−1485.

Kiens, B., Raben, A.B., Valeur, A-K. & Richter, E.A. (1990) Benefit of dietary simple carbohydrates on the early postexercise muscle glycogen repletion in male athletes. *Med. Sci Sports Exerc.* **22**, A524.

Kirsch, K.A. & Von Ameln, H. (1981) Feeding pattern of endurance athletes. *Eur. J. Appl. Physiol.* **47**, 197−208.

Kirwan, J.P., Costill, D.L., Mitchell, J.B. *et al.* (1988) Carbohydrate balance in competitive runners during successive days of intense training. *J. Appl. Physiol.* **65**, 2601−2606.

Lamb, D.R. & Brodowicz, G.R. (1986) Optimal use of fluids of varying formulations to minimize exercise-induced disturbances in homeostasis. *Sports Med.* **3**, 247−274.

Manore, M.M., Leklem, J.E. & Walter, M.C. (1988) Effect of carbohydrate and vitamin B_6 on fuel substrates during exercise in women. *Med. Sci. Sports Exerc.* **20**, 233−241.

Meredith, C.N., Zackin, M.J., Frontera, W.R. & Evans, W.J. (1989) Dietary protein requirements and body protein metabolism in endurance-trained men. *J. Appl. Physiol.* **66**, 2850−2856.

Meyer, T.W., Anderson, S. & Brenner, B.M. (1983) Dietary protein intake and progressive glomerular sclerosis: the role of capillary hypertension and hyperperfusion in the progression of renal disease. *Ann. Intern. Med.* **98**, 832−838.

Neufer, P.D., Costill, D.L., Fink, W.J., Kirwan, J.P., Fielding, R.A. & Flynn, M.G. (1986) Effects of exercise and carbohydrate composition on gastric emptying. *Med. Sci. Sports Exerc.* **18**, 658−662.

Nielsen, B. (1974) Effects of changes in plasma volume and osmolarity on thermoregulation during exercise. *Acta Physiol. Scand.* **90**, 725−730.

Nielsen, B. & Krog, P. (1989) Optimal fluid replacement during long lasting exercise in 18°C and 32°C ambient temperature. In: *International Congress of Physiological Science XXXI*, p. 5587. Helsinki (abstract).

Nilsson, L.H. & Hultman, E. (1974) Liver and muscle glycogen in man after glucose and fructose infusion. *Scand. J. Clin. Lab. Invest.* **33**, 5−10.

Poty, P., Olagnier, H., Metafiot, H., Denis, C. & Lacour, J.R. (1982) Courses cyclistes par étapes. Etude des problèmes alimentaires. *Médicine du Sport* **56**, 264−269.

Rennie, M.J., Edwards, R.H.T., Krywawyck, S. *et al.* (1981) Effect of exercise on protein turnover in man. *Clin. Sci.* **61**, 627−639.

Richter, E.A., Mikines, K.J., Galbo, H. & Kiens, B. (1989) Effect of exercise on insulin action in human skeletal muscle. *J. Appl. Physiol.* **66**, 876−885.

Saltin, B. (1964) Aerobic work capacity and circulation at exercise in man: with special reference to the effect of prolonged exercise and/or heat exposure. *Acta Physiol. Scand.* **62** (Suppl. 230), 1−52.

Velar, O. (1969) *Nutrient losses through sweating.* Thesis, University of Oslo.

Selected reading

Consolazio, C.F. (1983) Nutrition and performance.

Progr. Food Nutr. Sci. **7**, 1–187.

Costill, D.L. (1988) Carbohydrates for exercise: dietary demands for optimal performance. *Int. J. Sports Med.* **9**, 1–18.

Hickson, J.F. & Wolinsky, I. (1989) *Nutrition in exercise and sport.* CRC Press, Boca Raton, Florida.

Horton, E.S. & Terjung, R.L. (eds) (1988) *Exercise, Nutrition and Energy Metabolism.* Macmillan, New York.

Lemon, P.W.R. (1987) Protein and exercise: update 1987. *Med. Sci. Sports Exerc.* **19** (Suppl. 5), S179–S190.

Chapter 31

Psychology and Endurance Sports

LARS-ERIC UNESTÅHL

Introduction

This chapter identifies the mental factors behind peak performance in endurance sports and shows how they can be used in the training of mental skills and in the preparation for special events like sport competitions.

Mental training is defined as a systematic, long-term and developmental training of mental skills and attitudes. Mental preparation is defined as pretrained mental procedures, which are intended to become effective on certain predetermined occasions.

In order to discuss methods and techniques such as mental training in a more meaningful way, the goals and objectives have to be decided. Thus, a qualitative and quantitative evaluation of the proposed techniques can be made only in relation to specific and measurable objectives. As a basis for that, the definition of mental training is complemented as follows: mental training is the use of systematic, long-term and scientifically evaluated training in order to achieve peak performance and wellness.

Research background

The systematic training of mental skills in endurance sports is based on two areas of research:

1 Identification of the objectives and contents of mental training. What skills and attitudes are important for peak performance (identifi-cation and analysis of the ideal performance state).

2 Investigation of a state of consciousness appropriate for optimal change and growth.

Identifying peak performance

Peak performance or ideal performance in endurance sport (as well as other sports) was investigated during the early seventies:

1 Inter- and intraindividual variations in sport performance were examined and related to mental factors and preparation procedures.

2 Athletes were asked to describe their 'performance states' after good and bad performances.

3 The factors identified were varied in athletes with the help of posthypnotic suggestions, and the effect on performance was measured.

Mental skills for peak performance

Terms such as success and progress are more easily defined in sports, compared with life in general. Individual sports have a clear advantage compared with team sports. Thus, individual sports have been the most important area of investigation in order to find the relevant dimensions behind good performance. The Swedish national teams in track and field, shooting, swimming, judo, alpine and cross-country skiing were investigated and compared with athletes of a lower calibre (Uneståhl, 1979).

The four most important mental factors were:

1 *Self-image*: a combination of self-evaluation, self-confidence and self-esteem.

2 *Goal images*: images of the future, directing and energizing the present.

3 *Attitude*: reality testing and reality interpretation.

4 *Moods and feelings*: concentration, relaxation, arousal, satisfaction — the 'ideal performing feeling'.

Descriptions of the ideal performance state (IPS)

To investigate the IPS, athletes were interviewed after good and bad performances. Many of their comments point to the IPS as an alternative state of consciousness (ASC), like hypnosis. Some of the most typical similarities are described below (Unestähl, 1986a,b).

Amnesia: Athletes often seem to have selective or even sometimes total amnesia after perfect performance. This makes it difficult to describe the IPS. 'The only thing I remember from my olympic race is what I have seen on video afterwards. It was a perfect race. I was as in a trance.' 'For me it is a clear relation between the amount of memories from a race and the quality of the race. The better the race the less I remember afterwards.'

Concentration — dissociation: A more intensive attentiveness to a limited number of relevant stimuli (concentration) is accompanied by a general inattentiveness to all non-relevant stimuli (dissociation). Expressions such as 'another world', 'glass room', 'shell', 'tunnel' and 'trance' are common in the descriptions.

Pain detachment: A spontaneous increase of pain tolerance seems to occur in the IPS in much the same way as it does in hypnosis. The athletes do not experience the common feelings of exhaustion, pain and tiredness. 'I beat the record but I did not feel at all as tired as last time when the run was slower.' 'The

pain must have been there, but I didn't notice it this time.'

Perceptual changes: Trance-like perceptual changes such as time distortion (slow motion in fast sports), tunnel vision (decrease of peripheral vision in shooting), enlargement of objects (the golf-hole looks very big) have the purpose of performance enhancement. The most common change in endurance sport seems to be 'alteration of the relation objective—subjective time or a decreased dependence of the time dimension'.

Summary: Here is one athlete who nicely summarized his experience: 'I can't describe any details because now afterwards I see the whole race as a wonderful, natural and holistic experience, which cannot be divided and where words are an inappropriate means to describe this experience. The whole race went by itself, it was as if someone else was borrowing my body. I didn't have to think or worry about what to do, it came by itself. I watched what my body was doing and enjoyed it but at the same time I was as one with the body and the race. It was a trance-like state, which I naturally would like to experience in every race from now on.'

Lack of control: Most athletes seem to have little control over the IPS. 'Of course I would like to have it [IPS] every competition, but unfortunately it comes very seldom. And when it comes it often appears as a surprise. It can also disappear as suddenly as it came.' Thus, one goal for mental training and mental preparation is to increase control over the IPS.

Alternative states of consciousness

In order to increase athletes' control over the IPS, the dominant systems of control (DSC — voluntary effort) have to be replaced by 'alternative systems of control' (ASC-2). Very soon it became clear that these control systems had to be based on 'alternative states of consciousness' (ASC-1).

BACKGROUND RESEARCH

Below is a short summary of research findings from 46 research reports from Uppsala University, which have been summarized by Unestähl (1973; 1975).

1 Regular, systematic and long-term self-hypnotic training is superior to heterohypnosis in a variety of dimensions.

2 Audio-taped hypnotic inductions are as effective as inductions given by a present hypnotizer, measured on a standardized scale of hypnotic susceptibility (the Stanford scales).

3 Long-term imagery training gives a significant increase in imagery skills, measured by standardized scales for imagery vividness and control.

4 Long-term training in relaxation and imagery gives a significant increase in hypnotic skills, measured by the Stanford scales of hypnotic susceptibility.

5 Hypnotic alterations of bioelectric, cardiovascular, respiratory, vasomotor, gastro-intestinal, endocrine and metabolic functions are larger and more precise in comparison with non-hypnotic alterations, when the same techniques are used with or without hypnosis.

6 Hypnosis and self-hypnosis are often described as a state of increased concentration on a limited number of selected stimuli, accompanied by a dissociation from non-relevant stimuli.

7 Relaxation is a common, and sometimes the basic, element in hypnotic induction procedures. It is also a common feature of the hypnotic experience. In spite of this, relaxation is neither a necessary element in induction nor is it a necessary dimension of the hypnotic state.

8 Hypnotic susceptibility scores had a significant positive correlation with ideomotor skills, but a zero correlation with secondary suggestibility (gullibility).

9 A statement, common in textbooks, that the effects of posthypnotic suggestion could last for life turned out to be a false mixture of two things. Posthypnotic suggestion normally has a short duration (minutes or hours) but the signal-value (a trigger's capacity to release a certain effect) could last for years or (probably) throughout a lifetime.

10 Any simple or complex stimulus, for instance a word, movement, behaviour or situation, but also a thought or even a hallucination, can receive signal-value during hypnosis or self-hypnosis, after which it will serve as a trigger, releasing those posthypnotic effects that have been programmed in.

11 A trigger, signal-value or conditioning can be established in just one single hypnotic or self-hypnotic session.

12 Recognition thresholds for words are significantly lowered when the words have been given signal-value.

13 When a stimulus has become a trigger, it works even in those situations where the subject is unaware of the presence of the trigger. Such a trigger cannot be changed by voluntary effort.

14 A positive emotion, such as the ideal performance feeling, can be separated (borrowed) from a previous event and then conditioned to a future event (for instance a future competition)

15 Positive emotions, released by a pre-decided behaviour, are effective reinforcers of this behaviour.

Mental training: philosophy

1 The principles of peak performance and wellness can be explored, controlled and developed.
2 Mental skills can and should be looked at and treated in the same way as physical skills.
3 Human growth and development is directed by trainable factors in the human mind.
4 The sport-related growth model (SGM) starts with visions, missions and performance goals.
5 SGM uses history, accepts and enjoys the

present, and is oriented to and energized by the future.

6 SGM uses training as the main tool in order to proceed from knowledge to skills.

7 The ideal performing state, the ideal healing state and the ideal reality state are most easily reached, maintained and developed through a hypnotic-like state, where the reality testing is weakened.

Inner mental training

Inner mental training is divided into three phases, which are trained in the following order:

1 *Mental conditioning*: Learning muscular and mental relaxation and a special *state of mind*, an *alternative state of consciousness* (ASC), which provides a base for control and positive change.

2 *Mental technique training*: Learning alternative systems of self-control and self-directing techniques such as suggestion, autogenic formula or imagery techniques, all of which are more effective if combined with ASC.

3 *Mental strength training*: The mental skills described above are combined and applied to areas such as motivation, emotional reactions and mood states, attitudes, concentration, etc.

Mental conditioning

Experiments by Jansson (1990) have shown that the antagonistic muscles of élite athletes are more relaxed during competition than those of lower level athletes. This seems to occur independent of the type of sport, and the finding can also be generalized to other areas such as music (for example, violinists; Jansson, 1990).

In order to achieve *differential relaxation* (optimal tension in the appropriate muscles and relaxation in the antagonists) the athletes have to learn to start from a baseline of complete relaxation. The method is initially based upon directing the perception of the athletes to the differences in the experiences of tense and relaxed muscles. In the first week of training

the contraction–relaxation process is initiated by means of a prolonged contraction of the left fist in conjunction with an inspiration and a breath-hold for approximately 5 s, followed by expiration and relaxation. This accentuated form of tension building acts as a concrete physical 'trigger' which increases the induction speed of the relaxation process. An accelerated form of contraction–relaxation is progressively and differentially used with the other parts of the body. In that most athletes already have experience of these forms of building and releasing muscular tension, the normal learning process can be shortened.

Together with the perception of the differences between tension and relaxation due to muscular contraction, the athletes' attention is also directed to the state of relaxation that accompanies exhalation. This is later used as another trigger to induce the relaxation process.

The second week of training is also directed to physical relaxation, but in an abbreviated form. Using the inhalation and fist contraction as a trigger, the rest of the body is induced to relax simply by visualizing the body parts in a progressive order. The associated psychological states that accompany the warm, heavy sensations of physical relaxation, such as calmness, security, confidence, certitude and comfort, are introduced and reinforced.

In the third training programme (third week) the attention of the athletes is directed still more to the psychological effects of the relaxation by using suggestions and reassuring verbal cues in order to achieve a desired deep state of mental relaxation. Dissociative and 'deepening' techniques are used and the feeling of liberty, floating and gliding is introduced. A melting of barriers between mind–body and surroundings is noticed.

Mental training

The induced relaxation state is most profound when the concept of the 'inner mental room' is introduced. An enticing image of a warm, comfortable inner room is built up and shaped according to individual needs and desires. This sheltered spot provides the athletes with an inner place where the rest of the mental training can be carried out.

The mental room is intended to serve as a rest and recovery place, where meditative techniques are learned in order to achieve a state of deep relaxation and rest. An open fire serves as a trigger for new energy. However, the 'room' is also an 'inner working place' where skill learning and mental preparation for special events (like competition) can occur. For that reason the mental room is equipped with a screen and a blackboard, to be used later for mental rehearsal and self-suggestion.

Further training occurs over 3 weeks, during which the state of mental relaxation is attained with increased speed and depth of effect.

Parts of the fifth and sixth weeks are devoted to dissociation and detachment training. Mental relaxation is attempted in unprotected environments in which distractions can occur. Basic mental training may be carried out in noisy situations or in uncomfortable body positions. Athletes are taught techniques that allow them mentally to detach or isolate themselves, for instance by setting up thick mental walls that prevent the distractions from entering their mental room. Or they are taught to allow the entry of all stimuli, but to treat the irrelevant or disturbing stimuli passively by means of emotional dissociation.

By the end of this period, the athlete should be able to exhibit physical and mental self-control in most environments through physical and mental relaxation. It should again be emphasized that this training process is long term in nature and must be given sufficient time to be mastered. The basic mental training not only provides the necessary base and preparation for the next steps in the training, but also has considerable value in itself as a means of self-control. These learned skills, when practised five times a week for 6 weeks, provide useful means for athletes to deal with the chronic pressures of training, travel or extended competitions. Sleep facilitation, energy conservation and recovery from competitions are some goals for learning these basic coping skills. Basic mental training also becomes a healthy substitute for other common, but harmful, coping techniques such as drinking, eating, smoking and use of drugs.

CONCENTRATION TRAINING

Concentration is a passive process that can be seen as an optimization of the ratio between signal and noise. Concentration training requires an increased focusing of the athletes' attention upon the relevant performance cues as well as an increased dissociation from distracting cues. Attentiveness can vary in intensity. It can be directed towards something external or internal and the attention area can be broad or narrow (Nideffer & Sharpe, 1978). A state of deep relaxation results in a narrowing of attention as well as a shift from an external to an internal focus (Nideffer, 1981). These changes in attentional breadth and focus are useful for sports like running, since the task demands are relatively straightforward.

In many closed-skill sports, the desired type of concentration is characterized by intense attentiveness to a narrow attention area. This type of concentration, however, has a rather limited duration. In sports such as golf, where the ratio between performance time and competition time is very small, the limited duration of intense concentration can be solved through a 'trigger concentration'. In sports where this ratio = 1, variations are directed more to the contents and targets of attention.

Triggers

The athletes select two cues, which are to serve as triggers. The first one should be a part of their normal preparation for a race, such as the call to the start or preselected cues along the track. The second trigger is based on a special movement, position, word or image, which is not normally a part of their prestart or competitive routines.

In the inner mental room, a conditioning is shaped between the selected cues and the athlete's former experience of optimal concentration, in order to turn the cues into two triggers, which can release this concentration in future competitions. The first trigger will act automatically because it is part of the 'normal' procedure, while the second trigger is a kind of safety mechanism, to be used only if needed.

Meditation

Prolonged passive concentration is learned through demystified meditative techniques, which include taking sounds and objects as well as bodily processes as the focus of attention.

Emotional detachment

The athletes are asked to carry out the training in 'unprotected' environments, in which various distractions occur. These can include loud sounds, other people watching, or uncomfortable body positions. The athletes are then introduced to various techniques that allow them to decrease the 'noise-value' by mental detachment, passive observation or re-interpretation. This increase of the noise-tolerance level can serve as an effective way of coping with negative stress and disturbances in and outside sport.

MOTIVATION

Motivation directs and energizes behaviour. It creates persistence and single mindness. However, the goals have to be selected with great care in order to provide these effects. The athletes are taken through a 6-week motivational process where appropriate visions and long-term and short-term goals are selected, after which they are programmed into the mind. Of the important rules for appropriate goal-setting, two examples can be mentioned:

1 *Self-decided, self-controlled, concrete, specific and measurable goals.* Competition is defined as a fight between me and goals which I decide and which I control. Thus, the goal of winning has to be transferred to objectives like specific times. When a runner or swimmer approaches a competition with time-related goals, they feel certain because they:

(a) know what they intend to do;

(b) know that they are able to do it;

(c) do not worry about other competitors;

(d) are not negatively influenced by the type of competition.

Goals of this type also make it possible to follow individual improvements in a much better way.

2 *Optimal goal-probability.* The perceived probability of reaching a certain goal can vary from zero (very high task-difficulty) to one (low task-difficulty). Too low or too high a probability results in a poor performance. For many athletes maximum performance is related to a probability level of 40–60%. The relation between performance and goal-probability consists of a compromise between two relations — between performance and task-difficulty and between performance and believability. Athletes must be certain that they have the potential of reaching their selected goals. Here are some examples of practices that increase the believability in bold goals, which in turn give access to a higher performance level:

(a) Athletes can make a progression (in their mental room) 20 years into the future and experience the results that athletes will accomplish at that time. This mental imagery will adjust and accustom the mind to such results. This will make their own long-term goals bolder and more believable.

(b) Another progression, 3–5 years ahead, involves looking at the athlete's own results at that time, based on the rate of improvement they have had in the past. The athlete then asks whether it is necessary to wait for 3–5 years in order to achieve those results.

(c) General self-image training will also affect the question of how high goals can be and still be realistic. An increase in confidence and self-esteem will reduce impeding and blocking self-images and increase the awareness and belief in the athlete's own resources.

(d) An alternative state of consciousness (inner mental room) will reduce the 'reality testing' and make every goal-image, even very bold ones, more realistic.

Examples of goals in endurance sports

During the 1970s, it became more and more popular among top Swedish athletes to replace goals of winning, because winning was difficult or impossible to prepare for. Diffuse and abstract goals such as winning were changed to more specific and controllable goals. This was easier in individual sports like track and field and swimming than in soccer and other team sports.

It was important to have specific and measurable outcome goals which could then be translated to process goals. These pictures of the process (performance) were then programmed in during a deep relaxed state (goal-images).

In running, the most natural outcome goal became final time (for some athletes, final and intermediate times). With such a goal it was possible to start the mental preparation for important competitions months or even years in advance.

Time goals also made it easier to measure personal development and to give a winning feeling to every athlete (winning = achieving personal goals). In the translation of time goals to process goals, feelings played an important role. Some athletes worked with the ideal performing feeling as the only goal, and did not have to include any outcome goal in their preparation.

Goal-images

All positive changes (personal growth) are based on an awareness of the goal and the starting point. 'Where am I today? Where do I want to go?' However, these more 'intellectual' goals have to be translated into concrete images. Outcome goals must be transfered to process goals. What does a race with this final time look like?

Thus, it is important for all improvement to bring together two self-images. The first one is an image of the present situation, my present level of sport. The second one is an image about my future sport. 'What are the differences in my sport 1 year from now compared with the sport today?'

Goal programming

When the athletes have selected their short- and long-term goals for their sport career, these selected goals have to be integrated by means of a deep mental state. In a 'self-hypnotic' state, where the 'reality testing' is absent or reduced, the concrete and situation-related goal-images are programmed in and integrated. These future images or developmental pictures serve as directing mechanisms behind 'automaticity' in life, but also give the necessary energy for the hard training on the way to the goals.

Attitude training

'Self-fulfilling prophecies' work independently, whether the prophecy is positive or negative. The differences between good and poor athletes are not in the number of self-images and goals, but in the quality and content of images. The fear of failure has a stronger impact on 'problem athletes'.

Some athletes will clarify that they are aware about the importance of positive thinking, but will at the same time complain about lack of control. 'Of course I like to have positive and developmental thoughts and images, but as soon as I don't think of my thoughts, negative thoughts appear.' One important reason for this has been shown to be the emotional component of a certain thought or image. The stronger the feeling, the more the thought catches the mind. Because fear is a strong emotion, the fear of failure will direct thoughts towards failure. Mental training handles that question by teaching the athletes how they can get rid of fear. The five main mental training methods for achieving this are:

1 *Systematic desensitization*: a conditioning procedure in which the athletes in their mind (in the mental room) connect previous fearful situations with feelings of calmness and safety.

2 *Analysis of the real consequences of different outcomes*.

3 *Cognitive restructuring*: the selective perception, the 'frame of reference' is reprogrammed in a four-step process:

    (a) Awareness about previous ways of 'interpreting reality.'

    (b) Identification, analysis and selection of alternative interpretation principles: 'What is the advantage of this?' 'How can I become mentally stronger through this problem?' 'Turning threat into challenge.' 'There are no endings, only beginnings.'

    (c) Applications of these alternative interpretation principles in specific situations.

    (d) Generalization and automatization of situation-related learning.

4 *Autonomic restructuring*: if athletes notice that their heart starts to beat hard and fast before a competition, they will probably interpret this as nervousness. This 'flight' response will most likely be a negative factor, as the effects of a certain arousal level on performance are related to the interpretation of the situation. Thus, with automatic restructuring they can learn and automate a positive interpretation of high arousal ('Very good that my heart beat increases. I can now feel the loading of energy, as my body prepares for a good performance. . . .') The athletes are also asked to sit down twice a day for 3 min and repeat the keyword for the day with every pulse beat. Five 'C' words, which are important for a good competition, are chosen as key words — calm, committed, concentrated, confident, consistent.

5 *Mastery training*: an important difference between élite athletes and others is their attitude to mistakes. Lower level athletes have a bigger tendency to accept failure not as an occasional exception but as something typical or symp-

tomatic. They will start to blame themselves (inner talk) and their concentration on the task will diminish or disappear. Because this causes still more mistakes to follow, they often become more and more desperate. They sometimes begin to change things in a way that brings them still more out of rhythm. Mastery-oriented athletes, on the other hand, can analyse performance deterioration in a more objective way; they can continue after a mistake with the same self-image. They have even learned to use mistakes for development and further improvement in performance level. 'I feel calm and confident when I think of the future because I will use whatever happens for my personal development. The more "problems" I get, the better possibility I have of becoming mentally strong.' Such an attitude will take away worries and fears for things that could happen in the future.

Inner mental preparation

The mental training should proceed for at least 3–5 months in a regular (5 days a week) and systematic way, changing the training programme every week. Training should be conducted outside the competitive season in order not to interfere with competitive preparation. The training is intended to continue for only a couple of months, even if it might need some repetition and 'brushing up' later. The main intention, however, is to automate the learned mental skills in such a way that athletes do not have to analyse their mental processes at the time of the competition ('paralysis by analysis'). It will be so integrated and automated that it becomes a natural part of their way of being.

This takes time. Even if mental training programmes do not take more than 3–9 months to complete, the maximal effects of the mental training are often seen much later. One study was made of 100 bowlers from the élite level (national team) and down (Unestähl, 1985). This group was compared with a control group of 100 matched bowlers. After 3 months of mental training there were significant differences in the subjective ratings but not in performance scores. Three years later, however, there were significant and important intergroup differences in performance levels, in spite of the fact that the experimental group had only been training mentally during these 3 months.

In one way, mental training could be regarded as the first part of mental preparation for competition. Some of the effects of mental training are intended to appear automatically before and during a competition. This means that the athletes will derive benefits from the mental training without having to do anything different from before. For instance, the first trigger for increased concentration is merely picked out of the athletes' normal prestart routines.

The mental training also serves as a background for the special techniques of preparation which are described in this chapter. Improved self-confidence makes it easier to believe in the goal-programming for a certain competition. Increased visualization makes it easier to tell the body what to do in its own language (images). The acquired self-regulating skills make it easier to reach an optimal state of arousal, activation, tension and motivation at the time of competition. Inner mental preparation for sport, however, is directed more towards competition, either a specific event or competitions in general. It comprises the following five steps: model training, preseasonal training, precompetitive rehearsal, countdown mental preparation and competitive strategies.

Model training

The first kind of inner mental preparation concerns mental aspects of physical training in general. High level athletes have often reached a quantity of training which cannot be increased much more. However, it is important to differentiate between maximum and optimum quantities of training. Athletes have reached their optimum level of training when they will not benefit by an increase in training dose. On the contrary, additional training will often bring about various problems (such as overtraining and staleness).

Another variable where optimum level is probably equated more with maximum level, is model training or quality training. Model training is based on similarities between training and the competitive situation, such as including competitive elements in the training situation. It can be related to a law of psychology called 'state bound learning'. This law says that the use and benefits of learning are greater if the external situation and/or the state of mind during recall are similar to that of the learning situation. Competitive elements can be included in an athletes's regular training in many ways. Let us look at some suggestions (Unestähl, 1983).

GENERAL MODEL TRAINING

1 External conditions:
   (a) handicaps, time restrictions, task-difficulty;
   (b) fixed situations, tight situations, mistakes, bad performance, being behind or ahead;
   (c) optimal speed/effort.
2 Internal conditions: optimal level of tension, arousal, activation and motivation achieved by:
   (a) mental simulation;
   (b) in vivo simulation.

SPECIFIC MODEL TRAINING

1 Time of the year, time of day.
2 Location (photos, films).
3 Climate.
4 Type of competition.
5 'Mental atmosphere'.

Preseasonal preparation

Mental preparation for the next competitive season should start simultaneously with, or even somewhat before, other kinds of preparation. Seasonal goal-setting, for example, will give an additional flavour to physical workouts.

If athletes have earlier gone through the 3–9-month 'career training system' (basic mental training), the preseasonal preparation can be limited to 3 weeks.

Week 1. Repetition of earlier training: Dependent on their specific needs, the athletes select five of the career training programmes for practice during the first week.

Week 2. Seasonal goal setting: The athletes select a long-range goal and one or two intermediate goals as checkpoints for the next season. When these goals have been approved as clear and concrete objectives, the athletes have to specify the consequences of the goals and which requirements and demands they must fulfill in order to reach them. An investigation of seasonal goals (Unestáhl, 1983) showed that in 1980 a common goal among élite athletes was to qualify for the Olympics. If athletes prepare themselves (physically and mentally) for such a goal, the risk is that performance will drop for a while after having reached the goal. The time is often too short to prepare for the most important goal (peak performance at the Olympics) and the risk is that the athlete will achieve less good results at the Olympics.

Week 3. Goal programming: The athletes now use the same techniques of goal programming as they learned during career-training (contract, autogenic formula, hypnotic programming with suggestions and images). Other useful things that can be combined with goal programming are mental rehearsal of important sport-specific situations and mental rehearsal of key competitions during the season ahead.

Precompetitive preparation

The overwhelming majority of the literature about preparation for competition in endurance sports deals with physical preparation, while mental preparation procedures have rarely been addressed. Orlick (1980) has written one of the few 'practical' guides, in which he cites a number of strategies. These include self-assessment, listening to the body, talking to the body, relaxation, imagery and strategies to deal with pain (associative as well as dissociative).

Pelletier and Sachs (1981) tested and interviewed 20 runners. Their subjects reported that preparation for a marathon was at least 50% psychological and they emphasized the importance of mental factors for successful running.

The mental rehearsal of a future competition can start as soon as the athletes know about the competition. For a less important club event it can be enough to begin this training a few days in advance, while a more important competition can require one or more months of mental preparation. For big events like the Olympics, the mental preparation should preferably be extended to more than 1 year. In order to increase the vividness and reality of the rehearsal it is wise to obtain as much information as possible about the competition, the arena (photos, film, video) and other local conditions. One of the training programmes in the cassette 'Mental preparation for competition' has the following content:

1 To reactivate the 'ideal performing feeling' by reliving a 'model competition' in the past and to familiarize body and mind with the future competition (goal orientation).

2 To condition 'the winning feeling' to the coming competition. The programme is used differently, depending on the type of sport. Pär Arvidsson, an Olympic champion (1980) and world record-holder in an individual, closed-skill sport, namely swimming, states 'I sit down about 9 months before an important race and try to figure out what time I would need to swim to win the race. Then I decide what intermediate times I must have in order to make this final time. I then translate these times to a corresponding swimming speed, after which I start my mental rehearsal of the race. I increase the intensity as time goes on until I reach a maximum about 2–3 weeks before the race. I usually take the programme at night just before going to sleep. During training I often obtain "the winning feeling", "the ideal state".'

Countdown mental preparation

How does an athlete who has to dress in a particular way and in a particular order before a competition differ from a compulsive patient who must begin with the same leg every time a staircase is climbed? Very little. Athletes, like patients, can be very dependent on certain compulsive behaviours.

What purposes do prestart routines have? First of all, they create safety and security and serve as goal programming ('I do the same things that I used to do in good competitions'). Prestart routines also help athletes to enter an automated form of behaviour even before the competition. 'No need to think, just follow the old routines and habits, which makes it easier to hook on to the automaticity in the competition'.

There are, however, some important rules in the choice of prestart routines:

1 They should consist of an appropriate combination and integration of physical and mental preparation.
2 The routines should be of such a character that they can be carried out in all kinds of settings and circumstances.
3 It is advisable to have one normal set of prestart routines and one or two alternatives to be used in cases of under-motivation or over-motivation.
4 The routines should be automated.
5 They should be self-directed and if possible should not include anyone else.
6 They should be self-controlled (no interference from the surroundings).

Mental rehearsal during the prestart routine should be based on internal images having the purpose of starting the competition (mentally) in advance in order to evoke kinaesthetic feelings.

Competitive strategies

One main purpose of mental training and mental preparation is to improve a particular competitive performance; another is to increase consistency. Many of the parameters behind these goals are supposed to appear automatically, without any special competitive strategies. The competitive strategies that could be used in endurance sports can be divided into two categories. First are strategies that are planned and practised with the purpose of becoming an integral part of every competition. Runners, for example, usually develop all kinds of enhancing images. Morgan distinguished betweens two groups of marathoners: 'the associaters', who focused predominantly on the race and on their bodies, and the 'dissociaters', who used various mental devices to take their minds off the race and off their pains (Morgan & Pollock, 1977). The kind of strategies differ between élite athletes and lower class athletes. Fun-racers and middle class athletes seem to adopt more dissociation techniques, while élite athletes stay more in contact with their body (scanning).

The second kind of strategy is also preplanned and pretrained, but is used only if needed. When things go wrong, mistakes appear and performance deteriorates. Effective strategies are then needed to bring the performance back to normal (i.e. good performance). Such strategies have to be identified and practised in advance, in order to be ready for a quick intervention in situations of crisis. The training of effective competitive strategies gives a feeling of safety and the resulting decrease in fear of failure even helps to prevent mistakes. A marathon runner should have a pretrained pain plan and a plan of how to maintain the ideal performing feeling.

MAINTAINING IPF

An ideal performance (IP) creates an ideal performing feeling (IPF) but this relationship also works in the other direction (IPF gives an IP). In the same way that a mistake or a bad response creates a bad feeling, a bad feeling increases the probability of another bad response.

Here are some possible strategies that athletes can learn in order to continue with a good feeling in spite of isolated mistakes:

1 See a mistake as an exception (and a good performance as normal).

2 Return to normal = good performance, without letting mistakes lower self-esteem.

3 Prevent analysis (and inner talk criticism), for example by placing the incident in a 'problem bag' which is not opened and analysed until after the competition.

4 Repeat the performance mentally in a successful way in order to reinstate IPF immediately.

5 See the 'mistakes' as an opportunity to learn and grow (attitude training).

6 The critical part of the athlete (analysis and reality testing) can be silenced by engaging in another positive activity (thoughts about something else, about a positive part of the performance, an activity which gives a good feeling like whistling or humming).

Injuries

Prevention and rehabilitation of injuries is a new and promising field for the application of mental training. Mental factors seem to be involved in injury proneness, in recovery speed and in athletes' reactions to injury (pain tolerance, etc). The speed and quality of the healing process are also affected by psychological factors, although opinions differ as to the extent of their influence.

Injured athletes can be recommended to use mental training in the following ways:

1 They can work in general with inner mental programmes. This counteracts the inactivity feeling and the feeling of coming behind. Instead of physical training, they increase the intensity and frequency of the mental training.

2 They can use relaxation to increase peripheral blood flow and can also learn hypnotic methods to increase blood flow to specific injured parts.

3 They can apply goal-setting and goal-programming techniques in the recovery process.

4 They can detect and work with subconscious reasons for delaying recovery (secondary gains).

5 Additional possibilities, like using ideomotor training to stimulate NGF (nerve growth factors), are still under investigation.

The effects of the suggested methods vary in magnitude but not in quality, giving larger or smaller positive effects. The possibility of being able to train, the feeling of being active and of taking part in recovery mean a lot to many athletes. Even after complete recovery there are sometimes psychological after-effects which have to be eliminated. Mental training techniques, such as desensitization for the fear of injuries, are of value here.

Mental training for life

Many people today practise and use relaxation and other mental training techniques for different purposes, such as improving physical and creative performance, getting rid of phobic problems or influencing psychosomatic diseases. The same principles and methods lie behind all of these applications of mental training — in sport, education or health.

That principles of mental training are valid far beyond the sport area can be seen in the evaluation studies of 'inner mental training'. In a study of 5000 Swedish inner mentally trained athletes in 1980 (Unestål, 1985), many reports of the effects of training were taken from everyday life. Here are some examples:

'Better sleep, calmer, easier to concentrate and my competitive results have increased very clearly.'

'So far no improvement in the competitions but I have seen many positive effects in my everyday life.'

'I am functioning much better as a human being now, but I have also beaten the Swedish record.'

'More harmonious now, both in sport and everyday life. Never give up. Earlier I was out if I got behind. I now enjoy sport much more.'

'Of course I am satisfied with my Olympic gold, which has been the content in my goal-programming during recent years, but I have learned to appreciate and enjoy the way to this goal still more.'

Concluding remarks

Much has happened since the beginning of applied mental training a few decades ago. However, much remains to be done — in research as well as in areas of application. Because mental training is based on experiences that most people have had, the theory and practice are easy to grasp. It also means that everyone can take part in a fascinating development of mental training, not only as a spectator but as a participant.

Another interesting area is the philosophy that has developed around mental training. Mental training today is not only a training system. It is a way of thinking, feeling and behaving — a lifestyle. Let me finish with principle no. 10, which is related to 'attitude'. It reads as follows: 'The term "impossible" can only be used about the past, never about the future!'

References

Jansson, L. (1990) *Differential relaxation in elite sports.* Unpublished manuscript. Scandinavian International University, Örebro.

Morgan, W.P. & Pollock, M.L. (1977) Psychological characterization of the elite distance runner. *Ann. N. Y. Acad. Sci.* **301**, 383–403.

Nideffer, R. (1981) *The Ethics and Practice of Applied Sport Psychology.* Mouvement Publications, Ithaca, New York.

Nideffer, R. & Sharpe, R. (1978) *ACT: Attention Control Training.* Wyden Books, New York.

Orlick, T. (1980) *In Pursuit of Excellence.* Coaching Association of Canada, Ottawa.

Pelletier, D. & Sachs, M. (1981) *La motivation et la préparation psychologique des marathoniens.* Unpublished manuscript, University of Quebec.

Unestähl, L.-E. (1973) *Hypnosis and Posthypnotic Suggestions.* Veje Publishing, Örebro.

Unestähl, L.-E. (1975) *Hypnosis in the Seventies.* Veje Publishing, Örebro.

Unestähl, L.-E. (1979) *Självkontroll genom Mental Träning.* Veje Publishing, Örebro.

Unestähl, L.-E. (1983) *The Mental Aspects of Gymnastics.* Veje Publishing, Örebro.

Unestähl, L.-E. (1985) *Inner Mental Training.* Veje Publishing, Örebro.

Unestähl, L.-E. (1986a) *Sport Psychology in Theory and Practice.* Veje Publishing, Örebro.

Unestähl, L.-E. (1986b) *Contemporary Sport Psychology.* Veje Publishing, Örebro.

Chapter 32

Prevention of Injuries in Endurance Athletes

PER RENSTRÖM AND PEKKA KANNUS

Introduction

Interest in sports participation has increased tremendously during recent decades. There is a great interest among people in general to improve their health and body composition. Regular aerobic exercise has been linked to a decreased risk of vascular disease (Paffenbarger *et al.*, 1986) and has assisted in weight reduction (Lewis *et al.*, 1976). In addition, fitness and exercise have been claimed to decrease the morbidity of ageing and mortality (Bortz, 1982). Sporting activities have, therefore, been described as beneficial for society as a whole as well as for the individual. A certain amount of physical activity is considered to be an important element in health promotion, as noted in position statements by the American College of Sports Medicine (ACSM) in 1978 and 1990 and by the International Federation of Sports Medicine (FIMS) in 1989 (FIMS, 1989a).

Top-level competitive participation has, with increasing mass media attention, also become more common. Higher intensity has demanded more intense and longer duration training. The training has also become more specialized. Serious and specialized training starts at younger ages and continues until an older age, which means that there is an increased risk time for sustaining an injury. Sports were earlier carried out mostly by amateurs, but the increasing mass media and commercial interests have resulted in more participation by professionals. Vince Lombardi's philosophy that 'winning isn't everything, it is the only thing' has been accepted as the holy grail among athletes, especially in the USA. This attitude has resulted in increased exploitation and abuse of athletes. The pressure is often so high that drug abuse has become a problem and attention to injury prevention is often neglected.

With the increased interest in sports activities and sports participation at all levels, there has been an increase in the frequency and severity of sports injuries, both from acute accidents and from overuse trauma. An acute injury is defined as a single impact macrotrauma (for example, a blow to a leg resulting in a fracture, a rotational injury of a joint resulting in a ligament sprain, or a direct blow to the muscle resulting in muscle strain). An overuse injury is defined as a longstanding or recurring orthopaedic problem, starting during training or performance due to repetitive tissue overload, and resulting in microtrauma.

Numerous epidemiological studies of sports injuries are available (Sandelin, 1988). In the Netherlands, the overall incidence has been calculated as 3.3 injuries per 1000 h spent on sports (Galen *et al.*, 1990). However, because the population at risk is extremely difficult to identify, the actual incidence of sports injuries in one society, or in more specific sub-groups, is still almost unknown. Studies that analyse sports injuries have not been able to identify athletes at risk or the risk factors, and aetiological factors have not yet been fully assessed (Ekstrand, 1982).

The number of acute sports injuries treated in hospitals is, on the other hand, rather well known. Forty years ago, sports injuries formed 1.4% of all injuries seen in an emergency room. During the 1970s this figure varied between 5% and 7%, and today about 10% of all traumatic injuries treated in the emergency rooms of hospitals in industrialized countries are sustained in sports (Galen *et al.*, 1990).

The exact incidence rates of overuse injuries are even more difficult to calculate. Due to the general increase in sport participation, the absolute number of overuse injuries has probably increased dramatically during recent decades. The claim that the incidence has increased remains, however, without scientific evidence.

Both acute and overuse sports injuries are generally considered to be relatively benign. It is estimated that up to 75% of all sports injuries can be classified as mild to moderate, requiring only a short absence from sports and a short sick leave. The number of patients requiring further treatment as inpatients because of a sports injury appears to be around 10%. The number of patients who need operative treatment for an acute or overuse injury varies from 5% to 10% (Kannus *et al.*, 1989).

The cost to society is large. In the Netherlands, the total cost of treatment and sick leave has been estimated at US $350 million per year (Toom & Schuurman, 1988).

Despite the fact that most sports injuries are mild or moderate in character, the treatment of injured athletes often requires special evaluation and experience. The treating physician not only needs special knowledge in sports medicine, but should also be familiar with the particular sport and its rules, techniques, mechanics and demands. A correct diagnosis, adequate immediate and continuous treatment, and effective rehabilitation are prerequisites for return to full sports participation.

Despite adequate treatment based on advanced knowledge, modern technology and improved skills in sports medicine, some athletes fail to return to preinjury level and intensity of activity. Injuries are usually ex-perienced as a disaster by the athletes. Most injuries are unnecessary. The prevention of injuries should, therefore, be a major goal for every physician, physiotherapist, trainer, nurse, coach, parent, athlete and others active in sports and sports medicine.

Strategies in the prevention of sports injuries

Sports injury prevention should include efforts at individual, group and societal levels.

Direct or indirect sports injury prevention at an individual level can be called *primary prevention*, as is often the case in the prevention strategies of general medicine and health education. Medical preseason examination of a subject, warming up before the competition, and use of protective equipment (helmets, face masks, knee, shoulder and elbow paddings, safety-release ski bindings, braces, tape, etc.) are typical examples of primary prevention (Table 32.1).

Sports injury prevention at the group level can be called *secondary prevention*. The most common tactic is group information and education. Lectures to athletes and coaches about the importance of proper warming up and cooling down, careful following of the rules

Table 32.1 Strategies in the prevention of sports injuries. From Renström & Kannus (1991).

Primary prevention (prevention at individual level)
Medical screening
Protective equipment
Flexibility and strength training
Nutrition

Secondary prevention (prevention at group level)
Rules
Agreements
Information
Education

Tertiary prevention (prevention at societal level)
Societal planning
Legislation
Budget
Investments

(fair play), the disadvantages of drugs, alcohol and tobacco, and known risk factors of injuries are typical examples. Any decision within an individual sport event which makes that particular sport safer can also be considered as secondary prevention.

All efforts undertaken at a societal level to prevent sports injuries can be called *tertiary prevention*. Normally, tertiary prevention looks far forward, and any benefits will not be seen for years after the strategies were planned and made effective. Societal planning is often seen as a tool in tertiary prevention. An example might be a political decision to build new, safe cycling routes and to separate them completely from motor vehicle traffic. A legislative decision by one country or state to forbid all blows to the head in boxing can also be seen as tertiary prevention. Table 32.1 summarizes the three different levels of sports injury prevention.

These three levels can also apply to one individual (Hlobil *et al.*, 1987). Using this strategy, prevention of an injury before its occurrence can be called *primary* prevention. Efforts that are designed to prevent reinjury, or to prevent existing injuries from becoming chronic can be termed *secondary* prevention. Finally, *tertiary* prevention limits the progression of irreversible loss of function from a chronic injury.

Extrinsic factors predisposing to injury

Injury mechanisms

It is important to identify the risk factors and injury mechanisms that play an important role in the aetiology of injuries. *Acute injuries* are common in many sports, especially contact sports. Large impact traumas such as collision against another player, a fall against the ground, a tackling against the boards of a rink, or a blow by the club or puck in ice hockey are common. An acute impact injury is caused by deformation of tissues beyond their recoverable limit, resulting in damage to the anatomical structures or an alteration in normal function. The risk of injury is related to the energy delivered to the body by the impacting object as well as to the shape of the object (Viano *et al.*, 1989). The individual's capacity to withstand the trauma is of importance. For example, an osteoporotic bone will fracture more readily than a normal bone subjected to the same trauma. It is important to identify and define the mechanism of impact injury, to quantify the biomechanical response to such impact, to determine the impact tolerance level, and to develop injury assessment devices and techniques for evaluating injury prevention. It would also be of value if the resulting forces from the impact could be decreased and dispersed, to avoid deformation and severe damage to tissues.

Repeated overload in running and jumping activities is often associated with *overuse injuries*. In running, a force in the range of three to five times the body weight ascends the lower extremity at heel strike. This force has a short duration (20–40 ms) and rapid dissipation. Considering an impact of only 250% of body weight, a runner absorbs at ground contact a force of 110 Mg (110 tons) on each foot per mile (1.6 km) (Mann, 1981). The cumulative effect can be imagined in a long-distance runner, who runs 100 miles (160 km) per week and plants each foot about three million times a year.

These forces are so large it is not surprising that they contribute to injuries. Accordingly, it is possible that reduction of these forces may reduce the frequency and extent of injury.

A possible way of decreasing the load on the body is to change the type of motion. For example, one can run by landing on the heel or landing on the forefoot. In landing on the heel, the point of application of the ground reaction force and the line of action of that force are both behind the ankle joint. Therefore, structures on the anterior part of the leg are loaded on first contact and the Achilles tendon is unloaded. Heel landing, therefore, can be used to unload the Achilles tendon, for example during the recovery period of an Achilles tendinitis or peritendinitis.

Another possibility is to decrease the speed of the motion. By decreasing the speed of heel—toe running from 6 m·s^{-1} to 3 m·s^{-1}, the decreases in vertical impact and active forces are 40% and 20%, respectively (Nigg, 1988). A change in the speed of motion also changes the speed of the involved limbs and can therefore influence the forces acting on the athlete's body.

Little is known about the number of repetitions and their effects with respect to the load on the human body. Biological materials can have a positive response to the applied stress, provided that the stress increase is sufficiently slow. If the response is stronger than the effect of mechanical fatigue, the tissue becomes stronger. Generally, bones and muscles have high and fast responses, while cartilage and tendons show a smaller and slower response because of a low nutritional blood flow. Fatigue injuries such as stress fractures occur frequently. It is thus of importance to increase the number of repetitions slowly — the slow progression principle.

Training errors

Overuse injuries are associated with extrinsic and/or intrinsic factors. The most common extrinsic factors are excessive loads on the body, training errors, bad environmental conditions, poor equipment, and ineffective rules (Table 32.2). Training errors are probably present in 60—80% of reported injuries to runners (James *et al.*, 1978). The most common errors are too long a distance, too high an intensity, too fast a progression, and too much hill work. Monotonous, asymmetric and specialized training is a great risk factors in most sports. Running on the edge of the road means running with one leg short and one long, resulting in overuse injuries such as trochanteric bursitis and iliotibial band friction syndrome. By varying the exercise method (cycling, swim-

Table 32.2 Extrinsic factors related to injuries in sports. From Renström & Kannus (1991).

Excessive load on the body
type of movement
speed of movement
number of repetitions
footwear
surface
Training errors
excessive distances
fast progression
high intensity
hill work
poor technique
monotonous or asymmetric training
fatigue
Poor environmental conditions
dark
heat/cold
humidity
altitude
wind
Poor equipment
Ineffective rules

ming and cross-country skiing in addition to running), a much larger amount of total work can be carried out with less risk of injury.

In addition, poor technique and fatigue play a role. Even minor technical faults, continuously repeated, can cause overuse injuries. A minor fault in the throwing of a javelin may cause synovitis located to the medial side of the elbow after numerous repetitions. The same problem applies to baseball pitching. Fatigued muscles have a decreased ability to absorb repetitive shock or stress, leading to overuse injuries such as stress fractures, tennis elbow, and medial tibial stress syndrome.

Sports surface adjustment

During each contact of the foot with the ground, the ground acts on the foot with a ground reaction force and the foot acts on the ground with a force of the same magnitude but in an opposite direction. The forces during landing and take-off can be quite different on different surfaces. The impact force is much higher for running on asphalt than for running on grass or sand (Nigg, 1988). However, the active part of the ground reaction force remains about the same when comparing running on grass with running on asphalt. High impact forces are one cause of many running injuries, as well as injuries in other sports. In tennis, adolescents often sustain overuse injuries such as medial tibial stress syndrome and Achilles tendinitis on surfaces with a high friction. These problems are rarely seen on clay courts (Renström, 1988). It is therefore very important that people who are responsible for the development of sports facilities know the possibilities of reducing forces through the appropriate selection of sports surfaces.

Shock absorption can be achieved by the use of proper orthotics and shoes (see below).

Poor equipment

Equipment can be divided into instrumental and protective. Poorly instrumented equipment can cause overuse injuries, especially if used in combination with poor technique. One of the few areas where research has been carried out is in tennis, where the equipment can be of importance, for example the size of the racket. Oversized rackets absorb vibrations better from tennis balls that are hit off centre along the vertical axis (Elliott *et al.*, 1980). The frequency of tennis elbow is thus lower in players who use oversized rackets. Tennis elbow is also more likely to occur in players who use a heavy racket than in those who use a light one (Kulund *et al.*, 1979), but there are studies indicating that the mass of the racket does not influence the incidence of tennis elbow (Carroll, 1986). The material from which the racket is made may be an important factor in the incidence of tennis elbow: tennis elbow may result from using oversized aluminium rackets. Muscle activity generated in the forearm and shoulder muscles of players using rackets with different grip sizes showed that the force change in the muscles was not significant enough to suggest the need for a change of grip size (Adelsberg, 1986).

Gut stringing has been shown to provide better control, higher ball velocities, lower levels of vibration transmission to the hand, and improved player characteristics (Groppel, 1984). Gut stringing should thus be used when a player has tennis elbow. String tension has also been indicated as a factor in the occurrence of tennis elbow. The looser the strings, the higher the positive impact velocity. In general, tightly strung rackets give better control, whereas loosely strung rackets generate more force. The racket should be strung at around 50–55 lbs (220–250 N) tension in order to avoid tennis elbow. Heavy balls should be avoided, as well as 'dead', wet or pressureless balls, because the use of these will increase the impact against the tennis racket, thereby increasing the risk of tennis elbow. The use of slow courts is also suggested for athletes with tennis elbow problems.

Since 1972, an extensive prospective study of downhill skiing injuries has been carried out by the Department of Orthopaedics and Rehabilitation at the University of Vermont under the leadership of Robert J. Johnson. Between 1972 and 1987, all 5701 injuries reported to the injury clinic operating in the base lodge have been evaluated prospectively. During that time, approximately 1 690 000 skier visits have been made to the ski area. Virtually all injuries below the knee have decreased dramatically, in some groups by more than 80% (Johnson *et al.*, 1989). However, knee injuries involving the anterior cruciate ligament have increased. This decrease in lower extremity injuries appears to be equipment related. Proper use of ski bindings with sophisticated release mechanisms has played an important role (Fig. 32.1). Information concerning the importance of setting ski bindings at a proper release level has been effective in preventing ski injuries (Eriksson & Johnson, 1980).

These examples indicate that it is important to use the proper equipment in different sports.

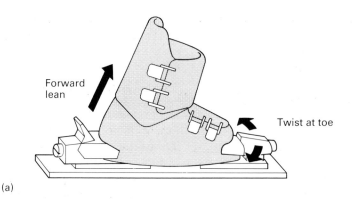

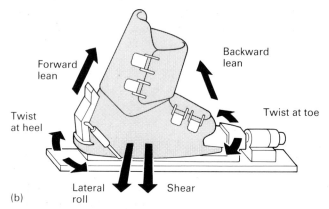

Fig. 32.1 Modern, well-adjusted and functioning ski bindings are essential. (a) Two-mode release capability; (b) multimode release capability. From Peterson & Renström (1986), with permission.

The equipment should also be used in a prescribed and tested fashion. The importance of avoiding poor equipment is part of the basic strategy in preventing all kinds of sports injuries. In addition, the efficacy of equipment can be increased significantly by secondary and tertiary preventive efforts, such as information, education, legislation and planning.

Ineffective rules

One extrinsic predisposing factor that is not well known is the inefficacy of many of the rules in sports. Improvement of the rules to make sports safer is a key factor in reducing the number of sports injuries. Interest in the improvement of rules has, however, developed rather late. Rules are becoming more and more concerned with facilities, environmental circumstances such as weather, personal equipment and tactics or practices demonstrated to

be unsafe (Ryan & Stoner, 1989). Coaches and athletes have shown considerable resistance to changing the rules, because frequently these place restrictions on a special style of play, which is popular even though it may be quite dangerous.

Rules that prevent contact activities likely to produce injuries have been instituted in American football. The clipping injury and the down field blocking below the waist are now forbidden (Peterson, 1970). Other rule changes have resulted in a dramatic decrease in both the total number of cervical spine injuries and of those resulting in quadriplegia (Torg et al., 1990).

Rules for safety have gradually been developed as, for example, in American football where the helmet is now compulsory. In ice hockey it has become compulsory to use a helmet in university and junior hockey as well as to use face masks. These rule changes have reduced the number of facial and eye injuries dramatically. Amateur boxers must, in several countries, use a protective head cover. In junior baseball there is a restriction on the number of pitchings per season, to avoid little leaguer's elbow. In volleyball, stepping on the net line is prohibited in order to avoid ankle sprains.

Sports techniques are developing rapidly and will force changes of existing rules; so will improved technology. It is, therefore, necessary to review and revise the rules continuously. In the future, rule changes may be a very important way of reducing the number of sports injuries since both the number of new sports, often with high risk for injury, and the number of participants seem to increase exponentially.

Poor environmental conditions

Weather may have an effect on the frequency of injury during sports. The rules provide that a baseball game be called off in the event of rain because wet fields increase the risk of injury. Darkness, too high or low a temperature or humidity, high altitude and a strong wind may also play a key role in injury pathogenesis. Darkness has to be taken into account when planning orienteering competitions. High temperature and humidity without wind restrict the cooling of marathon runners with potentially serious consequences (heat exhaustion, heat stroke or death). Low temperatures with a strong wind may produce frostbite, hypothermia and other cold injuries in sports such as downhill or cross-country skiing, ski jumping and mountain climbing.

It is essential to have clear rules about when training or competition must be cancelled because of poor environmental conditions. In cross-country skiing, there is a cancellation of the competition if the temperature is below $-20°C$ ($-4°F$) to avoid cold injuries. Other weather factors should also be taken into consideration. For example, the wind chill factor is critical in many winter sports, since the wind has a marked effect on heat loss. If the thermometer reads $-7°C$ ($20°F$) and the wind velocity

is 32 km·h^{-1} (20 miles·h^{-1}) the rate of cooling is comparable to $-23°C$ ($-10°F$) (Boswick et al., 1983).

Intrinsic factors predisposing to injury

The most common intrinsic factors related to overuse injuries are alignment abnormalities, leg length discrepancy, muscle weakness and imbalance, decreased flexibility, joint laxity, female sex, young or old age, overweight and some pre-disposing diseases (Table 32.3) (Renström & Johnson, 1985). In 40% of cases of running injury, intrinsic predisposing factors were present, but in only 10% were they the only demonstrable factor (Lysholm & Wiklander, 1987).

Malalignments

James et al. (1978) noticed that increased pronation was present in 60% of a group of injured runners. Hyperpronation of the foot is often physiological, but compensatory hyperpronation may occur for anatomical reasons (tibia vara, forefoot varus, leg length discrepancy or ligamentous laxity) or because of muscular

Table 32.3 Intrinsic factors related to overuse injuries in sports. From Renström & Kannus (1991).

Malalignments:
  foot hyperpronation/hypopronation
  pes planus/cavus
  forefoot varus/valgus
  hindfoot varus/valgus
  tibia vara
  genu valgum/varum
  patella alta/baja
  femoral neck anteversion
Leg length discrepancy
Muscle weakness/imbalance
Decreased flexibility
Joint laxity and instability
Female sex
Young/old age
Overweight
Predisposing diseases

weakness or tightness in the gastrocnemius and soleus muscles. Hyperpronation may, in turn, have secondary effects such as increased internal rotation of the tibia, resulting in lower leg and knee problems (Fig. 32.2). Several overuse injuries seem to be caused by, or associated with, this foot malalignment: medial tibial stress syndrome, tibialis posterior tendinitis, Achilles bursitis or tendinitis, plantar fasciitis, patellofemoral pain syndrome, iliotibial band friction syndrome and lower extremity stress fractures (Lorentzon, 1988).

If excessive or prolonged pronation occurs in an athlete with associated pain in the lower extremity, orthotics to be used in the shoes may be indicated. In hyperpronation, the medial side of the sole and forefoot is elevated. If hyperpronation is found in an asymptomatic person, shoe corrections are seldom necessary. The same principles can be followed in the prevention and treatment of other injuries associated with malalignments.

In the patellofemoral pain syndrome, some additional predisposing (risk) factors may be present, such as patella alta and excessive lateral displacement or tilting of the patella. Patellar bracing or taping may be beneficial in the

prevention of reinjury. Activity modification and quadriceps muscle training are, however, the most common route to success.

The occurrence of these proposed biomechanical alterations, their magnitude and, above all, their clinical significance are not well known. There are some indirect clinical associations between malalignments and injuries, but so far little direct scientific evidence exists. Correction of training errors may thus be warranted more often than orthotics.

Leg length discrepancy

Leg length discrepancy is a commonly discussed factor in orthopaedics and sports medicine. The orthopaedic view has been that discrepancies of less than 20 mm are largely cosmetic (Friberg *et al.*, 1985). In élite athletes, however, a discrepancy of more than 5–6 mm may be symptomatic, and for a discrepancy of 10 mm or more a built-up shoe or insert type of orthotics may be indicated (Lysholm & Wiklander, 1987).

As in foot hyperpronation, many biomechanical alterations have been proposed to result from leg length discrepancy: pelvic tilt to the shorter side followed by compensatory lumbar scoliosis and compression of the intervertebral disc on the concave (inner) side of the curve, increased abduction of the hip (longer leg), excessive pronation of the foot (on the longer or shorter side), secondary increased knee valgus, and outward rotation of the leg. As a result, leg length discrepancy has been suggested as a causal factor in the development of lower back pain, hip osteoarthritis, trochanteric bursitis, patellar tendinitis, iliotibial band friction syndrome and stress fractures.

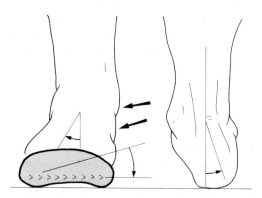

Fig. 32.2 Hyperpronation causes secondary effects such as increased tension on the medial aspect of the ankle and foot, valgus deviation of the calcaneus, oblique traction of the calcaneus tendon and increased internal rotation of the tibia. This hyperpronation can be prevented by use of orthotics. From Renström (1988).

Muscle weakness and imbalance

The significance of muscle weakness and imbalance in injury prevention is also a matter for discussion. Muscle imbalance implies an asymmetry between the agonist and antagonist muscles in one extremity, asymmetry between the extremities, or a differential with an anticipated normal value (Grace et al., 1984; Grace, 1985). An athlete with over 10% difference in quadriceps or hamstring strength between the right and left side is felt to be at a greater risk of muscular tendon injury. An athlete who has a hamstring-to-quadriceps strength ratio of 60% or less in one leg is believed to have a propensity to sustain a muscle injury (Safran et al., 1989). Heiser et al. (1984) showed that the University of Nebraska football team sustained a 7.7% incidence of hamstring injury with a 31.7% recurrence rate, but after these imbalances had been recognized and corrected the team had a 1.1% incidence of hamstring strains without any recurrences.

Muscle weakness due to scarring from previous injury predisposes to recurrent injury because the scar tissue is not as strong or elastic as the other components of the musculotendinous unit. There is an increased risk of muscle injury, not only because of inadequate muscle strength but also because there may be an inadequate corelaxation of the antagonist muscle.

It is well documented that athletes with previous joint injury have persistent and long-lasting muscular strength, power and endurance deficits in their affected extremity and that those joints are at greater danger of reinjury than uninjured joints (Kannus et al., 1987a). Many athletes feel fully rehabilitated and return to their sport too early. There is a persistent 20% loss of muscle strength in the affected leg for 5−10 years after knee surgery, although the athletes resume sports, believing themselves to be completely rehabilitated (Grimby et al., 1980). The same loss is observed after conservatively treated anterior cruciate ligament injuries of the knee. It is not clear how important muscle imbalance per se is as a causative factor for reinjury, since persistent joint instability, pain, swelling and impairment of neuromuscular coordination are also involved.

There is some evidence that multifactorial conditioning programmes can reduce the injury rate (Hlobil et al., 1987), while other studies have not found any direct relationship between muscle weakness or imbalance and injury (Grace, 1985). Thus, the question of any relationship between these variables remains open. However, rehabilitation after an injury is a tool not only to increase muscle strength, but also to improve the dynamic stability of the joint and coordination of the whole extremity. Therefore, it should always be a most important step in an athlete's way back to sports.

Decreased flexibility

Joint flexibility is an important part of physical performance (Corbin, 1984) and is probably important in the prevention of certain sports injuries such as muscle rupture, tendinitis, apophysitis and patellofemoral pain syndrome.

The available studies do not allow any conclusion on whether musculotendineal tightness is the cause or the consequence of injury. Prospective follow-up studies are needed. In the meantime, flexibility training must be regarded as an important tool in the prevention of muscle and tendon injuries.

A steady state value of the stretched musculotendineal tissue will ultimately be achieved. In other words, there is an optimal length of tissue beyond which further stretch is of no anatomical or physiological value. It is, however, important to preserve this optimal length with regular stretching.

Joint laxity and instability

In some people, especially in women, joints can be hypermobile. This means that the range of movement of the joint may be excessive in normal, physiological directions of movement, in abnormal directions, or in both (Fig. 32.3). Joint hypermobility is often genetic (Grahame, 1990). As a rule this does not require special attention in injury prevention, but more research is needed.

However, a ligamentous injury may lead to joint instability and residual problems,

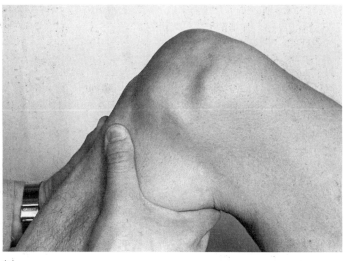

(a)

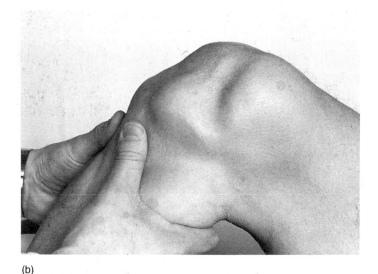

(b)

Fig. 32.3 Unstable joints resulting from untreated or maltreated ligamentous injury may result in osteoarthritis, for example of the knee. Correct initial treatment is of importance in the prevention of future complications. The figure shows the knee of a 27-year-old male athlete who had been conservatively treated for rupture of the anterior cruciate ligament; 10 years after injury the knee shows a major anterior laxity with a soft endpoint indicating insufficiency of the ligament. (a) shows the starting position of the drawer test, and (b) shows the end position of the test.

especially in the knee, ankle and shoulder joints. Athletes with post-traumatic instability often complain of fear of 'giving way', recurrent sprains, and pain or swelling during activity. Serious long-term consequences, such as post-traumatic osteoarthritis, may follow complete ligament tears when the joint has become unstable (Fig. 32.4) (Kannus, 1988; Kannus & Jarvinen, 1989).

In the prevention of reinjury to these unstable joints, specific muscle strengthening exercises are of great value. Good muscle function can to some extent compensate for ligamentous instability (Fig. 32.5). Joint braces and taping may be of value in the prevention of abnormal movements and reinjuries (AAOS, 1984).

Women in sport

There is an increase in female sport participation and in physical activity in general. There is also an increased female interest in sports

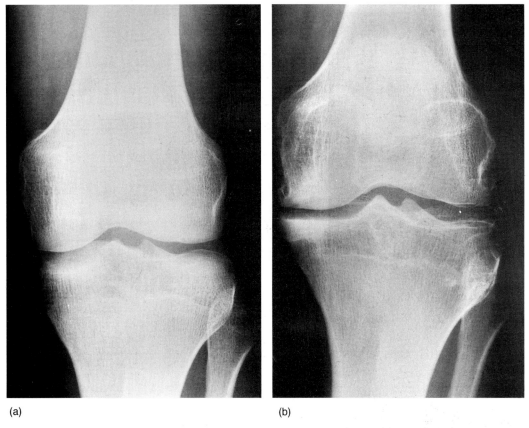

(a)   (b)

Fig. 32.4 Good muscle function developed through proper muscle exercises can, to some extent, compensate for ligamentous instability and prevent future problems. (a) Radiographs of a normal knee in a 34-year-old male who sustained complete anterior cruciate and medial–collateral ligament injuries in 1973. These injuries were treated conservatively. (b) 15 years later osteoarthritis has developed in the injured knee, which is now unstable.

events with a high risk of injury, such as gymnastics, soccer and team handball.

Injuries are therefore increasingly common. A recent, prospective study showed that 31% of injured athletes were female (Kannus *et al.*, 1987b). There is a high incidence of overuse injuries among women. The reason for this may be that the repetitive impact of the body weight is absorbed by a weaker musculoskeletal system in women compared with men of equal body mass (Lloyd *et al.*, 1986). Women have less muscle mass per kg of body mass (20–25%) than equally trained men (40%), and their overall muscle strength averages about

two thirds that of men (Drinkwater, 1988). Men also have greater bone mass than women. These factors, together with known female risk factors such as wider hips and more mobile joints, predispose women to overuse injuries.

Menstrual irregularities, which are much more common among female athletes than among non-athletes, constitute a risk factor for certain overuse injuries. There is an increased incidence of stress fractures among amenorrhoeic athletes compared with eumenorrhoeic athletes participating in the same sport (Marcus *et al.*, 1985) (Fig. 32.6). A prolonged hypo-oestrogenic state may result in a loss of bone

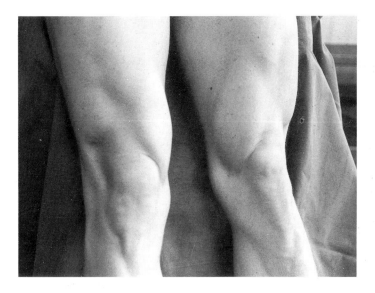

Fig. 32.5 Good muscle function may, through proper muscle exercise, to some extent compensate for ligamentous instability and prevent future problems. The figure shows a 21-year-old ice hockey player who 6 years earlier had sustained a grade 2 injury (partial tear) of the anterior cruciate ligament of his left knee. After 6 years, there were no strength deficits in his left thigh muscles and both quadriceps were extremely well developed. The left knee was still partially unstable during ligament stress tests, but the patient was asymptomatic.

mass (especially in trabecular bone areas), and may, therefore, increase the risk of osteoporotic acute fractures. In strenuous endurance sports, continuous recording of menstrual cycles and follow-up of dietary habits (sufficient protein, calcium and vitamin D) should be compulsory.

Young age

Regular training of children and young adults is becoming ever more common in sports. Competitive sports are carried out with increasing intensity and at lower ages. In some sports, such as figure skating, swimming and gymnastics, children start regular training at 4–5 years of age; training from 2–4 h for 5–6 days a week is not unusual. As a result, the risk of an acute or overuse injury increases.

Before puberty, a child's body seems to withstand repeated voluntary stress amazingly well. During the growth spurt, which occurs in most girls at about 12 years of age and in boys at about 14 years (see Chapters 28 & 35), there is a gross imbalance between muscle strength, tightness, joint mobility and coordination. In addition, during that phase the growth plates are extremely vulnerable to external forces, with an increased risk of acute and overuse injuries

(Micheli, 1983). Well-known examples of injuries during the growth spurt include traumatic epiphysiolyses of the hip joints and traction apophysitis of the tibial tubercle in jumpers (Osgood–Schlatter disease) or of the humeral medial epicondyle in young pitchers (little leaguer's elbow). The incidence of little leaguer's elbow has been decreased by restricting the number of pitching competitions allowed in the growing athlete.

Adaptation as a result of prolonged one-sided training in childhood can cause permanent asymmetric changes. An example of this is the so-called tennis shoulder, in which the end-result is an increased laxity in the joint capsule, ligaments and tendons, and an increased bone growth, resulting in a dropping of the shoulder and a relative lengthening of the racket arm (Fig. 32.7). In gymnastics, intensive training over a long period of time may produce hypermobility of the vertebral column and other joints, and the end-result may be early osteoarthritis (Sward, 1990). In competitive gymnastics, hyperextension (Fig. 32.8) is stimulated by the award of high scores. These rules should be analysed by sports medicine expertise.

It is essential that regular hard training

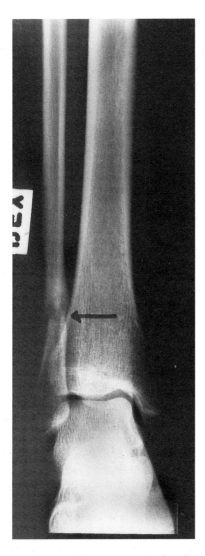

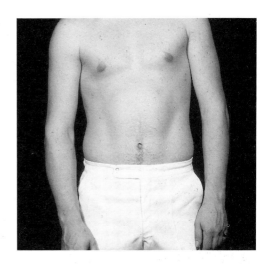

Fig. 32.7 Repetitive one-sided isometric tennis training can cause laxity in the joint capsule, ligament and tendons, and result in dropping of the shoulder — tennis shoulder.

Fig. 32.6 Stress fractures can occur in females with amenorrhoea or osteoporosis. The figure shows a 26-year-old female who had worked for 1 year as an aerobic dance teacher. She sustained simultaneous bilateral stress fractures of the fibula. When the stress fractures occurred, her menstrual cycle was very irregular due to hard training.

Old age

With ageing, various functions of the body gradually deteriorate, including the musculoskeletal system. Musculoskeletal disability deteriorates more slowly in long-distance runners aged 50–72 years than in non-running control groups (Lane *et al.*, 1987). Runners have less physical disability, maintain a better functional capacity, and have fewer physician visits per year.

In elderly athletes, sports injuries are more frequently overuse related than acute. In addition, compared with the injuries of young adults, elderly athletes' injuries more commonly have a degenerative basis (Kannus *et al.*, 1989). In a study of veteran élite athletes competing in the world master championships, the most common injuries were muscle and tendon strains in the lower leg (Peterson & Renström, 1980). Prevention of sports injuries in master athletes should, therefore, be concentrated on these areas. Maintenance of flexibility and neuromuscular coordination through daily stretching and calisthenics is recommended. Long warm-up and cooling down periods should be the rule. Slow progression is es-

during adolescence is carried out under supervision. Secondary and tertiary preventive measures such as protective rules, information and education are also of great importance.

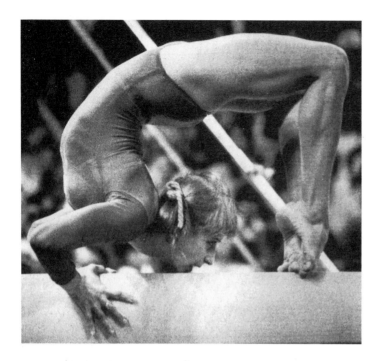

Fig. 32.8 Hyperextension in gymnasts is a risk factor for injury to the spinal vertebrae, especially in very young athletes. (Olga Korbut, winner of many gold medals in the 1972 Olympic games; photo courtesy of Pressens Bild.)

pecially important for elderly people. Participation in sports such as swimming, cycling or rowing, in which the whole body weight is not supported by the lower extremities, is recommended in most cases. Postmenopausal women need, on the other hand, to load their skeleton to prevent osteoporosis. Common sense must be used when planning long-term exercise programmes for the elderly. Racket sports such as tennis are of low risk and are therefore suitable for elderly people. Regular medical checkups are recommended.

Overweight

In sports injury prevention, overweight may be a problem in weight-bearing recreational physical activities, because the development of knee and hip symptoms and osteoarthritis are associated with overweight (Hartz *et al.*, 1986; Felson *et al.*, 1988). Physical activity may accelerate the osteoarthritic process. Interestingly,

a recent prospective study has shown that weight reduction in severely obese individuals leads to a significant relief of their musculoskeletal symptoms (McGoey *et al.*, 1990). A reduced energy intake and participation in sports events in which the whole body weight does not stress the lower extremities are recommended for overweight people.

Predisposing diseases

An athlete may have a predisposing disease making him or her prone to injury. A diabetic patient involved in long-distance running competition needs special care, since a patient with low blood sugar levels may lose his or her concentration and coordination capability. Children who have had Perthes' disease may have a major loss of the rotatory function of the hip and may develop secondary hip or knee swelling and irritation in strenuous physical activities. Children with Osgood–Schlatter's disease of their knees have an increased risk of patella alta in adulthood and of patellofemoral subluxation or chondromalacia problems during physical activity.

General preventive methods

The general prevention of sports injuries includes activities that concern everyone involved in physical activity.

Basic physical fitness

Good physical fitness is of the utmost importance in avoiding injury. Athletes whose basic fitness level is below normal are more prone to injury, both from acute trauma and from overuse (Peterson & Renström, 1986).

A basic physical fitness level can be achieved by regular exercise and general physical activity throughout the year. General conditioning and training of large muscle groups are of great importance in most sports. Training should progress gradually, especially in those who are no longer young.

Inactivity and immobilization have deleterious effects on the musculoskeletal tissues. Bones become decalcified, tendons and ligaments lose their tensile strength, muscle tissue atrophies and becomes weaker, and cartilage loses its elasticity (Jarvinen, 1976; Akeson et al., 1980; Jozsa et al., 1988a; 1988b). Therefore, during the period of rehabilitation following illness or injury, or after a break in training, it is important that a reasonable level of basic physical fitness is reached before competition is resumed.

Warm-up

Warm-up exercises are designed to prepare the body for the ensuing sporting activity. They have two functions: to prevent injury and to enhance performance.

At rest, the blood flow to the skeletal muscles is relatively low, and most of the small blood vessels (capillaries) supplying them are closed.

When activity begins, the blood flow to these muscles increases as the vessels open. At rest, 15–20% of the blood flow is directed to the skeletal muscles, while the corresponding figure after 10–12 min of all-round exercise is 70–75%. A muscle can achieve maximum aerobic performance only when all its blood vessels are functional and maximally open.

The elastic components of muscle are more susceptible to injury when a muscle is cold (Zarins & Ciullo, 1983). The increase in muscle temperature is thought to enhance the chemical reactions of contraction and to increase the elasticity of intramuscular connective tissue. The warm-up speeds up the metabolic processes, allowing faster and more forceful contractions (Safran et al., 1989). Muscle viscosity drops with an increase in temperature, making the contractions smoother. This thermally dependent increase in connective tissue elasticity may be the reason why warmed up muscles stretch to a greater length before tearing and require application of a greater force for failure. The most common and important injuries to be prevented by warm-up are not only muscle strains, but also tendon, ligament and other soft tissue injuries.

Warm-up is also a way of preparing an athlete's mind for physical activity. A proper warm-up may relax the athlete and aid concentration. There is also an improved brain–muscle coordination and cooperation, with less likelihood of uncontrolled muscle activity and strain.

Warm-up can be passive or active. A passive warm-up may use a sauna, a warm shower, warm clothes or a massage. The circulation is somewhat increased, but is lower than that achieved with active warm-up. Active warm-up is both general and sport-specific. The general part includes jogging or stationary cycling in order to involve the large muscle groups. After this general warm-up the more sport-specific exercises can begin. Runners, for example, should concentrate this further warm-up on the muscles, tendon, joints and ligaments of the lower extremities. Stretching is also essential, but application of heavy loads at the outer limits of joint movements should be avoided.

The final stage of warm-up concentrates on technique, or on practising sport-specific movements. The pace of the exercises can be gradually increased, and the whole warm-up session should last for at least 15–20 min, depending on the sport involved. The effect of the warm-up soon starts to wear off and, therefore, mild exercise should be continued. Ideally, the delay before competition should be no longer than 10 min. During this time the athlete also prepares psychologically.

Cooling down

After training or competition, cooling down exercises are desirable. Cooling down enhances the washout of the products of muscle metabolism (lactic acid, etc.), shortening the recovery time. It also offers a unique possibility for stretching exercises, since the muscle temperature is still high and stretching can be performed safely and easily.

Cooling down is normally performed in two phases. The first phase includes aerobic sport-specific movements at 50–70% of maximal aerobic power. For example, after cross-country skiing competition, the athlete should ski an additional 1–3 km at mild or moderate speed. The second phase consists of general large muscle exercise, such as gentle jogging, performed at 30–50% of maximal aerobic power. Stretching for 5–15 min, depending on the sport, is included in this phase.

Slow progression

The musculoskeletal system must be allowed to adapt gradually to increasing loads. At least 50% of all overuse injuries are caused by training errors. The majority of these errors are due to breaking this principle of slow progression.

A male competitive runner, who has increased his weekly mileage slowly but steadily every year, is able after 10 years' progression to run more than 200 km (130 miles) per week without musculoskeletal problems. At the same time, a colleague who has increased the mileage faster is much more prone to overuse troubles while running the same amount per week.

Musculoskeletal adaptation to stress is a slow but very reliable process. Therefore, to avoid injury to muscle (e.g. pain, soreness, strain and compartment syndromes), tendons (tendinitis, peritendinitis, tenoperiostitis, tendinous and partial or complete ruptures), joints (cartilage softening or avulsion, meniscal ruptures, ligament sprains, synovitis and osteoarthritis) and bones (stress fractures, osteoporotic fractures and apophysitis), athletes and their coaches must understand the importance of slow progression. This is of particular concern to children and adolescents.

Preventive training

Training of the musculoskeletal system is the key to both the prevention of injury and to a successful recovery after an injury. Repeated, slowly progressive exercises will improve the mechanical and structural properties of the muscles, tendons, joints, ligaments and bones by increasing their mass and tensile strength. Preventive training includes muscle training, flexibility training, coordination and proprioceptive training, and sport-specific training.

MUSCLE TRAINING

Muscle training can be isometric, concentric or eccentric. Isometric exercise is an effective method to increase strength, but the response is greatest around the angle at which the training is carried out. Isokinetic training is a form of concentric or eccentric training, performed at a constant angular velocity throughout the range of motion; it is a very effective method of increasing muscle strength, power and endurance. However, this type of motion is not used in sports.

In many exercises, for example in running, there is a stretch-shortening cycle where the stretch (eccentric action) proceeds shortening (concentric action) (Komi, 1984). Eccentric exercises combined with stretching can be used in the preventive as well as rehabilitative phases of overuse injuries (Curwin & Stanish, 1984). It is, however, important to realize that eccentric contractions may sometimes contribute to the production of both acute and chronic overuse tendon and muscle problems (e.g. muscle soreness) as a part of the deceleration forces. Therefore, eccentric exercises are not recommended for elderly athletes as a part of their regular training.

FLEXIBILITY TRAINING

Strength training has a negative effect on joint flexibility (Moller, 1984). This can be counteracted by flexibility training. The flexibility of a particular joint is primarily limited by the tightness of the connective tissue. Flexibility exercises should be started after the growth spurt, when there is a rapid increase in muscle volume and power. Flexibility decreases with age, and flexibility training should therefore be emphasized more and more with increasing age.

Flexibility training aims to maintain and/or improve joint mobility, to reduce the risk of joint over-loading at extreme joint angles, to increase muscle and tendon strength, to enhance coordination between the various parts of the musculoskeletal system, and to adapt the musculoskeletal system to the specific demands of a particular sport.

Stretching is one of the most important methods of flexibility training. It should be preceded by a 3–5-min warm-up. *Dynamic (or ballistic, spring, bounce or rebound) stretching* implies repeated muscle extension to its limit followed by immediate relaxation. This type of stretching is not effective as it activates protective reflexes and, therefore, is seldom used nowadays.

Static (or hold or prolonged) stretching involves slowly stretching the muscle as far as possible and then holding that position, held for 20–60 s. This technique is commonly used.

Static contract–relax–hold stretching includes first a slow stretch to the limit of motion and then a maximum isometric contraction at that position, held for 4–6 s. This is then followed by a relaxation for 2–3 s, and thereafter a passive stretch is made to the extreme position and that position is held for 10–60 s. This technique is a modification of the PNF (proprioceptive neuromuscular facilitation) technique frequently used by physical therapists.

3S system (scientific stretching for sport) is a fourth type of stretching. The muscle is passively stretched and then exposed to an isometric contraction. This technique is effective but requires a partner to hold and stretch the leg.

COORDINATION AND PROPRIOCEPTIVE TRAINING

This involves training the interaction between the nervous system and muscles, tendons, joints and ligaments. In many sports, good technique and coordination are essential in prevention of acute and overuse injuries.

After an ankle ligament injury, during which the nerves in the joint capsule are often injured, proprioceptive training is performed periodically on a tilt board for 6–8 months to regain full function, and then continued to prevent recurrent injuries (Tropp, 1985) (Fig. 32.9).

SPORT-SPECIFIC TRAINING

Sport-specific conditioning can usually be achieved by training within the sport itself. For example, many soccer and tennis coaches prefer training carried out on the soccer field or tennis court, respectively. If the sports event is, however, dangerous by nature (boxing, motor sports, aerial freestyle skiing, etc.) or involves a high risk of injury (gymnastics, American football, etc.), simulating exercises should be performed before taking part in the sport itself. In freestyle skiing this involves training and jumping into a water pool.

Sport-specific training often includes all the other parts of preventive training, and is there-

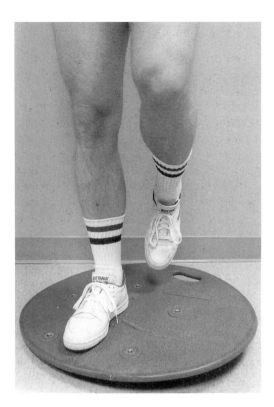

Fig. 32.9 Tilt board exercises can improve proprioceptive capacity and strength in ankle joints with functional instability, and thereby prevent recurrence of ankle sprains.

fore one of the most effective approaches to the primary prevention of sports injuries. After an injury, the sport-specific exercise programme should be the final step in rehabilitation before returning to the sports arena.

Medical examinations

Some sports require a medical examination just before the competition (e.g. boxing or ultra-marathon running) to prevent injury or general medical complications. For middle-aged and older people (35 years and over) who have decided to start a regular exercise programme, a medical screening examination is rec-

ommended (International Federation of Sports Medicine, 1989a). Such screening should include a complete orthopaedic evaluation to discover possible risk factors for injury.

Nutrition and diet

In injury prevention, nutrition becomes important in longlasting training and competition situations during which the body's carbohydrate stores are emptying. The performance level, reactions and coordination of the subject become impaired, and the athlete is then prone to injury. To avoid complete emptying of the glycogen stores, a carbohydrate loading technique can be used (Costill, 1988) (see Chapters 12 & 33).

In injury prevention, other nutritional elements of food (fat, proteins, vitamins and minerals) are of secondary value, although they do have a tremendous effect on general well-being. A well-balanced diet is therefore recommended for every active individual.

Drugs, medication and doping

Athletes taking part in competitions should not be under medication of any kind. However, if the medication used is needed, for example in asthma or diabetes, is not a banned substance and is prescribed by the athlete's own physician, it will enhance the athlete's general well-being and allows her or him to take an enjoyable part in sports.

From the point of view of injury prevention, stimulants, narcotics, anabolic steroids, diuretics, alcohol, local anaesthetics and corticosteroids are dangerous.

Pain is a warning signal and a guide to correct diagnosis and treatment and, therefore, pain inhibition of any kind is dangerous in combination with sports injuries. If pain has been reduced by local anaesthetics or corticosteroids, the athlete should not participate. Corticosteroid injections may cause hypoxia and degenerative alterations in the tendon tissue, weakening the tensile strength of the tendon (Kamian, 1989).

Hygiene

The skin secretes sweat and grease in which dust and dirt may adhere and become a breeding ground for bacteria, producing unpleasant odours, rashes, irritation and pimples. Inadequate foot care allows dirt to collect between the toes again providing a breeding ground for bacteria and fungi.

General preparation for sports

An athlete preparing for regular hard training and competition should lead a well-regulated daily life with regular food habits, enough sleep, and avoidance of drug abuse. The importance of regular, sound living habits cannot be overemphasized for an athlete with aspirations to reach or to stay at the top.

The athlete needs not only to be physically well prepared for training and competition but mentally prepared as well. This means that the athlete should be aware of the requirements of the sport and what it takes to complete a race or competition. The degree of mental tension varies from sport to sport. Too much mental tension can cause reactions such as lack of appetite, headaches and, occasionally, defective coordination which can lead to an increased risk of injury. If mental tension is excessive, it is the responsibility of the coach to find a way back to an optimal level. Discussion with the athlete and gradually increasing the competitive element of the training have often been used to prepare the athlete. An athlete usually learns quickly what is her or his optimal level of mental tension for competitive performance.

Preventive equipment

Preventive equipment is of the utmost importance in sports, and includes the use of protective equipment, braces, tapes, shoes and orthotics.

Protective equipment

Protective equipment plays an important role in the safe participation in sports, especially in contact sports such as American football, ice hockey, lacrosse, team handball, volleyball, football (soccer), etc. This is also true in some popular racket sports such as squash.

The protective equipment for an athlete must be chosen carefully and should be fitted by a knowledgeable individual. The player's acceptance is also necessary. Players must be made aware that modifying the equipment for more comfort may sacrifice its protective effect, thereby increasing the risk of injury.

Protective head equipment is used in many sports, especially in ice hockey and American football. No helmet is designed well enough to prevent a head injury completely, but they can reduce the magnitude of a blow while dispersing its force over as large an area as possible (Gieck, 1990). The American football helmet and the ice hockey helmet, have been well tested. Chin straps and face masks may be added to the helmet. Face masks are compulsory in junior and university ice hockey (Fig. 32.10). The number of facial and eye injuries has decreased drastically with adoption of this rule.

There are sports with a high risk of eye injury when *protective eye devices* are not worn, for example ice hockey, racket sports (such as racquetball and badminton), lacrosse and baseball. Adequate eye protective devices are now available according to a position statement from the International Federation of Sports Medicine (1989b). Protective eye wear in low risk sports can consist of normal eye glass frames with polycarbonate lenses. Moulded polycarbonate frames and lenses are suggested for athletes who ordinarily do not wear glasses, but participate in moderate to high risk non-contact sports. Face masks or helmets with face protection are required for use in sports with a high risk of contact of collision. Some basketball players have begun wearing protective eye guards as well.

Ear guards are often worn by water polo

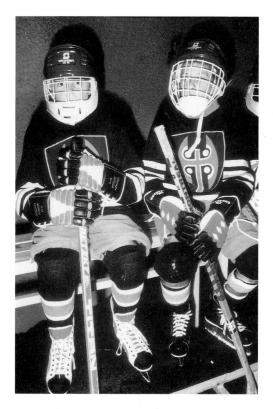

Fig. 32.10 Helmets with face masks are now compulsory in junior ice hockey. The use of these protective device prevents many injuries.

players and wrestlers and should be well fitted to the head and not come off during competition. These protective devices have partially eliminated the cauliflower ear that was earlier common among wrestlers.

Mouthpieces have been mandatory in American football since the 1960s, as well as in boxing. Participants in other sports, for example lacrosse, field hockey and ice hockey, have also begun to wear them.

Well-designed *shoulder and elbow pads* are used in ice hockey and in American football (Fig. 32.11), as well as other protective pads over the thorax.

Protective equipment for the lower extremities is also worn in American football. Ice hockey goalkeepers wear special padding to protect themselves against the puck. *Shin protective padding* is compulsory in soccer.

Protective equipment should be designed to absorb and distribute impact forces. The equipment is continuously being developed and improved to meet the increasing requirements of sports.

Role of braces in injury prevention

Braces are commonly used to prevent injuries, to protect against reinjury and to aid in rehabilitation after injury. Braces are specially designed to be used on ankle, knee, elbow and wrist joints. The most commonly used braces are knee stabilizing braces, which have been classified by the American Academy of Orthopaedic Surgeons (1984) into three types: prophylactic, rehabilitative and functional braces.

Prophylactic knee braces are designed to prevent or reduce the severity of damage to the knee joint caused by an injury. These braces are not commonly used in Europe, because they cannot be used in soccer, but they can be used in American football. They usually have one lateral hinge. Prophylactic braces have a limited capacity to protect the medial collateral ligament from direct lateral stress when the knee is in full extension. The efficacy of these braces, as well as their future role in sports medicine, is unclear.

Rehabilitative knee braces are designed to immobilize the knee or allow limited and controlled flexion motions after injury or operative procedures. They provide accurate control over motion and avoid excessive loading of the healing tissue. They may provide some stability, but they cannot duplicate the function of the undamaged ligaments (Hofman *et al.*, 1984). Biomechanical investigations of rehabilitative knee braces have shown that most braces reduce both translations and rotations relative to the unbraced limb under static test conditions (Cawley, 1989). The loads were, however, well below those expected in normal physiological loading conditions, indicating

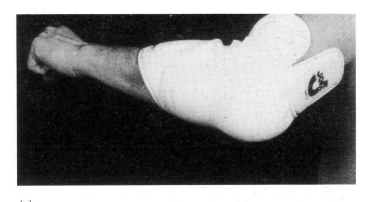

(a)

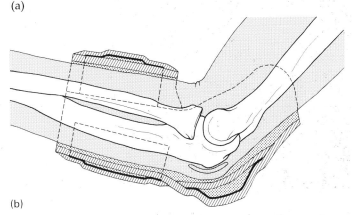

Fig. 32.11 Protective padding devices should take up and distribute impact forces correctly. The figure shows an elbow protective device in ice hockey (a) and the principles of distribution of shock absorption (b). From Peterson & Renström (1986), with permission.

(b)

that the data may be clinically relevant only in patients who are not fully weightbearing. These braces will be more commonly used as surgical techniques improve and as the importance of early mobilization is stressed.

Functional knee braces are designed to assist the functional stability of unstable knee joints. There are many designs, but they are limited in their direct control of the rotation of the tibia and femur by the soft tissues covering the limbs, which is the principal mechanical interface for the brace. Functional braces therefore attempt to control secondary rotation by blocking the principal components of instability, which are translations in multiple planes. Many patients are satisfied with this type of brace and feel it to be of some value (Colville *et al.,* 1986). Biomechanically, the braces have been

shown to decrease anterior translation, but only at low loads and slow speeds. There is limited research available to support the efficacy of these braces. Continued research will be of great value as there is a clinical need for more effective knee braces.

Braces for patellofemoral pain syndromes have been developed with the aim of preventing lateral subluxation of the patella. These braces seem to have limited value, but are used as some patients experience a reduction in pain.

Ankle stability bracing is used more and more instead of tape (Fig. 32.12). The most effective support of the ankle, producing the lowest incidence of ligament injuries, is a combination of high-top shoes and laced ankle stabilizers (Rovere *et al.,* 1988). *Tennis elbow braces* are used more and more. They are applied to relaxed muscles, thereby preventing the lower arm extensor muscles from full contraction and protecting the insertion of the extensor muscles at the lateral epicondyle. Electromyographic studies have verified the effect of these braces (Groppel & Nirschl, 1983).

The role of braces in injury prevention is still controversial because of the lack of scientific data. Biomechanically, braces seem to have a limited effect, but the injured athletes often experience some relief while wearing them.

Heat retainers or neoprene sleeves have been used in the treatment of overuse injuries and in the rehabilitation of most injuries for many years. They have also been used by, for example, many alpine skiers to prevent injury in cold weather. The idea behind these braces is that heat enhances the circulation around the injured area, facilitating the healing process. Heat also enhances elasticity, with potential value in the prevention and rehabilitation of muscle tendon injuries (Fig. 32.13).

Role of tape in injury prevention

Medical tape is used extensively to support different joints, especially the ankle. Taping of the ankle is of value in the prevention of ankle injuries. Ekstrand (1982) showed that the number of ankle sprains in soccer could be reduced 75% by a preventive programme including prophylactic taping, stretching, player education, etc. A combination of prophylactic taping and the use of high-top shoes in basketball reduced the number of ankle sprains (Garrick, 1977). Tape was also shown to have a significantly prophylactic effect against injuries of the lateral ligaments of the ankle in a 2-year prospective randomized study of team handball players (Lindenberger *et al.*, 1990).

Tape is also used at other locations and seems to have an effect on joints with little soft tissue between the skin and the joint, such as the ankle, wrist and finger joints. Morehouse (1970) found that after 5 min of intense physical activity, the effect of knee joint taping on side stability had completely disappeared.

The role of taping is decreasing because of associated skin problems, because the effects of taping are not long lasting, and because tape is expensive. It often requires trained application and use of a sharp instrument for removal.

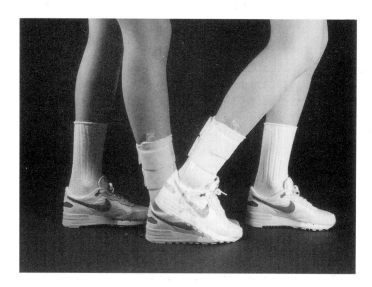

Fig. 32.12 Ankle braces help to prevent recurrence of ankle injuries. Their support is increased when they are used in combination with a sport shoe.

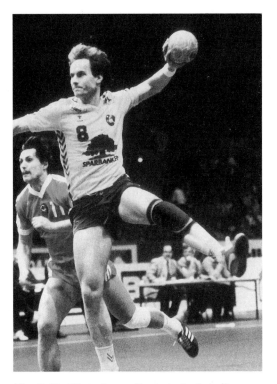

Fig. 32.13 Heat plays an important role in the prevention of sports injuries as it increases the circulation and improves the elasticity of the collagen in tendons, muscles and ligaments. Heat retaining braces are, therefore, increasingly used in both prevention and rehabilitation after injury.

Role of shoes in injury prevention

In the reduction of impact forces, shoes are of great importance. There has been a revolution in the development and design of shoes during the last 15 years. Most modern shoes are designed to give both stability and shock absorption. Good running shoes should absorb and/or reduce impact forces, and should provide medial–lateral stability, avoiding excessive pronation and over-supination of the foot. It is a question of cushioning, support and friction. There are appropriate shoes availables for almost every sport event.

The ideal shoe should hold the foot so that it functions much as when barefoot. Shock-absorbing characteristics are important and shoe design has a great influence on the shock absorption at heel strike (Jorgenssen & Ekstrand, 1988). Shoes also have a stabilizing function, and hyperpronation can be prevented by stable shoes with a firm and high heel counter. Running shoes should control the rolling movement at push-off (Pforringer & Segesser, 1986). Shoes should be very flexible in the forefoot, or they can cause forefoot over-use problems during push-off. An ideal shoe should not wear out within the first few months of use. It is more important to buy good shoes than expensive clothing.

The importance of choosing the correct shoe for different sports activities cannot be overemphasized. Correct shoe wear plays a very important role in injury prevention, particularly in avoidance of overuse injuries.

Role of orthotics in injury prevention

During the past 10 years, custom-made orthotic devices have been used increasingly as sports physicians have come to understand the role of malalignments in the genesis of overuse injuries.

The biomechanical goals of orthotic devices have been summarized by Doxey (1985):
1 To prevent abnormal movements of the subtalar and metatarsal joints.
2 To rebalance the malaligned foot to a more neutral position.
3 To resist or normalize the foot's abduction to the ground at heel strike.
4 To resist or normalize the foot's propulsive function as a rigid lever at push-off.
5 To maximize hallux function.
6 To maximize toe function in propulsion.
7 To allow normal foot movements and muscle activity at the proper time.

The failure of orthotic treatment experienced by some people may have occurred because the orthotics were not adjusted as needed. Support diminishes owing to the person's progressive pronation or the compression of the orthotic appliance material. The orthotic control of pronation is satisfactory for daily activities, but may not be adequate for the increased pronation in running, which can gradually be resumed when the athlete is asymptomatic.

There is a lack of scientific support for the use of orthotics. Orthotic treatment has been especially successful in typical running injuries, with a success rate of 70% (Smith *et al.*, 1986). There are some clinical reports which imply that orthotics are effective in the treatment of stress injuries and pain syndromes of the lower limbs (Darrigan & Gauley, 1985). Orthotics have mostly been prescribed to control excessive pronation. It has been shown that both maximum pronation and the initial maximal velocity of pronation can be reduced this way (Clarke *et al.*, 1983), while the total movement is maintained. Orthotics for pronation can significantly decrease abduction of the foot during walking and running, as well as correcting leg length discrepancy. There are no prospective randomized studies available, but there is a vast experience in sports medicine concerning the value of orthotics in compensating and neutralizing different malalignments.

Custom-made orthotics has made it possible for the sports physician to treat the cause of injuries and not only the symptoms. The use of orthotics should be encouraged if there are clear biomechanical indications for such treatment.

References

Adelsberg, S. (1986) The tennis stroke: an EMG analysis of selected muscles with rackets and increasing grip size. *Am. J. Sports Med.* **14**, 139–142.

Akeson, W.H., Amiel, D. & Woo, S.Y. (1980) Immobility effects on synovial joints: the pathomechanics of joint contracture. *Biorheology* **17**, 95–100.

American Academy of Orthopaedic Surgeons (1984) *Knee braces.* Seminar report, 18–19 August, Chicago.

American College of Sports Medicine (1978) Position statement on the recommended quantity and quality of exercise for developing and maintaining fitness in healthy adults. *Med. Sci. Sports* **10**, VII.

American College of Sports Medicine (1990) Position statement on the recommended quantity and quality of exercise for developing and maintaining cardiorespiratory and muscular fitness in healthy adults. *Med. Sci. Sports Exerc.* **22**, 265–274.

Bortz, W.M. (1982) Disuse and aging. *J.A.M.A.* **248**, 1203.

Boswick, J.A. Jr., Danzl, D.F., Hamlet, M.P. & Schultz, A.L. (1983) Helping the frostbitten patient. *Patient Care* **17**, 90–115.

Carroll, R. (1986) Tennis elbow and tennis rackets: case studies of club tennis players. In: MacGregor & Moncur (eds) *Sports and Medicine*, pp. 281–288. E. & F.N. Spon, London.

Cawley, P. (1989) Factors which influence choice of functional knee brace for skiing. *Idrottsmedicin. (J. Sports Med.) (Stockholm)* **1**.

Clarke, T.E., Frederick, E.C. & Hlavac, H.F. (1983) Effects of a soft orthotic device on rear foot movement in running. *Pediatr. Sports Med.* **1**, 20–23.

Colville, M.R., Lee, C.L. & Ciullo, J.V. (1986) The Lennox Hill brace. An evaluation of effectiveness in treating knee instability. *Am. J. Sports Med.* **14**(4), 257–261.

Corbin, C.B. (1984) Flexibility. *Clin. Sports Med.* **3**, 101–117.

Costill, D.L. (1988) Carbohydrates for exercise: dietary demands for optimal performance. *Int. J. Sports Med.* **9**, 1–18.

Curwin, S. & Stanish, W.D. (1984) *Tendinitis: Its Etiology and Treatment.* The Collamore Press, Lexington, Massachusetts.

Darrigan, R.D. & Ganley, J.V. (1985) Functional orthoses with intrinsic rear foot post. *J. Am. Podiatr. Med. Assoc.* **75**, 619–624.

Doxey, G.E. (1985) Clinical use and fabrication and molded thermoplastic foot orthotic devices. Suggestion from the field. *Phys. Ther.* **11**, 1679–1682.

Drinkwater, B. (1988) Training of female athletes. In: Dirix, A., Knuttgen, H.G. & Tittel, K. (eds) *The Olympic Book of Sports Medicine*, pp. 309–327. Blackwell Scientific Publications, Oxford.

Ekstrand, J. (1982) *Soccer injuries and their prevention.* Academic dissertation. Linkoping University, Linkoping, Sweden.

Elliott, B.C., Blanksby, B.A. & Ellis, R. (1980) Vibration and rebound velocity characteristics of conventional and oversized tennis rackets. *Res. Q. Exerc. Sport* **51**, 608–615.

Eriksson, E. & Johnson, R. (1980) The etiology of downhill ski injuries. *Exerc. Sports Sci. Rev.* **8**, 1–17.

Felson, D.T., Anderson, J.J., Naimvk, A., Walker, A.M. & Meenan, R.F. (1988) Obesity and knee osteoarthritis. The Framingham Study. *Ann. Intern. Med.* **109**, 18–24.

Friberg, O., Kvist, M., Aalto, T. & Kujala, V. (1985) Leg length inequality in the etiology of low back pain and low limb overuse injuries in young athletes. *Idrottsmedicin* **3**, 5–7.

Galen, W.Ch.C. van & Diederiks, J.P.M. (1990) *Sport-blessures breed uitgemeten* (English summary). Publ. Comp. De Vrieseborvh, Haarlem, The Netherlands.

Garrick, J.G. (1977) The frequency of injury, mechanism of injury and epidemiology of ankle sprains. *Am. J. Sports Med.* **5**, 241–242.

Gieck, I. (1990) Protective equipment for sports. In: Ryan, A. & Allman, F. (eds) *Sports Medicine*, pp. 211–242. Academic Press, San Diego.

Grace, T.G. (1985) Muscle imbalance and extremity injury. A perplexing relationship. *Sports Med.* **2**, 77–82.

Grace, T.G., Sweetser, E.R. & Nelson, M.A. (1984) Isokinetic muscle imbalance and knee-joint injuries. *J. Bone Joint Surg.* **66A**, 734–740.

Grahame, R. (1990) The hypermobility syndrome. *Ann. Rheum. Dis.* **49**, 199–200.

Grimby, G., Gustafsson, E., Peterson, L. & Renström, P. (1980) Quadriceps function and training after knee ligament surgery. *Med. Sci. Sports* **12**, 70–75.

Groppel, J.L. (1984) *Tennis for Advanced Players and Those Who Would Like To Be.* Human Kinetics, Champaign, Illinois.

Groppel, J.L. & Nirschl, R.P. (1983) A mechanical and electromyographical analysis of the effects of various joint counterforce braces on the tennis player. *Am. J. Sports Med.* **14**, 195–200.

Hartz, A.J., Fischer, M.E., Bril, G. *et al.* (1986) The association of obesity with joint pain and osteoarthritis in the HANES data. *J. Chron. Dis.* **39**, 311–319.

Heiser, T.M., Weber, J., Sullivan, G., Clare, P. & Jacobs, R.R. (1984) Prophylaxis and management of hamstring muscle injuries in intercollegiate football players. *Am. J. Sports Med.* **12**, 368–370.

Hlobil, H., van Mechelen, W. & Kemper, H.C.G. (1987) *How Can Sports Injuries be Prevented?*, pp. 1–236. NISGZ Publication 25E, Oosterbeek.

Hofman, A.A., Wyatt, R.W., Bourne, M. & Daniels, A.U. (1984) Knee stability in orthotic knee braces. *Am. J. Sports Med.* **12**, 371–374.

International Federation of Sports Medicine (1989a) Physical exercise — an important factor for health. A position statement. *Int. J. Sports Med.* **10**, 460–461.

International Federation of Sports Medicine (1989b) Eye injuries and eye protection in sports. *Aust. Sports Med. Fed.* **7**(2), 19–20.

James, S.L., Bates, B.T. & Osternig, L.R. (1978) Injuries to runners. *Am. J. Sports Med.* **6**, 40–50.

Jarvinen, M. (1976) *Healing of a crush injury in rat striated muscle with special reference to treatment of early mobilization and immobilization.* Academic dissertation, University of Turku, Turku, Finland.

Johnson, R.J., Ettlinger, C.F. & Shealy, J.E. (1989) Skier injury trends. In: Johnson, R.J., Mote, C.D. Jr.

& Binet, M.-H. (eds) *Skiing Trauma and Safety: Seventh International Symposium*, ASTM STP 1022, pp. 25–31. American Society for Testing and Materials, Philadelphia.

Jorgenssen, U. & Ekstrand, J. (1988) Significance of heel pad confinement for the shock absorption at heel strike. *Int. J. Sports Med.* **9**, 468–473.

Jozsa, L., Reffy, A., Jarvinen, M., Kannus, P., Lehto, M. & Kvist, M. (1988a) Cortical and trabecular osteopenia after immobilization. A quantitative histological study of the rat knee. *Int. Orthop.* **12**, 169–172.

Jozsa, L., Thoring, J., Jarvinen, M., Kannus, P., Lehto, M. & Kvist, M. (1988b) Quantitative alterations in intramuscular connective tissue following immobilization: an experimental study in the rat calf muscles. *Exp. Mol. Pathol.* **49**, 267–278.

Kamian, M. (1989) A rational management of tennis elbow. *Sports Med.* **9**(3), 173–191.

Kannus, P. (1988) *Conservative treatment of acute knee distortions — long-term results and their evaluation methods.* Academic dissertation, Tampere, Finland.

Kannus, P. & Jarvinen, M. (1989) Posttraumatic anterior cruciate ligament insufficiency as a cause of osteoarthritis in a knee joint. *Clin. Rheumatol.* **8**, 251–260.

Kannus, P., Latvala, K. & Jarvinen, M. (1987a) Thigh muscle strengths in the anterior cruciate ligament deficient knee: isokinetic and isometric long-term results. *J. Orthop. Sports Phys. Ther.* **9**, 223–227.

Kannus, P., Niittymaki, S. & Jarvinen, M. (1987b) Sports injuries in women: a one-year prospective follow-up study at an outpatient sports clinic. *Br. J. Sports Med.* **21**, 37–39.

Kannus, P., Niittymaki, S., Jarvinen, M. & Lehto, M. (1989) Sports injuries in elderly athletes: a three-year prospective, controlled study. *Age Ageing* **18**, 263–270.

Komi, P.V. (1984) Physiological and biomechanical correlates of muscle function: effects of muscle structure and stretch-shortening cycle on force and speed. *Exerc. Sports Sci. Rev. (ACSM)* **12**, 81–121.

Kulund, D.N., McCue III, F.C., Rockwell, D.A. & Gieck, J.H. (1979) Tennis injuries: prevention and treatment, a review. *Am. J. Sports Med.* **7**, 249–253.

Lane, N.E., Bloch, D.A. & Wood, P.D. (1987) Aging, long-distance running, and the development of musculoskeletal disability: a controlled study. *Am. J. Med.* **82**, 772–780.

Lewis, S., Haskell, W.L., Wood, P.H., Monoogian, N., Bailey, J.E. & Pereira, M. (1976) Effects of physical activity on weight reduction in middle-aged women. *Am. J. Clin. Nutr.* **29**, 151–156.

Lindenberger, U., Reese, D., Renström, P., Andreasson, G. & Peterson, L. (1990) A prospective study of the effect of ankle taping. *FIMS Proceedings of* the XXIV World Congress of Sports Medicine, Amsterdam.

Lloyd, T., Traintafyllou, S.J., Baker, E.R. et al. (1986) Women athletes with menstrual irregularity have increased musculoskeletal injuries. Med. Sci. Sports 18, 374–379.

Lorentzon, R. (1988) Causes of injuries: intrinsic factors. In: Dirix, A., Knuttgen, H.G. & Tittel, K. (eds) The Olympic Book of Sports Medicine, pp. 376–390. Blackwell Scientific Publications, Oxford.

Lysholm, J. & Wiklander, J. (1987) Injuries in runners. Am. J. Sports Med. 15, 168–171.

McGoey, B.V., Deitel, M., Saplys, R.J.F. & Kliman, M.E. (1990) Effect of weight loss on musculoskeletal pain in the morbidly obese. J. Bone Joint Surg. 72B, 322–323.

Mann, R.A., Baxter, D.E. & Lutter, L.D. (1981) Symposium. Foot Ankle 1, 190–224.

Marcus, R., Cann, C., Madvig, P. et al. (1985) Menstrual function and bone mass in élite women distance runners. Ann. Intern. Med. 102, 158–163.

Micheli, L.J. (1983) Overuse injuries in children sports: the growth factor. Orthop. Clin. North Am. 14, 337–360.

Moller, M. (1984) Athletic training and flexibility. A study on range of motion in the lower extremity. Medical Dissertation, Linkoping University, Linkoping, Sweden.

Morehouse, C.A. (1970) Evaluation of knee abduction and adduction, the effects of selected exercise programs on knee stability and its relationship to knee injuries in college football. Project report, Pennsylvania State University, USA.

Nigg, B. (1988) Causes of injuries: extrinsic factors. In: Dirix, A., Knuttgen, H.G. & Tittel, K. (eds) The Olympic Book of Sports Medicine, pp. 363–375. Blackwell Scientific Publications, Oxford.

Paffenbarger, R.S., Hyde, R.T., Wing, A.L. & Hsieh, C. (1986) Physical activity, all-cause mortality, and longevity of college alumni. New Engl. J. Med. 314, 605–613.

Peterson, L. (1970) The cross body block: the major cause of knee injuries. J.A.M.A. 211, 449–452.

Peterson, L. & Renström, P. (1980) Varldsmasterskapen for veteraner – en medicinsk utmaning (Championships for veterans – a medical challenge). Lakartidningen (Stockholm) 77, 3618.

Peterson, L. & Renström, P. (1986) Sports Injuries. Their Prevention and Treatment. Martin Dunitz, London.

Pforringer, W. & Segesser B. (1986) The sports shoe.

Orthopade 15, 260–263.

Renström, P. (1988) Diagnosis and management of overuse injuries. In: Dirix, A., Knuttgen, H.G. & Tittel, K. (eds) The Olympic Book of Sports Medicine, pp. 446–468. Blackwell Scientific Publications, Oxford.

Renström, P. & Johnson, R.J. (1985) Overuse injuries in sports. A review. Sports Med. 2, 316–333.

Renström, P. & Kannus, P. (1991) Chapter 21. In: Strauss, R.H. (ed.) Sports Medicine. W.B. Saunders, Philadelphia.

Rovere, G.D., Clarke, T.J., Yates, C.S. & Burley, K. (1988) Retrospective comparison of taping on ankle stabilizers in preventing ankle injuries. Am. J. Sports Med. 16(3), 228–233.

Ryan, A.J. & Stoner, C.J. (1989) Role of skills and rules in the prevention of sports injuries. In: Ryan, A.J. & Allman Jr, F.L. (eds) Sports Medicine, 2nd edn, pp. 263–278. Academic Press, San Diego, California.

Safran, M., Seaber, A. & Garnett, W. (1989) Warm-up and muscular injury prevention. An update. Sports Med. 8(4), 239–249.

Sandelin, J. (1988) Acute sports injuries: a clinical and epidemiological study. Academic dissertation, Yliopistopaino, Helsinki.

Smith, L.S., Clarke, T.E., Hamill, C.L. & Santopietro, F. (1986) The effects of soft and semi-rigid orthoses upon rear foot movement in running. J. Am. Podiatr. Med. Assoc. 76, 227–233.

Sward, L. (1990) The back of the young top athlete; symptoms, muscle strength, mobility, anthropometric and radiological findings. Thesis, Göteborg, Sweden.

Toom, P.J. den & Schuurman, M.I.M. (1988) Een model voor de berekening van kosten van ongevallen in de privesfeer (English summary). Consumer Safety Institute, Amsterdam.

Torg, J.S., Vegso, J.J., O'Neill, M.J. & Sennett, B. (1990) The epidemiologic, pathologic, biomechanical, and cinematographic analysis of football induced cervical spine trauma. Am. J. Sports Med. 18(1), 50–57.

Tropp, H. (1985) Functional instability of the ankle joint. Medical Dissertation, Linkoping University, Linkoping, Sweden.

Viano, D., King, A., Melvin, J. & Weber, K. (1989) Injury biomechanics research; an essential element in the prevention of trauma. J. Biomech. 22(5), 403–417.

Zarins, B. & Ciullo, J. (1983) Acute muscle and tendon injuries in athletes. Clin. Sports Med. 2(1), 167–182.

Chapter 33

Biochemical Causes of Fatigue and Overtraining

ERIC A. NEWSHOLME, EVA BLOMSTRAND, NEIL McANDREW
AND MARK PARRY-BILLINGS

Introduction

Fatigue is defined physiologically as the inability to maintain power output; to the athlete it is the insuperable need to reduce pace. Experienced athletes should be able to judge their power output so that they finish *just* within limits set by their own susceptibility to fatigue. Training extends the limits but never abolishes them. Fatigue prevents dramatic changes in metabolism that could result in irreversible damage to muscles and even to other organs such as the brain. So what are the causes of fatigue? At the molecular level of the myofibril and the excitation–contraction coupling process, several theories have been put forward. At the next upper level of biochemistry it is possible to suggest metabolic reasons for fatigue. These may be easier for the athlete to understand since they relate to factors such as fuel supply or oxygen provision and there may be simple nutritional means of influencing them.

In general, we consider that there are five main metabolic causes of fatigue in physical activity: the first two causes relate directly to the muscle but the last two, and possibly the last three, involve the brain. This organ may be able to detect changes in the levels of normal constituents of the blood which can then act as a specific signal and increase the *sensitivity* of the runner to fatigue, that is, it makes the runner give up more easily than otherwise.
1 Depletion of phosphocreatine in the muscle.
2 Accumulation of lactic acid in the muscle.
3 Depletion of glycogen in the muscle.
4 Depletion of blood glucose.
5 Increase in the concentration ratio of tryptophan to branched chain amino acids in the blood stream.

To understand fully these causes of fatigue, it is necessary to appreciate the fuels used by muscle and the fuels used in different physical activities. In this chapter we use running races as examples for discussion of both fuels and fatigue. The marathon and ultramarathon races are used as examples of endurance activities which presumably could also include such activities as cycling (the Tour de France is an excellent example of an endurance event) and cross-country skiing; for middle-distance and sprint races, such activities as rowing, canoeing, kayaking and swimming could also be used. The nutritional and metabolic principles that apply to Olympic running events also apply to other activities.

Fuels for the athlete

Energy for the contractile unit in the muscle fibre (the myofibrils) is obtained from the hydrolysis of adenosine triphosphate (ATP) to adenosine diphosphate (ADP) and phosphate. However, the amount of ATP in the muscle is limited: the total amount of ATP in the muscles of the sprinter would support the energy requirement for only 2 s. To continue running, ATP must be regenerated from ADP and phosphate; this occurs due to the oxidation of fuels. Thus ATP is produced in energy-yielding reactions and is utilized in energy-requiring processes: this constitutes the ADP/ATP cycle (Fig. 33.1). Although the chemical details of the use of ATP by muscle and its production in the mitochondria interest many biochemists and physiologists, it is the fuels whose metabolism provides energy for the synthesis of ATP that are of much more relevance to the scientifically interested athlete (Newsholme & Leech, 1983a; 1983b).

This subject appears to be straightforward since only two major fuel reserves exist in the body — carbohydrate and fat, or more specifically glycogen and triglyceride. Glycogen is composed of many thousands of glucose units, polymerized into a gigantic tree-like molecule. The importance of this structure is that it can be *rapidly* broken down to release large numbers of molecules of glucose (glucose-1-phosphate) from the ends of its branches. Most of the glycogen in the body is in the muscles; the precise amount will depend upon the amount of muscle and the previous exercise and dietary history of the person. For the 70-kg man who has rested for 1–2 days and eaten a high carbohydrate diet (at least 70% of the energy intake as carbohydrate) the total musculature should contain about 500 g glycogen. This fuel is used in all track events and is the most important fuel for the athlete.

There is, however, one additional fuel, phosphocreatine, which acts as a short-term buffer for ATP in muscle. It is a particularly important fuel in the 100 and 200-m track events and in sprinting to the tape in other races.

One hundred grams of glycogen is stored in the liver, where its main purpose is to provide glucose to maintain the blood level, for example between meals. A number of tissues require glucose. Paramount among these is the brain which uses about 5 g·h^{-1}. This is supplied from liver glycogen, for example during the overnight fast, and usage of hepatic stores will continue if breakfast is missed. Some of the glucose released from the glycogen in the liver can also be used by muscles; this is particularly important in marathon and ultramarathon runs. But it also means that the main glucose store of the body may be depleted in the marathon runner and especially the ultramarathon runner, which can jeopardize the function of the brain and hence cause fatigue (see below).

Triglyceride is stored in special cells called adipocytes, each of which contains a droplet of triglyceride which occupies almost the whole cell. An adult male may contain 10^{11} such cells. The adipocytes cluster together to form discrete depots of adipose tissue, the primary function of which is to store chemical energy. Compared with glycogen, the quantities of triglyceride stored are large; on average, a 70-kg male stores about 8 kg triglyceride and an average woman of 60 kg stores nearly twice as much. However, to be used by muscle, triglyceride must be hydrolysed in the adipocyte to fatty acids which are released into the blood stream, where they

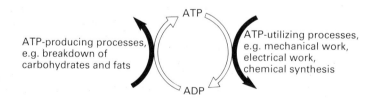

Fig. 33.1 The ATP/ADP cycle. ATP links energy-producing processes to those that require energy. As both take place at the same rate, the concentration of ATP remains constant except for transient periods when, for example, muscle activity increases or decreases. At these times, changes in ATP concentration initiate other changes which modify the rate of ATP generation to match that of utilization.

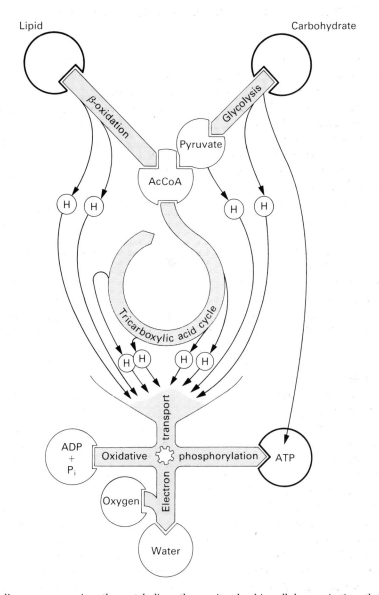

Fig. 33.2 This diagram summarizes the metabolic pathways involved in cellular respiration; these pathways generate ATP, using energy made available through the oxidation of fuels. The central feature is a series of reactions known as oxidative phosphorylation, in which ATP is made from ADP and phosphate (Pi), using energy provided by the electron transfer pathway. In this pathway, reducing equivalents, denoted H, are oxidized by oxygen to form water and at the same time regenerate the oxidizing agent needed for further fuel breakdown. Reducing equivalents, mostly in the form of the molecule NADH, are produced as a result of triglyceride and carbohydrate breakdown. The pathways involved each consist of a series of reactions catalysed by enzymes. The pathway of triglyceride breakdown, known as β-oxidation, results in the splitting of long fatty acid molecules into short acetate units. These become temporarily attached to a coenzyme A 'handle' to form acetyl coenzyme A (AcCoA) which enters the tricarboxylic acid (Krebs) cycle. In this cyclic sequence of reactions, the acetate group is transferred to an acceptor and is oxidized to yield more reducing equivalents and to release carbon dioxide. The acceptor then picks up another acetate unit and the process continues. Through operation of the pathway known as glycolysis, carbohydrates (glucose and glycogen) are also broken down to produce acetyl coenzyme A. As well as contributing reducing equivalents, this glycolysis also produces a little ATP directly. This is of vital importance under anaerobic conditions, when lack of oxygen precludes operation of the electron transfer pathway.

are carried to the muscle bound to albumin. This causes a serious limitation for the athlete (see below).

In summary, the athlete has two main fuel tanks. A small one containing glycogen can be mobilized and used very rapidly and a much larger one containing fat can be utilized more slowly. These equip humans with fuel reserves for a very wide range of physical activities, from short periods of explosive effort to prolonged endurance events. The important question for the athlete is how far these stores of fuel limit performance. Can any limitation be overcome by diet and/or training?

Converting fuel into ATP

Glucose, glucose-contained-in-glycogen or fatty acid, can be oxidized to carbon dioxide and water to release energy in the cell. This conversion is achieved by the action of a large number of enzymes working sequentially (Fig. 33.2). Since it requires oxygen, the process is known as aerobic metabolism. Of importance to the athlete, the pathway for glycogen oxidation can be divided into two separate sequences and the initial part can be used to generate ATP anaerobically. The first 12 or so steps of glucose metabolism produce a compound known as pyruvate which, when oxygen is available, enters the mitochondria for complete oxidation to carbon dioxide and water by the Krebs cycle and the electron transfer chain. However, in the absence, or at a very low concentration, of oxygen the pyruvate is converted into lactic acid, a process known as glycolysis. The significance of this process is enormous since the oxygen supply can be a major factor limiting the performance of most athletes during both competition and intense training. Although the flow of blood to the muscles during exercise is increased dramatically, it is logistically impossible to deliver enough oxygen to the muscles to support a high aerobic power output. Anaerobic glycolysis can *then* be used, in addition to the aerobic process (the Krebs cycle plus electron transfer

process) to generate more ATP. But there is a price to pay.

First, the amount of ATP that can be generated anaerobically in comparison with that generated aerobically is quite small, less than 10%: three molecules of ATP are produced from ADP as one glucose molecule in glycogen is converted to lactic acid, whereas 39 are produced if the same glucose molecule was converted to carbon dioxide and water. But in muscle (even in aerobically trained subjects) the activities of the enzymes that catalyse the reactions of glycolysis are so great that this more than compensates for the reduced 'efficiency'. Thus the rate of ATP generation from glycolysis can be very high, with a high power output (Table 33.1). However, this can for only a very short time be sustained, because glycogen is used at a very rapid rate and this fuel store would be rapidly depleted, resulting in fatigue.

Second, whereas aerobic metabolism produces the relatively innocuous carbon dioxide and water as end products, anaerobic metabolism produces lactate plus protons, and the protons can be dangerous. The accumulation of protons in a muscle rapidly decreases its pH: a decrease in pH > 1.0 unit (i.e. a > 10-fold increase in proton concentration) jeopardizes the biochemical life of the cell. The change of pH normally restricts the sprint more than the amount of glycogen in the muscle. The latter *could* support near-maximal sprinting for 1000 m, but this is not possible due to the damage which a decrease in pH would cause in the muscle. Fatigue occurs well before 1000 m have been covered.

Anaerobic metabolism is important for all track events. This is because aerobic and anaerobic processes are not mutually exclusive: in track events longer than 100 or 200 m, both processes are used. Complete oxidation of glycogen (aerobic metabolism) and glycogen conversion to lactic acid (anaerobic metabolism) both play a role in generating energy to satisfy the power output. But the proportion of aerobic and anaerobic metabolism occurring in each event differs (Table 33.2). It is, in part, the

Table 33.1 Calculated maximum rates of ATP formation in human muscle, based on maximal activities of key indicator enzymes under aerobic and anaerobic conditions.

| Group | Sex | Calculated maximum rate of ATP formation from glucose or glycogen (μmol·min^{-1}·g^{-1} fresh weight at 25°C) | |
		Anaerobic glycolysis	Oxidation via Krebs cycle
Untrained	Male	104	13
	Female	87	16
Medium trained	Male	91	21
	Female	89	19
Well trained	Male	72	26
	Female	61	29

Maximum rates of ATP formation are calculated as follows: for anaerobic glycolysis 6-phosphofructokinase activity is multiplied by 3; for oxidation by the Krebs cycle, oxoglutarate dehydrogenase activity is multiplied by 18. Enzyme activity data from Blomstrand *et al.* (1986). It is well established that the capacity for anaerobic glycolysis is decreased by endurance training but the significance and value of this response is unknown.

trade-off between aerobic and anaerobic metabolism that makes middle-distance running such a skilled activity. On the basis of the information given in Table 33.2, and other information, a suggestion is given of the fuels that are used to provide ATP in various events (Table 33.3).

Metabolic causes of fatigue

Examination of world sprint records indicates that fatigue occurs very early in these events, even for Olympic champions. This fatigue is due, we believe, to a depletion of a fuel found in each muscle fibre — phosphocreatine. A

Table 33.2 Proportion of ATP derived from aerobic metabolism in various events and suggested causes of fatigue.

Event (metres)	Percentage of ATP derived from aerobic metabolism*	Possible major causes of fatigue
100	0	Phosphocreatine depletion
200	10	Phosphocreatine depletion
400	25 }	Phosphocreatine depletion and H$^+$ accumulation
800	50 }	
1500	65	H$^+$ accumulation
5000	87 }	
10 000	97 }	Glycogen depletion
Marathon	100 }	

* It should be noted that these values are 'guesstimates' based on available biochemical information and they will undoubtedly vary from athlete to athlete.

Table 33.3 An estimate of percentage contribution of various fuels to ATP generation in different events.

	Percentage contribution to ATP generation				
		Glycogen		Blood glucose	Triglyceride
Event (metres)	Phosphocreatine	Anaerobic	Aerobic	(liver glycogen)	(fatty acids)
100	50	50	—	—	—
200	25	65	10	—	—
400	12.5	62.5	25	—	—
800	*	50	50	—	—
1500	*	25	75	—	—
5000	*	12.5	87.5	—	—
10 000	*	3	97	—	—
Marathon	—	—	75	5	20
Ultramarathon (84 km)	—	—	35	5	60
24-h race	—	—	10	2	88

* In these events phosphocreatine is used for the first few seconds and, if it has been resynthesized during the race, in the sprint to the tape.

best time for the 200-m race cannot be predicted simply by doubling the best time for the 100-m race, since the 100-m race includes an acceleration phase which does not occur in the second 100 m of the 200-m race. What we need is a time for the best 'flying' 100 m, and this is then added to the 100-m record. Carl Lewis's achievement in the 1984 Los Angeles Olympics provides the necessary data since he clocked 8.91 s in his leg of the 100-m relay; this is 100 m with the acceleration period largely removed. Adding this to Ben Johnson's unofficial world record for the 100 m gives a best possible predicted time of 18.84 s, nearly a whole second ahead of the current world record for 200 m. It should be noted that this fatigue does not result in a dramatic decrease in performance — it causes about a 10% decrease in power output — but this is sufficient to cause a potential victor to finish last in the 200-m race. This knowledge is, therefore, of the utmost importance to the sprinter. The scientific evidence that the fatigue can be caused by phosphocreatine comes from the work of E. Hultman. Electrical stimulation of the muscle of volunteers (to avoid any fatigue due to the brain) decreased power output very quickly and the loss of function occurred in

concert with a decrease in phosphocreatine levels (Hultman & Sjoholm, 1986). This suggests that the maximal power output in sprinting can only be achieved if both anaerobic glycolysis and phosphocreatine are used for ATP generation. When phosphocreatine stores are depleted, the power output must fall by about 10% since glycolysis cannot provide enough ATP to satisfy the maximal rate of ATP utilization by muscle (Table 33.2). Anything that preserves or increases the phosphocreatine level in muscle is important to the sprinter. Power training may increase the level of phosphocreatine slightly and rest for 10–20 min before the sprint event may be important in restoration of levels after warming up.

Protons in muscle

Lactate and protons (not lactic acid as most textbooks suggest) are produced from the anaerobic breakdown of glycogen. When the athletics commentator describes the sprint to the tape by saying that the athlete finishes in 'a sea of lactic acid', this is not strictly chemically correct — it is 'a sea of protons'. The problem with protons is that they can associate with bases to produce acids. The 'bases' in question are the enzymes that carry out all the chemical reactions in cells. Enzymes are proteins and as such bear a number of basic (as well as acidic) groups. Indeed their catalytic activity depends on such groups. Some of these key basic groups disappear when they acquire protons, so that they perform much less well as catalysts. Larger increases in protons can destroy their three-dimensional structure permanently.

Precisely how acidity causes fatigue is not known, but the mechanism of fatigue is of less importance to the athlete than how to overcome or, more correctly, to delay it. One answer to the 'proton problem' lies in buffers which mop-up protons by combining with them as follows:

$$Buffer^- + H^+ \rightarrow Buffer-H$$

The problem for the athlete is that there is a limited amount of buffering capacity within the muscle, enough to absorb protons for only about 10−15 s of maximal sprinting. But in addition to buffering in muscle, protons can leave the muscle, probably in the form of lactic acid. This dissociates into lactate and a proton in the blood stream; once in the blood, the protons encounter a much larger buffering system, that based on the hydrogen carbonate ion. This absorbs protons according to the equation:

$$HCO_3^- + H^+ \rightarrow H_2CO_3 \rightarrow CO_2 + H_2O$$

The beauty of the hydrogen carbonate buffer is that the carbonic acid decomposes into water and carbon dioxide, and carbon dioxide is then lost from the body via the lungs. This allows more carbonic acid to form and so extends the buffering capacity. An increase in blood acidity stimulates the rate of breathing so that yet more carbon dioxide is lost. The main source of hydrogen carbonate ion in the blood is the kidney, so that the kidney and lungs between them operate a push−pull system to rid the body of excess acid (protons). This, to a large extent, is what happens in track races longer than 100−200 m. One means of trying to improve the performance of 400-m sprinters, for example, is to ingest a solution of sodium bicarbonate before the event in order to increase the buffer capacity (this is known as 'soda loading'). There is some evidence that this does improve sprinting performance (Jones et al., 1977; Sutton et al., 1981). But the side-effects can be dramatic — vomiting and diarrhoea! It may also contravene the 'doping' regulations.

For the athlete, the efficacy of the buffering system in the blood depends on just how quickly protons escape from muscles into the blood. Thus, improving the blood supply to the muscle not only provides more oxygen for aerobic metabolism (improving the efficiency of ATP generation) but also allows lactic acid to escape rapidly from the muscle into the blood stream for better buffering. This allows 'extra energy' to be produced from anaerobic metabolism. This is important in middle-distance running since power output is limited by oxygen availability (Tables 33.2 and 33.3).

Muscle glycogen levels

From the above discussion we can see that in distances longer than 100 or 200 m a compromise is possible between the aerobic and anaerobic systems within the muscle. The blood that flows through the muscle not only provides oxygen for the much more efficient complete oxidation of glycogen (i.e. more ATP is produced) but the protons produced from anaerobic glycolysis can readily escape into the blood stream (as lactic acid) and be carried away from the muscle into the blood stream where they will be buffered and effectively lost to the body as carbon dioxide (see above). Hence the athlete can use the aerobic system towards its maximum capacity and further ATP can be produced from the anaerobic glycolysis. So what causes fatigue in this situation? The answer is either the amount of glycogen in the muscle or the accumulation of protons in the muscle. If the rate of anaerobic conversion of glycogen to lactate is greater than the capacity to lose lactic acid from the muscle, protons will accumulate to cause fatigue as in the 400-m sprinter. But even if the protons can be lost from the muscle, a high rate of anaerobic metabolism could also rapidly result in fatigue due to depletion of muscle glycogen. Anaerobic metabolism normally provides about 3% of the energy in a 10-km race, but it consumes almost one third of the glycogen store. If an athlete increases the pace, a greater emphasis on anaerobic metabolism would lead to glycogen depletion and hence fatigue well before the end of the event.

The balance of aerobic/anaerobic energy generation will vary from athlete to athlete but the following factors play a role: (i) the fibre composition of the athlete's muscle; (ii) the blood supply to the muscle; (iii) the pace at which the athlete runs; and (iv) the distance of the event.

The importance of glycogen as a fuel for both aerobic and anaerobic metabolism in middle-distance running emphasizes the need to maintain the level of this fuel in the muscle before each training event and before the competition itself. This demands sensible nutrition for each athlete: diets must contain a very high proportion of the energy as carbohydrate (at least 60% of the energy should be carbohydrate; Costill & Miller, 1980; see Chapter 12).

An understanding of evidence for the role of depletion of glycogen in causing fatigue requires consideration of the limit for rates of fatty acid oxidation by muscle. When a muscle runs out of glycogen, why is it not possible to switch to fat as a fuel and maintain the power output of the muscles and hence the pace? Because the store of fat is enormous, this would delay fatigue in, for example, the marathon dramatically. The marathon pace could then be maintained for several days! Why is this not possible?

Let us assume that the energy required for maximum sprinting speed could be produced sufficiently rapidly from complete aerobic metabolism. How long would muscle glycogen last? The answer is about 40 min. (This rate of ATP utilization for maximum sprinting is 3

$\mu mol \cdot s^{-1} \cdot g^{-1}$ wet muscle. For aerobic metabolism, this will require $3/36$ $\mu mol \cdot s^{-1} \cdot g^{-1}$ glycogen untilization; 200 $\mu mol \cdot g^{-1}$ glycogen is present in muscle, so this will last for $200 \div 3/36$ s or 40 min.) But we know that the running speed in the marathon is just about 50% of maximum sprinting speed (i.e. about 5 $m \cdot s^{-1}$). This means that the use of muscle glycogen as a fuel would be extended to about 80 min. This is further extended by the ability to use glycogen stored in the liver (about 100 g) via blood glucose, which could provide energy for another 20 min of marathon running. Hence the total energy from glycogen stores would be about 100 min or about 75% of the time required to run the marathon. It might be possible to increase the muscle glycogen content further by dietary manipulation (see Chapter 12), but the glycogen content taken for these calculations is probably close to maximal, so that we could guess that glycogen will provide aerobic fuel for no more than 80% of the marathon. Hence the marathon can be run only if there is another fuel to supplement the glycogen — that is fat, in the form of fatty acids in the blood.

Fatigue in the marathon occurs long before all the fat is consumed because fatty acid oxidation alone cannot support the high rate of energy production required by the athlete. It can satisfy only about 50% of the maximum (the maximum aerobic capacity, not the maximum total capacity). This means that when the glycogen stores are depleted in the muscles of the runner, the pace must fall by about 50%; for an élite marathon runner this will mean a drop in pace to just above a fast walking pace! The probable limiting factor for ATP formation from the oxidation of fatty acids is their rate of uptake by the muscle. Fatty acids are available in the blood stream but, unlike glucose, they are almost insoluble in the aqueous medium of the plasma. Hence, they are transported in the blood in association with a plasma protein, albumin. This means that the free concentration of fatty acids in the plasma (i.e. that not bound to albumin) is very low; but it is this free concentration that governs the rate of diffusion of fatty acids from the blood stream into the muscle. The rate of diffusion of fatty acids across the interstitial space from capillaries to muscle fibre probably limits the rate of ATP generation when fatty acids are the major fuel. This re-emphasizes the importance of using both glycogen and fatty acids in the marathon. Although some fatty acid may be made available within the muscle from stored triacylglycerol, the rate at which this can provide ATP is limited by the capacity of the β-oxidation system in the mitochondria.

It is likely that élite marathon runners obtain most of their energy (perhaps > 80%) from the oxidation of glycogen and < 20% from fat; but the percentage of fat oxidation will not be fixed at 20% throughout the entire race. It will start at close to zero and will probably increase towards 50% as the glycogen stores are used up. However, it is vitally important that the athlete does not run out of glycogen before the end of the race. This precise balance between use of carbohydrate and fat can only be 'learnt' by experience of running long distances — one of the reasons, perhaps, why the marathon runner must include at least one long training run (30+ km) each week during 'peak' training. The specific pieces of evidence in support of this hypothesis are as follows (see Newsholme & Leech, 1983b):

1 If carbohydrate stores of the body are depleted, for example by feeding subjects a high fat diet for 3 days before exercise, a given level of exercise produces exhaustion considerably more quickly than for subjects on a normal diet and especially in comparison to those on a high carbohydrate diet.

2 If the carbohydrate store in the muscle is elevated, a given level of exercise can be maintained for a longer period of time.

3 If the fatty acid concentration in the blood is artificially elevated before exercise, a given intensity of exercise can be maintained for a longer period of time: this manipulation ensures that the plasma fatty acid concentration is elevated at the beginning of exercise rather than 30 min or more later.

4 In élite ultradistance runners, running for 24 h, the power output declined towards 50% of $\dot{V}_{O_2 max}$ during the race, while the respiratory exchange ratio decreased to about 0.7 indicating mainly lipid oxidation (Davies & Thompson, 1979; Noakes, 1986). This suggests that, even in élite distance runners, lipid oxidation could only provide perhaps about 50% of the energy required for maximum power output towards the end of the event.

5 P. Cerretelli (personal communication) has investigated the $\dot{V}_{O_2 max}$ of a patient with muscle 6-phosphofructokinase deficiency. The rate of glucose oxidation would be minimal in the patient so that fatty acid oxidation would provide all the energy; Cerretelli found that the $\dot{V}_{O_2 max}$ was approximately 60% of that which he would expect from other physiological characteristics of the patient.

Blood glucose level

Ultramarathon runners are able to mobilize and utilize fatty acids to provide the energy to run continuously for many hours. During this time, their oxygen consumption gradually falls to about 50% of their maximum aerobic power. This corresponds to a complete dependence on fatty acids once their glycogen reserves are exhausted. The limited store of glycogen in muscle explains why it is not possible for the same athletes to run from London to Brighton (87 km) at the same pace as the London marathon (42 km): there is a much greater dependence on fatty acid oxidation in the longer runs.

In such long runs, it becomes important that blood glucose is strictly conserved for the brain (which can use no other fuel under these circumstances). Thus an important characteristic of ultradistance runners (and presumably one that is enhanced by training) is their ability to prevent high rates of utilization of glucose, transported from liver to muscle in the blood. Nevertheless, hypoglycaemia remains a major hazard. To avoid this, it is advantageous for the ultramarathon runner to take glucose or other carbohydrate-containing drinks, especially in the later stages of the race (Noakes, 1986; see Chapter 30).

What causes the fatigue due to hypoglycaemia? Although the muscle may well be involved, it would appear that fatigue in such events can also be due to the brain. This latter form of fatigue is generally known as *central fatigue*. The brain interprets the decrease in blood glucose level as a danger signal and steps are taken to decrease power output. The fatigue, however, may be quite different from that which occurs in a 400-m sprint, when the muscles will simply not carry out the high demands for power output and the pace slows. In central fatigue, the runner finds it progressively harder mentally to maintain the power output: the perceived effort, becomes progressively greater so that only the tough — mentally and physiologically — can perform such feats of endurance.

Amino acids and fatigue

One important role of some amino acids is that they act as precursors for certain brain neurotransmitters, the chemicals that carry out specific messenger roles in the brain. One of these amino acids is tryptophan, which is converted in the brain to a neurotransmitter known as 5-hydroxytryptamine (5-HT). There is evidence that tiredness and sleep may be, in part, influenced by the brain level of 5-HT; it is possible, therefore, that this neurotransmitter may be involved in central fatigue.

There are two important additional facts. First, branched chain amino acids (leucine, isoleucine and valine) are not taken up by liver but they are used by muscle primarily for energy formation; their rate of oxidation is increased during exercise (Wagenmakers *et al.*, 1989). Second, both branched chain amino acids and tryptophan enter the brain upon the same amino acid carrier. Hence there is competition between the two types of amino acids for entry into brain.

A decrease in the level of branched chain amino acids (leucine, isoleucine and valine) in the blood, due to an increased rate of utilization by muscle, will increase the ratio of tryptophan to branched chain amino acids in the blood stream and favour the entry of tryptophan into the brain. This will increase the rate of formation of 5-HT and hence increase the level of this neurotransmitter in the brain (Fig. 33.3). This could result in fatigue originating in the brain. As with hypoglycaemia, it might make the mental effort to maintain the pace of running that much more difficult. The blood level of fatty acids may play an additional role in this type of fatigue. Tryptophan is unique amongst the amino acids in that it is bound to plasma albumin; it exists as a bound and a free form which are in equilibrium. This equilibrium is changed in favour of free tryptophan by fatty acids, which also bind to albumin. Thus an increase in the plasma fatty acid level above about 1 mM increases the free concentration of tryptophan, and it is probable that the free concentration rather than the total concentration of tryptophan influences the rate of entry of tryptophan into the brain. Hence an increase in the plasma fatty acid level plus a decrease in that of branched chain amino acids could markedly influence the plasma concentration ratio of free tryptophan to branched chain amino acids. This has been shown to be the case in endurance activity, particularly in the marathon (Blomstrand *et al.*, 1988) (Table 33.4). Animal experiments have shown that the concentration of 5-HT is increased in two areas of the brain after endurance exercise (Blomstrand *et al.*, 1989; Barry-Pillings *et al.*, 1990).

It seems likely that muscle will use branched chain amino acids for energy when its glycogen level becomes depleted. Similarly, it is possible that as the glycogen level falls, the blood level of fatty acids will increase above 1 mM and hence influence the plasma level of free tryptophan. Thus the fatigue that is caused by the depletion of muscle glycogen could be due to an increase in the level of 5-HT in a specific area of the brain. Failure of the motor centre to

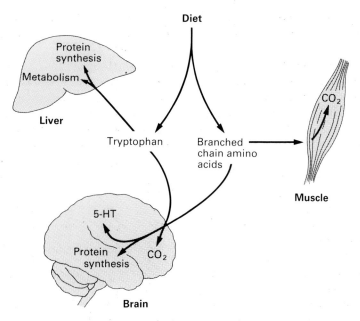

Fig. 33.3 The interrelationships between muscle, liver and brain in relation to metabolism of branched chain amino acids and tryptophan. Most amino acids are metabolized in the liver, except for the branched chain amino acids valine, leucine and isoleucine, which are taken up and may be oxidized by muscle. Branched chain amino acids and tryptophan are both taken up by the brain. Competition occurs between amino acids for a single type of carrier to transport them from the blood into brain cells. Exercise can lower the blood concentrations of branched chain amino acids since these amino acids are oxidized by muscle. Consequently, the competition for the entry of tryptophan into the brain will be decreased and the rate of uptake of this amino acid into the brain will increase, resulting in a faster rate of manufacture and hence in higher concentrations of the neurotransmitter 5-hydroxytryptamine (5-HT); this *may* result in central fatigue.

stimulate muscle would necessitate a fall of power output; fatigue would be due to a change in the balance of concentrations of key amino acids in the blood but initiated by a large fall in the muscle glycogen level!

The overtraining syndrome

A syndrome is a set of symptoms that occur together, usually, it is assumed, as a consequence of one underlying cause. The term is legitimately applied to overtraining (Table 33.5).

Exercise elicits a 'stress' response and results in a degree of short-term fatigue, from which the athlete recovers. If exercise is performed on a regular basis, *adaptation* occurs and the athlete's performance improves. This is the *training* effect. However, if exercise periods are too frequent, too intense and/or too prolonged, recovery after each exercise bout is not complete; less adaptation and hence less improvement in performance occurs. If continued, this can lead to a decrease in performance. This is the overtrained state.

The overtraining syndrome is a complex clinical condition, which has been described not only in human athletes, but also in racehorses. The mechanism responsible may be involved in other conditions of stress; some of the symptoms of athletic overtraining have been reported, for example, in stressed business-people or students taking exams.

The overtraining syndrome can be caused by too much exercise: it can also be caused by a combination of too much exercise with some other form of stress (Kuipers & Keizer, 1988).

Table 33.4   Plasma concentrations of fatty acids, branched chain amino acids and tryptophan before and after the Stockholm marathon.

Conditions	Plasma concentrations (µM)				
	Fatty acids	Branched chain amino acids	Tryptophan Total	Free	Ratio of free tryptophan: branched chain amino acids
Before the run	350	470	55	7·7	1.6
After the run	1550*	380*	57	18.0*	4·7

* Indicates $p < 0.001$ as compared with the pre-exercise value (Student's t test). Data from Blomstrand *et al.* (1988).

There is considerable interindividual variability with regard to the development of overtraining. Verma *et al.* (1978) put a group of 15 male subjects through a common training programme with the result that 10 subjects improved and five became overtrained. What determines the variability in susceptibility to this condition is not known. There is, however, a possible common mechanism to account for many of the signs and symptoms of overtraining which might explain this variability.

Table 33.5   Some signs and symptoms of the overtraining syndrome. From Noakes (1986).

Increased early morning heart rate
Slow recovery of heart rate after exercise
Postural hypotension
Increased resting blood pressure
Slow return of blood pressure to basal after exercise
Fall in haematocrit
Decreased performance
Amenorrhoea
Decreased $V_{O_2 max}$
Weight loss
Increased incidence of infections
Poor healing of wounds
Loss of libido
Disturbed sleep
Decreased appetite
Depression
Loss of drive and enthusiasm
Increased fluid intake at night
Muscle and joint pains: heavy leggedness
Increased serum creatine phosphokinase activity

The imbalanced amino acid hypothesis

It is proposed that excessive exercise can alter chronically the balance between the plasma concentrations of branched chain amino acids and free tryptophan. As explained above this could lead to chronic increases in the levels of tryptophan and 5-HT in the brain and peripheral nerve cells. This chronic change in the plasma concentration may be caused by a prolonged increase in the rate of use of branched chain amino acids by muscle and perhaps an elevation in the plasma fatty acid level. Could this lead to behavioural changes other than and in addition to the fatigue described above?

CENTRAL 5-HT AND THE OVERTRAINING SYNDROME

5-HT-containing cells occur in several large clusters in the pons and upper medulla in the central nervous system, within groups of cells known as the raphe nuclei. Projections from these cells pass rostrally to most areas of the brain via the medial forebrain bundle: the cortex, hippocampus, limbic system and hypothalamus all receive 5-HT terminals (Rang & Dale, 1987). Projections from the caudal nuclei run to the medulla and spinal cord. With such wide-ranging projections to areas involved in motor, neuroendocrine and 'emotive' functions, interpretation of changes in levels of 5-HT is difficult, but prolonged changes in the concentration of this neurotransmitter in these areas of the brain could account for the wide-ranging effects of overtraining (Table 33.5).

The physiological functions of 5-HT in the brain can be grouped into three areas: sleep, wakefulness and mood; motoneuron excitability; autonomic and endocrine function.

Sleep: Lesions in the raphe nuclei or the administration of *p*-chlorophenylalanine, an inhibitor of the synthesis of 5-HT, abolish sleep in animals; the microinjection of 5-HT in specific medullary areas of the brain induces sleep.

Motoneuron excitability: Descending 5-HT neurons increase motoneuron excitability and in so doing increase monosynaptic reflexes and decrease polysynaptic reflexes. Inhibition of polysynaptic reflexes may include those involved in exercise such as running and may contribute to the decreased maximal work capacity in the overtrained state.

Autonomic and endocrine: From the medulla oblongata (brainstem) 5-HT neurons project to the hypothalamus which is considered to be the major centre for autonomic, endocrine and neuronal integration. Rang and Dale (1987) observed that 5-HT inhibits the release from the hypothalamus of factors that control the rate of release of pituitary hormones. A low rate of secretion of gonadotrophin releasing hormone (GnRH) by the hypothalamus would decrease the rate of release of luteinizing hormone (LH) and follicle stimulating hormone (FSH) from the pituitary: this would in turn decrease the plasma levels of LH and FSH. Nash (1987) has reported a decrease in the secretion of LH in overtrained humans. This would be expected to lower the rate of testosterone synthesis and release, with a subsequent decline in plasma levels of testosterone. In the female, such a decrease would interfere in the complex endocrine system that controls the menstrual cycle and could thus lead to irregular menses or amenorrhoea. Lightman and Everitt (1986) provide some evidence to suggest that 5-HT

plays a role in GnRH rhythmicity; the latter is inhibited by high levels of 5-HT, and if central levels of 5-HT are elevated pharmacologically, the preovulatory LH surge is lost and amenorrhoea develops.

Lesions in the ventromedial hypothalamus, which decreases the level of 5-HT, lead to hyperphagia. Hence an elevation in the level of 5-HT could explain the loss of appetite in overtrained subjects.

PERIPHERAL 5-HT AND THE OVERTRAINING SYNDROME

Similar considerations regarding entry of tryptophan and its conversion pathway to 5-HT apply to peripheral nerves (Rang & Dale, 1987). Hence peripheral 5-HT levels could be elevated in the overtrained state. 5-HT stimulates sympathetic afferent nerves in the heart which would cause an increase in heart rate, a well-established sign of overtraining. In contrast, 5-HT inhibits noradrenaline release from sympathetic nerve endings on blood vessels; this would be expected to have a general vasodilatory effect and could explain changes in blood pressure in the overtrained state.

Conclusion

An increase in the level of 5-HT in the brain and in some peripheral nerves and tissues could explain many of the signs and symptoms of overtraining. But why should an increase in intensity or duration of exercise above normal lead, over a short period of time, to a change in 5-HT in nerves and perhaps other cells? The mechanism might be as simple as a disturbance in the normal plasma amino acid concentration balance, in particular an increase in the ratio of plasma free tryptophan to branched chain amino acids. In addition, the immunosuppression that occurs in overtraining (Keast *et al.*, 1988), with the resultant increase in risk from upper respiratory tract infections may be due to a decrease in the plasma concentration of another amino acid, glutamine. If this hypothesis is correct, many of the problems of over-training could be overcome by ingestion of sufficient branched chain amino acids to restore the plasma concentration ratio to normal, and sufficient glutamine or glutamine peptides to restore this level to normal. Experiments to test this hypothesis are currently in progress.

References

Blomstrand, E., Celsing, F. & Newsholme, E.A. (1988) Changes in plasma concentrations of aromatic and branched chain amino acids during sustained exercise in man and their possible role in fatigue. *Acta Physiol. Scand.* **133**, 115–121.

Blomstrand, E., Ekblom, B. & Newsholme, E.A. (1986) Maximum activities of key glycolytic and oxidative enzymes in human muscle from differently trained individuals. *J. Physiol.* **381**, 111–118.

Blomstrand, E., Perrett, D., Parry-Billings, M. & Newsholme, E.A. (1989) Effect of sustained exercise on plasma amino acid concentrations and on 5-HT tryptamine metabolism in six different brain regions in the rat. *Acta Physiol. Scand.* **136**, 473–481.

Costill, D.L. & Miller, J.M. (1980) Nutrition for endurance sport: carbohydrate and fluid balance. *Int. J. Sports Med.* **1**, 2–14.

Davies, C.T.M. & Thompson, M.W. (1979) Aerobic performance of female marathon and male ultra-marathon athletes. *Eur. J. Appl. Physiol.* **41**, 233–245.

Hultman, E. & Sjoholm, H. (1986). Biochemical cause of fatigue. In: Jones, N.L., McCarney, N. & McComas, A.J. (eds) *Human Muscle Power*, pp. 215–238. Human Kinetics, Champaign, Illinois.

Jones, N.L., Sutton, J.R., Taylor, R. & Toews, C.J. (1977) Effects of pH on cardiorespiratory and metabolic responses to exercise. *J. Appl. Physiol.* **43**, 959–964.

Keast, D., Cameron, K. & Morton, A.R. (1988). Exercise and the immune response. *Sports Med.* **5**, 248–267.

Kuipers, H. & Keizer, H.A. (1988) Overtraining in elite athletes; review and directions for the future. *Sports Med.* **6**, 79–92.

Lightman, S.L. & Everitt, B.J. (1986) *Neuroendocrinology*. Blackwell Scientific Publications, Oxford.

Nash, H.L. (1987) Can exercise suppress reproductive hormones in men? *Phys. Sports Med.* **15**(1), 180–189.

Newsholme, E.A. & Leech, A.R. (1983a) *The Runner: Energy and Endurance*. Oxford Books, Somerton, Oxford.

Newsholme, E.A. & Leech, A.R. (1983b) *Biochemistry for the Medical Sciences*. John Wiley, Chichester.

Noakes, T. (1986) *Lore of Running*. Oxford University Press, Cape Town.

Parry-Billings, M., Blomstrand, E., McAndrew, N. & Newsholme, E.A (1990) A communication link between skeletal muscle, brain and cells of the immune system. *Int. J. Sports Med.* **11**, S122–S128.

Rang, H.P. & Dale, M.M. (1987) *Pharmacology*. Churchill, Livingstone, London.

Sutton, J.R., Jones, N.L. & Toews, C.J. (1981) Effect of pH on muscle glycolysis during exercise. *Clin. Sci. Mol. Med.* **6**, 331–338.

Verma, S.K., Makindroo, S.R. & Kansal, D.K. (1978) Effect of four weeks of hard physical training on certain physiological and morphological parameters of basketball players. *J. Sports Med.* **18**, 379–384.

Wagenmakers, A.J.M., Brookes, J.H., Coakley, J.H., Reilly, T. & Edwards, R.H.T. (1989). Exercise-induced activation of the branched-chain 2-oxo-acid dehydrogenase in human muscle. *Eur. J. Appl. Physiol.* **59**, 159–167.

Chapter 34

Reversible Reproductive Changes with Endurance Training

JERILYNN C. PRIOR

Introduction

In the past 20 years there has been an explosion of information about the interrelationships between exercise and reproduction, particularly in women. The pendulum has swung from a total lack of attention to any effect of athletics on reproduction (except the notion that women must be protected from exertion), to the belief that strenuous exercise causes disease states such as amenorrhoea, osteoporosis and stress fractures. In contrast, very little attention has been paid to the reproductive changes occurring in men with exercise training.

Data which are methodologically valid (for studies of dynamic, steady state endocrine systems, this means data from prospective clinical trials) indicate that *both* men and women experience reproductive adaptations to the metabolic and hormonal demands of endurance exercise training. Furthermore, data suggest that any reproductive changes related to exercise are *always reversible*.

This chapter reviews the evidence that exercise is *causally* related to reproductive change in men and women. Rather than simply cataloguing data from numerous cross-sectional reports, the review seeks to place the compiled evidence in a critical, scientific framework, using an epidemiological approach. This approach is necessary because research on exercise and reproductive function may be biased by one's view of gender roles and sexuality, both of which are culturally defined as well as biologically related. To decrease this potential bias, only prospective data from clearly defined populations will be used as evidence in this analysis.

Evidence for a causal association between exercise and changes in reproductive fuction

What scientific data are necessary before the conclusion can be drawn that exercise *causes* reproductive change? What will we consider a reproductive *change*? The answer to the second question, obviously, hinges on what we define as normal. For women, cyclic menstrual flow at intervals of 21–36 days is considered normal (Abraham, 1978). In clinical practice, the assumption is made that such a 'regular' cycle is an ovulatory cycle and further documentation of ovulation is omitted. However, recent studies show that the major changes in reproduction, in sedentary as well as exercise-training women, involve changes in *ovulation* (Prior *et al.*, 1988). Entry criteria for potential women subjects in a study of exercise-related menstrual cycle changes, at a minimum, would require documentation of premenstrual molimina in addition to monthly flow before subjects could be considered normal.

Therefore, a careful preselection of volunteers for exercise-training studies would require that women subjects have normal ovulatory function before study entry, and that men have normal gonadal function and semen quality. In

365

addition, Sackett (1981) has outlined eight epidemiological questions that must be answered affirmatively before causality is confirmed:

1 Is there evidence from human experiments?
2 How strong is the association?
3 Do other investigators consistently find the same results?
4 Is there a dose−response gradient?
5 Does the association make epidemiological sense?
6 Is the association biologically sensible?
7 Is the association specific?
8 Is the relationship analogous to other, well-accepted relationships?

The first of the epidemiological criteria for causality has been met for women, and probably for men. Clear evidence from prospective, observational or experimental studies documents that reproductive changes occur with training in ovulatory women. The initial change is a decrease in premenstrual symptoms (molimina or observable post-ovulatory physical and emotional changes), especially decreases in fluid retention and breast tenderness (Prior et al., 1987). These decreasing premenstrual symptoms occur both in sedentary women

who begin a mild exercise programme (Fig. 34.1) and in ovulatory runners training for a marathon (Fig. 34.2).

Prospective exercise-training studies in women have shown varying degrees of suppression of ovulatory function during increased training (Shangold et al., 1979; Bonen et al., 1981; Prior et al., 1982a; 1982b; Bullen et al., 1985; Ronkainen et al., 1985). The menstrual cycle may remain ovulatory, with a shortened luteal phase (Shangold et al., 1979; Prior et al., 1982a; 1982b), or it may become anovulatory (Prior et al., 1982a; 1982b) with a normal cycle interval. A population of sedentary women followed prospectively also demonstrated a similar variability in ovulatory function (Prior et al., 1990a).

If prospective training studies in women document changes in ovulatory function, do these studies also document the development of amenorrhoea (in other words, loss of flow for ≥6 months)? The answer is no. Although hundreds of articles imply amenorrhoea is caused by sport or exercise participation, based on cross-sectional differences between sedentary and exercising subjects, no prospective

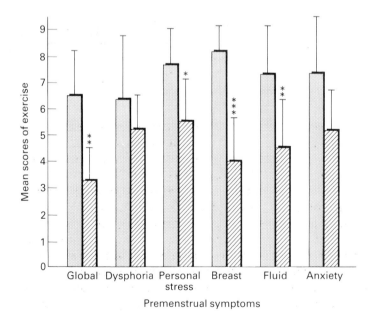

Fig. 34.1 Mean ± standard deviation of menstrual cycle questionnaire scores (reported days 2−5 of the cycle) during the last sedentary (■) and sixth exercise-training (▨) cycle in eight women serving as their own controls. The data were analysed with the Wilcoxon paired signed ranks test. *, $p = 0.025$; **, $p = 0.01$; ***, $p = 0.005$. From Prior et al. (1987), with permission.

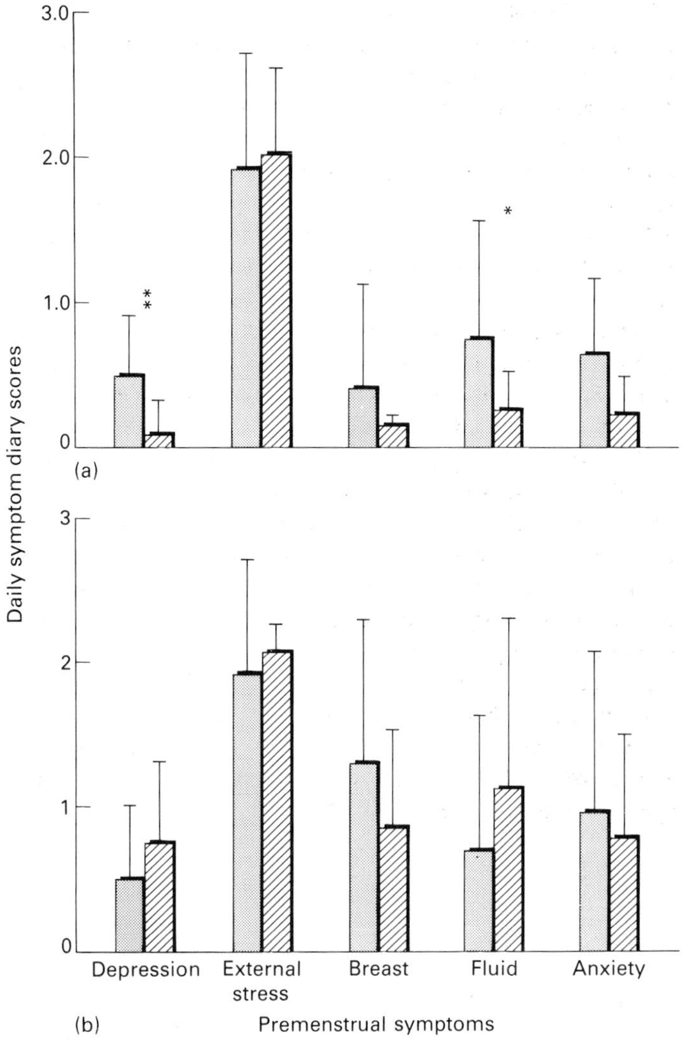

Fig. 34.2 Mean ± standard deviation of daily symptom diary scores during the 14 days preceding menstrual flow, with the first (▥) and sixth (▨) consecutive menstrual cycles in (a) seven women runners who intensified exercise before a marathon race, and in (b) six non-training women. The data were analysed with the Wilcoxon paired signed ranks test. Intergroup analysis (Mann–Whitney *U* test) showed that training women had significantly lower breast symptoms during cycle 1 ($p = 0.019$). At cycle 6, the two groups differed in depression ($p = 0.045$), fluid, ($p = 0.019$) and breast symptoms ($p = 0.006$). *, $p < 0.05$; **, $p < 0.02$. From Prior *et al.* (1987), with permission.

study has shown the development of amenorrhoea when exercise-training is the single, potentially causal factor.

The hypothalamus adapts to exercise training as it does to other stressors such as a decrease of body mass, emotional stress, or illness (Prior, 1990). Because women with gynaecological immaturity, in association with a decrease of body mass, travel, a move away from home, or situational stress, may develop amenorrhoea, these factors must be absent before exercise can be considered as causing amenorrhoea. The closest any prospective study has come to describing the development of amenorrhoea was a 55-day delay in flow in a young woman (in her early 20s) who was stressed by a restricted energy intake and a move to a residential camp, in addition to undertaking strenuous exercise training (Bullen *et al.*, 1985).

Why, then, is there an almost universal acceptance of a causal association between exercise and amenorrhoea? The most simple answer is that, unlike exercise, documentation of previous reproductive maturity, emotional stress or restricted energy intake is subtle and difficult to quantify. The answer also relates to the roles of women and men in our Western, urban society. Numerous authors write about the stresses of life which lead a vulnerable person to need to feel in control. If a person's environment, relationships and future appear to be beyond his or her control, then at least personal control can be achieved over diet and exercise (Mitchell, 1987).

The interrelationships that lead to amenorrhoea are shown diagrammatically in Fig. 34.3. If emotional stress leads to restrictive eating patterns and compulsive exercise, reproductive changes will not be reversed until the emotional problems have been resolved. Exercise-related menstrual cycle changes, however, are reversible with decreases in training, or maintenance of the same level of training, as though the reproductive system, like the cardiorespiratory system, can become 'conditioned' to exercise (Prior, 1982).

We have answered affirmatively that reversible reproductive changes are causally related to exercise for women. Is the same true for men? Evidence suggests that parallel suppression of reproductive function occurs in men. A recent review concluded: 'The chronic effects of endurance training on the HPG (hypothalamic–pituitary–gonadal) axis in men are clear and it seems likely that the mechanism of inhibition is central, and analogous to that described in women' (Cumming et al., 1989).

The early reproductive changes in men have not been scientifically studied, but are probably subtle changes in libido and morning erections. No prospective training studies of men are currently published except in abstract (Wheeler et al., 1987). Both cross-sectional (Hackney et al., 1988; McColl et al., 1989) and prospective data for endurance training (Wheeler et al., 1987) suggest suppression of testosterone, decreases in luteinizing hormone (LH) pulsatility, decreased semen quality (Ayers et al., 1985) and decreased fertility (Baker et al., 1984). Compulsive running and anorexia-like exercise behaviour have also been reported in men. Although we do not have a good sense of the variance of these changes over time in sedentary normal men all the data are consistent with the hypothesis, that there is hypothalamic suppression of reproductive function during training for men, as well as women.

Epidemiological evidence for a strong association between exercise training and changes of reproductive function is not available. The strength of the association arises, at present, from the frequency of case reports or cross-sectional studies. What is needed is a prospective observational study of reproductively mature sedentary, training and non-training

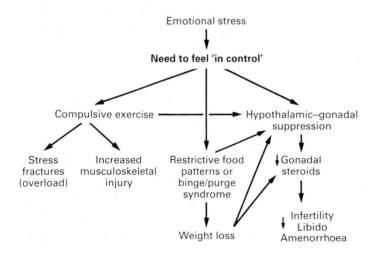

Fig. 34.3 Diagram illustrating interrelationships between stress, compulsive exercise, restrictive eating and amenorrhoea. Multiple factors are thus causally related to the development of amenorrhoea.

(but regularly exercising) men and women across 1 year. Diaries for recording the subtle changes in libido, molimina and emotional symptoms, and prospective documentation of training duration and intensity, sexual activity, lipids, diet, body mass, fat reserves and bone metabolism, are needed. Then reproductive changes can be correlated to potential causal factors.

A third epidemiological criterion for causality is the inconsistency of data from centre to centre. The bulk of data are consistent. Any discrepancies arise from the experimental conditions — testing after 36 h, rather than 12−24 h, without exercise, thus allowing recovery of the hypothalamus and higher LH levels (Hackney et al., 1988), or failure to test subjects in a parallel basal (non-exercise) state (Rogol et al., 1984).

The fourth epidemiological criterion concerns the presence of a dose−response gradient. The gradient relating exercise to reproductive effect is largely 'subclinical' (Cumming et al., 1989) and subtle. The gradient would be demonstrable only in prospective studies, since the reproductive system seeks to return inexorably to the optimum (fertile) steady state. The phenomenon of adaptation is difficult to document, because statistical methods are not suitable its quantitative analysis (Prior, 1985). However, a gradient has been documented in animals, depending on the rapidity with which an exercise load is introduced (Selye, 1939). Figure 34.4 shows that rats forced to run on a motorized treadmill continued to have normal oestrus if a gradual onset of training was allowed. Data from a human subject showed that one woman runner had a short luteal phase and anovulatory changes before her first marathon run. Such changes were not present during similar training for her second marathon (Prior, 1990).

The fifth criterion for a causal association is that the association makes epidemiological sense. Yes — temporary suppression of reproductive function during intense condition saves 'resources' for the training rather than spending them on current reproductive needs.

This is the easiest of the criteria to satisfy, because the reproductive system can be seen as adapting to the 'stress' of exercise, as it would to other stresses such as food deprivation, emotional threat or illness (Selye, 1939; Prior, 1982).

For the reasons listed above, reproductive change with exercise meets the necessary criterion that it is biologically sensible. In times of emergency, fertility becomes secondary to survival. This means that the adrenal stress hormones are oversecreted and the reproductive hormones are temporarily suppressed. When this emergency hormonal response becomes permanent, then detrimental effects may occur, for example, in bone metabolism (Bilanin et al., 1989), and reversibility is lost.

The seventh causal criterion is specificity of the association. Evidence suggests some degree of specificity. Reproductive changes do not occur with sports that require no endurance conditioning (such as golf or croquet). They may also occur less with some aerobic sports (such as swimming) than they do with running or bicycling.

The final criterion of causality is that the relationship be analogous to other, well-accepted relationships. It appears that, at least for women, the changes in reproduction with a decrease of body mass, or with emotional stress, are similar to those occurring with exercise-training. The notion of adaptation (Selye, 1939; Prior, 1982) suggests that several stressors can have the same final path of reproductive change. It is likely that all reverse to normal in the same way.

Therapeutic approach to exercise-related reproductive changes

An appropriate approach to changes in reproduction in active men and women requires that normal reproductive function be sought. This means that despite regular cycles, we must ask about molimina, and despite lack of complaint, we must ask about normal libido and morning erections as evidence of normality. If alterations

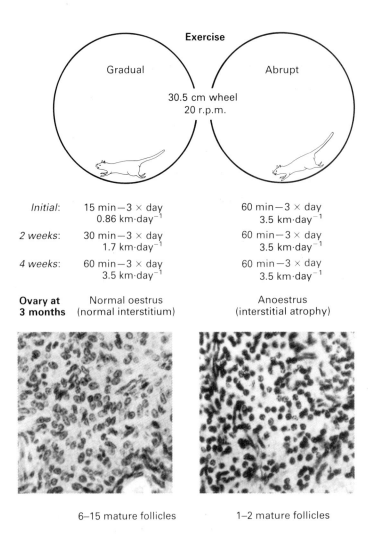

	Exercise	
	Gradual	Abrupt

30.5 cm wheel
20 r.p.m.

Initial:	15 min−3 × day 0.86 km·day^{-1}	60 min−3 × day 3.5 km·day^{-1}
2 weeks:	30 min−3 × day 1.7 km·day^{-1}	60 min−3 × day 3.5 km·day^{-1}
4 weeks:	60 min−3 × day 3.5 km·day^{-1}	60 min−3 × day 3.5 km·day^{-1}
Ovary at 3 months	Normal oestrus (normal interstitium)	Anoestrus (interstitial atrophy)

6–15 mature follicles   1–2 mature follicles

Fig. 34.4 To illustrate the concept of 'general adaptation' developed by Hans Selye. Exercise was introduced abruptly or gradually in rats. The photomicrographs show normal compared with atrophic interstitium in rat ovaries. From Selye (1939), modified with permission.

in reproductive function are suspected in an exercising person, do not assume they are *caused* by exercise if they are persistent. Figure 34.5 outlines the stepwise approach to the exercising woman. This approach, and a parallel one for men, requires cooperation between the athlete and the physician or trainer. It requires few expensive hormone tests, but relies on careful documentation of exercise, body mass and symptoms, along with reproductive signs and symptoms. For women, the daily symptom diary (Prior *et al.*, 1987a), with or without a basal temperature list, quantitatively analysed (Prior *et al.*, 1990b) will give the necessary data.

Similar helpful tools are not presently available for male athletes.

The major detrimental effect of prolonged hypothalamic−pituitary−gonadal suppression with exercise is accelerated loss of trabecular bone mineral (Marcus *et al.*, 1985; Bilanin *et al.*, 1989). As discussed above, persistently abnormal male hormone levels or menstrual cycles are not caused by exercise, but may be associated with an 'exercise lifestyle' (see Fig. 34.3). Elevated cortisol levels, reported in both men (Barron *et al.*, 1985) and women (Ding *et al.*, 1988), are not only detrimental to bone directly by decreasing osteoblastic bone synthesis, but

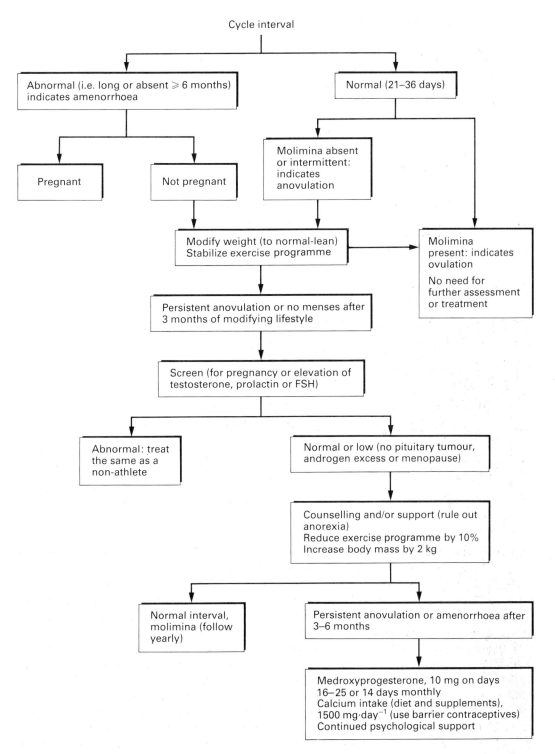

Fig. 34.5 Therapeutic approach to the establishment of normal reproductive cycles in the female athlete. From Prior (1987), modified with permission. FSH, follicle-stimulating hormone.

also indirectly because lower gonadal steroids increase bone loss (Fisher *et al.*, 1986).

Medroxyprogesterone treatment can reverse the negative effects of glucocorticoids and allow trabecular bone formation in steroid-dependent asthmatic men (Grecu *et al.*, 1970). Since progesterone is missing or decreased in the common reproductive changes with exercise in women, therapy with cyclic medroxyprogesterone acetate (Provera®, 10 mg·day^{-1} from day 16 through day 25 of the menstrual cycle) will replace the abnormally low or missing hormone, and may promote bone formation. Restoration of body mass close to the normal level, an adequate intake of calcium (1000 mg·day^{-1}) and vitamin D (400 units daily, or the amount in a normal multiple vitamin pill) and dealing with emotional stress are all essential parts of therapy.

Summary

Apparent exercise-related amenorrhoea confirms the cultural bias that sport is not good for women, yet parallel, but less visible, changes occur in men. We now know that conditioning exercise-training *is* associated with reproductive changes and that these changes are reversible. Reproductive system changes which persist are always compounded by additional suppressors such as loss of body mass, illness or psychological stress.

For gynaecologically mature women (menstruation for 10 years or longer), the most prevalent change with increased exercise is a decrease in normal premenstrual symptoms, followed by luteal phase shortening. If exercise intensification is continued, anovulation may occur. The young woman (within 12 years of menarche) or the woman who has not established ovulatory cycles may develop oligomenorrhoea (cycle interval ≥ 36 days). She may even become amenorrhoeic (cycle interval ≥ 180 days) if there is associated loss of body mass or situational stress.

No prospective studies of men have evaluated changes in reproductive function during training. Documented decreases in serum testosterone and prolactin levels and lower LH pulse frequency reflect reversible hypothalamic suppression.

Reproductive changes are important physiological adaptations, similar to those occurring in the heart, lungs, muscle and skeleton. The end result is normal function at a higher level of fitness. Overtraining, or too rapid an increase in exercise, involves maladaptation of the neuroendocrine system to excessive loads of exercise (as can also be seen in the musculoskeletal and cardiovascular systems). Amenorrhoea associated with exercise may be one manifestation of overtraining in women. Overtraining is reversible with rest, nutritional and emotional support.

The potentially detrimental effects of exercise-related reproductive changes, with the exception of overtraining, have less to do with exercise and more to do with loss of body mass, stress, young age or reproductive immaturity. Bone loss is a concern. Anovulatory and short-lived phase cycles are associated with trabecular bone loss (Prior *et al.*, 1990a), although cortical bone may be benefited by non-compulsive mechanical loading.

Finally, appropriate evaluation and therapy of reproductive change in an exercising person must be individualized. An adaptive approach would initially involve stabilization of exercise and restoration of lost body mass to encourage return of normal function.

References

Abraham, G.E. (1978) The normal menstrual cycle. In: Givens, J.R. (ed.) *Endocrine Causes of Menstrual Disorders*, pp. 15–44. Year Book Medical Publishers, Chicago.

Ayers, J.W., Komesu, Y., Romain, T. & Ansbacher, R.A. (1985) Anthropometric, hormonal and psychological correlates of semen quality in endurance trained male athletes. *Fertil. Steril.* **43**, 917–921.

Baker, E.R., Leuker, R. & Stumpf, P.G. (1984) Relationship of exercise to semen parameters and fertility success of artificial insemination donors. *Fertil. Steril.* **41**, 107S.

Barron, J.L., Noakes, T.D., Levy, W., Smith, C. &

Millar, R.P. (1985) Hypothalamic dysfunction in overtrained athletes. *J. Clin. Endocrinol. Metab.* **60**, 803–806.

Bilanin, J.E., Blanchard, M.S. & Russek-Cohen, G. (1989) Lower vertebral bone density in male long distance runners. *Med. Sci. Sports Exerc.* **21**, 66–70.

Bonen, A., Belcastro, A.N. & Simpson, A.A. (1981) Profiles of menstrual cycle hormones in teenage athletes. *J. Appl. Physiol.* **50**, 545–551.

Bullen, B.A., Skrinar, G.S., Beitins, I.Z., von Mering, G., Turnbull, B.A. & McArthur, J.W. (1985) Induction of menstrual disorders by strenuous exercise in untrained women. *N. Engl. J. Med.* **312**, 1349–1353.

Cumming, D.C., Wheeler, G.D. & McColl, E.M. (1989) The effects of exercise on reproductive function in men. *Sports Med.* **7**, 1–17.

Ding, J.H., Sheckter, C.B., Drinkwater, B.L., Soules, M.R. & Bremner, W.J. (1988) High serum cortisol levels in exercise-associated amenorrhea. *Ann. Intern. Med.* **108**, 530–534.

Fisher, E.C., Nelson, M.E., Frontera, W.R., Turksoy, R.N. & Evans, W.J. (1986) Bone mineral content and levels of gonadotropins and estrogens in amenorrheic running women. *J. Clin. Endocrinol. Metab.* **62**, 1232–1236.

Grecu, E., Weinshelbaum, A. & Simmons, R. (1970) Effective therapy of glucocorticoid osteoporosis with medroxyprogesterone acetate (MPA) and calcium. *Calcif. Tissue Int.* **46**, 294–299.

Hackney, A.C., Sinning, W.E. & Bruot, B.C. (1988) Reproductive hormone profiles of endurance-trained and untrained males. *Med. Sci. Sports Exerc.* **20**, 60–65.

McColl, E.M., Wheeler, G.D., Gomes, P., Bhambhani, Y. & Cumming, D.C. (1989) The effects of acute exercise on pulsatile LH release in high-mileage male runners. *Clin. Endocrinol.* **31**, 617–621.

Marcus, R., Cann, C.E., Madvig, P., Minkoff, J., Goddard, M. & Bayer, M. (1985) Menstrual function and bone mass in élite women distance runners. Endocrine and metabolic features. *Ann. Intern. Med.* **102**, 158–163.

Mitchell, J. (1987) Going for the burn. Pumping iron: What's healthy about the current fitness boom? In: Lawrence, M. (ed.) *Fed Up and Hungry: Women, Oppression and Food*, pp. 156–174. Perter Bedrick Books, New York.

Prior, J.C. (1982) Endocrine 'conditioning' with endurance training: a preliminary review. *Can. J. Appl. Sport Sci.* **7**, 149–157.

Prior, J.C. (1985) Luteal phase defects and anovulation: adaptive alterations occurring with conditioning exercise. *Sem. Reprod. Endocrinol.* **3**, 27–33.

Prior, J.C. (1987) Exercise in women. *Med. N. Am.*, Fall, 16–23.

Prior, J.C. (1990) Reproduction: exercise-related adaptations and the health of women and men. In: Bouchard, C., Shephard, R.J., Stephens, T., Sutton, J.R. & McPherson, B.D. (eds) *Exercise, Fitness and Health.* pp. 661–675. Human Kinetics, Champaign, Illinois.

Prior, J.C., Cameron, K., Ho Yeun, B. & Thomas, J. (1982a) Menstrual cycle changes with marathon training: anovulation and short luteal phase. *Can. J. Appl. Sport Sci.* **7**, 173–177.

Prior, J.C., Ho Yeun, B., Clement, P., Bowie, L. & Thomas, J. (1982b) Reversible luteal phase changes and infertility associated with marathon training. *Lancet* **ii**, 269–270.

Prior, J.C., Vigna, Y.M., Alojado, N., Sciarretta, D. & Schulzer, M. (1987) Conditioning exercise decreases premenstrual symptoms: a prospective controlled six month trial. *Fertil. Steril.* **47**, 402–409.

Prior, J.C., Vigna, Y.M., Burgess, A.E. & Cunningham, N. (1988) Marathon training, in the absence of luteal phase change, is not a risk factor for trabecular bone loss. *J. Bone Min. Res.* **3**, S85.

Prior, J.C., Vigna, Y.M., Schechter, M.T. & Burgess, A.E. (1990a) Spinal bone loss and ovulatory disturbances. *New Engl. J. Med.* **323**, 1221–1227.

Prior, J.C., Vigna, Y.M., Schulzer, M., Hall, J.E. & Bonen, A. (1990b) Determination of luteal phase length by quantitative basal temperature methods: validation against the midcycle LH peak. *Clin. Invest. Med.* **13**, 123–129.

Rogol, A.D., Veldhuis, J.D., Williams, F.A. & Johnson, M.L. (1984) Pulsatile secretion of gonadotropins and prolactin in male marathon runners. *J. Androl.* **5**, 21–27.

Ronkainen, H.R., Pakarinen, A.J., Kirkinen, P. & Kauppila, A.J. (1985) Physical exercise-induced changes and season-associated differences in the pituitary-ovarian function of runners and joggers. *J. Clin. Endocrinol. Metab.* **60**, 416–422.

Sackett, D.L. (1981) Evaluation: requirements for clinical application. In: Warren, K.S. (ed) *Coping with Biomedical Literature*, pp. 123–156. Praeger Publishers, New York.

Selye, H. (1939) The effect of adaptation to various damaging agents on the female sex organs in the rat. *Endocrinology* **25**, 615–624.

Shangold, M.M., Freeman, R., Thysen, B. & Gatz, M. (1979) The relationship between long-distance running, plasma progesterone, and luteal phase length. *Fertil. Steril.* **31**, 130–133.

Wheeler, G.D., Williamson, S., Singh, M., Pierce, W.D. & Epling, W.F. (1987) Decreased serum total and free testosterone and LH pulse frequency with endurance training in men. *Endocr. Soc. Abstr.* **69**, 767.

PART 5

SPECIFIC POPULATION GROUPS AND ENDURANCE TRAINING

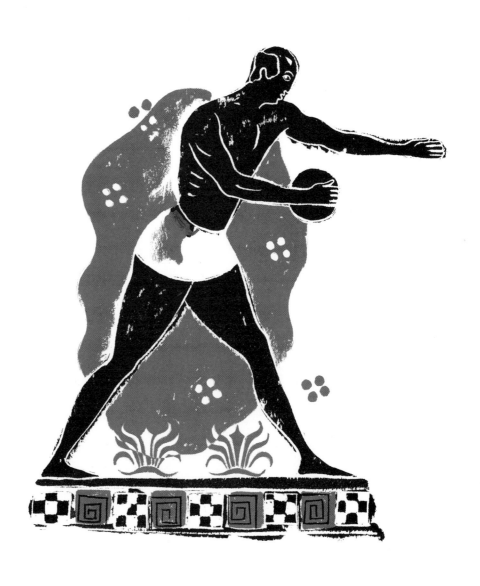

Chapter 35

Aerobic Responses to Physical Training in Children

THOMAS W. ROWLAND

Introduction

Sustained exercise is not characteristic of the usual daily physical activities of children, yet considerable attention has been focused on endurance fitness and trainability in the paediatric age group. This interest stems from several considerations.

First, regular physical activity, particularly as it relates to endurance fitness, yields benefits to health that include prevention of obesity, emotional wellbeing, and reduction of risks for atherosclerotic vascular disease. It is of concern, then, that mass testing results in children have been interpreted as indicating that youngsters in developed nations possess suboptimal levels of aerobic fitness. While demands for improved physical education programmes have ensued, there is a clearcut need to determine the proper design of exercise programmes in children that will improve aerobic fitness — if this effect can be achieved at all.

Second, aerobic exercise regimens have been utilized in rehabilitation programmes for children with cardiac, pulmonary and muscular disease. Knowledge concerning the efficacy of training to improve aerobic function would help clarify the role of endurance activities in these programmes.

Third, prepubertal athletes have been increasingly evident in world-class competitions. These children are training with intensive regimens with little information regarding the safety and benefits involved. Information per-

taining to physiological training responses in children would help create guidelines for these young competitors.

Lastly, normal physiological development as children grow closely resembles that of the changes expected in response to endurance training programmes. An understanding of aerobic developmental and training responses in children might therefore provide insight into the mechanisms responsible for physiological adaptations to exercise at all ages.

The fitness effect

The physiological effects of endurance training have been discussed in other chapters. The following represents a summary of these changes as a preliminary to examining the effects of training in prepubertal children.

Participation by a previously sedentary young adult in a regular programme of endurance activities of specific intensity, frequency and duration produces a predictable constellation of physiological, metabolic and anatomical changes which have collectively been termed the fitness effect. Gains in aerobic function are manifest by improvements in both absolute and weight-relative maximal oxygen uptake ($\dot{V}_{O_2 max}$), generally by 5–20% above that of pretraining levels. Increased $\dot{V}_{O_2 max}$ is a manifestation of greater maximal cardiac output, as well as an effect of peripheral factors such as augmented oxygen extraction by exercising muscle, a rise in blood volume and greater muscle vascular supply.

Improvements in maximal cardiac output reflect the ability of the heart to generate a greater peak stroke volume, since maximal heart rate does not change appreciably after training. At rest and during submaximal exercise (in activities such as walking, running or cycling), the heart rate is lower and stroke volume is higher in the trained compared with the untrained adult, while oxygen intake and cardiac output are unchanged or somewhat reduced.

The mechanisms that stimulate these alterations are not clear, but changes in autonomic influences, energy substrate utilization and aerobic enzyme activity related to differential muscle fibre function may all be involved. The physiological fitness effect is a response to stress; the adaptations resulting from a period of physical training appear favourable from the standpoint of improvements in system efficiency and functional reserve capacity. These changes in turn are manifest by associated improvements in athletic performance.

The extent to which children before the age of puberty demonstrate similar physiological adaptations to endurance training has long been questioned. Indeed, several early studies indicated that a programme of physical training could not significantly improve maximal aerobic power in prepubertal subjects. Two possible explanations for this finding were proposed. First, during exercise training, certain hormonal responses (sex steroids? growth hormone?) may be required to trigger physiological and metabolic adaptations. Because such hormonal influences are blunted in prepubertal subjects, children are incapable of demonstrating a physiological training effect (Katch, 1983). According to this concept, there is a critical point (presumably the time of puberty) before which few physiological adaptations to training can be expected. However, the influence of age-related differences in hormone levels on physiological adaptations to repetitive exercise is currently unknown.

Alternatively, improvements in oxygen in-take after training would not be expected if children are already operating at peak aerobic function. It has been suggested that children are trainable, but for most youngsters the typically high level of daily physical activity in effect maintains them in a constant trained state anyway. If so, further improvement in physiological function following an aerobic training programme would not be expected.

More recent studies have provided evidence that, given the proper training regimen, improvements in aerobic function can be expected to occur in prepubertal subjects. These reports, although marred by methodological flaws, appear to indicate that the extent of the training response in children may, be less than that observed in young adults. The following sections will review these conflicting data as well as the questions of critical periods for an optimal training effect and the relationship between habitual daily activity and fitness in prepubertal children. In the many studies addressing these issues, 'prepubertal' has been defined variously by chronological age, absence of secondary sexual characteristics, or age relative to maximal height velocity. Before presenting this information, it is important to note those technical and ethical considerations that confound an understanding of training responses in children.

Developmental, methodological and ethical considerations

The normal developmental progression of physiological determinants of endurance exercise bears a striking resemblance to features of the fitness effect. A sedentary child who participates in no physical activity at all will demonstrate, as he or she grows, a fall in resting and submaximal heart rate, an increased absolute maximal oxygen intake and cardiac output, a stable maximal heart rate, and lower oxygen intake at a given submaximal running speed (Bar-Or, 1983). Changes in weight-relative $\dot{V}_{O_{2\,max}}$ are less predictable. In population studies, mean $\dot{V}_{O_{2\,max}}$ per kg in boys does not change between 6 and 16 years of age (while declining after the preteen years in girls), but given individuals may show a rise or fall in serial testing.

Given this parallel, the difficulty of separating maturation from training effects during an exercise programme for children becomes obvious. Including untrained controls in such studies helps to identify the presence or absence of a true training effect. But considering the strong genetic influence on aerobic trainability (as well as potential developmental and motivational differences), even 'matched' untrained controls may not provide a valid means of accomplishing this (short of using identical twins). It follows that the results of aerobic training programmes without control subjects are particularly difficult to interpret.

The valid measurement of maximal aerobic power requires a true maximal effort on the part of the subject and — particularly crucial in studies involving different ages — techniques and equipment that are not affected by subject size. These factors may significantly influence oxygen intake values reported in training studies. Whether the reproducibility of $\dot{V}O_{2\,max}$ (based on motivation and attention span, for instance) is the same in 6-year-old as in 12-year-old subjects, or in active and sedentary children, is unknown. Likewise, the effects of valve dead space, tubing diameter and gas mixing chamber sizes on $\dot{V}O_{2\,max}$ in children of different sizes has not been well evaluated. Whether the type of exercise protocol will affect maximal oxygen intake variability also needs investigation, as do the effects of staff or family encouragement and ambient conditions during testing.

Studies of physiological adaptations to training in children are also hampered by ethical considerations. Invasive procedures (muscle biopsies, central vascular catheters), methodology that involves radiation (nuclear ventriculography) and use of non-therapeutic drugs are improper in healthy paediatric subjects. Most information on physiological responses to training in children has therefore been re-stricted to traditional gas exchange parameters and heart rate. Increasing use of non-invasive methodologies (carbon dioxide rebreathing, cardiac output, echocardiography) may provide new useful information in the paediatric age group.

In adults, oxygen intake expressed per kilogram of body mass is the traditional marker of both cardiovascular functional capacity and endurance performance fitness. Doubt has been cast, however, on both of these relationships in growing children. It would appear inappropriate to expect $\dot{V}O_{2\,max}$ per kg to closely indicate capabilities in endurance sports, for instance, because performance improves dramatically during the childhood years, while $\dot{V}O_{2\,max}$ per kg is typically constant. The average 14-year-old boy can run 1.5 km almost twice as fast as a 5-year-old, but $\dot{V}O_{2\,max}$ per kg values for the two youngsters will be similar. Also, some data suggest that cardiac functional reserve (relative to body mass) may be less in children than young adults. And metabolic scope, the ratio of maximal to resting oxygen intake, increases steadily during childhood, implying that the reserve capacity for oxygen delivery improves despite stable $\dot{V}O_{2\,max}$ per kg (Rowland, 1989).

Habitual activity as a training stimulus

The concept has been advanced that children may not respond physiologically to aerobic training programmes because their innately high physical activity levels serve as a continuous training stimulus. According to this argument, children are already at a genetically determined limit of maximal cardiovascular function and cannot further increase $\dot{V}O_{2\,max}$ with exercise training.

Data examining the typical heart rates of children during their daily lives immediately cast doubt on this concept. While the training intensity/frequency stimulus that might be necessary to improve aerobic fitness in children is unknown, adults have been recommended to exercise for 15–60 min three times a week at a heart rate of 60–90% maximum. If these guidelines were to apply to children, a sustained heart rate of at least 160 beats·min^{-1} would be necessary to stimulate physiological adaptations and, as noted in a later section, target heart rates for the training of children probably need to be above even this level.

Studies of heart rates during the daily activities of children show that youngsters do not typically exceed 160 beats·min^{-1} for more than a total of 10–20 min daily, this being in sporadic rather than sustained bursts of activity. Heart rates are usually higher in boys than in girls. Thus it would not be expected (at least from the standpoint of adult norms) that children would be able to improve cardiovascular fitness above that resulting from growth alone as a result of their usual daily physical activities.

The argument that children are already highly trained by daily physical exercise would be strengthened if a connection were observed between a child's level of habitual physical activity and $\dot{V}o_{2\,max}$ seen during exercise testing. Still, even if such an association could be demonstrated, one would not be able to discern whether regular activity created greater levels of fitness or whether those with inherently high aerobic fitness were more likely to engage in physical activities.

Research data supporting a relationship between habitual activity level and maximal oxygen intake are not as strong as one might intuitively expect. Of seven such reports, only four have indicated a positive association between the two variables (Rowland, 1990). Conflicting data in these studies may reflect the lack of a precise tool to measure daily exercise activity as well as the confounding influence of factors such as body habitus and composition, motivation, family support and previous athletic experience.

Based on these two lines of evidence, it appears unlikely that the daily physical activity of children is of sufficient intensity to maximize aerobic power and thereby render youngsters 'untrainable'.

Physiological profiles of élite child athletes

A comparison of the cardiovascular profiles of élite prepubertal athletes with those of non-athletic children might serve to assess the adaptability of physiological mechanisms to early training. Unfortunately, regular athletic training is not the only factor that might differentiate the two groups. Differences might also result if (1) prepubertal athletes were developmentally more mature than their non-athletic colleagues, and/or (2) child athletes were attracted to sports participation by their innate genetic capacity for superior endurance performance. Current research information unfortunately offers little means of differentiating the effects of training, genetic preselection and advanced developmental maturity to explain physiological differences between child athletes and non-athletes.

With this caveat in mind, reports describing the physiological characteristics of élite child athletes can be examined. Profiles of child competitors in several endurance sports have been described (distance runners, swimmers, cyclists), with little indepth investigation into any particular activity. The physiological picture of these athletes is, however, reasonably consistent.

Highly trained prepubertal endurance athletes demonstrate a greater $\dot{V}o_{2\,max}$ per kg than non-athletic children. For male distance runners typical values are 60–65 ml·kg^{-1}·min^{-1}, about 20–30% greater than that expected in the general paediatric population. This contrasts with values in élite adult runners, who can exhibit a $\dot{V}o_{2\,max}$ per kg as high as 70–80 ml·kg^{-1}·min^{-1}, which is about 70% greater than non-athletic males of the same age group. This discrepancy has been cited as evidence that prepubertal children cannot develop aerobic capacity with training to the extent expected in adults. Alternative explanations are possible, however, particularly the fact that adult runners have had the benefit of many more years of training than the child athlete.

Gender does not affect this phenomenon. Values for maximal oxygen intake are lower in prepubertal female runners compared with male competitors (about $55-60$ ml·kg^{-1}·min^{-1}), but these figures are again approximately 30% greater than those of sedentary girls.

Most studies indicate that child endurance athletes have lower resting and submaximal heart rates than non-athletes, but maximal heart rates during exercise testing are similar. Submaximal blood pressure and oxygen intake have been less among athletes in some studies.

A comparison of prepubertal hockey players with inactive children showed no differences in the relationship of submaximal heart rate and stroke volume between the two groups (Hamilton & Andrew, 1976). In the same study, postpubertal players indicated the expected fitness effect: lower heart rate and higher stroke volume at a given submaximal rate of work than that observed in untrained controls. The authors suggested the apparent lack of a fitness effect in the prepubertal subjects might reflect the high habitual activity levels of the control subjects. Differences in postpubertal subjects could then be explained by a 'detraining' effect on the more sedentary control subjects as they entered adolescence.

For the most part, then, child endurance athletes exhibit features of a training effect, although differences from non-athletes appear to be less than those observed between endurance athletes and non-athletes in the adult population. It is impossible to decide, however, whether these characteristics are indeed an effect of training or whether they reflect inherited qualities or evidence of accelerated biological maturation.

Training studies

The most direct means of assessing the ability of prepubertal children to respond physiologically to endurance training is the measurement of maximal aerobic power before and after a period of regular training. Since 1986, at least 31 such studies have been reported, so it is surprising that the answer to the question of the trainability of children continues to be unclear (Sady, 1986). These studies have varied widely in design and have utilized a number of exercise programmes, including distance and interval running, cross-country skiing, biking, swimming and bench stepping. Duration has ranged from 1 week to 7 years.

Results of these training programmes have not been consistent, some showing improvements in $\dot{V}o_{2\,max}$, and others not. Attempts to compare studies is difficult, because they encompass such a wide variety of types of exercise as well as differences in programme frequency, duration and intensity. Many also suffer from small numbers of subjects, lack of untrained controls and inadequate documentation of exercise intensity (Rowland, 1985; Vaccaro & Mahon, 1987; Bar-Or, 1989; Pate & Ward, 1990). Accepting the multiplicity of programme structure and methodological weaknesses of these studies, most of these authors agree that an aerobic training effect can probably be achieved in both prepubertal boys and girls given an appropriate exercise regimen.

Rowland (1985) examined nine training studies in children which were felt to follow criteria for improving aerobic fitness in adults (continuous activity of large muscle groups, from three to five sessions per week, for $15-60$ min, at an intensity producing a heart rate $60-90\%$ of maximum). Six such studies demonstrated a training-induced rise in $\dot{V}o_{2\,max}$ per kg ranging from 7% to 26%, similar to improvements noted in adults after aerobic training. The author was hesitant to conclude that these data indicated expected trainability in children, however, because of several methodological flaws common to these reports (small subject numbers, absence of controls, non-representative samples, failure to document exercise intensity, variable pretraining fitness levels). Still, this analysis appears to have two implications: (1) most data indicate that $\dot{V}o_{2\,max}$ can be improved by training in children; and (2) guidelines for improving aerobic power in adult subjects may also be appropriate for prepubertal children.

Bar-Or (1989) listed nine studies in which prepubertal children responded to training with little or no improvement in $\dot{V}O_{2\,max}$. Five of these did not involve endurance activities in the training regimen. It cannot be concluded, however, that such programmes need to involve aerobic activities to cause a change in maximal oxygen intake. Several studies have indicated improvements in $\dot{V}O_{2\,max}$ utilizing resistance forms of exercise (Pate & Ward, 1990). Of the studies reviewed by Bar-Or (1989) that failed to demonstrate a significant aerobic training effect, all but one indicated improvements in exercise performance (better running times).

Vaccaro and Mahon (1987) presented a selected summary of studies on the effects of endurance training of children. Many of these reports involved athletically inclined subjects who were more likely to volunteer for exercise studies. It was concluded that cardiorespiratory capacity can be expected to improve following such training if the programme is of sufficient intensity, frequency and duration. However, the optimal levels for each of these factors could not be defined.

Pate and Ward (1990) reviewed the paediatric training literature that complied with stringent pre-established criteria. In this analysis, reports were included only if: (1) a well-matched control group was included; (2) the training protocol was easily interpreted regarding frequency, duration and intensity of the programme; (3) physiological measures were employed; (4) statistical analysis was performed; and (5) the results were published in a peer-reviewed scientific journal.

Twelve training studies involving prepubertal subjects were analysed which complied with these criteria. In eight reports, a rise in $\dot{V}O_{2\,max}$ per kg was observed that ranged from 1.3% to 20.5% (average 10%), while in control subjects $\dot{V}O_{2\,max}$ per kg changed from −3.3% to +9.9% (average 2.7%). The mean improvement in maximal aerobic power was

at the low end of values reported in adult programmes.

The authors attempted to identify those factors that might be involved in determining the magnitude of aerobic response. Using age as a marker of developmental status, they noted that of the 12 studies reviewed, $\dot{V}O_{2\,max}$ per kg failed to change in two of the four studies involving the youngest subjects, but in only one of eight studies involving 10−13-year-olds. In addition, the magnitude of improvement in the younger subjects was only about one half that in the older group. Appreciating the small number of studies as well as the difficulty of testing young subjects maximally, these data suggest that younger children may be not as trainable as older.

Gender-related differences in trainability could not be evaluated, because almost all studies involved males. The few reports of girls in training programmes have indicated typical improvements in $\dot{V}O_{2\,max}$. Initial fitness levels have been found to correlate negatively with aerobic responses to training in adults, but the analysis of Pate and Ward (1990) failed to indicate such a relationship in paediatric studies.

The authors were unable to identify any clearcut contributions of mode, pattern, frequency, duration or intensity of training to the extent of improvement in $\dot{V}O_{2\,max}$. Failure to improve maximal aerobic power in three studies was attributed to possible inadequate intensity and short exercise periods.

Because this analysis failed to indicate pre-training fitness as a predictor of aerobic responses to training, it is of interest that $\dot{V}O_{2\,max}$ per kg does not usually increase in longitudinal studies of well-trained prepubertal athletes. Of four such studies (all in runners), only one reported a substantial improvement in weight-relative $\dot{V}O_{2\,max}$, and in that study the girl runners had only an average level of aerobic fitness at the beginning of the study (mean $\dot{V}O_{2\,max}$ 46 ml·kg^{-1}·min^{-1}). These observations suggest that as in adults, paediatric subjects with high initial fitness levels might not demonstrate large improvements in $\dot{V}O_{2\,max}$ per kg with training.

Four studies have compared responses to training in separate groups of pre- and post-pubertal subjects. A 14-week programme of running and bench stepping (without quantification of intensity) resulted in a 17.6% increase in $\dot{V}O_{2\,max}$ in 12–13-year-old girls (prepubertal?) and a 16.1% response in 18–21-year-old girls. These changes were both significantly greater than those observed in untrained controls.

A comparison of aerobic responses to run/walk training in prepubertal boys and adult men over 10 weeks showed no significant differences. Both groups experienced improvements (3–8% increase in $\dot{V}O_{2\,max}$) that were greatest with more intensive training. A study in Japan indicated that training of postpubertal subjects demonstrated greater gains of aerobic fitness than those trained during the prepubertal years (Kobayashi et al., 1978). However, an investigation of pre- and postpubertal subjects using twins as controls could find no differences in trainability (Weber et al., 1976).

There is little information on physiological responses to endurance training in children other than gains of maximal oxygen intake. Several studies have reported a decline in submaximal heart rate. Limited information suggests that maximal cardiac output can also be improved. Peak stroke volume in prepubertal boys has been shown to improve by 20% after 4 months of regular endurance exercise (Eriksson, 1972). Increased function of both anaerobic and aerobic enzymes in muscle has also been demonstrated after endurance training in children.

Training intensity and aerobic responses

In adults sufficient intensity of training, as indicated by exercise heart rate, is a vital prerequisite to improvements in aerobic power. Target heart rates for improvement of aerobic fitness have been identified as 65–85% of

maximum, or 60% of heart rate reserve (the difference between resting and maximal heart rate) added to the resting rate.

It is not known whether such formulae are equally appropriate as threshold markers for aerobic training in children. Indeed, there is virtually no information available to serve as appropriate guidelines for improving aerobic function in the paediatric age group. One study indicated that a heart rate of 170–180 beats·min^{-1} was necessary to increase $\dot{V}O_{2\,max}$ during a 6-week cycle training programme in 11–13-year-old boys.

The heart rate at the anaerobic threshold (AT) has been suggested as a valid marker of intensity of exercise appropriate to improve aerobic power. In children the average heart rate at AT is usually 165–170 beats·min^{-1}, equal to 85% of maximal heart rate or 75% of heart rate reserve. The formulae for estimating target heart rates in adults would therefore underestimate heart rate at AT in children. This suggests the possibility that studies which have failed to show an improvement of maximal oxygen intake in children following training may have adopted an insufficient exercise intensity.

Critical period for trainability

If the physiological response to aerobic training is diminished in children compared with adults, there is presumably a certain point when the ability to improve aerobic power matures. This has long been postulated to occur at the time of puberty, when physiological and anatomical changes occur that might have a bearing on responses to exercise training (increased anaerobic capacity, improved muscle power in males, greater sweating rates and a rise in sex steroids). The research studies addressing this question have, however, generally failed to support such a conclusion.

The best means of relating trainability to puberty is by longitudinally examining $\dot{V}O_{2\,max}$ responses to a training programme in relationship to an individual's age at peak height velocity. A controlled study of this nature has not yet been reported. Most studies that have compared training responses in separate groups of prepubertal and post-pubertal subjects have found no significant differences. A non-training longitudinal study of Canadian boys indicated that the greatest acceleration in maximal oxygen intake occurred just after the time of peak height velocity, but a similar study failed to find any significant improvements in $\dot{V}_{O_2\,max}$ per kg at puberty.

Summary

Considerable research effort has been expended in attempts to decipher the physiological responsiveness of children to aerobic training. Firm conclusions have been hampered by the multiplicity of programme design, methodological flaws and confounding influences of normal growth and development. However, certain tentative conclusions can be drawn from the available information:

1 Prepubertal children appear to be capable of responding to endurance training with improvements in maximal aerobic power. Such adaptations are qualitatively similar, but probably quantitatively less compared with those in adults.

2 Improvements in aerobic function through training in children are presumably contingent upon a programme of adequate mode, intensity, frequency and duration. The threshold levels for improvement of aerobic function in children are unknown. Limited data suggest that guidelines identified for adults are also appropriate for children, except that target heart rates as indicators of training intensity may be underestimated if adult-oriented formulae are utilized.

3 The concept of a critical time for optimal improvement in maximal aerobic power with training has not been confirmed.

4 The inability to draw firm conclusions regarding aerobic trainability of children reflects the need for improved research. In particular, there is a need to investigate the aerobic responses of children with a broad range of initial fitness, participating in a training programme of appropriate design, with comparison of physiological responses to those in both untrained controls and postpubertal subjects.

References

Bar-Or, O. (1983) *Pediatric Sports Medicine for the Practitioner*. Springer-Verlag, New York.

Bar-Or, O. (1989) Trainability of the prepubescent child. *Phys. Sportsmed.* **17**, 65−81.

Eriksson, B.O. (1972) Physical training, oxygen supply, and muscle metabolism in 11−13 year old boys. *Acta Physiol. Scand. Suppl.* **384**, 1−48.

Hamilton, P. & Andrew, G.M. (1976) Influence of growth and athletic training on heart and lung function. *J. Appl. Physiol.* **36**, 27−38.

Katch, V.L. (1983) Physical conditioning of children. *J. Adol. Health Care* **3**, 241−246.

Kobayashi, K., Kitamura, K., Miura, M. *et al.* (1978) Aerobic power as related to body growth and training in Japanese boys: a longitudinal study. *J. Appl. Physiol.* **44**, 666−672.

Pate, R.R. & Ward, D.S. (1990) Endurance exercise trainability in children and youth. In: Grana, W.A., Lombardo, J.A., Sharkey, B.J. & Stone, J.A. (eds) *Advances in Sports Medicine and Fitness*, Vol. 3, pp. 37−55. Yearbook Medical Publishers, Chicago.

Rowland, T.W. (1985) Aerobic response to endurance training in prepubescent children: a critical analysis. *Med. Sci. Sports Exerc.* **17**, 493−497.

Rowland, T.W. (1989) Oxygen uptake and endurance fitness in children: a developmental perspective. *Ped. Exerc. Sci.* **1**, 313−328.

Rowland, T.W. (1990) *Exercise and Children's Health*. Human Kinetics Publishers, Champaign, Illinois.

Sady, S.P. (1986) Cardiorespiratory exercise training in children. *Clin. Sports Med.* **5**, 493−514.

Vaccaro, P. & Mahon, A. (1987) Cardiorespiratory responses to endurance training in children. *Sports Med.* **4**, 352−363.

Weber, G., Kartodihardjo, W. & Klissouras, V. (1976) Growth and physical training with reference to heredity. *J. Appl. Physiol.* **44**, 666−672.

Chapter 36

Pregnant Women and Endurance Exercise

DONALD C. McKENZIE

Introduction

Pregnancy represents a physiological stress that, in theory, has potential benefits to the endurance athlete. During the first and second trimesters, when prolonged aerobic exercise is still possible, stroke volume, ejection fraction and cardiac output are augmented, blood volume is significantly increased, and absolute $\dot{V}o_{2\,max}$ could rise accordingly. These adaptations are similar to those induced by cardiovascular training and there exists a theoretical possibility that the pregnant athlete has, albeit transiently, a physiological advantage over her non-pregnant counterpart. Unfortunately, participation in prolonged endurance events, particularly when the environmental conditions favour the development of hyperthermia, may have a detrimental effect on the development of the fetus.

This chapter reviews the adaptations that occur with pregnancy with specific reference to those variables that influence performance in endurance activities. The potential negative effects of such activities are presented and, finally, a summary of issues pertinent to the élite female athlete is outlined.

Maternal adaptations to pregnancy

The physiological changes that occur in the resting pregnant woman are well documented (Table 36.1). In our present context, the cardiorespiratory changes that take place in the first two trimesters are of importance. Cardiac output and stroke volume are increased as a result of endocrine changes, reduced peripheral vascular resistance, and an increased venous return (Roy et al., 1966). The blood volume is increased by some 50% relative to non-pregnant levels, but this is partially offset by

Table 36.1 Physiological adaptations to pregnancy (at rest).

Variable	First trimester	Second trimester	Third trimester
Heart rate (beats·min^{-1})	↑	↑ ↑	↑ ↑
Stroke volume (ml)	↑	↑ ↑	– or ↑
Cardiac output (l·min^{-1})	↑	↑ ↑	– or ↑
Ejection fraction (%)	– or ↑	– or ↑	– or ↑
$\dot{V}_E/\dot{V}o$	↑	↑ ↑	↑ ↑
$\dot{V}o_2$ (l·min^{-1})	↑	↑ ↑	↑ ↑
$\dot{V}o_2$ (ml·kg^{-1}·min^{-1})	–	↓	↓
Blood volume (litres)	↑ ↑	↑ ↑ ↑	↑ ↑ ↑

–, No change; ↑, ↑ ↑, ↑ ↑ ↑, degree of increase; ↓, decrease.

an increased capacity of the venous system (Pritchard, 1965). The ventilatory equivalent for oxygen ($\dot{V}_E/\dot{V}_{O_2}$) is augmented due to a progressive increase of respiratory minute volume that reaches 50% above non-pregnant values late in gestation. The enhanced ventilatory response to exercise leads to a small increase in arterial P_{O_2}, with a reduction of P_{CO_2}. The resultant respiratory alkalosis is only partially compensated by bicarbonate excretion, leaving an arterial pH of approximately 7.47. The mild alkalosis facilitates placental gas exchange and may protect against fetal acidosis (Liberatore et al., 1984).

Maternal responses to submaximal and maximal exercise

The circulatory response to exercise of moderate intensity reflects the 'hyperkinetic' condition of the cardiovascular system (Table 36.2). The cardiac output and stroke volume are increased until 20–24 weeks' gestation and then fall towards term (Veland et al., 1969). The decrease observed near term is due to greater peripheral pooling of blood and an obstruction of the venous return by the enlarged uterus. The hyperkinetic circulation is balanced by a reduction in peripheral resistance, so that the systemic blood pressure remains within normal limits for non-pregnant females (Artal et al., 1981).

The heart rate response to a given intensity of submaximal exercise increases progressively during pregnancy (Knuttgen & Emerson, 1974; Morton et al., 1985). This has important implications for the exercise scientist, coach and athlete. Coaches and exercise physiologists who deal with élite athletes routinely use the exercise heart rate as a method to prescribe an appropriate intensity for a training session. The progressive increase in heart rate during pregnancy complicates both the exercise prescription and the interpretation of field data. Coaches often use the early morning pulse as an indicator of overtraining; however, the rise in this parameter due to physiological processes unrelated to exercise invalidates this monitoring strategy in pregnant women. Although the determination of maximal aerobic power in élite athletes should involve direct measurement, some researchers still use values predicted from the heart rate response to submaximal exercise. The increase in heart rate associated with pregnancy further reduces the validity of such tests; the error of such predictions is already up to 15% in the non-pregnant subject; the pregnancy-induced increase in the submaximal heart rate makes any such test of very limited value.

Studies of maximal heart rate during pregnancy have yielded conflicting results, reported values being either unchanged from prepregnant levels or reduced. It is difficult to determine whether the values obtained from such testing represent true maximal scores. The criteria for establishing maximal values in this population have not been determined, but

Table 36.2 Physiological adaptations to pregnancy during submaximal exercise.

Variable	First trimester	Second trimester	Third trimester
Heart rate (beats·min^{-1})	↑	↑↑	↑↑
Stroke volume (ml)	↑	↑↑	− or ↑
Cardiac output (l·min^{-1})	↑	↑↑	− or ↑
$\dot{V}_E/\dot{V}_{O_2}$	↑↑	↑↑	↑↑
$\dot{V}_{O_2}$ (l·min^{-1})	− or ↑	− or ↑	− or ↑
$\dot{V}_{O_2}$ (ml·kg^{-1}·min^{-1})	↓	↓↓	↓↓↓

−, No change; ↑, ↑↑, degree of increase; ↓, ↓↓, ↓↓↓, degree of decrease.

would undoubtedly be different than in non-pregnant élite athletes. For example, volitional fatigue is likely to occur at a lower relative work rate in an athlete who knows that she is pregnant.

The oxygen consumption required for a standardized non-weight-bearing task remains unaltered during pregnancy. This implies that the mechanical efficiency of exercise remains unchanged. Due to the potential risks involved and the lack of an accurate tool to monitor the fetal response, few studies have reported the physiological changes associated with maximal exercise in pregnant women. Only one research group has measured the maximal oxygen intake directly and they reported no significant changes in this parameter or the maximal heart rate of eight healthy females at 25 ± 3 weeks of gestation (Sady et al., 1988). These individuals demonstrated no significant changes of aerobic power in the first 6 months postpartum. However, the subjects were not athletes ($\dot{V}o_{2\,max} = 1.99\ l\cdot min^{-1}$) and the results cannot be generalized to a physically more active population. Other studies reporting predicted maximal oxygen intake suffer from the possible error introduced by heart rate changes during pregnancy; such studies have generally observed no significant changes of maximal aerobic power during pregnancy.

None of the studies cited tested élite athletes. The physiological changes introduced by years of endurance training would presumably be modified by the circulatory, respiratory and endocrine alterations associated with pregnancy. The relative inactivity imposed by pregnancy and the gain of body mass would also influence performance-related variables. There are anecdotal reports of impressive athletic achievements during the early stages of pregnancy and during the postpartum period. However, there are no controlled studies and the mechanisms involved in such changes remain speculative. This is clearly an area that requires further investigation.

Fetal response to maternal exercise

The physiological adaptations to pregnancy have, as their primary purpose, the provision of a suitable environment that will allow an optimal development of the fetus. Exercise presents an additional physiological stress to the mother and the cumulative effect of the two processes raises concerns about increased maternal/fetal core temperature, alterations in uterine blood flow with associated changes in acid–base status, and changes in substrate utilization by the mother and the fetus.

Studies that have examined the interaction between maternal hyperthermia and fetal wellbeing have, for the most part, utilized animal models. The resultant data are not always comparable to findings in humans. In animals, there is a strong relationship between a rise of core temperature and teratogenic effects, the major abnormalities being found in the central nervous system. Human studies concerned with heat exposure and fetal wellbeing have been, for ethical reasons, largely retrospective. One study discussed data from 915 women who had developed a core temperature $> 38.9°C$. Most of the women concerned had developed hyperthermia in response to a fever-inducing disease process in the first trimester of pregnancy. There was a significant increase in the number of births with major central nervous system abnormalities (Smith et al., 1978). Another study examined the pregnancies of 24 women who had developed hyperthermia in the first trimester of pregnancy. In every case, there was evidence of fetal central nervous system defects (Pleet et al., 1981). In contrast to these reports, data from the Collaborative Perinatal Project demonstrated that the incidence of fetal central nervous system abnormalities (including low IQ scores), was no greater in women who had developed core temperatures above $38.9°C$ than in a control group (Clarren et al., 1979). The important difference between these apparently conflicting studies seems to be the duration of hypothermia. The likelihood of teratogenic effects is lower with shorter, intermittent, exposure to hyperthermia (1–3 days). Recommendations based on these studies limit the increase in maternal core temperature to 38.9°C (102°F), the theoretical threshold for teratogenesis.

There are some prospective data on Finnish women who are frequently exposed to sauna baths during pregnancy (Vaha-Eskeli & Erkkola, 1988). The highest recorded core temperature in such individuals was 38.1°C; this gave rise to no significant endocrine changes, and the fetal heart rate, although elevated, was normal when fetal movements were considered. Thus, exposure to sauna baths or hyperthermia of this magnitude may not represent a significant stress to the fetus.

The majority of studies of uterine blood flow during exercise have used an animal model; such data support the hypothesis that uterine blood flow is reduced in proportion to the intensity and duration of exercise. Oxygen delivery to the uterus, however, is maintained due to the haemoconcentration associated with the exercise (Lotgering *et al.*, 1984).

Changes of the fetal heart rate have been used as an indicator of fetal distress and an exercise test has been proposed to detect uteroplacental insufficiency. The value of exercise testing as a method of assessing fetal condition and the integrity of the uteroplacental unit require further research. The fetal heart rate is moderately increased soon after the start of maternal exercise, but recovers to pre-exercise levels within 20 min of recovery. Transient fetal bradycardia has been reported soon after the onset of exercise, with readings returning to normal as the exercise bout continues. The physiological significance of the bradycardia is controversial; it may merely represent a normal response to moderate fetal hypoxia.

The fetus depends on carbohydrate as an energy source, and the avoidance of maternal hypoglycaemia during or following exercise is thus an important consideration. Human data are scarce but there is work that suggests the ability of pregnant women to metabolize carbohydrate during strenuous exercise may be lim-ited, perhaps as an adaptive response to protect the fetus. Animal studies have reported a reduction in fetal glucose uptake after maternal exercise. More research on this important performance-related topic is required.

Pregnancy and the élite athlete

The majority of the studies on élite endurance athletes have lacked reliability, due to the small number of women under investigation or the anecdotal nature of the report. Retrospective studies on the outcomes of pregnancy have generally noted favourable consequences of exposure to chronic exercise. Shorter periods of labour, less obstetrical complications, and normal fetal development in élite competitive or Olympic athletes have been reported (Erdelyi, 1962; Zaharieva, 1972). Such retrospective studies suffer from the use of questionnaires and memory recall, and lack objective medical data.

Prospective studies of élite athletes with pre-pregnancy data plus information on their training programmes and physiological profiles during pregnancy are needed, because there have been anecdotal reports of improved performance in such individuals following pregnancy. Some prospective data exist on women who have maintained a regular fitness programme during pregnancy. Wong and McKenzie (1987) suggested that women with high levels of aerobic fitness have a shorter labour than women who are not as fit. Other studies have reported a lower maternal weight gain and babies with lighter birth weights in subjects who sustained a high level of physical activity during pregnancy (Clapp & Dickstein, 1984). In a study of 845 women, Hall and Kauffman (1987) found that women who maintained an exercise programme throughout pregnancy reported an improved self-image, decreased discomfort and a relief of tension. A shorter hospital stay was also noted in women with the highest index of fitness.

Practical advice

There is very little information about the effects of chronic exercise in élite female athletes during pregnancy. Several of the cardiovascular adaptations to pregnancy, plus the significant increase in blood volume, would favour an improved aerobic performance, particularly before a large gain in body mass.

Pregnancy is not a time to increase training substantially. Approximately 60% of pregnant women voluntarily reduce their level of physical activity by the 28th week of gestation. The athlete should be allowed to control her training programme at this stage, and the coach must be sympathetic to her wishes if she should elect to reduce her level of physical activity or even withdraw from competitive sport.

The addition of new forms of training to compensate for a lack of normal endurance activity is not justifiable, with the exception of 'running-in-water', which can provide an equivalent physiological stress with the obvious benefit of being in a non-weight-bearing environment.

The avoidance of hyperthermia is recommended intuitively although the literature suggests that a mild, transient hyperthermia is well tolerated by the fetus. Nevertheless, caution must be shown in prescribing endurance training programmes for pregnant athletes when sustained hyperthermia has a potential to cause permanent fetal injury.

References

Artal, R., Platt, L.D., Sperling, M., Kammula, R.K., Jilek, J. & Nakamma, R. (1981) Exercise in pregnancy I. Maternal cardiovascular and metabolic responses in normal pregnancy. *Am. J. Obstet. Gynecol.* **140**, 123–127.

Clapp, J.F.I. & Dickstein, S. (1984) Endurance exercise and pregnancy outcome. *Med. Sci. Sports. Exerc.* **16**, 556–562.

Clarren, S.K., Smith, D.W., Harvey, M.A.S., Ward, R.H. & Myrianthopoulos, N.C. (1979) Hyperthermia — a prospective evaluation of a possible teratogenic agent in man. *J. Pediatr.* **95**, 81–83.

Erdelyi, G.J. (1962) Gynecological survey of female athletes. *J. Sports Med. Phys. Fitness* **2**, 174–179.

Hall, D.C. & Kaufman, D.A. (1987) Effects of aerobic and strength conditioning on pregnancy outcomes. *Am. J. Obstet. Gynecol.* **157**, 1199–1203.

Knuttgen, H.G. & Emerson, K.J. (1974) Physiological response to pregnancy at rest and during exercise. *J. Appl. Physiol.* **36**, 549–553.

Liberatore, S.M., Pistelli, R., Patalano, F., Moneta, E., Incalzi, R.A. & Ciappi, G. (1984) Respiratory function during pregnancy. *Respiration* **46**, 145–150.

Lotgering, F.K., Gilbert, R.D. & Longo, L.D. (1984) The interactions of exercise and pregnancy. *Am. J. Obstet. Gynecol.* **149**, 560–568.

Morton, M.J., Paul, N.S., Compos, G.R., Hartz, M.V. & Metcalfe J. (1985) Exercise dynamics in late gestation: effects of physical training. *Am. J. Obstet. Gynecol.* **152**, 91–97.

Pleet, H., Graham, J.M. & Smith, D.W. (1981) Central nervous system and facial defects associated with maternal hyperthermia at four to 14 weeks gestation. *Pediatrics* **67**, 785–789.

Pritchard, J.A. (1965) Changes in the blood volume during pregnancy and delivery. *Anesthesiology* **26**, 393–399.

Roy, S.B., Malkani, P.K., Ranjit, V. & Bhatia, M.L. (1966) Circulatory effects of pregnancy. *Am. J. Obstet. Gynecol.* **96**, 221–225.

Sady, M., Haydon, B., Sady, S., Carpenter, M., Coustan, D. & Thompson, P. (1988) Maximal exercise during pregnancy and postpartum. *Med. Sci. Sports Exerc.* **20**, 511 (abstract).

Smith, D.W., Clarren, S.K. & Harvey, M.A.S. (1978) Hyperthermia as a possible teratogenic agent. *J. Pediatr.* **92**, 878–883.

Veland, K., Novy, M.J., Peterson, E.N. & Metcalfe, J. (1969) Maternal cardiovascular dynamics IV. The influence of gestational age on the maternal cardiovascular response to posture and exercise. *Am. J. Obstet. Gynecol.* **104**, 856–864.

Vaha-Eskeli, K. & Erkkola, R. (1988) The sauna and pregnancy. *Ann. Clin. Res.* **20**, 279–282.

Wong, S.C. & McKenzie, D.C. (1987) Cardiorespiratory fitness during pregnancy and its effect on outcome. *Int. J. Sports Med.* **8**, 79–83.

Zaharieva, E. (1972) Olympic participation by women. *J.A.M.A.* **221**, 992–995.

Chapter 37

The Elderly and Endurance Training

MICHAEL L. POLLOCK, DAVID T. LOWENTHAL,
JAMES E. GRAVES AND JOAN F. CARROLL

Introduction

The population in North America and most industrialized countries is living longer. The US Census Bureau data show that since 1980 the US population has increased by 11% in the age range of 65–74 years, 17.1% for 75–84 years, and 24.8% above 85 years. Beck (1989) reported that the number of persons in the USA over 65 years of age was 29.8 million in 1987 and is projected to be 34.9 million by the year 2000, an increase of 17.1%. With increased life expectancy, persons who reached 65 years of age in 1985 will live an average of 17 additional years (Beck, 1989).

Stephens (1987) reported that the activity levels of elderly persons have increased over the past two decades. Even so, it was estimated that at most 10% of elderly individuals participate in regular vigorous physical activity (defined as activity that involves an energy expenditure 12.5 kJ·kg^{-1} body mass, three times per week for a minimum of 20 min per session) (Haskell *et al.*, 1985). Further, up to 50% of North Americans over 60 years of age rate themselves as having a sedentary lifestyle (Stephens, 1987).

There is a dramatic increase in health problems and physical limitations associated with ageing. The physical and physiological limitations that will be discussed here are related to changes in aerobic power/maximal oxygen intake ($\dot{V}o_{2\,max}$), body composition, muscular strength, activities of daily living and

a variety of chronic diseases. It is well established that many health problems and physical limitations are related to lifestyle. Thus, sedentary living may have a significant adverse effect on health and physical wellbeing. With the elderly population living longer, the importance of leisure-time activity and regular exercise-training is apparent. The purpose of this chapter is to discuss the various health problems and physical/physiological limitations that are associated with ageing, to review studies dealing with endurance training in the elderly, and to give recommendations for exercise prescription in such individuals. Special concerns and contraindications to exercise in the elderly will also be addressed.

Physiological and pathological changes related to ageing and exercise

Physical capacity declines with age (Dehn & Bruce, 1972; Raven & Mitchell, 1980). The loss of physical capacity has been attributed to age, medications, diseases and/or a sedentary lifestyle. The majority of the elderly do not exercise, nor have they been encouraged to participate in regular exercise. It is unclear, therefore, whether the reduced state of physical conditioning associated with ageing is a result of deconditioning (sedentary lifestyle), age, or both. Several reports have suggested that the age-associated decline in physical performance can be minimized by regular endurance training

(Ordway & Wekstein, 1979; Buskirk & Hodgson, 1987; Pollock & Wilmore, 1990).

Age-associated changes in organ and tissue function such as a decline in fat-free mass, total body and intracellular water and an increase in fat mass (Sidney *et al.*, 1977; Suominen *et al.*, 1977a) may alter the physiological responses to exercise and influence drug dynamics and kinetics (Richey & Bender, 1975; 1977; Epstein, 1979).

Changes in cardiac function

Cardiac performance undergoes direct and indirect age-associated changes. With increasing age, there is a small reduction in the contractility of the myocardium (Becklake *et al.*, 1965; Dock, 1966; Gerstenblith *et al.*, 1976) which may be due to a decrease in myocardial catecholamine responses (Gerstenblith *et al.*, 1976). Plasma noradrenaline concentrations of the elderly are increased, but the cardiovascular responses are diminished (Palmer *et al.*, 1978; Eisdorfer, 1980). The myocardium increases in stiffness, which impairs ventricular diastolic relaxation and increases end diastolic pressure (Templeton *et al.*, 1979; Weisfeldt, 1981). This suggests that exercise-induced increases in heart rate would be less well tolerated in older individuals than in younger populations. The age-associated decline in maximal heart rate is well established (Åstrand & Rodahl, 1986). The cause of this alteration is multifactorial, but is mostly related to a decrement in sympathetic nervous system (adrenergic) reactivity. Reductions in $\dot{V}_{O_{2\,max}}$, cardiac output, stroke volume and stroke index have all been observed with increasing age (Brandfonbrenner *et al.*, 1955; Becklake *et al.*, 1965; Dehn & Bruce, 1972; Gerstenblith *et al.*, 1976; Raven & Mitchell, 1980), especially in those individuals with heart disease. The healthy elderly human heart tends to maintain cardiac output, increasing stroke volume through the Starling effect (Weisfeldt, 1981).

In a young adult, acute exercise results in a redistribution of the cardiac output from in-

active to active tissues (Clausen, 1977); in particular, there is a reduction in resting splanchnic flow in order to increase perfusion of the exercising muscle. In the elderly, the resting splanchnic blood flow is reduced to a greater extent than cardiac output, thereby allowing other tissues to be adequately perfused (Bender, 1965). This reduction in resting splanchnic blood flow limits the availability of blood for redirection to skeletal muscle and the skin during exercise.

Older persons do not tolerate high ambient temperatures as well as younger persons (Shock, 1977), because decreases in cardiovascular and hypothalamic function compromise heat dissipating mechanisms (Irion *et al.*, 1984). The dissipation of heat is further compromised by the decrease in fat-free mass, intracellular and total body water, and an increase in body fat.

Regular endurance exercise favourably alters coronary artery disease (CAD) risk factors, including hypertension, triglyceride and high density lipoprotein (HDL)-cholesterol concentrations, glucose tolerance and obesity. In addition, regular exercise raises the angina threshold (Pollock & Wilmore, 1990).

CAD and graded exercise testing

In spite of a downward trend in CAD mortality rates over the past two decades, cardiovascular disease is still the leading cause of death in older North Americans; CAD accounts for 80% of all cardiovascular deaths. Fifty per cent of US citizens aged over 70 years show coronary artery stenoses of 75% or more at autopsy (Gersh *et al.*, 1983).

Disease has many atypical manifestations in the elderly. Silent ischaemia may present as confusion, a disturbance of mobility or dizziness. However, angina pectoris remains the most common presenting symptom of CAD. Dyspnoea is also a common presenting symptom in elderly people who have either a myocardial infarction or transient ischaemia (Gottlieb *et al.*, 1988).

Fifty per cent of North Americans over the age of 65 years have a diagnostically abnormal resting electrocardiogram (ECG). This may reflect age-related changes in the heart, such as mild thickening of the ventricular wall and fibrosis of the conduction system. Electro-cardiographic observation of deep Q waves, 1–2 mm of ST segmental depression or T wave changes when associated with symptoms of ischaemia remain classical features of clinically significant disease (Gottlieb et al., 1988).

The aforementioned ECG changes may be interpreted as a false negative graded exercise test, especially if no further ischaemic changes are noted because of a lack of adequate exercise effort. However, further ST segmental depression to 3–4 mm, superimposed on a baseline resting ECG of 1–2 mm depression, may connote ischaemia (Bruce, 1985). Interpretation of the baseline resting ECG and the pattern observed during graded exercise testing must be made with knowledge of the confounding effects of ageing and underlying conditions, including CAD, hypokalaemia, hypomagnesaemia, hypercalcaemia and hypoxaemia.

Musculoskeletal abnormalities and disease may also compromise exercise test performance. Individualization of the graded exercise test (treadmill or cycle ergometer) is important, and protocol selection must depend on each patient's capabilities.

The use of radionuclide scintigraphy and thallium in graded exercise testing may improve the sensitivity of the test over that of the ECG alone at lower levels of intensity. However, some decrease in specificity is found due to other concomitant illnesses that may produce abnormalities of heart function or perfusion. The gold standard for the diagnosis of CAD remains coronary arteriography.

Changes in blood pressure

Systolic blood pressure usually rises with advancing age (Kannel, 1976; Amery et al., 1978). Longitudinal data from the Framingham Study (Kannel, 1976; Kannel et al., 1987) showed a mean increase of 20–25 mmHg between the ages of 36 and 74 years in both men and women. In the same study, the diastolic blood pressure tended to fall in both men and women older than 60 years of age.

Ageing is associated with a progressive increase in the rigidity of the aorta and peripheral arteries (Dustan, 1974; Hollander, 1976), due to a loss of elastic fibres, an increase in the collagenous materials, and calcium deposition in the media. As aortic rigidity increases, the pulse generated during systole is transmitted to the arterial tree relatively unchanged. Therefore, systolic hypertension predominates in elderly hypertensive patients.

Because of the rise in diastolic blood pressure with isometric or dynamic resistance exercise (Lewis et al., 1985; MacDougall et al., 1985), the elderly with poorly controlled hypertension and/or left ventricular dysfunction should limit their strength training and concentrate more on moderate endurance exercise (Sheldahl et al., 1983; MacDougall et al., 1985). Hagberg and Seals (1986) noted that aerobic training resulted in an 8-mmHg reduction in both systolic and diastolic blood pressure in elderly hypertensive subjects.

Baroreceptor reflex function

Baroreceptor sensitivity decreases with age (Gribbin et al., 1971; Pickering et al., 1972) and (independently) with hypertension (Bristow et al., 1969; Gribbin et al., 1971). Therefore, rapid adjustment of the cerebral circulation to changes in posture may be impaired in the elderly. Adrenergic-blocking agents should be carefully titrated, and blood pressure should be checked in the supine, sitting and standing positions. Regular endurance training does not seem to rectify the gradual deterioration in orthostatic blood pressure regulation with age.

Renal function

Glomerular filtration rate (GFR) and renal plasma flow are well maintained up to the fifth decade. Even so, a linear decrease in GFR and renal plasma flow after the age of 20 years lead to a loss of 4 ml·min^{-1} per decade in GFR and 35 ml·min^{-1} per decade in renal plasma flow (Slack & Wilson, 1976).

Exercise results in an acute yet reversible reduction in GFR and renal plasma flow. There is a need to investigate whether these changes become superimposed on the alterations associated with ageing, adversely affecting renal function.

A defect in renal concentrating ability and sluggish renal conservation of sodium intake make elderly patients more liable to dehydration (Papper, 1973; Epstein & Hollenberg, 1976). Therefore, diuretic agents should be used cautiously and elderly participants in endurance events should be encouraged to drink plenty of fluids. Hyponatraemia and oversecretion of antidiuretic hormone further compromise normal salt, water and electrolyte homoeostasis in the elderly, a problem that can be compounded by overzealous diuretic administration.

Renin−angiotensin−aldosterone system

Plasma renin activity and plasma aldosterone concentration decrease with age in normotensive subjects, and are even lower in elderly hypertensives (Hayduck et al., 1973; Amery et al., 1978; Ogihara et al., 1979). Sympathetic nervous system deterioration with ageing is due, in part, to a decrease in β-receptor reactivity; on the other hand, plasma catecholamine levels are elevated. This is reflected in a gradual decrease of renin−angiotensin−aldosterone activity. As a result, patients have high-normal or slightly elevated resting serum potassium concentrations. This tendency is clinically augmented by the administration of potassium-sparing diuretics, β-adrenergic blocking drugs, angiotensin-converting enzyme inhibitors, and non-steroidal anti-inflammatory drugs. The hyperkalaemia may be further exacerbated if the patient is an

insulin-dependent diabetic with a degree of renal insufficiency.

As a result of vigorous endurance exercise, serum potassium increases. The elderly have some protection against a lethal hyperkalaemia because skeletal muscle mass, the major source of intracellular potassium, is reduced. After endurance training, exercise-induced increases in potassium are not as large as in the untrained (Braith et al., 1990).

Hepatic function

Senescence affects hepatic function, with a decrease in the production of albumin, its molecular alteration or changes in receptor affinity. This affects many drugs that are bound to albumin and also decreases phase I (oxidation, methylation, hydroxylation) pathways of drug biotransformation (Lowenthal, 1990). Exercise, acutely and reversibly, decreases hepatic blood flow. However, it is not known whether the changes with age plus exercise exaggerate pharmacodynamic changes.

Musculoskeletal changes

Manifestations of disease are at times difficult to distinguish from age-related changes (Cummings et al., 1985; Lane et al., 1986). A decrease in muscle mass relative to total body mass starts in the fifth decade and becomes marked in the seventh decade of life. This change leads to a decrease in muscle strength, endurance, bulk and a reduction in the number of muscle fibres.

Glycolytic energy metabolism is reduced more than those enzymes involved in oxidative metabolism. The diaphragm and cardiac muscle do not seem to incur age changes.

Hyaline cartilage on the articular surface of various joints shows degenerative changes and clinically represents the fundamental alteration in degenerative osteoarthritis (Lane et al., 1986).

Bone loss is a hallmark of ageing (Cummings et al., 1985; Heidrich & Thompson, 1987). The rate of bone loss is highly individual and is greatly augmented in postmenopausal women. A decrease in bone mass (osteoporosis) can reduce body stature as well as predispose the individual to spontaneous fractures. Dynamic weight-bearing exercise can slow the decrement in bone mass. Older women are more prone to osteoporosis than older men; this may reflect hormonal differences affecting bone (Lane *et al.*, 1986).

Exercise in preventive geriatrics

Health in older people is best measured in terms of function, mental status, mobility, continence and a range of activities of daily living. Primary preventive strategies can forestall the onset of disease. Whether exercise can prevent the development of atherosclerosis, delay the occurrence of clinical CAD or prevent the evolution of hypertension is at present debatable. But moderate endurance exercise (leisure-time activity or physical training) significantly decreases cardiovascular mortality (Paffenbarger *et al.*, 1986; Leon *et al.*, 1987; Blair *et al.*, 1989). Risk factors associated with CAD are still relevant for the elderly and should be taken into consideration (Kannel *et al.*, 1987). Secondary prevention is aimed at the early diagnosis and treatment of subclinical disease. Endurance exercise can alter the contributions of stress, sedentary lifestyle, obesity and diabetes to the development of CAD (Kannel *et al.*, 1987). Tertiary prevention focuses on maintaining or improving functional status, the latter making a useful contribution in the elderly (Williams, 1984).

Special concerns related to medical clearance for exercise

Exercise for the healthy elderly person needs to be addressed in the same manner as that for a younger individual. A physician must perform a comprehensive history, physical and mental status examination, basic laboratory studies and a dynamic graded exercise test. In clearance for graded exercise testing the absolute and relative contraindications to exercise are similar for elderly and younger participants (Table 37.1). However, the considerations shown in Table 37.2 are special concerns for the elderly.

The graded exercise test needs to include careful attention to changes in cardiac rhythm compatible with ischaemia and changes in blood pressure. Abnormalities in patient response and/or symptomatology cannot be taken as signs of ageing, but must be interpreted as signs of disease. Careful observation during recovery from the graded exercise test is also critical, since arrhythmias and sudden changes of blood pressure may occur during this phase. Older patients may need a short, active, walking recovery period after both testing and training sessions in order to decrease venous pooling and attenuate abrupt increases in intravascular volume that would occur if they were placed promptly supine. Once the formal test recovery period is completed, the patient needs to be observed while upright for at least an additional 5 min and to have the blood pressure

Table 37.1 Contraindications to exercise testing in 35–64-year-olds.

Recent acute myocardial infarction
Unstable angina pectoris
Uncontrolled hypertension
Uncontrolled arrhythmia
Symptomatic left ventricular dysfunction
Acute myocarditis
Acute pericarditis
Thrombophlebitis and/or recent pulmonary embolus
Tertiary heart block
Psychotic mental illness

Table 37.2 Contraindications to exercise testing or training unique to the elderly population.

Dementia
Frailty
Global cerebrovascular accident with no evidence
  of reversibility
Multiple pressure sores
Idiopathic gait disturbances and falls
Urinary incontinence

---

checked before being allowed to resume normal activity.

Effects of endurance training in the elderly

Even though endurance training has a favourable effect on blood pressure (Hagberg & Seals, 1986), glucose tolerance (Holloszy et al., 1986), HDL-cholesterol (Wood et al., 1983; Haskell, 1986), cardiovascular mortality (Paffenbarger et al., 1986; Leon et al., 1987; Blair et al., 1989), bone density (Smith et al., 1981; Chow et al., 1987), and other physical and health-related factors, this section focuses on the effects of endurance training on aerobic power and body composition (body mass, percentage fat, and fat-free mass). The importance of resistance training and its effect on strength and fat-free mass will also be discussed. The important question is no longer whether elderly participants can make improvements with exercise, but to what extent training-induced adaptations can improve their fitness and wellbeing. Also, how do their training results compare with the responses of middle-aged and younger participants?

Aerobic power

$\dot{V}O_{2\,max}$ decreases with age (Robinson, 1938; Dehn & Bruce, 1972; Buskirk & Hodgson, 1987). Heath et al. (1981) estimated a 9% reduction in $\dot{V}O_{2\,max}$ for each decade after the age of 30 years. Longitudinal studies on average participants (Kasch & Wallace, 1976; Kasch et al., 1985; Åstrand & Rodahl, 1986) and athletes (Pollock et al., 1987) have shown that lifestyle (chronic endurance training) significantly attenuates this decline. When such training is maintained, there may be little or no decline in $\dot{V}O_{2\,max}$ over 10–20-year follow-up evaluations. Thus, it has been concluded that the decline in $\dot{V}O_{2\,max}$ is less than 5% per decade for active individuals (Buskirk & Hodgson, 1987).

Early studies showed moderate to no improvement in $\dot{V}O_{2\,max}$ with endurance training in persons over 60 years of age (Benestad, 1965; deVries, 1970) (Table 37.3). This led many to suggest that elderly participants did not adapt to endurance training to the same extent as middle-aged and younger subjects. However, the short duration of the Benestad study and the relatively low intensity of training used by deVries may have limited improvements.

Recent reviews (American College of Sports Medicine (ACSM), 1990; Pollock & Wilmore, 1990) have shown that aerobic power is increased by 15–30% in most populations with 3–12 months of endurance training. The ACSM's position stand (1990) on 'The recommended quantity and quality of exercise for developing and maintaining cardiorespiratory and muscular fitness in healthy adults' is shown in Table 37.4.

Intensity and duration of training are interrelated. Lower intensity exercise requires a longer duration to elicit results that are comparable to those found with higher intensity training. Within this framework the total amount of energy expended appears to be the important factor (ACSM recommends 1050–1260 kJ (250–300 kcal) per exercise session for a 70-kg person). Thus, activities with an intensity similar to moderate walking require a training duration of 40–50 min and jogging/running requires 20–30 min.

Table 37.3 shows the effects of endurance training on $\dot{V}O_{2\,max}$ in the elderly. Even though several investigations did not report precise information on intensity of training, it does appear that elderly participants who meet the guidelines for fitness recommended by the ACSM increase their $\dot{V}O_{2\,max}$ to the same magnitude as younger participants. For example, Sidney and Shephard (1978) showed that subjects who trained at 60% or 80% of maximal heart rate reserve (HRR_{max}) for 30 min more than 2 days per week had a 14% and 29% increase in $\dot{V}O_{2\,max}$ respectively, while a group who trained at 60% of HRR_{max} for less than 2 days per week showed no change.

Table 37.3 Effect of exercise training on improvement of $\dot{V}o_{2\,max}$ in the elderly.

Study	n	Mean age (years)	Training (weeks)	Type	Intensity (% HRR_{max})	Frequency (days·week^{-1})	Duration (min)	Δ $\dot{V}o_{2\,max}$ (%)
Sidney &	14	62	14	W	60	>2	30	14*
Shephard	8	64	14	W	80	>2	30	29*
(1978)	8	65	14	W	80	<2	30	19*
	12	71	14	W	60	<2	30	−1
Cunningham et al. (1987)	100	63	52	W/J	60 + max METS‡	3	30	11*
Seals et al. (1984)	11	63	26	W	40–50	3	20–30	12*
			26	W/J, B, WG	85	3	30–45	17*
Schwartz (1988)	10	65	12	W/J	80–85	3	40	10*
Meredith et al. (1989)	10	65	12	B	70	3	45	20*
Niinimaa &	10	65	11	W/J, C	HR 125–145	3	10–15	0.5
Shephard (1978)	9	65	11	W/J, C	HR 145–155	3	10–15	10
Chow et al. (1987)	19	66	54	W,D,C	80% HR_{max}	3	30	72*
Adams & deVries (1973)	17	66	12	W/J, C	60	3	15–20	21*†
Badenhop et al.	14	66	9	B	30–45	3	25	16*
(1983)	14	68	9	B	60–75	3	25	15*
deVries (1970)	68	69	6	W/J, C	n.r.	3	30–45	5*†
deVries (1970)	8	69	42	W/J, C	n.r.	3	30–45	8†
Souminen et al. (1977b)	26	69	8	W/J, S BG, G	n.r.	3	60	11*†
Barry et al. (1966)	8	70	12	B-INT	n.r.	3	40	38*
Hagberg et al. (1989)	16	72	26	W/J	75–85	3	35–45	20*
Benestad (1965)	13	75	5–6	WG-INT	n.r.	3	10–22	0

* Significantly different from baseline measurement at $p \leqslant 0.05$ or less.
† $\dot{V}o_2$ predicted by Åstrand Ryhming submaximal cycle test.
‡ 1 MET = resting metabolic equivalent, usually 3.5 ml oxygen·kg^{-1}·min^{-1}.
B, bicycling; BG, ball games; C, calisthenics; D, dance; G, gymnastics; HR, heart rate; HRR_{max}, maximal heart rate reserve; INT, intervals; n.r., not reported. S, swimming; W, walk; WG, walking on an uphill grade; W/J, walk/jog.

Muscular strength

Resistance training does little to promote aerobic fitness, although it is an effective means of developing and maintaining fat-free mass. As was mentioned earlier, muscular strength and fat-free mass decrease with age, with more dramatic changes occurring after 50–60 years of age (Forbes, 1976; 1987). Thus, some type of strength training can benefit most elderly people.

Body composition

Changes in body composition (body mass, percentage fat and fat-free mass) associated with aerobic training are shown in Table 37.5. Although body mass is reported in most studies, body fat and fat-free mass are mentioned infrequently. Many of the aerobic training programmes that met the aerobic fitness guidelines of the ACSM (see Table 37.4) showed a modest, but significant decrease of body mass

Table 37.4 The American College of Sports Medicine's position stand on 'The recommended quantity and quality of exercise for developing and maintaining cardiorespiratory and muscular fitness in healthy adults' (ACSM, 1990).

Factor	Recommendation
Frequency of training	3–5 days per week
Intensity of training	60–90% of maximal heart rate or 50–85% of $\dot{V}O_{2\,max}$ or maximal heart rate reserve
Duration of training	20–60 min of continuous aerobic activity. Duration depends on the intensity of the activity; thus lower intensity activity should be conducted over a longer period of time. Because of the importance of the 'total fitness' effect, more readily attained in longer duration programmes, and because of the potential hazards and compliance problems associated with high intensity activity, low to moderate intensity activity of longer duration is recommended for the non-athletic adult
Mode of activity	Any activity that uses large muscle groups, can be maintained continuously, and is rhythmic and aerobic in nature, e.g. walking–hiking, running–jogging, cycling–bicycling, cross-country skiing, dancing, rope skipping, rowing, stair climbing, swimming, skating and various endurance game activities
Resistance training	Strength training of a moderate intensity, sufficient to develop and maintain fat-free weight, should be an integral part of an adult fitness programme. One set of 8–12 repetitions of 8–10 exercises that condition the major muscle groups on at least 2 days per week is the recommended minimum

(from 0.0 to −2.8 kg, $\bar{x} = 1.1$ kg) (note, one study showed no loss of mass). The average loss (Table 37.5) was less than the average of 1.5 kg found in 32 studies on young and middle-aged subjects (Wilmore, 1983; ACSM, 1990). The percentage fat changes in the elderly ranged from −0.9 to −2.6% ($\bar{x} = 1.4\%$), again less than the −2.2% fat reported by the ACSM (1990) from Wilmore's review (1983). A valid comparison of reductions in body mass and fat with aerobic training between elderly and younger participants is not yet possible, but it appears that elderly exercisers make similar modest changes.

Most studies have not reported fat-free mass data in regard to aerobic training.

Exercise prescription in the elderly

Most elderly men and women can benefit from a regular and appropriately designed exercise programme. Like middle-aged and younger participants, exercise prescription for the elderly is dependent on their needs, goals, physical and health status, available time, equipment and facilities, and personal preference (Larson & Bruce, 1987; Pollock & Wilmore, 1990). Shephard (1990) adds that when prescribing exercise for the elderly, safety of the programme, compliance and potential effectiveness should be considered. Lower intensity exercise programmes aid participants in avoiding injury and a potential cardiovascular event, both of which are related to higher intensity exercise (Waller, 1987; Pollock & Wilmore, 1990). Because elderly subjects vary more in health status and level of fitness than middle-aged participants, the art of prescribing safe and adequate training regimens becomes more challenging.

Guidelines for exercise in the elderly

In general, the prescription needed to develop and maintain cardiorespiratory fitness in the elderly does not differ much in principle from that used for middle-aged or younger partici-

Table 37.5 Effect of aerobic training on body composition in the elderly.

Study	n	Mean age (years)	Weeks	Type	Intensity (%HRR$_{max}$)	Frequency (days·week^{-1})	Duration (min)	Criterion	Δ BM (kg)	Δ BF (%)	Δ SF (mm)	Δ FFM (kg)
Cunningham et al. (1987)	102	63	52	W/J	60 + max MET‡	3	30	Σ8 SF[1]	−0.4		+1.1	
Seals et al. (1984)†	11	63	26	W	40	3	20–30	Σ6 SF[2]	−0.5		−5.0	
			26	W/J, B, WG	75–85	3	30–45		−1.2*			
Schwartz (1988)	10	65	12	W/J	80–85	3	40	HW	−2.8*	−2.6*	−17.0*	+0.08
Meredith et al. (1989)	10	65	12	B	70	3	45	HW	+0.1	−1.3		
Niinimaa & Shephard (1978)	10	65	52	W/J, C	HR125–145	3	10–15		−1.1			
	9	65	52	W/J, C	HR145–155	3	10–15		+0.4			
Adams & deVries (1973)	17	66	12	W/J, C	60	3	15–20 W/J 20–25 C	Σ2 SF[3]	−0.5[n.a.]		−1.8[n.a.]	
deVries (1970)	68	69	6	W/J, C	n.a.	3	30–45	Σ3 SF[4]	−0.9*	−0.9*		
	8	69	42	W/J, C	n.a.	3	30–45		−1.0	−0.9		
Souminen et al. (1977b)	26	69	8	W/J, S, BG, G	n.a.	3	60		−0.3			
Graves et al. (in press)	17	72	26	W/J	85	3	35–45	Σ7 SF[5]	−1.0*	−1.5*	−12.5*	

* Significantly different from baseline measurement at $p < 0.05$ or less.

† Complete study was 52 consecutive weeks of training, same subjects throughout.

‡ See Table 37.3

B, bicycling; BF, body fat; BG, ball games; BM, body mass; C, calisthenics; FFM, fat-free mass; G, gymnastics; HR, heart rate; HRR$_{max}$, maximal heart rate reserve; HW, hydrostatic weighing; n.a., no statistics available; S, swimming; SF, skinfolds; W, walk; WG, walking on an uphill grade; W/J, walk/jog.

[1] Chest, triceps, biceps, subscapular, umbilical, suprailiac, anterior thigh and medial calf.

[2] Triceps, subscapular, pectoral, umbilical, suprailiac and anterior thigh.

[3] Triceps and suprailiac.

[4] Triceps, subscapular and chest.

[5] Chest, axilla, triceps, subscapular, abdominal, suprailiac and anterior thigh.

pants (see Table 37.4). The major difference is in how these guidelines are applied to the elderly. Programmes most often recommended are similar to those prescribed for the unfit, obese, cardiac or more fragile participant. Thus, it is typically suggested that old people exercise at a lower intensity, for a longer duration, use activities that avoid high impact on the joints, and progress in training at a slower rate than younger individuals (deVries, 1979; Lampman, 1987; ACSM, 1990; Pollock & Wilmore, 1990; Shephard, 1990).

The programme should include warm-up, some muscular conditioning, a substantial aerobic phase, and a cool-down period. The total programme should not last for more than 1 h for an average individual (Pollock & Wilmore, 1990). Programmes of longer duration usually have high dropout rates.

The elderly participant should place more emphasis on the warm-up and cool-down periods. The warm-up should include stretching, low-level calisthenics, and low-level aerobic activity such as slow walking, cycling or swimming. The muscular conditioning period could come before or after the main endurance aerobic period, depending on personal preference. The muscular conditioning period includes moderate intensity calisthenics and/or weight training. The aerobic period would normally be specific to the participant's needs and sport, and could include any of a variety of endurance activities such as fast walking, swimming, cycling, stair stepping or rowing.

The biggest difference between endurance training programmes for the elderly and those prescribed for younger participants is the intensity/duration component (Pollock & Wilmore, 1990). For the average elderly person, the intensity of training would be more moderate (50–70% of HRR_{max}) and the duration would be longer (40–50 min). Younger participants may benefit from high intensity interval training (short duration sprints and rest periods), but this is not usually recommended for the elderly, due to the increased risk of injury and potential of precipitating a cardiac event. If the subject has not recently been active in sports, an initial training intensity of 30–45% of HRR_{max} is appropriate for many elderly participants during the first weeks of endurance training. The starting programme is usually conducted for a duration of 15–20 min. It is important to increase intensity and duration gradually to minimize the risk of injury or untoward event. Thus, progression of training may take several weeks or months to achieve the maintenance level. Our experience suggests that the duration of training should be increased by 5 min and the intensity by increments of 5% of HRR_{max} approximately every 2 weeks. The unfit subject should progress first by increasing duration and then by increasing intensity (Pollock & Wilmore, 1990).

The training intensity for each workout can easily be monitored by determining heart rate at the midpoint and end of each training session, and making the appropriate calculation of the percentage of HRR_{max}. More recently, the rating of perceived exertion (RPE) scale (Borg, 1982) has been used to help monitor exercise intensity (Birk & Birk, 1987; ACSM, 1990; Pollock & Wilmore, 1990). The RPE scale relates well to heart rate, $\dot{V}O_2$, pulmonary ventilation and blood lactate (Borg, 1982). Thus, knowledge of the RPE will allow the participants to regulate their training programme perceptually. Exercising at an intensity that produces a training effect is important and, at the same time, regulating the programme at a perceptually acceptable level (moderate to somewhat hard) will aid in long-term adherence (Table 37.6).

Is the training intensity for exercise prescription calculated and interpreted in the same manner for elderly participants as for young and middle-aged adults? In our experience with healthy elderly subjects and cardiac patients, the percentage of HRR technique and RPE scale are acceptable (Pollock et al., 1986; Pollock, 1988). Table 37.6 shows the recommended classification of exercise intensity based on endurance exercise programmes lasting for

Table 37.6 Classification of intensity of exercise based on 30–60 min of endurance training. Adapted from Pollock & Wilmore (1990).

Relative intensity ($V_{O_{2\,max}}$ or HRR_{max})	Rating of perceived exertion	Classification of intensity
< 30%	< 10	Very light
30–49%	10–11	Light
50–74%	12–13	Moderate (somewhat hard)
75–84%	14–16	Heavy
< 85%	> 16	Very heavy

HRR_{max}, maximal heart rate reserve.

30–60 min (Pollock & Wilmore, 1990). The table lists the relationship between the percentage of HRR_{max} and RPE. Based on the elderly participants' individualized exercise test results, these markers of intensity have similar value and meaning in the training and progression of training in elderly as in younger participants.

Because of the strong relationship between high-impact activities, such as jogging/running and aerobic dance, and musculo-skeletal injuries, low-impact activities should be emphasized where possible (Kilbom et al., 1969; Mann et al., 1969; Oja et al., 1974; Pollock et al., 1977; 1991; Richie et al., 1985). Injuries related to high-impact activity are also related to ageing (Table 37.7; Pollock, 1988). The programmes listed were conducted with healthy, previously sedentary volunteers, who trained for 5–6 months by walking (W) and walk/jogging (W/J) for 30–40 min, for 3 days (W/J) or 4 days (W) per week (Pollock et al., 1971; 1976; 1977; 1991). In the experiments conducted by Pollock et al. in 1976 and 1977, training began with equal amounts of W/J and progressed to more continuous jogging as adaptation to training occurred. In our recent investigation (Pollock et al., 1991), jogging was not introduced until after 3 months of moderately paced walking (40–60% of HRR_{max}, RPE 11–12) to fast walking (60–70% of HRR_{max}, RPE 12–13) training.

It was surprising that even after 3 months of preliminary training (W), the injury rate was high when the 70-year-old subjects began to walk/jog. Injuries occurred within the first 2 weeks of W/J, and in all cases but one were resolved within 3 weeks of training on a stationary cycle or slow walking on a treadmill. One woman had a stress fracture of the tibia and could not continue in the study. Eventually, all subjects could develop a training heart rate of 75–85% of HRR_{max} (RPE 14–15). The injured subjects continued to walk on the treadmill at an elevation that elicited the desired heart rate response. All of the six women who began to W/J were injured, but only two of eight men were affected. We realize that this is a small sample, but it appears that elderly females are more susceptible to injury than elderly males.

In the above mentioned W/J study on 70–79-year-old participants (Pollock et al., 1991), the average increases in $V_{O_{2\,max}}$ were 16% and 22%, after 3 and 6 months' training, respectively (Hagberg et al., 1989). The W/J programme that was prescribed was not limited by the cardiorespiratory system, but by the musculoskeletal system (orthopaedic limitations). Further, since a 16% increase in $V_{O_{2\,max}}$ was attained by moderate intensity walking during the first 3 months of the programme, the additional 6% increase in $V_{O_{2\,max}}$ found with W/J was probably not worth the additional risk of injury.

The fast walking study reported in Table 37.7 (Pollock et al., 1971) produced a 30% increase in $V_{O_{2\,max}}$ and had the lowest injury (12%) and

Table 37.7 Comparison of injuries by age.*

Study	n	Age range (years)	Mode	Injuries (%)
Pollock *et al.* (1977)	50	20—35	W	18
Pollock *et al.* (1971)	19	40—56	W	12
Pollock *et al.* (1976)	22	49—65	W/J	41
Pollock *et al.* (1991)	14	70—79	W, W/J	57

* All programmes were conducted with healthy, previously sedentary individuals. Except for Pollock *et al.* (1971), all programmes had a walk/jog (W/J) component; the 1971 study included only walking (W) as the mode of training. Injuries occurred mainly in the foot, ankle, leg, or knee and led to withdrawal from training for at least 1 week.
From Pollock (1988).

dropout rate of any of the 25 endurance training studies conducted by Pollock and colleagues since 1968. These data and others have clearly shown that walking is an effective programme for developing a moderate level of aerobic fitness and improving body composition (Sharkey & Holleman, 1967; Pollock *et al.*, 1975; Leon *et al.*, 1979; Rippe *et al.*, 1988). Walking is simple to carry out and requires little in terms of skill, special facilities or equipment. Its lower intensity and impact forces make it safe and easily adaptable to elderly participants.

If exercise-training cannot be sustained for the required length of time, low-level interval-training may be necessary. This would include periods of slow to moderate walking interspersed with periods of very slow walking or sitting. As adaptation occurs, longer periods of moderate to fast walking are used. The RPE scale is useful in rating peripheral discomfort/pain. Our experience has shown that when the discomfort level reaches 13 (moderate—somewhat hard) on the RPE scale, a rest period should begin. Boyd *et al.* (1984) reported significant improvements of performance in intermittent claudication patients who were trained relatively pain-free for 12 weeks. Shephard (1990) recommends circuit training whereby 1—2-min bouts of light activity are interspersed with short bouts of exercise using different tasks/exercise stations.

Strength training

A well-rounded stretching and muscle conditioning programme is particularly useful in the elderly, because of a loss of muscle mass and functional capacity of various body segments (Forbes, 1976; 1987; Åstrand & Rodahl, 1986; Pollock & Wilmore, 1990). For example, Pollock *et al.* (1987) completed a 10-year follow-up study on master runners whose ages ranged from 50 to 82 years. The study was designed to assess the runners' ability to maintain their aerobic power over a 10-year time span. Eleven of the 25 subjects evaluated continued to train at the same level over the 10-year period, and their $\dot{V}O_{2\,max}$ did not change (54.2 vs. 53.3 ml·kg^{-1}·min^{-1}), whereas the group who reduced their training showed a significant decrease (52.5 vs. 45.9 ml·kg^{-1}·min^{-1}). The striking finding in the investigation was the significant loss of fat-free mass in both groups. As a whole they showed a slight loss of body mass, an increase in body fat, and a 2.0 kg decline in fat-free mass over this time span. Considering their low body fat (13.2%) and continued training, this last change was a surprising finding. Short-term studies with younger individuals show that fat-free mass is usually maintained with endurance training (Pollock & Wilmore, 1990), while weight/resistance training activities generally increase muscle mass (Gettman & Pollock, 1981; Fleck & Kraemer, 1987).

Although ageing is an important consideration, the manner in which the runners trained (just by running) also contributed to the loss of fat-free mass. The training mode shows significant specificity (Åstrand & Rodahl, 1986). Specificity of training was supported by response circumference measurements on the upper arm and thigh. The upper arm girth showed a significant reduction, while the thigh remained constant. An interview with each athlete revealed that most of them only trained aerobically and did little strength training. Three of the 25 subjects included upper-body training as part of their regular regimen. Two weight-trained and one was an avid cross-country skier. These three athletes were the only ones who maintained their fat-free mass. Age did not seem to be a factor, because there was one athlete for each decade of age from 50 to 80 years. These data illustrate the need for a well-rounded exercise programme. It is also one of the reasons for the ACSM adding a strength component to their Position Stand (see Table 37.4).

Although calisthenics can provide enough overload to increase strength in the elderly, moderate weight-training can be safe and can produce better results (Fleck & Kraemer, 1987). The eight to ten exercises recommended by the ACSM (see Table 37.4) should be adequate to train the major muscles of the body (arms, shoulders, trunk, hips and legs). The development of new equipment such as variable resistance exercise devices makes this type of training particularly suitable and safe for the elderly population (Pollock, 1988; Pollock & Wilmore, 1990).

Summary

After maturation, aerobic power and muscular strength decline. These declines in physiological function are associated with a reduction in muscle mass, a concomitant increase in relative body fat and an increased incidence of disease.

Although traditionally considered a direct consequence of the ageing process, recent studies have shown that many age-related declines in functional capacity and health status can be reduced by regular physical activity. This suggests that reduced physiological function is related to a sedentary lifestyle and that elderly men and women would benefit from exercise training.

The needs and goals of an exercise programme for elderly persons should emphasize fitness development, but the maintenance of functional capacity and quality of life are equally important. The basic guidelines of frequency, intensity, and duration of training and mode of activity recommended by the ACSM are appropriate for the elderly. The big difference is the manner in which these guidelines are applied.

Given that the elderly person is more fragile and has more physical–medical limitations than the middle-aged participant, the intensity of the programme is lower, while training frequency and duration are increased. High-impact activities should be avoided and progression of training should be more gradual. The calculation of the training heart rate, 50–85% of HRR_{max}, and its relationship to relative metabolic work and rating of perceived exertion, are similar to those found for younger participants. Because of the importance of maintaining muscle mass and bone density in middle and old age, a well-rounded endurance training programme should include some strength/resistance exercise of the major muscle groups. Finally, exercise prescription for most elderly persons should emphasize moderate-intensity, low-impact activities; it should avoid heavy static–dynamic lifting, and allow for a slow, gradual adaptation period.

References

Adams, G. & deVries, H. (1973) Physiological effects of an exercise training regimen upon women aged 52 to 79. *J. Gerontol.* **28**, 50–55.

American College of Sports Medicine (ACSM) (1990) The recommended quantity and quality of exercise for developing and maintaining cardiorespiratory and muscle fitness in healthy adults. *Med. Sci. Sports Exerc.* **22**, 265–274.

Amery, A., Wasir, H., Bulpitt, C. *et al.* (1978) Aging and the cardiovascular system. *Acta. Cardiol. (Brux)* **6**, 443.

Åstrand, P. & Rodahl, K. (1986) *Textbook of Work Physiology*, 3rd edn. McGraw-Hill, New York.

Badenhop, D., Cleary, P., Schaal, S., Fox, E. & Bartels, R. (1983) Physiological adjustments to higher- or lower-intensity exercise in elders. *Med. Sci. Sports Exerc.* **15**, 496–502.

Barry, A., Daly, J., Pruett, E. *et al.* (1966) The effects of physical conditioning on older individuals. I. Work capacity, circulatory–respiratory function and work electrocardiogram. *J. Gerontol.* **21**, 182–191.

Beck, J. (1989) General principles of aging: demography of aging. In: Beck, J. (ed.) *Geriatrics Review Syllabus: A Core Curriculum in Geriatric Medicine*, pp. 1–5. American Geriatrics Society, New York.

Becklake, M., Frank, H., Dagenais, G., Ostiguy, G. & Guzman, C. (1965) Age changes in myocardial function and exercise response. *Prog. Cardiovasc. Dis.* **19**, 1–21.

Bender, A. (1965) The effect of increasing age on the distribution of peripheral blood flow in man. *J. Am. Geriatr. Soc.* **13**, 192–198.

Benestad, A. (1965) Trainability of old men. *Acta Med. Scand.* **178**, 321–327.

Birk, T. & Birk, C. (1987) Use of ratings of perceived exertion for exercise prescription. *J. Sports Med.* **4**, 1–8.

Blair, S., Kohl, H., Paffenbarger, R., Clark, D., Cooper, K. & Gibbons, L. (1989) Physical fitness and all-cause mortality: a prospective study of healthy men and women. *J.A.M.A.* **262**, 2395–2401.

Borg, G. (1982) Psychophysical bases of perceived exertion. *Med. Sci Sports Exerc.* **14**, 377–381.

Boyd, C., Bird, P., Charles, C., Wellons, H., MacDougall, M. & Wolfe, L. (1984) Pain free physical training in intermittent claudication. *J. Sports Med.* **24**, 112–122.

Braith, R., Lowenthal, D., Graves, J., Leggett, S., Wilcox, C. & Pollock, M. (1990) The influence of exercise training on the renin–aldesterone system of the elderly. *Med. Sci. Sports Exerc.* (abstract) **22**, S33.

Brandfonbrenner, M., Landowne, M. & Shock, N. (1955) Changes in cardiac output with age. *Circulation* **12**, 557–566.

Bristow, J., Honour, A., Pickering, G., Sleight, P. & Smith, H. (1969) Diminished baroflex sensitivity in high blood pressure. *Circulation* **39**, 48.

Bruce, R. (1985) Functional aerobic capacity, exercise and aging. In: Andres, R., Bierman, E. & Hazzard, W. (eds) *Principles of Geriatric Medicine*, pp. 87–103. McGraw-Hill, New York.

Buskirk, E. & Hodgson, J. (1987) Age and aerobic power: the rate of change in men and women. *Fed. Proc.* **46**, 1824–1829.

Chow, R., Harrison, J., Sturtridge, W. *et al.* (1987) The effect of exercise on bone mass of osteoporotic patients on fluoride treatments. *Clin. Invest. Med.* **10**, 59–63.

Clausen, J. (1977) Effect of physical training on cardiovascular adjustments to exercise in man. *Physiol. Rev.* **57**, 779–815.

Cummings, S., Kelsey, J., Nevitt, M. *et al.* (1985) Epidemiology of osteoporosis and osteoporotic fractures. *Epidemiol. Rev.* **7**, 178–208.

Cunningham, D., Rechnitzer, P., Howard, J. & Donner, A. (1987) Exercise training of men at retirement: a clinical trial. *J. Gerontol.* **42**, 17–23.

Dehn, M. & Bruce, R. (1972) Longitudinal variations in maximal oxygen intake with age and activity. *J. Appl. Physiol.* **33**, 805–807.

deVries, H. (1970) Physiological effects of an exercise training program upon men aged 52 to 88. *J. Gerontol.* **24**, 325–336.

deVries, H. (1979) Tips on prescribing exercise regimens for your older patient. *Geriatrics* **75–77**, 80–81.

Dock, W. (1966) How some hearts age. *J.A.M.A.* **195**, 442–444.

Dustan, H. (1974) Atherosclerosis complicating chronic hypertension. *Circulation* **50**, 871.

Eisdorfer, C. (1980) Neurotransmitters and aging: clinical correlates. In: R. Adelman *et al.* (eds) *Neural Regulatory Mechanisms During Aging*, pp. 53–69. Alan R. Liss, New York.

Epstein, M. (1979) Effects of aging of the kidney. *Fed. Proc., Fed. Am. Soc. Exp. Biol.* **38**, 168–173.

Epstein, M. & Hollenberg, N. (1976) Age as a determinant of renal sodium conservation in normal man. *J. Lab. Clin. Med.* **87**, 411.

Fleck, S. & Kraemer, W. (1987) *Designing Resistance Training Programs*. Human Kinetics, Champaign, Illinois.

Forbes, G. (1976) The adult decline in lean body mass. *Hum. Biol.* **48**, 161–173.

Forbes, G. (1987) *Human Body Composition. Growth, Aging, Nutrition and Activity.* Springer-Verlag, New York.

Gersh, B., Kronmal, R., Frye, R. *et al.* (1983) Coronary arteriography and coronary artery bypass surgery: morbidity and mortality in patients age 65 years or older: a report from the coronary artery surgery study. *Circulation* **67**, 483.

Gerstenblith, G., Lakatta, E. & Weisfeldt, M. (1976) Age changes in myocardial function and exercise response. *Prog. Cardiovasc. Dis.* **19**, 1–21.

Gettman, L. & Pollock, M. (1981) Circuit weight training: a critical review of its physiological benefits. *Phys. Sportsmed.* **9**(1), 44−60.

Gottlieb, S., Gottlieb, S., Ashuffsc, *et al.* (1988) Silent ischemia on Holter monitoring predicts mortality in high risk post infarction patients. *J.A.M.A.* **259**, 1030−1035.

Graves, J., Panton, L., Pollock, M., Hagberg, J. & Leggett, S. (1990) Effect of aerobic and resistance training on strength and body composition of men and women 70−79 years of age. *J. Gerontol. Med. Sci.* (in press).

Gribbin, B., Pickering, T., Sleight, P. & Peto, R. (1971) Effect of age and high blood pressure on baroflex sensitivity in man. *Circ. Res.* **29**, 424.

Hagberg, J. & Seals, D. (1986) Exercise training and hypertension. *Acta. Med. Scand.* **711**(Suppl.), 131−136.

Hagberg, J., Graves, J., Limacher, M. *et al.* (1989) Cardiovascular responses of 70−79 year old men and women to exercise training. *J. Appl. Physiol.* **66**, 2589−2594.

Haskell, W. (1986) The influence of exercise training on plasma lipids and lipoproteins in health and disease. *Acta. Med. Scand. Suppl.* **711**, 25−37.

Haskell, W., Montoye, H. & Orenstein, D. (1985) Physical activity and exercise to achieve health-related physical fitness components. *Public Health Rep.* **100**, 202−212.

Hayduck, K., Krause, D., Kaufmann, W., Huenges, R., Schillmoeller, U. & Unbehaun, V. (1973) Age dependent changes of plasma renin concentration in humans. *Clin. Sci. Mol. Med.* **45** (Suppl. 1), 273.

Heath, G., Hagberg, J., Ehsani, A. & Holloszy, J. (1981) A physiological comparison of young and older endurance athletes. *J. Appl. Physiol.* **51**, 634−640.

Heidrich, F. & Thompson, R. (1987) Osteoporosis prevention: strategies applicable for general population groups. *J. Fam. Pract.* **25**, 33−39.

Hollander, W. (1976) Role of hypertension in athero-sclerosis and cardiovascular disease. *Am. J. Cardiol.* **38**, 786.

Holloszy, J., Schultz, J., Kusnierkiewicz, J., Hagberg, J. & Ehsani, A. (1986) Effects of exercise on glucose tolerance and insulin resistance. *Acta. Med. Scand.* **711**(Suppl.), 55−65.

Irion, G., Wailgum, T., Stevens, C., Kendrick, Z. & Paolone, A. (1984) The effect of age on the hemodynamic response to thermal stress during exercise. In: Cristafalo, V., Baker, G., Adelman, R. & Roberts, I. (eds) *Altered Endocrine States During Aging*, pp. 187−195. H.A. Liss, New York.

Kannel, W. (1976) Blood pressure and the development of cardiovascular disease in the aged. In: Caird, F., Dahl, J. & Kennedy, R. (eds) *Cardiology in Old Age*, pp. 143−175. Plenum Press, New York.

Kannel, W., Doyle, J., Shephard, R., Stamler, J. & Vokonas, P. (1987) Prevention of cardiovascular disease in the elderly. *J. Am. Coll. Cardiol.* **10**, 25A−28A.

Kasch, F. & Wallace, J. (1976) Physiological variables during 10 years of endurance exercise. *Med. Sci. Sports* **8**, 5−8.

Kasch, F., Wallace, J. & van Camp, S. (1985) Effects of 18 years of endurance exercise on physical work capacity of older men. *J. Cardiopulm. Rehab.* **15**, 308−312.

Kilbom, A., Hartley, L., Saltin, B., Bjure, J., Grimby, G. & Åstrand, I. (1969) Physical training in sedentary middle-aged and older men. *Scand J. Clin. Lab. Invest.* **24**, 315−322.

Lampman, R. (1987) Evaluating and prescribing exercise for elderly patients. *Geriatrics* **42**, 63−76.

Lane, C., Bloch, D., Jones, S. *et al.* (1986) Long distance running, bone density, and osteoarthritis. *J.A.M.A.* **255**, 1147−1151.

Larson, E. & Bruce, R. (1987) Health benefits of exercise in an aging society. *Arch. Intern. Med.* **147**, 353−356.

Leon, A., Connett, J., Jacobs, D. & Rauramaa, R. (1987) Leisure-time physical activity levels and risk of coronary heart disease and death: the multiple risk factor intervention trial. *J.A.M.A.* **258**, 2388−2395.

Leon, A., Conrad, J., Hunninghake, D. & Serfass, R. (1979) Effects of a vigorous walking program on body composition, and carbohydrate and lipid metabolism of obese young men. *Am. J. Clin. Nutr.* **32**, 1776−1787.

Lewis, S., Snell, P., Taylor, W. *et al.* (1985) Role of muscle mass and mode of contraction in circulatory responses to exercise. *J. Appl. Physiol.* **58**, 146−151.

Lowenthal, D. (1990) Geriatric clinical pharmacology. In: Asrams, W. & Berkow, R. (eds) *Merck Manual of Geriatrics*. Merck & Co., Rahway, New Jersey.

MacDougall, J., Tuxen, D., Sale, D., Moroz, J. & Sutton, J. (1985) Arterial blood pressure responses to heavy resistance exercise. *J. Appl. Physiol.* **58**, 785−790.

Mann, G., Garrett L., Farhi, A. *et al.* (1969) Exercise to prevent coronary heart disease. *Am. J. Med.* **46**, 12−27.

Meredith, C., Frontera, W., Fisher, E. *et al.* (1989) Peripheral effects of endurance training in young and old subjects. *J. Appl. Physiol.* **66**, 2844−2849.

Niinimaa, V. & Shephard, R. (1978) Training and oxygen conductance in the elderly. *J. Gerontol.* **33**, 354−361.

Ogihara, T., Hata, T., Maruyama, A. *et al.* (1979) Studies on the renin−angiotensin aldosterone system in elderly hypertensive patients with an angiotensin II antagonist. *Clin. Sci.* **57**, 461–463.

Oja, P., Teraslinna, P., Partanen, T. & Karava, R. (1974) Feasibility of an 18 months' physical training program for middle-aged men and its effect on physical fitness. *Am. J. Public Health* **64**, 459–465.

Ordway, G. & Wekstein, D. (1979) The effect of age on selected cardiovascular responses to static (isometric) exercise. *Proc. Soc. Exp. Biol. Med.* **161**, 189–192.

Paffenbarger, R., Hyde, R., Wing, A. & Hsieh, C. (1986) Physical activity and all-cause mortality, and longevity of college alumni. *N. Engl. J. Med.* **314**, 605–613.

Palmer, G., Ziegler, M. & Lake, C. (1978) Response of norepinephrine and blood pressure to stress increases with age. *J. Gerontol.* **33**, 482–487.

Papper, S. (1973) The effects of age in reducing renal function. *Geriatrics* **28**, 83–87.

Pickering, T., Gribbin, B. & Oliver, D. (1972) Baroflex sensitivity in patients on long-term hemodialysis. *Clin. Sci.* **43**, 645–657.

Pollock, M. (1988) Exercise prescriptions for the elderly. In: Spirduso, W. & Eckert, H. (eds) *Physical Activity and Aging* pp. 163–174. Human Kinetics, Champaign, Illinois.

Pollock, M., Dawson, G., Miller, H. *et al.*, (1976) Physiologic responses of men 49 to 65 years of age to endurance training. *J. Am. Geriatr. Soc.* **24**, 97–104.

Pollock, M., Dimmick, J., Miller, H., Kendrick, Z. & Linnerud, A. (1975) Effects of mode of training on cardiovascular function and body composition of middle-aged men. *Med. Sci. Sports* **7**, 139–145.

Pollock, M., Foster, C., Knapp, D., Rod, J. & Schmidt, D. (1987) Effect of age and training on aerobic capacity and body composition of master athletes. *J. Appl. Physiol.* **62**, 725–731.

Pollock, M., Gettman, L., Milesis, C., Bah, M., Durstine, L. & Johnson, R. (1977) Effects of frequency and duration of training on attrition and incidence of injury. *Med. Sci. Sports Exerc.* **19**, 31–36.

Pollock, M., Graves, J., Leggett, S., Braith, R. & Hagberg, J. (1991) Injuries and adherence to aerobic and strength training exercise programs for the elderly. *Med. Sci. Sports Exerc.* (in press).

Pollock, M., Jackson, A. & Foster, C. (1986) The use of the perception scale for exercise prescription. In: Borg, G. & Ottoson, D. (eds) *The Perception of Exertion in Physical Work*, pp. 161–176. MacMillan, London.

Pollock, M., Miller, H., Janeway, R., Linnerud, A., Robertson, B. & Valentino, R. (1971) Effects of walking on body composition and cardiovascular function of middle-aged men. *J. Appl. Physiol.* **30**, 126–130.

Pollock, M. & Wilmore, J. (1990) *Exercise in Health and Disease: Evaluation and Prescription for Prevention and Rehabilitation*, 2nd edn. W.B. Saunders, Philadelphia.

Raven, P. & Mitchell, J. (1980) The effect of aging on the cardiovascular response to dynamic and static exercise. In: Wisfeldt, M. (ed.) *The Aging Heart*, pp. 269–296. Raven Press, New York.

Richey, D. & Bender, A. (1975) Effects of human aging on drug absorption and metabolism. In: Goldman, R. & Rockstein, M. (eds) *Physiology and Pathology of Human Aging*, pp. 59–71. Academic Press, New York.

Richey, D. & Bender, A. (1977) Pharmacokinetic consequences of aging. *Ann. Rev. Pharmacol. Toxicol.* **17**, 49–65.

Richie, D., Kelso, S. & Bellucci, P. (1985) Aerobic dance injuries: a retrospective study of instructors and participants. *Phys. Sportsmed.* **13**(2), 114–120.

Rippe, J., Ward, A., Porcari, J. & Freedson, P. (1988) Walking for health and fitness. *J.A.M.A.* **259**, 2720–2724.

Robinson, S. (1938) Experimental studies of physical fitness in relation to age. *Arbeitsphysiol.* **10**, 251–323.

Schwartz, R. (1988) Effects of exercise training on high density lipoproteins and apolipoprotein A-I in old and young men. *Metabolism* **37**, 1128–1133.

Seals, D., Hagberg, J., Hurley, B., Ehsani, A. & Holloszy, J. (1984) Endurance training in older men and women. I. Cardiovascular responses to exercise. *J. Appl. Physiol.* **57**, 1024–1029.

Sharkey, B. & Holleman, J. (1967) Cardiorespiratory adaptations to training at specified intensities. *Res. Q.* **38**, 698–704.

Sheldahl, L., Wilkie, N., Tristani, F. & Kalbfleisch, J. (1983) Responses of patients after myocardial infarction to carrying a graded series of weight loads. *Am. J. Cardiol.* **52**, 698–703.

Shephard, R. (1990) The scientific basis of exercise prescribing for the very old. *J. Am. Geriatr. Soc.* **38**, 62–70.

Shock, N. (1977) Systems integration. In: Finch, C. & Hayflick, L. (eds) *Handbook of the Biology of Aging*, pp. 639–665. Van Nostrand Reinhold, New York.

Sidney, K. & Shephard, R. (1978) Frequency and intensity of exercise training for elderly subjects. *Med. Sci. Sports Exerc.* **10**, 125–131.

Sidney, K., Shephard, R. & Harrison, J. (1977) Endurance training and body composition in the elderly. *Am. J. Clin. Nutr.* **30**, 326–333.

Slack, T. & Wilson, D. (1976) Normal renal function: C_{in} and C_{PAH} in healthy donors before and after nephrectomy. *Mayo Clin. Proc.* **51**, 296–300.

Smith, E., Reddan, W. & Smith, P. (1981) Physical activity and calcium modalities for bone mineral increase in aged women. *Med. Sci. Sports Exerc.* **13**, 60−64.

Stephens, T. (1987) Secular trends in adult physical activity: exercise boom or bust? *Res. Q.* **58**, 94−105.

Suominen, H., Heikkinen, E., Leisen, H., Michel, D. & Hollman, W. (1977a) Effects of 8 weeks' endurance training on skeletal muscle metabolism in 56−70 year old sedentary men. *Eur. J. Appl. Physiol.* **37**, 173−180.

Suominen, H., Heikkinen, E. & Parkatti, T. (1977b) Effect of eight weeks' physical training on muscle and connective tissue of the m. vastus lateralis in 69-year-old men and women. *J. Gerontol.* **32**, 33−37.

Templeton, G., Platt, M., Willerson, J. & Weisfeldt, M. (1979) Influence of aging on left ventricular hemodynamics and stiffness in beagles. *Circ. Res.* **44**, 189−194.

Waller, B. (1987) Sudden death in middle-aged conditioned subjects: Coronary atherosclerosis is the culprit. *Mayo Clin. Proc.* **62**, 634−636.

Weisfeldt, M. (1981) Left ventricular function. In: Weisfeldt, M.L. (ed.) *The Aging Heart*, pp. 297−316. Raven Press, New York.

Williams, T. (1984) *Rehabilitation in the Aging*. Raven Press, New York.

Wilmore, J. (1983) Body composition in sport and exercise: directions for future research. *Med. Sci. Sports Exerc.* **15**, 21−31.

Wood, P., Haskell, W., Blair, S. *et al.* (1983) Increased exercise level and plasma lipoprotein concentrations: a one-year, randomized, controlled study in sedentary, middle-aged men. *Metabolism* **32**, 31−39.

PART 6

CLINICAL ASPECTS OF
ENDURANCE TRAINING

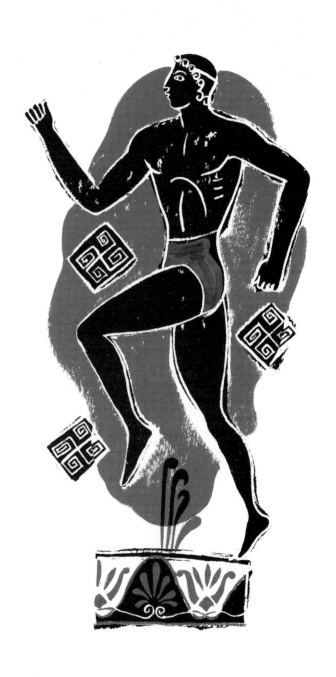

Chapter 38

Medical Surveillance of Endurance Sport

ROY J. SHEPHARD

Introduction

From the standpoint of medical surveillance, endurance activities fall into three broad categories: international endurance competitions such as a 10 000-m run or the 'Tour de France' cycle race, mass participation events (marathon races, 'fun runs', triathlons and ski-hikes such as the Vasa Loppet), and epic expeditions such as an ascent of Mount Everest or a transpolar ski trek. Differing principles govern the provision of medical coverage for each of these categories of activity.

International competition

Most international competitions include some endurance events, and the general arrangements made for medical screening, preparation and care of the participants (Dirix *et al.*, 1988) need only slight modifications to accommodate the special needs of the endurance competitor.

Preliminary screening

Preliminary medical screening should focus particularly upon the function of the cardio-respiratory system, looking for evidence of exercise-induced bronchospasm and conditions that might be harbingers of sudden death (Shephard, 1990a). A watch must also be kept for other previously unrecognized medical disorders, for example early diabetes and (in winter sport contestants) unusual sensitivity to

cold. Finally, note should be taken of musculo-skeletal problems that might be exacerbated by prolonged training (for example, differences of leg length or a poor limb alignment).

Respiratory allergies and exercise-induced bronchospasm are likely to impair endurance performance if they remain untreated (Shephard, 1977). Moreover, poor counselling may cause the athlete unwittingly to take medication that will lead to disqualification from competition. Permitted treatments of exercise-induced bronchospasm include cromoglycate, theophylline, beclomethasone dipropionate, and such β_2-agonists as salbutamol, terbutaline and metaproterenol, but adrenaline, ephedrine and isoprenaline are all prohibited drugs (Fitch & Morton, 1988).

In the young competitor, disorders that are of particular concern (Shephard, 1990a; see Chapter 40) include conditions increasing myocardial oxygen demand (pulmonary stenosis, aortic stenosis or regurgitation, Marfan's syndrome, mitral valve prolapse and regurgitation, hypertension, phaeochromocytoma and hypertrophic cardiomyopathy), impairments of coronary blood flow (anomalous origin of a coronary artery or coronary atheroma), anaemia (related to poor nutrition or sickle cell disease), abnormalities of cardiac rhythm (conduction block, premature ventricular contractions, Wolff−Parkinson−White syndrome), and episodes of syncope (hypoglycaemia, hypocapnia, epilepsy, reversal of intracardiac shunt, hypertrophic cardiomyopathy, Stokes−Adams attack). In Masters competitions, many of the same considerations will arise; dominant causes of myocardial ischaemia are coronary atherosclerosis, cardiomyopathy, hypertension, and aortic stenosis or regurgitation. Additional potential disturbances of rhythm include atrial fibrillation and flutter. Syncope may arise from poor venous tone (varicosities or the use of hypotensive drugs), malfunction of a prosthetic valve, the sick sinus syndrome, and supraventricular or ventricular tachycardias, while excessive dyspnoea during exercise may reflect poor myocardial function. Standard clinical examination of the heart will be complemented as necessary by resting and stress electrocardiography, echocardiography to assure normal dimensions of the ventricular cavities and an absence of septal hypertrophy, an evaluation of the blood pressure response during a symptom-limited treadmill test, and Holter monitoring for significant arrhythmias (Venerando *et al.*, 1988).

Many endurance and ultraendurance events, including some team sports, tend to carry normal participants close to hypoglycaemia (Ekblom, 1986; Shephard, 1990b). Problems of blood glucose regulation will naturally be more severe if there is a tendency to diabetes. If insulin is already being administered to the athlete, there is a danger that the metabolic demands of prolonged exercise may provoke a hypoglycaemic crisis by reducing the need for insulin, while at the same time increasing the rate of absorption of the hormone from an intramuscular depot.

Frostbite is always a potential danger in prolonged winter sports events, and a person who has an unusual vascular sensitivity to cold must be advised to take extra precautions on days when the wind chill is high.

Finally, endurance events subject certain segments of the musculoskeletal system to extended strain, and a thorough history and examination of the active parts is needed. Older competitors are more likely to have musculoskeletal problems than their younger counterparts.

Preparation

During the phase of preparation for major competition, the physician can contribute advice leading to sound nutrition (Burke & Read, 1989) and the avoidance of over-training (Kuipers & Keizer, 1988). It is also important to establish a good rapport with the athlete, allowing both minor psychotherapy and the offering of appropriate counsel against doping.

NUTRITION

The physician should be prepared to offer advice on overall food needs and on more specific aspects of nutrition, including glycogen loading and the needs for supplementary minerals and vitamins.

Some endurance athletes (particularly young female contestants in distance running events) are at risk of an inadequate total food intake, and it is important to monitor body mass to be sure that an energy deficit does not develop during periods of intensive training (Wheeler *et al.*, 1986).

An energy expenditure as high as 83 MJ has been recorded over 24-h cycling events (White *et al.*, 1984). Others have noted expenditures of 31 MJ·day^{-1} over 7 days of walking (Thomas & Reilly, 1975) and 29 MJ over 7 h of cross-country skiing (Hedman, 1957). In some events such as cross-Canada runs, expenditures of 30–40 MJ·day^{-1} may continue for several months. It is then useful to increase body fat stores by perhaps 10 kg (this will provide a reserve approaching 300 MJ of food energy). If the activity is to continue over the entire day throughout several weeks, it becomes necessary to find (largely by trial and error) preparations that will allow the individual concerned to ingest a substantial amount of energy while exercising (Shephard *et al.*, 1977).

Glycogen loading provides fuel for the working muscle under both aerobic and anaerobic conditions (Costill, 1988; Hasson & Barnes, 1989). By sustaining blood glucose, it also contributes to cerebral performance, for example in orienteering (Kujala *et al.*, 1989) and prolonged dinghy sailing (Niinimaa *et al.*, 1977). The traditional approach to glycogen loading of muscle (Saltin & Hermansen, 1967) involved a bout of exhausting exercise, followed by 3 days on a low carbohydrate diet and then 3 days on a high carbohydrate diet; such tactics led to irritability, hypoglycaemia and an interruption of training. However, Sherman *et al.* (1981) have demonstrated that equally good 'super-compensation' of glycogen reserves is possible if the 3 days of low carbohydrate diet are omitted.

Because endurance events depend on oxygen transport, it is important to maximize the athlete's haemoglobin concentration. Endurance competitors are vulnerable to anaemia because of iron loss in sweat, intravascular haemolysis, occasional bleeding in the bladder and intestine, and a poor absorption of iron (Haymes & Lamanca, 1989; Miller, 1990). Iron therapy may be helpful for selected individuals, particularly if the iron saturation of ferritin is low, but it is important not to be misled by a pseudoanaemia associated with plasma volume expansion (Newhouse & Clement, 1988).

Body mineral stores are substantial, but if preparation of an athlete occurs in a hot and humid environment, substantial losses of other minerals may develop. Simple evidence of a cumulative depletion of mineral reserves can be obtained (Wyndham & Strydom, 1972) from a monitoring of body mass (as salt is lost, body fluid reserves become depleted).

The athlete's need for B-group vitamins is proportional to total energy consumption (Shephard, 1983). Nevertheless, if a good mixed diet is provided, the intake will also rise appropriately in an endurance athlete. Vitamin C has been argued to protect against injuries and/or to speed the healing of tendons, but again there seems no good evidence to support this view. There are thus no good medical reasons for recommending special mineral or vitamin supplements to the distance competitor.

Overtraining

On the principle that if a little training is good, more training must be better, many athletes reach a state of overtraining (O'Brien, 1988), with adverse consequences for both performance and health.

The affected individual feels fatigued and lacks motivation for further training or competition. There are complaints of loss of appetite, weight loss and disturbance of sleep. The waking pulse rate is often elevated, blood samples may show elevation of serum enzyme levels (creatine phosphokinase, lactate dehydrogenase and serum glutamic oxaloacetic transaminase; Noakes, 1987), and a predominance of catabolism is shown by a decrease in the ratio of testosterone to cortisone, associated with a high level of sex-hormone binding globulins (Adlercreutz *et al.*, 1986).

The athlete becomes accident prone, and overuse injuries of muscle and bone are common. Both the resting immune function and the immune response to exercise are also impaired, so that the affected individual becomes vulnerable to minor infections.

Before reaching a diagnosis of over-training, it is important to rule out any more serious cause, such as a haemolytic streptococcal infection or glandular fever. The condition is best prevented by developing an appropriate 'tapering' of precompetition training in discussion with the coach. Once the syndrome has developed, psychotherapy and a period of complete rest are desirable; sometimes, several weeks without training are required for full recovery.

Doping

The sports physician has a role to play in protecting the competitor against drug use through a combination of appeals to fair play and warnings against the dangers of self-prescribed medication. The medical adviser must also ensure that banned drugs are not taken accidentally during self-treatment of minor ailments (see above). Competitors and their coaches should thus be asked to present for checking any 'over-the-counter' medications that they may have purchased.

At one time, amphetamines were popular drugs of abuse among endurance competitors, being valued partly for their cerebral stimulating effects, and partly because they diverted blood flow from skin to muscle (Puffer, 1986). Reputedly, the illegal administration of such drugs caused a number of heat stroke fatalities in international events during the 1960s. Side-effects of the amphetamines include irregularities of heart rhythm, a dangerous rise of core temperature, and a masking of fatigue that predisposes to collapse, heat exhaustion and stroke (Bell & Doege, 1987). However, drugs of this class are readily detected by the doping control technology of modern competitions, and they are thus no longer used by endurance competitors.

Caffeine remains a popular stimulant, particularly for long-distance cyclists; it stimulates the brain, reduces cerebral and possibly muscular fatigue, and mobilizes fat. High blood concentrations were discovered in some athletes at the Montreal Olympic games. In 1984, the International Olympic Committee (IOC) prohibited urinary caffeine levels in excess of $15\ \mu g \cdot ml^{-1}$, and in 1986 this threshold was reduced to $12\ \mu g \cdot ml^{-1}$ (Bell & Doege, 1987). Permitted levels are nevertheless substantially higher than would be reached by the drinking of normal amounts of coffee.

A third abuse admitted by some long-distance competitors is blood doping (see Chapter 21). Recently, there have also been suspicions of the administration of synthetic preparations of erythropoietin in order to stimulate haemoglobin production. There are many risks associated with standard blood transfusions (Dirix et al., 1988), including allergic reactions, acute haemolysis leading to kidney damage, delayed transfusion reactions with fever and jaundice, transmission of diseases such as viral hepatitis and acquired immune deficiency syndrome, a possible over-load of the circulation and metabolic shock. Some of these dangers are avoided by an autologous transfusion of the competitor's stored blood, but the athlete then faces a substantial interval when training is disrupted by the loss of blood (Eichner, 1987). Unfortunately, there is as yet no good test for blood doping, although procedures are now being developed based upon concentrations of haemoglobin, bilirubin, iron and erythropoietin (Berglund, 1988).

Preliminary site visit

It is desirable that the team physician make an early preliminary site visit in order to inspect the sites of competition, to establish liaison with local medical committees (including accreditation of the medical team), to examine the available medical facilities, equipment and living quarters, to discuss the provision of medical insurance coverage for team members, to determine any specific environmental and sanitary hazards, and to relate the World Health Organization's recommended schedule of prophylactic therapy to the current experience of local public health agencies.

In IOC sponsored events, the basic standards for both athletic and medical facilities have been specified (Hannemann, 1988), but it is useful to ascertain local regulations governing the import and export of any additional equipment that the sports physician may desire.

Potential environmental hazards include extremes of heat and cold (see Chapter 42), together with pollution of air (see Chapter 44), water and ground. It may be necessary to exert pressure on local organizers to ensure that events do not proceed in the midday heat in order to provide television crews with good lighting and large crowds, and appropriate agreement should be reached on conditions calling for a cancelling of competition. On the basis of site observations, competitors can be advised on a suitable acclimatization schedule, and where and when to exercise, with a view to minimizing their exposure to environmental hazards.

Water can be a potent source of disease in a developing country (Diop Mar, 1988), with a potential for the spread of bacteria (leptospirosis, salmonella, shigella and cholera), viruses (particularly poliomyelitis and enteroviral infections), and parasitic infections such as amoebiasis and schistosomiasis. Drinking stations must use water of adequate quality (where necessary, bottled, boiled or chemically treated), and the athlete should be warned against eating seafood or other produce washed in dirty water. Ice and ice-cream of unknown quality must also be avoided. In events such as the triathlon and cross-country runs, there is a risk of swimming on polluted beaches or wading through polluted streams. If the competition takes place on contaminated ground, there is a potential for injuries to become infected with the organisms causing gas gangrene and tetanus. Finally, in some countries there are serious insect-borne hazards such as malaria and encephalitis. Measures to prevent tropical infections include a careful check on the nature and timing of required vaccinations and immunizations, ensuring that contestants take a full course of chloroquine during and following visits to those parts of the world where malaria is prevalent, and prescribing such other forms of chemoprophylaxis as may be recommended by local public health agencies (Diop Mar, 1988).

In practice, the most likely hazard remains infection with an unfamiliar strain of *Escherichia coli*. The resultant diarrhoea can cause marked fluid loss and a resultant deterioration of endurance performance. Care in the selection of clean, hygienic food can often prevent such infections. An affected individual should take soft drinks and soup *ad libitum* in order to restore fluid and salt loss, and an oral preparation containing trimethoprim (160 mg) and sulphamethoxazole (800 mg) administered twice daily will usually effect a rapid cure. However, prophylactic use of such medication is not recommended, since it alters the bacterial flora and can in itself cause diarrhoea.

Immediate preparation

The athlete should be examined briefly immediately before departure for an event. Such examination may reveal conditions such as an injury or an infection that requires close monitoring or precludes competition. The examination allows a further opportunity for confidence-building discussion between the doctor and the athlete. Medical records should be updated, and if the competition will take the athlete away from the main treatment facility a summary of the medical history, medication, vaccinations and immunizations, allergies and the like should be prepared, to travel with the athlete. Any medications that the athlete is currently receiving should be checked relative to the regulations of the particular competition and, where necessary, legitimate drug needs should be discussed with those responsible for the monitoring of doping.

Arrangements for immediate adaptation to the new environment should be reviewed, including the time needed for adjustment to any displacement of circadian rhythms, increase of altitude, or change of climate. Advice can also be offered on the provision of fluids and food immediately before and during competition (Costill, 1988). A carbohydrate-containing meal should be taken 3–4 h before an event. If large amounts of glucose are given in the hour before competition, this may provoke a massive secretion of insulin, with a fall of blood glucose and a deterioration of performance during competition (Costill, 1988; Hasson & Barnes, 1989). However, there may be some advantage in taking a small amount of glucose, fructose or some other snack 5 min before a race begins. Likewise, a limited pre-event loading with fluid (to perhaps 500 ml) may be helpful, although if larger amounts of fluid are ingested and the day is cold there may be an embarrassing diuresis. During competition, the endurance athlete must be reminded that thirst provides a poor guide to fluid needs. If the day is warm and the rules of competition allow, an attempt should be made to drink 150 ml of fluid every

15 min, either as pure water, or as a dilute glucose–electrolyte solution.

Medical supervision during competition

The medical requirements of the athlete during attendance at an even and actual participation are usually quite limited. The largest number of treatments are for minor gastrointestinal and respiratory infections, sunburn, minor skin complaints, minor psychological problems and minor musculoskeletal problems.

Nevertheless, the supervising physician must remain constantly vigilant, and must be prepared to treat more serious problems, including hyperthermia (in summer endurance events), hypothermia (in winter events) and cardiac catastrophes.

Medical supervision of mass participation events

In many respects, the potential medical problems associated with a mass participation event such as a marathon, a 'fun run', a triathlon, or a large-scale cross-country ski competition are greater than those associated with a major international competition. The number of participants to be supervised is very much larger; they cover a wide spectrum of ages from quite young children to senior citizens; they vary widely in their level of initial training and experience; and a number are affected by chronic medical conditions, sometimes unrecognized. At the same time, treatment must be offered from makeshift facilities, using limited equipment, and, because the event is less prestigious, the number of medical and paramedical personnel offering their time for emergency care is likely to be much smaller than in a major international event.

Nevertheless, many of the general principles of preparation for the event, both preventive and therapeutic, are similar to those already discussed for the top-level athlete (Tunstall-Pedoe, 1984; Dobbin, 1986; Robertson, 1988).

Initial preparations

A medical committee should be established at an early stage in preparations for the event. This should include not only interested local physicians, but also representatives of other paramedical disciplines whose help will be sought in dealing with casualties — physiotherapists, podiatrists, nurses, the St John's Ambulance Brigade and the Red Cross. A reasonable level of staffing (Tunstall-Pedoe, 1984) for a marathon run includes 20 first-aiders, three nurses, one physiotherapist, one podiatrist and one doctor for every 1000 registrants.

While the number of admissions to local hospitals is not likely to be large, contact should be made with appropriate emergency departments to be sure that they know of the event and are familiar with the treatment of possible emergencies, particularly hyperthermia and hypothermia. Training should also be offered to those of the paramedical team who have not had previous experience in dealing with a large-scale competition. All members of the team should advise disoriented individuals to withdraw from competition.

Liaison should be established with the race organizers and local ambulance and police units to ensure adequate control of crowds and traffic. Sufficient vehicles must be available to evacuate the anticipated number of casualties from treatment stations, to collect stragglers who are unable to complete the event because of thermal problems or general exhaustion, and to return all of these individuals to the finish line.

A waiver in the initial application form should clarify that competitors in an athletic event are competing at their own risk, and that it is their responsibility to seek medical advice if they have any uncertainty about their fitness to participate. Nevertheless, the early circulation of a medical advice sheet can substantially reduce the incidence of casualties during the event. In particular, registrants should be given information about minimal training requirements, techniques of heat acclimatization (Murphy, 1979), proper clothing, avoidance of musculoskeletal problems, general factors increasing cardiovascular risks, and such potentially serious dangers of the event as hypothermia, hyperthermia and hypoglycaemia. It should be stressed that thirst is not a good guide to fluid needs, that those who do not drink regularly are likely to drop out of competition (Holmich *et al.*, 1988), and that alcohol on the night before an event can lead to both dehydration and impaired thermal regulation (Maughan, 1984). Competitors should also be told categorically not to participate if they are unwell, and not to persist if they are feeling faint or exhausted. Because heat stress often impairs judgement, it is wise to assign a partner to each participant who will run at a similar pace and will monitor their condition. A brief record noting the participant's personal physician and medical history should be prepared and carried, as suggested for international competitors, since casualties may be too confused to indicate even their names after a collapse has occurred. The process of public education can be reinforced if the chairperson of the medical committee offers practical advice in prior presentations to the local newspaper, radio and television station.

Early decisions will need to be taken on any lower or upper age limits for participation, and on the desirability of admitting those with known disabilities. While quite young children can often complete an event such as a marathon run without harm, involvement of preadolescents in prolonged competition is to be discouraged. The prolonged training that is required can have adverse effects on immature bones, and an exhausted child may face excessive pressures to complete the actual event from ambitious parents or coaches.

Detailed planning

The route for the event should be surveyed in detail. Any obstacles and bottlenecks must be clearly marked or eliminated, and provision must be made for an adequate number of drink, first aid and toilet stations.

Drinks should be provided every 3–4 km in events that cover distances of 16 km and more. The design of a drink station needs some thought so that runners do not collide with others who have stopped, or slip on discarded paper cups and fruit peelings. Cups should be large enough that participants can drink about 150 ml of fluid from a cup that is no more than half-filled, thereby avoiding the spillage of fluid. Participants should also be told how drinks will be passed to them, and where to discard the cups after use. Some companies offer exotic beverages for the athlete, but the prime need is for water as a replacement fluid. It is better to have an adequate supply of clean water than a limited volume of a commercial drink that is exhausted by the first wave of competitors. On the other hand, an excessive intake of water over an ultramarathon can sometimes cause hyponatraemia (Frizzell *et al.*, 1986). If glucose–electrolyte solutions are used, these must be freshly prepared, as they provide an excellent culture medium for bacteria. Some commercially available preparations also contain too high a concentration of glucose ($>5\%$); this slows gastric emptying and thus limits the absorption of water. Sponging or hosing of participants is not recommended; while it gives a psychological boost, it often increases heat stress by causing vasoconstriction of the skin vessels (Bassett *et al.*, 1987).

First aid stations should be sited immediately beyond the drink stations. Tents or trailers may be used, but they should have protection from wet ground, and a minimum of telephone communication with a nearby ambulance. In cool conditions, there should be sufficient heating to prevent hypothermia in exhausted runners, and in warm weather, fans or air conditioners will be required.

Well-marked toilets should be provided at strategic points along the route, as some participants overhydrate before a race, and others may be affected by the 'runner's trots'.

Immediately beyond the finishing line, there should be a large recovery area, where all participants can change into warm dry clothing, eat, and sit until sufficiently recovered to make the homeward journey. The medical treatment section within the recovery area should be large enough to accommodate at least 5% of the anticipated number of participants (Tunstall-Pedoe, 1984; Robertson, 1988). Simple facilities for each sex should include reserves of dry clothing, camp beds, pillows and blankets, adequate fresh water and ice, dressings, waste buckets and vomit bowls. Medical equipment should include stretchers, splints, dressings, oxygen cylinders, blood pressure cuffs, stethoscopes, rectal thermometers, transfusion sets with drip stands, the standard array of emergency drugs and, if possible, a portable defibrillator.

If the wheelchair disabled are to be included as participants (Marshall, 1984), suitably adapted toilet facilities must be organized at appropriate intervals along the route. Wheelchairs can reach speeds of 60 km·h^{-1}. It is thus important that the course have no steep hills or sharp bends, and that there is adequate space to pass tired runners throughout. Notice also that because of their higher speeds, wheelchair participants are more vulnerable to hypothermia.

Immediate preparations

A substantial number of registrants themselves decide to withdraw some 2 weeks before an endurance event because of pregnancy, injury or infection (Clough et al., 1987). A much clearer idea of the size of the field can thus be obtained if participation is confirmed in the final week before competition.

The anticipated weather conditions along the route should be discussed with the local meteorological station on the morning of the event, and participants should be advised if particular care is needed to avoid heat stress, frostbite or hypothermia (Richards et al., 1979; Hanson, 1985). If conditions exceed a wet bulb temperature of 28°C, if the wind chill is more severe than −35°C, or if there is black ice, the race should be cancelled (American College of Sports Medicine, 1984; Tunstall-Pedoe, 1984). If conditions are warm, a slowing of pace should be commended to participants (England et al., 1982), and a clothing check should be instituted if starting temperatures are below 15°C (Robertson, 1988).

At the start of the race, participants should be reminded of the information given in the advice sheet, and warned against competing if they feel unwell. Registration in the following year should be offered to all who decide to withdraw from competition for health reasons.

Plan of treatment

The entrances to first aid and medical stations should be guarded, to allow the logging of casualties as they are admitted, and to exclude press, television crews and relatives. Authorized personnel should be given suitable identification badges.

The proportion of participants seeking medical help ranges widely between 0.1 and 12.5% (Williams et al., 1981; Tunstall-Pedoe, 1984; Robertson, 1988), depending largely upon weather conditions. A preliminary triage should divide casualties between those to be treated by podiatrists (mainly blisters and subungual haematomata), those appropriate to physiotherapists (for instance, cases of severe cramps), those with medical problems (such as diarrhoea or vomiting) and the rare cases needing immediate and intensive care (intravenous fluids or resuscitation).

Most of the complaints encountered during an event are minor in nature (Table 38.1); they include blisters, chafing and even nipple-bleeding from nylon running shorts and vests, muscle cramps and general exhaustion. Depending on environmental conditions, a proportion of competitors (mainly the less fit individuals) may develop various heat pathologies (Wyndham & Strydom, 1972; see Chapter 42) or hypothermia (Pugh, 1972; see Chapter 42). Rectal temperatures should thus be recorded immediately on all who have collapsed. Oral thermometers must not be used, since

Table 38.1 Distribution of casualties seeking medical aid during Seattle's Emerald City Marathon from 1983 to 1987. Data from Robertson (1988), with permission.

Injury*	%
Muscle cramps or strains	22
Blisters	20
Other orthopaedic injuries	23
Exhaustion or dehydration	17
Thermal injuries	14
Other medical problems	4

* Total injuries 2.0–5.5% of finishers.

gross errors can arise in an athlete due to cooling of the tongue by inspired air, and lack of control over the recent drinking of hot or cold fluids. In no circumstances should a participant who is dazed, disoriented or having problems of thermoregulation be allowed to return to the competition. Nevertheless, at the end of the event, many participants who seem confused and ill respond well to a monitored warm-down by slow walking and the administration of oral fluids (Robertson, 1988).

Major cardiac events are surprisingly rare in mass participation events; for instance, there is about one death per million person-hours of cross-country skiing (Vuori *et al.*, 1975; Williams *et al.*, 1981; Tunstall-Pedoe, 1983; Sadaniantz & Thompson, 1990). Nevertheless, it is important that aggressive participants be discouraged from denying prodromal symptoms (Northcote & Ballantyne, 1984), and that those providing medical care are thoroughly familiar with techniques of cardiac resuscitation. It is also important that hospitals receiving casualties do not confuse a race-induced release of serum creatine kinase from the active muscles with the cardiac enzyme release that accompanies myocardial infarction (Young, 1984; Noakes, 1987).

Many of the minor problems of mass competition can be avoided by simple preventive measures. Clothing should be comfortable, preferably of natural fibre that 'breathes', does not chafe, and can be adjusted to allow a variation of thermal protection over a long day. A hat should be added in bright sunlight, and most women will be more comfortable wearing a brassière. In cold weather, heat loss is substantially reduced by wearing a hat and gloves (Maughan, 1984). Shoes should have been 'broken in', but still provide adequate ankle support, and socks should be well-fitting woollen or cotton rather than nylon. The application of zinc oxide powder, plaster and possibly petroleum jelly at friction points will minimize skin problems (Holmich *et al.*, 1988).

Thermal emergencies will be less likely if events are cancelled in extreme conditions and care is taken with the hydration of participants when the weather is warm. Cardiac catastrophes are also less likely if participants are encouraged not to persist in an event beyond the point of exhaustion.

Most events are repeated on an annual basis. It is thus important to call a final meeting of the medical committee after the event, to review the success of prevention and treatment, and to learn any necessary lessons for future years. If the experience has been adverse because of apparent negligence, national associations may also wish to consider exercising some sanctions against the organizers of the event (Robertson, 1988).

Medical emergencies in wilderness expeditions

Where possible, those contemplating a mountain expedition, a long wilderness canoe trip or an arctic ski-trek should recruit a physician to their numbers. However, the extreme nature of the environment and the very limited facilities will only allow the provision of minimal emergency care during the trip.

The specific example of climbing is considered in Chapter 55. Prudence would suggest a thorough medical examination and extensive training before an expedition, but in practice some mountaineering and transarctic teams have included older individuals who were relatively unfit and had known medical problems such as hypertension (Pugh, 1962; Shephard, 1990c).

A physician joining a wilderness expedition must be thoroughly familiar with the likely problems of a particular habitat, but probably his or her most important function will be to decide when a casualty should be evacuated. Arrangements should be made for the airlifting of emergency supplies and for evacuation before the trip is begun, and radio communication with base should be maintained throughout.

References

Adlercreutz, H., Harkonen, M., Kuoppasalmi, K. et al. (1986) Effect of training on plasma anabolic and catabolic steroid hormones and their response during physical exercise. Int. J. Sports Med. 7, 27–28.

American College of Sports Medicine (1984) Prevention of thermal injuries during distance running. Sports Med. Bull. 19(3), 8.

Bassett, D., Nagle, F., Mookerjee, S. et al. (1987) Thermoregulatory response to skin wetting during prolonged treadmill running. Med. Sci. Sports Exerc. 19, 28–32.

Bell, A.J. & Doege, C.T. (1987) Athletes use and abuse of drugs. Phys. Sportsmed. 15(3), 99–108.

Berglund, B. (1988) Development of techniques for the detection of blood doping in sport. Sports Med. 5, 127–135.

Burke, L.M. & Read, R.S.D. (1989). Sports nutrition: approaching the nineties. Sports Med. 8, 80–100.

Clough, P.J., Dutch, S., Maughan, R.J. & Shepherd, J. (1987) Pre-race drop-out in marathon runners: reasons for withdrawal and future plans. Br. J. Sports Med. 21, 148–149.

Costill, D.L. (1988) Nutrition and dietetics. In: Dirix, A., Knuttgen, H. & Tittel, K. (eds) The Olympic Book of Sports Medicine, pp. 603–634. Blackwell Scientific Publications, Oxford.

Diop Mar, I. (1988) Infectious diseases in tropical climates. In: Dirix, A., Knuttgen, H. & Tittel, K. (eds) The Olympic Book of Sports Medicine, pp. 583–588. Blackwell Scientific Publications, Oxford.

Dirix, A., Knuttgen, H. & Tittel, K. (eds) (1988) The Olympic Book of Sports Medicine. Blackwell Scientific Publications, Oxford.

Dobbin, S. (1986) Providing medical services for fun runs and marathons in North America. In: Sutton,

J. & Brock, R.C. (eds) Sports Medicine for the Mature Athlete, pp. 193–203. Benchmark Press, Indianapolis.

Eichner, E.R. (1987) Blood doping: results and consequences from the laboratory and the field. Phys. Sportsmed. 15(1), 120–129.

Ekblom, B. (1986) Applied physiology of soccer. Sports Med. 3, 50–60.

England, A., Fraser, D., Hightower, A. et al. (1982) Preventing heat injury in runners: suggestions from the 1979 Peachtree road race experience. Ann. Intern. Med. 97, 196–201.

Fitch, K.D. & Morton, A.R. (1988) Respiratory disease. In: Dirix, A., Knuttgen, H. & Tittel, K. (eds) The Olympic Book of Sports Medicine, pp. 531–541. Blackwell Scientific Publications, Oxford.

Frizzell, R., Lang, G., Lowance, D. & Lathan S. (1986) Hyponatremia and ultramarathon running. J.A.M.A. 255, 772–774.

Hannemann, D. (1988) Standardization of medical care during international sports events. In: Dirix, A., Knuttgen, H. & Tittel, K. (eds) The Olympic Book of Sports Medicine, pp. 646–652. Blackwell Scientific Publications, Oxford.

Hanson, P. (1985) Marathon medicine. Emerg. Med. 17(15), 62–92.

Hasson, S.M. & Barnes, W.S. (1989) Effect of carbohydrate ingestion on exercise of varying intensity and duration. Practical implications. Sports Med. 8, 327–334.

Haymes, E. & Lamanca, J.J. (1989) Iron loss in runners during exercise: implications and recommendations. Sports Med. 7, 277–285.

Hedman, R. (1957) The available glycogen in man and the connection between rate of oxygen intake and carbohydrate usage. Acta Physiol. Scand. 40, 305–321.

Holmich, P., Darre, E., Jahnsen, F. & Hartvig-Jensen, T. (1988) The élite marathon runner: problems during and after competition. Br. J. Sports Med. 22, 19–21.

Kuipers, H. & Keizer, H.A. (1988) Overtraining in élite athletes. Review and directions for the future. Sports Med. 6, 79–92.

Kujala, U.M., Heinonen, O.J., Kvist, M. et al. (1989) Orienteering performance and ingestion of glucose and glucose polymers. Br. J. Sports Med. 23, 105–108.

Marshall, T. (1984) Wheelchairs and marathon road racing. Br. J. Sports Med. 18, 301–304.

Maughan, R.J. (1984) Temperature regulation during marathon competition. Br. J. Sports Med. 18, 257–260.

Miller, B.J. (1990) Haematological effects of running: a brief review. Sports Med. 9, 1–6.

Murphy, R. (1979) Heat illness and athletics. In:

Strauss, R. (ed.) *Sports Medicine and Physiology*, pp. 320–326. W.B. Saunders, Philadelphia.

Newhouse, I.J. & Clement, D. (1988) Iron status in athletes. An update. *Sports Med.* **5**, 337–352.

Niinimaa, V., Wright, G., Shephard, R.J. & Clarke, J. (1977) Characteristics of the successful dinghy sailor. *J. Sports Med. Phys. Fitness* **17**, 83–96.

Noakes, T.D. (1987) Effect of exercise on serum enzyme activities in humans. *Sports Med.* **4**, 245–267.

Northcote, R.J. & Ballantyne, D. (1984) Reducing the prevalence of exercise related cardiac death. *Br. J. Sports Med.* **18**, 288–292.

O'Brien, M. (1988) Over-training and sports psychology. In: Dirix, A., Knuttgen, H. & Tittel, K. (eds) *The Olympic Book of Sports Medicine*, pp. 635–645. Blackwell Scientific Publications, Oxford.

Puffer, C.J. (1986) The use of drugs in swimming. *Clin. Sports Med.* **5**(1), 77–89.

Pugh, L.G.C.E. (1962) Physiological and medical aspects of the Himalayan Scientific and Mountaineering Expedition 1960–1961. *Br. Med. J.* **2**, 621–627.

Pugh, L.G.C.E. (1972) Accidental hypothermia among hillwalkers and climbers in Britain. In: Cumming, G.R., Snidal, D. & Taylor, A.W. (eds) *Environmental Effects on Work Performance*, pp. 41–55. Canadian Association of Sport Sciences, Ottawa.

Richards, R., Richards, D., Schofield, P., Ross, V. & Sutton, J. (1979) Reducing the hazards in Sydney's the Sun-to-Surf runs 1971 to 1979. *Med. J. Aust.* **2**, 453–457.

Robertson, J.W. (1988) Medical problems in mass participation runs. Recommendations. *Sports Med.* **6**, 261–270.

Sadaniantz, A. & Thompson, P.D. (1990) The problem of sudden death in athletes as illustrated by case studies. *Sports Med.* **9**, 199–204.

Saltin, B. & Hermansen, L. (1967) Glycogen stores and prolonged severe exercise. In: Blix, G. (ed.) *Nutrition and Physical Activity*, p. 32. Almqvist & Wiksell, Uppsala.

Shephard, R.J. (1977) Exercise-induced bronchospasm — a review. *Med. Sci. Sports* **9**, 1–10.

Shephard, R.J. (1983) *Biochemistry of Exercise*. C.C. Thomas, Springfield, Illinois.

Shephard, R.J. (1990a) The cardiovascular system. In: Rians, C.B. (ed.) *Clinical Sports Medicine* (in press).

Shephard, R.J. (1990b) Meeting carbohydrate and fluid needs in soccer. *Can. J. Sport Sci.* **15**, 165–171.

Shephard, R.J. (1990c) Some consequences of polar stress: data from a transpolar ski trek. *Arct. Med. Res.* (in press).

Shephard, R.J., Conway, S., Thomson, M., Anderson, G.H. & Kavanagh, T. (1977) Nutritional demands of sub-maximum work: marathon and trans-Canada events. In: Pavluk, J. (ed.) *International Symposium on Athletic Nutrition*, pp. 42–58. Polska Federacja Sportu, Warsaw.

Sherman, W.M., Costill, D.L., Fink, W.J. & Miller, J.M. (1981) Effect of exercise-diet manipulation on muscle glycogen and its subsequent utilization during performance. *Int. J. Sports Med.* **2**, 114–118.

Thomas, V. & Reilly, T. (1975) Circulatory, psychological and performance variables during 100 hours of paced continuous exercise under conditions of controlled energy intake and work output. *J. Hum. Movement Stud.* **1**, 149.

Tunstall-Pedoe, D.S. (1983) Cardiological problems in sport. *Br. J. Hosp. Med.* **29**, 213–220.

Tunstall-Pedoe, D.S. (1984) Popular marathons, half-marathons and long distance runs: recommendations for medical support. *Br. Med. J.* **288**, 1355–1359.

Venerando, A., Zeppilli, P. & Caselli, G. (1988) Cardiovascular disease. In: Dirix, A., Knuttgen, H. & Tittel, K. (eds). *The Olympic Book of Sports Medicine*, pp. 505–530. Blackwell Scientific Publications, Oxford.

Vuori, I., Saraste, M., Vihava, M. & Pakkarinen, A. (1975) Feasibility of long distance ski hikes (20–90 km) as a mass sport. In: Toyne, A.H. (ed.) *Proceedings of 20th World Congress of Sports Medicine*, pp. 530–544. Australian Sports Federation, Melbourne.

Wheeler, G.D., Wall, S.R., Belcastro, A.N., Conger, P. & Cumming, D. (1986) Are anorexic tendencies prevalent in the habitual runner? *Br. J. Sports Med.* **20**, 77–81.

White, J.A., Ward, C. & Nelson, H. (1984) Ergogenic demands of a 24 hour cycling event. *Br. J. Sports Med.* **18**, 165–171.

Williams, R.S., Schocken, D.D., Morey, M. & Koisch, F.P. (1981) Medical aspects of competitive distance running. *Postgrad. Med.* **70**, 41–44.

Wyndham, C.H. & Strydom, N.B. (1972) Körperliche Arbeit bei hoher Temperatur. In: Hollmann, W. (ed.) *Zentrale Themen der Sportmedizin*, pp. 131–149. Springer Verlag, Berlin.

Young, A. (1984) Plasma creatine kinase after the marathon — a diagnostic dilemma. *Br. J. Sports Med.* **18**, 269–272.

Chapter 39

Cardiovascular Benefits of Endurance Exercise

AARON R. FOLSOM AND KRISTINE E. ENSRUD

Introduction

Diseases of the cardiovascular system, in particular arterial hypertension, coronary heart disease and stroke, are among the leading causes of morbidity and mortality in most industrialized countries. While there is no rigorous experimental proof that endurance exercise helps to prevent cardiovascular diseases, evidence from observational (non-experimental) epidemiological studies indicates convincingly that this is the case. This chapter summarizes the cardiovascular benefits of endurance exercise, the possible mechanisms of its effects, and the frequency, intensity, duration and type of exercise needed to produce such effects.

Methodological issues in research of exercise and health

The demonstration of a causal relation between lack of exercise and cardiovascular diseases has been hampered by several methodological issues. The strongest aetiological proof would be offered by experimental studies, in which healthy subjects would be randomized to either endurance exercise or no exercise and both groups would then be followed to observe the incidence of cardiovascular disease. Such experiments have not proven feasible, because of the long duration and large sample sizes required and the high proportion of controls who would be likely to take up exercise during

a trial. Several trials of endurance exercise in patients who have established hypertension or who have sustained a myocardial infarction have been carried out successfully, but these tertiary prevention trials offer only indirect information on disease aetiology. Medical scientists, therefore, have had to rely on evidence from observational studies, measuring cardiovascular disease incidence in relation to self-determined exercise patterns. Unfortunately, healthy or fitter individuals tend to select themselves more often to higher exercise levels and sicker individuals to lower exercise levels, potentially resulting in biased estimates of the association between exercise and prevention of disease. Another problem is the relatively homogeneous distribution of exercise in most industrialized populations. The small difference between 'high' and 'low' exercise categories hampers the detection of possible relationships between exercise and cardiovascular disease (LaPorte et al., 1984).

The measurement of habitual endurance exercise is another major methodological obstacle to epidemiological investigations. For reasons of safety, practicality and cost, objective measures of exercise or fitness have not been extensively used. Questionnaire estimates of habitual exercise have, at best, only moderate reliability and validity. This has led to misclassification of exercise levels in many studies. Misclassification is also likely if occupational exercise is based on job title alone, or if leisure exercise is estimated from a single questionnaire. Other errors arise in the diagnosis of cardiovascular disease.

Yet another methodological difficulty of epidemiological studies is the control of confounding factors related to both exercise and cardiovascular disease. Confounders are extraneous factors that can distort real associations. For example, in studies of coronary heart disease incidence, it is usually important to take into account other coronary risk factors to determine the 'independent' effect of exercise on disease. Fortunately, in recent years epidemiologists have paid more attention to these methodological issues, conducting studies with better design and analysis.

Exercise and hypertension

Arterial hypertension is a major risk factor for coronary heart disease and stroke. In many industrialized populations, it is a highly prevalent condition, with up to 25% of the adult population affected. Large clinical trials have demonstrated clearly that a pharmacological lowering of blood pressure significantly reduces cardiovascular morbidity and mortality rates (Cutler & Furberg, 1985). In recent years, there has been increasing interest in non-pharmacological modalities, including endurance exercise, weight loss and sodium restriction, as means both to prevent the development of hypertension and to control blood pressure in hypertensive individuals.

Cross-sectional epidemiological comparisons of athletes and non-athletes, active and inactive occupations, and groups active and inactive in their leisure time do not consistently support the hypothesis that habitual physical activity prevents the development of hypertension (Blackburn, 1986). Two recent well-designed prospective studies, however, suggest that regular exercise may reduce the incidence of hypertension. Paffenbarger et al. (1983) followed 14 998 Harvard alumni for 6–10 years, and reported that men who expended less than 8 MJ per week (2000 kcal) in leisure-time exercise had a 1.3-fold greater risk ($p < 0.05$) of

developing hypertension than men who expended 8 MJ or more per week. The association between exercise and a lower incidence of hypertension was not explained by body size index and, in fact, was stronger for overweight subjects. Similarly, Blair et al. (1984) assessed the physical fitness of healthy normotensives (4820 men and 1219 women aged 20–65 years) by treadmill testing and found low vs. high physical fitness (maximal treadmill time) was significantly associated with the 4 year incidence of hypertension. Both men and women benefited. After adjustment for sex, age, length of follow-up, baseline blood pressure and baseline body mass index, subjects with low levels of physical fitness had a relative risk of 1.5 for the development of hypertension.

Numerous experimental studies have attempted to determine whether regular dynamic exercise lowers blood pressure in hypertensive individuals. Detailed reviews can be found elsewhere (Seals & Hagberg, 1984; Tipton, 1984; Blackburn, 1986; Martin & Dubbert, 1987). Many experiments must be interpreted with caution due to inadequate study design, principally the absence of comparable, concurrent, non-exercising, hypertensive control groups. Uncontrolled studies typically have shown a greater effect of exercise on blood pressure levels than controlled studies.

Table 39.1 summarizes the results of published controlled clinical trials of exercise training as therapy for mild hypertension. The training regimen in these six trials typically consisted of walking, jogging or cycling for 30–60 min, three times a week. DePlaen and Detry (1980), in a small study of 10 hypertensive subjects, did not find any significant reduction in blood pressure in the exercise group; in fact, the blood pressure reduction was greatest in the non-exercising control group. Bonanno and Lies (1974) in an investigation of exercise in normotensives and hypertensives observed significant diastolic blood pressure reductions in both exercise and sedentary control groups, whereas systolic blood pressure declined sig-

Table 39.1 Controlled trials of exercise to reduce blood pressure in mild hypertensives.

Study	n	Sex	Age (years)	Baseline blood pressure (mmHg)	Intervention period (months)	Within-group blood pressure difference (mmHg/mmHg)	Between-group blood pressure difference (mmHg/mmHg)
DePlaen & Detry (1980)	6 (exercise) 4 (control)	M/F	44 (mean)	169/108 158/113	3	-1/+3 -4/-6	+3/+9
Bonanno & Lies (1974)	12 (exercise) 15 (control)	M	30–58	148/97 150/101	3	-13/-14 -3/-11	-10/-3
Kukkonen et al. (1982)	13 (exercise) 12 (control)	M	35–50	145/99 140/97	4	-9/-11 0/-7	-9/-4
Hagberg et al. (1983)	25 (exercise) 17 (control)	M/F	15–16	137/80 Not reported	6	-8/-5 n.s.	Unknown
Duncan et al. (1985)	44 (exercise) 12 (control)	M	21–37	146/94 145/93	4	-12/-7 -6/+3	-6/-10
Hagberg et al. (1989)	10 (moderate intensity exercise, 70–85% $\dot{V}o_{2\,max}$) 14 (low intensity exercise, 50% $\dot{V}o_{2\,max}$) 9 (control)	M/F	60–69	157/99 164/94 154/90	9	-9/-11 -21/-12 -1/-2	-8/-9 -20/-10

nificantly only in the exercise group. These results were duplicated in a later study conducted by Kukkonen et al. (1982). Between-group comparisons were not performed in either of these studies, but the results suggest a beneficial effect of exercise training on systolic blood pressure in individuals with mild hypertension. In a study of 42 adolescents with pressure above the 95th percentile for age and sex, Hagberg and colleagues (1983) concluded that both systolic and diastolic blood pressure decreased significantly with training. However, their sedentary controls were self-selected rather than randomly assigned and did not have baseline or follow-up blood pressures reported. Duncan and coworkers (1985) evaluated the effects of a 4-month exercise programme on blood pressure and plasma catecholamine levels in 56 patients with mild hypertension. At the end of the study, the exercise group had a decrease in diastolic blood pressure of 7 mmHg, while the control group had an increase of 3 mmHg. This difference was statistically significant ($p < 0.001$). In a recent study of 33 subjects with mild hypertension, Hagberg and colleagues (1989) noted a significant difference in diastolic blood pressure reduction between both low- and moderate-intensity exercise groups and a sedentary control group ($p < 0.05$). Systolic blood pressure reduction, however, was significantly different only between the low-intensity group and the control group, suggesting that the magnitude of blood pressure reduction was not directly related to the intensity of training.

Numerous mechanisms have been proposed for a potential antihypertensive effect of regular exercise. These include exercise-induced vasodilation; changes in body composition and diet; decreased extracellular blood volume through sweating, increased renal function, and consequently increased fluid and sodium excretion; exercise-mediated stress/catecholamine/renin reduction; reduced sympathetic activity; or some general effect of improved cardiovascular fitness (Martin & Dubbert, 1987). Any mechanism(s) must ultimately operate via Ohm's law, where mean blood pressure is the product of cardiac output and total peripheral resistance.

In summary, prospective and experimental studies generally support the belief that regular exercise reduces the future risk of hypertension by 25–35% and exerts a blood pressure lowering effect of 5–10 mmHg in mild hypertensives. Clinicians should recommend exercise to sedentary patients with hypertension, as an adjunct to therapy. Athletes with hypertension generally need not be discouraged from exercising, but appropriate attention must be paid to controlling the blood pressure and avoiding hypokalaemia. Additional research is needed to establish the benefit of exercise in individuals at risk for the development of hypertension; the duration, frequency and intensity of exercise that is effective in lowering blood pressure; the physiological mechanisms underlying the relationship between physical activity and blood pressure; and whether regular exercise is capable of lowering blood pressure independently of weight loss.

Exercise and coronary heart disease

Coronary heart disease is caused by atherosclerotic narrowing of the coronary arteries. Its ischaemic manifestations, angina, myocardial infarction and sudden death, result from a compromised coronary circulation, due to either direct obstruction by an atherosclerotic plaque or rupture of the plaque and attendant coronary arterial thrombosis (DeWood et al., 1980). Major risk factors for coronary heart disease include hypercholesterolaemia, arterial hypertension, cigarette smoking and diabetes mellitus.

The role of lack of exercise in causing coronary heart disease has been extensively investigated and frequently reviewed (Blackburn, 1983; Leon, 1983; Paffenbarger & Hyde, 1984; Blair & Oberman, 1987). The most thorough review has been written by Powell and colleagues (1987). These authors summarized 54 investigations of exercise and coronary heart disease incidence published through 1985. Since then, at least seven new studies have been reported (Lie *et al.*, 1985; Leon *et al.*, 1987; Scragg *et al.*, 1987; Sobolski *et al.*, 1987; Ekelund *et al.*, 1988; Siscovick *et al.*, 1988; Blair *et al.*, 1989), and results from some earlier studies have been extended (Kannel *et al.*, 1986; Donahue *et al.*, 1988; Salonen *et al.*, 1988). Taking all of these published data together leads fairly convincingly to the conclusion that lack of endurance exercise is a contributing cause of coronary heart disease.

Figure 39.1 summarizes the outcome of studies that Powell *et al.* (1987) concluded had satisfactory methodologies as well as new studies recently reported. Studies whose confidence intervals do not overlap unity or are labelled by an asterisk are statistically significant. The salient epidemiological features of the association between lack of exercise and coronary heart disease are as follows:

1 *Strength*: the risk of coronary heart disease is on average twofold higher in subjects who have low levels of exercise compared with those with high exercise levels (Fig. 39.1). This doubling of risk is not markedly lower than the relative risks of coronary disease ascribed to hypercholesterolaemia, arterial hypertension or cigarette smoking.

2 *Consistency*: the association between exercise and coronary disease is generally consistent. About two thirds of all studies show lack of exercise is associated with a significant elevation of risk (Powell *et al.*, 1987). Occupational and leisure-time exercise studies are approximately equally consistent in demonstrating an effect. The effect extends to both fatal and non-fatal coronary events. Powell and colleagues further concluded that studies with the best methodologies generally showed the strongest relations.

3 *Dose—response*: two thirds of the studies that measured exercise at two or more levels demonstrated a dose—response effect (Powell *et al.*, 1987); that is, the lower the level of exercise, the greater the risk of coronary heart disease.

4 *Temporality*: the majority of studies have been prospective, thereby demonstrating that

activity level appropriately predates the onset of coronary heart disease.

5 *Independence*: most studies that measured other coronary risk factors simultaneously have reported that lack of exercise was an independent risk factor for coronary heart disease.

6 *Generalizability*: most studies have focused on middle-aged, white men. Evidence is suggestive that exercise also protects older men (Morris *et al.*, 1980; Donahue *et al.*, 1988), women (Fig. 39.1) and non-whites (Cassel *et al.*, 1971; Garcia-Palmieri *et al.*, 1982; Donahue *et al.*, 1988).

The association between exercise and coronary disease also holds for studies that have measured coronary heart disease incidence or mortality rates in relation to endurance fitness (exercise capacity during treadmill or cycle ergometer exercise). Indeed, all prospective studies of fitness report elevated coronary heart disease incidence rates in unfit subjects (Fig. 39.1; Wilhelmsen *et al.*, 1981; Bruce *et al.*, 1983; Erikssen, 1986). The relative risk of coronary heart disease in unfit men is approximately two- to threefold greater than in fit men. However, the relative risk of being an unfit male may approach 8.0 (Ekelund *et al.*, 1988; Blair *et al.*, 1989) when compared to men with the highest fitness (e.g. the upper 20% of fitness).

In addition to reducing the incidence of coronary heart disease, endurance exercise also appears to reduce the risk of death following a myocardial infarction. Several randomized, controlled trials of exercise in postmyocardial infarction patients have been conducted. Unfortunately these tertiary prevention trials have all been small; they have been conducted only in men, and they have sometimes involved other interventions besides exercise. Although only one trial showed a significant benefit by itself, pooled data from postinfarction trials indicate that survival is improved among patients who exercise (Shephard, 1986; O'Connor *et al.*, 1989). O'Connor *et al.* (1989) performed a meta-analysis of 22 randomized exercise trials (Fig. 39.2) involving a total of

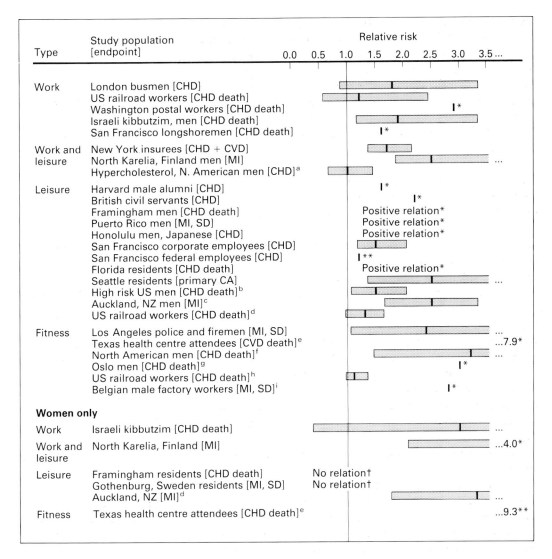

Fig. 39.1 Relative risk of coronary heart disease in non-exercisers versus exercisers. Results are either from studies having no 'unsatisfactory' ratings, as reviewed by Powell *et al.* (1987), or subsequently published studies. Only one 'hard' endpoint per study is depicted. Both the definition of exercise and the degree of confounder adjustment vary across studies. Short dark vertical lines indicate point estimates of relative risk; shaded areas depict the 95% confidence intervals. If relative risk or confidence intervals were unavailable statistical significance is depicted as *, $p < 0.05$; **, $p > 0.05$. CA, cardiac arrest; CHD, coronary heart disease; CVD, cardiovascular disease; MI, myocardial infarction; SD, sudden death.

[a] Siscovick *et al.* (1988); [b] Leon *et al.* (1987); [c] Scragg *et al.* (1987); [d] Slattery *et al.* (1989); [e] Blair *et al.* (1989); [f] Ekelund *et al.* (1988); [g] Lie *et al.* (1985); [h] Slattery & Jacobs (1988); [i] Sobolski *et al.* (1987).

4554 postinfarction patients followed for an average of 3 years after randomization. The relative risks in the pooled exercise group vs. the pooled comparison group were significantly reduced for *total mortality* (relative risk = 0.80), *cardiovascular mortality* (0.78) and *fatal reinfarction* (0.75). *Sudden death* was significantly reduced in exercisers at 1 year (relative risk = 0.63), but not at 2 and 3 years. There was no observable effect of exercise on the rate of *non-fatal reinfarctions*. Thus, existing data suggest that endurance exercise in patients who survive a myocardial infarction results in a 20% reduction in the overall mortality rate, due to a decreased risk of cardiovascular mortality, fatal reinfarctions and early sudden death. Recommendations have been published for prescribing exercise in the clinical setting to prevent cardiovascular disease (American College of Sports Medicine, 1978; 1986; Maskin, 1986; Harris *et al.*, 1989).

There are several hypothesized biological mechanisms by which endurance exercise may reduce coronary heart disease incidence or mortality rates (Table 39.2). The four most plausible are: (i) reduced coronary atherosclerosis; (ii) reduced coronary thrombosis; (iii) increased myocardial vascularity; and (iv) improved cardiac function and electrical stability. The latter three mechanisms may be especially important in preventing death in postmyocardial infarction patients.

Atherosclerosis is most likely reduced by the beneficial effects of exercise on coronary risk factors. Exercise clearly can improve blood pressure, reduce body mass, modify blood lipids and increase insulin sensitivity. The latter three effects are discussed later in this chapter. In addition, exercise may lead indirectly to reductions in psychological stress (Dishman, 1985; Taylor *et al.*, 1985) and smoking (Folsom *et al.*, 1985). Exercise might also reduce atherogenesis directly. Although difficult to demonstrate in humans, exercise has prevented the development of coronary atheroma in a controlled trial where non-human primates were fed an atherogenic diet (Kramsch *et al.*,

Table 39.2 Mechanisms by which endurance exercise may prevent coronary heart disease. Partly adapted from Leon (1983) and Powell *et al.* (1987).

Reduced coronary atherosclerosis
Improved risk factors
  decreased blood pressure
  decreased body mass
  improved blood lipid profile: increased high density lipoprotein cholesterol; decreased triglycerides
  improved insulin sensitivity and glucose tolerance
Possible direct effect on atherogenesis

Reduced coronary thrombosis
Increased fibrinolytic activity
Decreased platelet aggregation

Increased myocardial vascularity

Improved myocardial function and electrical stability
Improved cardiorespiratory function: increased stroke volume, reduced heart rate, increased muscle extraction and utilization of oxygen
Decreased adrenergic activity, increased resistance to ventricular fibrillation

---

1981). Exercise may reduce the risk of coronary thrombosis when atherosclerosis is present, by increasing fibrinolysis (Williams *et al.*, 1980) and reducing platelet aggregability (Rauramaa *et al.*, 1986). Platelet effects may be due to exercise-induced alterations of arachidonic acid metabolism (Rauramaa, 1984).

In animals, exercise can increase the calibre of the coronary arteries (Bove & Dewey, 1985) and enhance collateral circulation (Neill & Oxendine, 1979). However, such adaptations of the coronary vasculature are undocumented in humans. Exercise can reduce heart rate and blood pressure, both major determinants of myocardial oxygen demand (Maskin, 1986). These adaptations may lead to reduced circulating levels of noradrenaline (Cooksey *et al.*, 1978) and increased resistance to ventricular fibrillation (Billman *et al.*, 1984). Correspondingly, humans who exercise regularly appear to have a reduced risk of cardiac arrest compared with those who are sedentary, even though the overall risk of cardiac arrest is somewhat higher

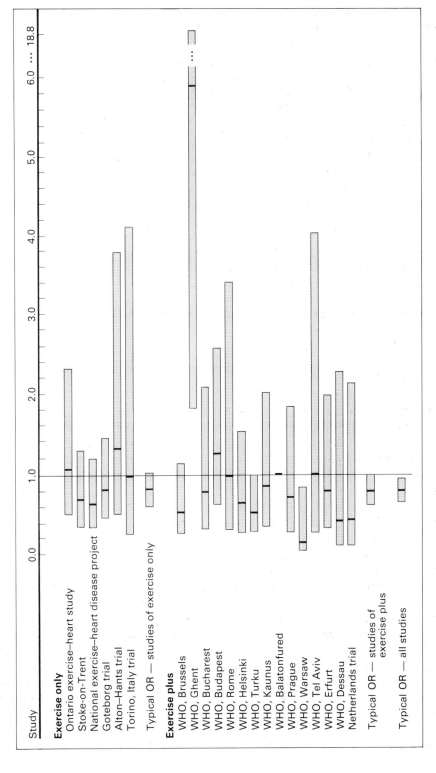

Fig. 39.2 Randomized trials of exercise for cardiac rehabilitation: effect on mortality 3 years after randomization. Short dark vertical lines indicate the relative odds of death in the exercise group compared with controls; shaded areas depict the 95% confidence intervals. 'Typical OR' refers to the odds ratio from the meta-analysis; 'exercise plus' refers to studies with additional interventions but primarily involving exercise. From O'Connor *et al.* (1989), modified with permission.

during exercise than during rest (Siscovick *et al.*, 1982; 1984).

Exercise and stroke

Cerebrovascular stroke is an important cause of disability and mortality, especially in the elderly. There are several aetiologies of stroke, the two most prevalent being thrombotic stroke, which results from atherosclerosis of the cerebral and precerebral arteries, and intra-cerebral haemorrhage. Arterial hypertension is the most important risk factor for stroke, but other risk factors for atherosclerosis also contribute (Dyken *et al.*, 1984).

Even though many of the risk factors for stroke and coronary heart disease are similar, the role of endurance exercise in reducing the risk of stroke is less well established. We identified nine published epidemiological studies of exercise and stroke, summarized in Table 39.3. About half of the studies reported that a lack of exercise was significantly associated with stroke occurrence, the median increase in risk being about 1.5-fold. This is neither as strong nor as consistent a risk as for coronary heart disease. Of three studies that could quantify exercise at two or more levels, two (Herman *et al.*, 1983; Paffenbarger *et al.*, 1984) observed a dose–response pattern of lower stroke occurrence at successively greater exercise levels. However, a dose–response relationship was not observed in the study of Menotti and Seccareccia (1985).

There are no studies of the relation of stroke to physical fitness. Likewise, few data are available for either women or non-whites.

In summary, existing evidence suggests that endurance exercise may reduce the risk of cerebrovascular stroke. The plausible mechanisms include reduced hypertension, reduced atherosclerosis, and/or reduced thrombosis of the cerebral and precerebral arteries. However, additional research is needed to clarify the causality and generalizability of these findings, as well as the duration, frequency and intensity of exercise required to prevent stroke.

Exercise and metabolic cardiovascular risk factors

Obesity

Obesity is a moderately important risk factor for atherosclerotic diseases (Barrett-Connor, 1985) and a strong risk factor for hypertension (Stamler *et al.*, 1978). Excess energy intake relative to energy utilization is the cause of obesity. Controlled trials show unequivocally that exercise programmes reduce overweight in obese patients (Epstein & Wing, 1980). Furthermore, reduction of body mass is more easily achieved and maintained when exercise is part of a weight-loss programme (Martin & Dubbert, 1982). Clinicians should certainly recommend exercise to overweight patients in whom there is no medical contraindication.

Blood lipids and lipoproteins

Incidence of coronary heart disease and thrombotic stroke are associated directly with plasma concentrations of total cholesterol, low density lipoprotein (LDL) cholesterol, and tri-glycerides, and inversely with high density lipoprotein (HDL) cholesterol (Castelli *et al.*, 1977). Recent clinical trials have demonstrated that lowering of elevated plasma LDL-cholesterol (Lipid Research Clinics Program, 1984) and possibly raising HDL-cholesterol (Manninen *et al.*, 1988) reduces the incidence of coronary heart disease. Whether the triglyceride level is truly an independent risk factor is disputed (Hulley *et al.*, 1980).

The numerous studies of the effects of acute and long-term exercise on lipid metabolism in normolipaemic and hyperlipaemic subjects have been thoroughly reviewed (Dufaux *et al.*, 1982; Haskell, 1984; Goldberg & Elliot, 1987; Superko & Haskell, 1987). Proper interpretation of the results of these studies is difficult due to the presence of many confounding factors that

Table 39.3 Epidemiological studies of exercise and stroke occurrence.

Study	Population	Relative risk (RR)
Paffenbarger et al. (1970)	Longshoremen	RR = 1.1 for stroke mortality, less active work vs. more active work
Kannel & Sorlie (1979)	Framingham men	Stroke incidence inversely but not significantly associated with a physical activity index
Kagan et al. (1980)	Hawaii Japanese men	Mean physical activity index not significantly different in thromboembolic or haemorrhagic stroke cases vs. subjects free of stroke
Salonen et al. (1982)	Finnish men	RR = 1.6* for stroke incidence, low vs. high work activity
	Finnish women	RR = 1.7* for stroke incidence, low vs. high work activity
Pomrehn et al. (1982)	Iowa men, 1964–70	RR = 1.12* for stroke mortality, non-farmers vs. farmers
	Iowa men, 1971–78	RR = 1.10 for stroke mortality, non-farmers vs. farmers
Herman et al. (1983)	Dutch men and women	In stroke cases vs. controls: RR = 2.0* for little leisure activity vs. regular light leisure activity RR = 4.2* for little leisure activity vs. regular heavy leisure activity
Paffenbarger et al. (1984)	Harvard male alumni	Stroke mortality trend* RR = 1.3 for < 500 kcal·week^{-1} (2100 kJ·week^{-1}) vs. 500–1999 kcal·week^{-1} (2100–8400 kJ·week^{-1}) leisure activity RR = 2.7 for < 500 kcal·week^{-1} (2100 kJ·week^{-1}) vs. 2000+ kcal·week^{-1} (8400+ kJ·week^{-1}) leisure activity
Menotti & Seccareccia (1985)	Italian men	RR = 1.5* for stroke mortality, sedentary vs. moderately active jobs RR = 1.0, sedentary vs. heavy jobs
Lapidus & Bengtsson (1986)	Swedish women	Stroke mortality, least active category vs. three higher activity categories for work (RR = 7.8*) and leisure (RR = 10.1*)

* Significant $p < 0.05$.

affect blood lipid values, including energy intake, dietary composition and changes of body mass.

Neither cross-sectional nor prospective studies have consistently supported a relationship between endurance exercise and total or LDL-cholesterol levels in normolipaemic or hyperlipaemic subjects (Goldberg & Elliot, 1987; Superko & Haskell, 1987). On the other hand, many cross-sectional studies have found lower levels of plasma triglycerides among more active individuals (Björntorp et al., 1972; Wood et al., 1976). Prospective studies in both normolipaemic subjects and patients with hypertriglyceridaemia have generally shown a significant reduction in serum triglycerides after exercise training (Lopez-S et al., 1974; Wood et al., 1988). The decrease in triglycerides has often been tied to exercise-induced weight loss.

Cross-sectional studies have frequently noted an association between the level of endurance fitness and HDL-cholesterol concentration (Wood *et al.*, 1976; Hartung *et al.*, 1980). The majority of these studies did not, however, consider confounding variables. A recent well-designed study (Nakamura *et al.*, 1983), which matched joggers with sedentary controls of similar age, sex, body mass index, and total cholesterol and triglyceride levels, found significantly higher HDL-cholesterol concentrations among joggers. Prospective investigations have generally supported the belief that regular exercise increases HDL-cholesterol (Huttunen *et al.*, 1979; Kiens *et al.*, 1980; Thompson *et al.*, 1988), although several investigators have reported negative findings (LaRosa *et al.*, 1982; Raz *et al.*, 1988). Differences among these studies, including the number and type of participants, the presence or absence of a control group, dietary changes, and the duration and intensity of the training programme, account in part for the variable results. In addition, the ratio of HDL subfractions, HDL_2/HDL_3, may beneficially increase with exercise without necessarily altering the total HDL-cholesterol concentration (Rauramaa *et al.*, 1984).

One of the best-designed experimental studies to date is that of Wood and colleagues (1983). In a randomized, controlled 1-year trial of running in 81 men, they found a correlation between exercise level and increased HDL-cholesterol, but there was a threshold effect: a significant increase in HDL-cholesterol was detected only in those men whose running distance during the last 7 months of the trial exceeded an average of 12.9 km (8 miles) per week. Furthermore, an exercise-induced loss of body mass was an essential element of the HDL-cholesterol response. Wood *et al.* (1988) subsequently showed that HDL-cholesterol and triglyceride changes with a decrease of body mass are comparable whether they are achieved through exercise or diet.

In summary, an independent relationship between endurance exercise and concentrations of plasma lipids has not been unequivocally established. However, evidence to date suggests that exercise training probably has beneficial effects on the levels of triglycerides and HDL-cholesterol, to a large degree through an exercise-mediated decrease of body mass. The most likely mechanisms for these effects are exercise-induced alterations in lipolytic enzymes, such as lipoprotein lipase and hepatic lipase (Lithell *et al.*, 1979; Herbert *et al.*, 1984; Kantor *et al.*, 1984). Clinicians may wish to recommend exercise as part of a complete regimen for control of dyslipidaemias.

Glucose intolerance and insulin sensitivity

Diabetes mellitus is an important coronary heart disease risk factor. There are no prospective data on the relation of exercise to the incidence of diabetes, but exercise and physical conditioning do appear to influence insulin and glucose regulation in patients with non-insulin-dependent diabetes (Björntorp, 1982; Kemmer & Berger, 1983; Rauramaa, 1984; Richter & Galbo, 1986). In non-insulin-dependent diabetics, exercise has been shown to increase insulin receptor density, enhance insulin sensitivity, and occasionally to improve glucose utilization (LeBlanc *et al.*, 1979; Soman *et al.*, 1979; Pedersen *et al.*, 1980; Schneider *et al.*, 1984; Ronnemaa *et al.*, 1986). The accompanying decrease of body mass and reduction of adiposity are important contributing factors, although exercise may also have a weak independent effect.

The effect of regular exercise may vary according to the subtype of non-insulin-dependent diabetes (Krotkiewski *et al.*, 1985). In diabetics with *high* insulin levels and marked insulin resistance, exercise decreases insulin secretion, with no improvement in glucose tolerance. In contrast, in non-insulin-dependent diabetics with *low* insulin levels, exercise increases insulin secretion (perhaps due to sensitization of the autonomic nervous system), thereby improving glucose tolerance. These reported effects are unrelated to weight change (Krotkiewski *et al.*, 1985).

In summary, exercise has important beneficial effects on glucose tolerance and insulin utilization. These may play an important role in the cardiovascular effects of exercise. Clinicians should consider recommending appropriate exercise to patients with non-insulin-dependent diabetes mellitus, especially those with obesity. Exercise, however, must be undertaken cautiously in diabetics at risk of hypoglycaemia, such as those who are insulin dependent.

Exercise recommendations for cardiovascular health

Only incomplete information is available about the optimal type, intensity, frequency and duration of exercise needed to prevent cardiovascular disease. Many types of exercise have shown a benefit, including work, leisure exercise, sports and non-specific 'exercise'. Beneficial exercise typically has involved endurance, that is dynamic movement of large muscle groups on a regular basis. There is no evidence that exercise to produce strength, flexibility or coordination prevents cardiovascular disease.

Even low to moderate intensity endurance activity offers some protection against coronary disease, relative to complete sedentariness. For example, Magnus and colleagues (1979) reported that walking, cycling or gardening, if habitual, was sufficient to reduce coronary heart disease risk by 55%. Low intensity exercise, such as walking, can also improve body composition.

Exercise duration does not need to be excessive to offer some benefit. Paffenbarger found that even 2–8 MJ (500–1999 kcal) per week of leisure-time exercise was associated with a 28% reduction in first heart attack rates among Harvard male alumni when compared with colleagues spending less than 2 MJ (500 kcal) per week (Paffenbarger et al., 1984; 1986). Leon et al. (1987) similarly found that intermediate levels of leisure-time exercise (2.5–5.7 MJ, 596–1373 kcal·week⁻¹) in high-risk men was

associated with a 63% reduction in fatal coronary heart disease and sudden deaths when compared with lower levels of exercise. No further reduction in risk was found with caloric expenditures > 5.7 MJ (1373 kcal) per week.

At least moderate exercise intensity or duration seems necessary to improve lipid profiles. For example, Haskell et al. (1985) estimated that the lower threshold of lipid effects is approximately 4 MJ (1000 kcal) per week of endurance-type exercise at moderate intensity. Wood et al. (1988) found HDL-cholesterol rose when the runners' distance exceeded 12.9 km per week. Beneficial changes in other metabolic factors associated with coronary heart disease risk, such as blood pressure and insulin sensitivity also seem to require at least moderate levels of exercise or a decrease in body mass.

However, the optimal cardiovascular and metabolic effects of exercise may require vigorous levels of physical activity and perhaps achievement of physical fitness. In many studies there has been a dose−response relationship between exercise and coronary disease prevention (see Fig. 39.1). Haskell (1984) estimated that there is a dose−response relationship between an energy expenditure of 4−19 MJ (1000−4500 kcal) per week and lipid or lipoprotein levels. Insulin sensitivity and glucose control also seem to be optimized at high levels of exercise. The coronary heart disease incidence in many studies was lowest in those who exercised vigorously, for example at 21−31 kJ (5−7.5 kcal) per minute (Paffenbarger et al., 1970; Morris et al., 1980; Garcia-Palmieri et al., 1982), or in those who achieved a leisure energy expenditure of at least 8 MJ (2000 kcal) per week (Paffenbarger et al., 1984). Haskell (1985) concluded that reduced coronary heart disease risk begins with exercise as low as 0.6 MJ (150 kcal) per day and that risks become lower as exercise increases up to 17 MJ (4000 kcal) per day. Exercise must be regular and long term to be beneficial, as evidenced by the high coronary heart disease risk in college athletes who became sedentary later in life (Paffenbarger et al., 1984).

Other evidence that regular vigorous exercise is optimal comes from studies of endurance fitness and coronary heart disease. Relative risks tend to exhibit a strong dose–response relationship in physical fitness studies, with the most fit subjects having up to an eightfold reduction in coronary heart disease (see Fig. 39.1). This implies that regular and vigorous activity sufficient to produce fitness results in the greatest cardiovascular benefit.

Exercise recommendations by health organizations

The available data on exercise and health have been translated into policy recommendations for both individuals and populations. One widely accepted set of exercise guidelines for individuals was proposed by the American College of Sports Medicine (1978). They recommended that exercise should involve large muscle groups in dynamic movement for periods of 20 min or longer, 3 or more days per week, and performed at an intensity of 60% or more of an individual's cardiorespiratory capacity. The US Preventive Services Task Force Report (1989) recommended that 'clinicians should counsel all patients to engage in a programme of regular physical activity, tailored to their health status and personal lifestyle'. Of concern in prescribing exercise are the possible risks. The three most common risks, injury, osteoarthritis and sudden death, are described elsewhere in this book. Methods to assess exercise risk, along with practical tips for individual exercise counselling in the clinical setting, have been published (American College of Sports Medicine, 1986; Harris et al., 1989).

Exercise recommendations from a population-wide perspective are also important. A large proportion of the population in most industrialized countries does not exercise regularly. In the USA at least 40% of the adult population is sedentary (Stephens et al., 1985). Of the 60% who claim to exercise, only about

10–20% regularly participate in vigorous endurance activity. As a result, the US Department of Health and Human Services (1980) has set population-wide exercise objectives for the USA for the year 1990 and, drafted recently, for the year 2000 (US Department of Health and Human Services, 1991). The Year 2000 goals are that at least 60% of US citizens aged 6 years and older will participate in light to moderate physical activities, and at least 20% of adults and 75% of children will engage in vigorous activities, 3 or more days per week, for 20 min or more per occasion. Population strategies for exercise promotion are reviewed elsewhere (Shephard, 1983; Iverson et al., 1985).

The estimated effect of increasing exercise on a population-wide basis can be predicted by attributable risk calculations (Lilienfeld & Lilienfeld, 1980). If it is assumed that a lack of vigorous exercise carries a relative risk for cardiovascular disease of 2.0, then a 20% increase in the population-wide prevalence of exercise (i.e. from 40–60%) might reduce cardiovascular disease rates by 17%. A 40% increase in exercise prevalence might reduce cardiovascular disease rates by a sizeable 29%.

Conclusion

Endurance exercise is clearly important in the primary, secondary and tertiary prevention of coronary heart disease. It also appears to contribute to the prevention and control of arterial hypertension and cerebrovascular stroke. Evidence on the frequency, intensity, duration and type of exercise required for cardiovascular benefits is incomplete. Exercise for cardiovascular health can certainly be recommended to most individuals, but additional research is needed to refine specific recommendations for subgroups of the population. How to motivate individuals to adopt endurance exercise as a lifelong habit remains a challenge.

References

American College of Sports Medicine (1978) Position statement on the recommended quantity and quality of exercise for developing and maintaining fitness in healthy adults. *Med. Sci. Sports Exerc.* **10**, vii–x.

American College of Sports Medicine (1986) *Guidelines for Graded Exercise Testing and Prescription*, 3rd edn. Lea & Febiger, Philadelphia.

Barrett-Connor, E.L. (1985) Obesity, atherosclerosis, and coronary artery disease. *Ann. Intern. Med.* **103**, 1010–1019.

Billman, G.E., Schwartz, P.J. & Stone, H.L. (1984) The effects of daily exercise on susceptibility to sudden cardiac death. *Circulation* **69**, 1182–1189.

Björntorp, P.M. (1982) Effects of physical training on diabetes mellitus, Type II. In: Bostrom, H. & Ljungstedt, N. (eds) *Recent Trends in Diabetes Research*, pp. 115–125. Almqvist & Wiksell International, Stockholm.

Björntorp, P.M., Fahlen, M., Grimby, G. *et al.* (1972) Carbohydrate and lipid metabolism in middle aged, physically well-trained men. *Metabolism* **21**, 1037–1044.

Blackburn, H. (1983) Physical activity and coronary heart disease: a brief update and population view. *J. Cardiac Rehab.* **3**, 101–111, 171–174.

Blackburn, H. (1986) Physical activity and hypertension. *J. Clin. Hypertension* **2**, 154–162.

Blair, S.N., Goodyear, N.N., Gibbons. L.W. & Cooper, K.H. (1984) Physical fitness and incidence of hypertension in healthy normotensive men and women. *J.A.M.A.* **252**, 487–490.

Blair, S.N., Kohl, H.W. III, Paffenbarger, R.S. Jr, Clark, D.G., Cooper, K.H. & Gibbons, L.W. (1989) Physical fitness and all-cause mortality. A prospective study of healthy men and women. *J.A.M.A.* **262**, 2395–2401.

Blair, S.N. & Oberman, A. (1987) Epidemiologic analysis of coronary heart disease and exercise. *Cardiol. Clin.* **5**, 271–283.

Bonanno, J.A. & Lies, J.E. (1974) Effects of physical training on coronary risk factors. *Am. J. Cardiol.* **33**, 760–764.

Bove, A.A. & Dewey, J.D. (1985) Proximal coronary vasomotor reactivity after exercise training in dogs. *Circulation* **71**, 620–625.

Bruce, R.A., Hossack, K.F., DeRouen, T.A. & Hofer, V. (1983) Enhanced risk assessment for primary coronary heart disease events by maximal exercise testing: 10 years' experience of Seattle Heart Watch. *J. Am. Coll. Cardiol.* **2**, 565–573.

Cassel, J., Heyden, S., Bartel, A.G. *et al.* (1971) Occupation and physical activity in coronary heart disease. *Arch. Intern. Med.* **128**, 920–928.

Castelli, W.P., Doyle, J.T., Gordon, T. *et al.* (1977) HDL cholesterol and other lipids in coronary heart disease. The Cooperative Lipoprotein Phenotyping Study. *Circulation* **55**, 767–772.

Cooksey, J.D., Reilly, P., Brown, S., Bromze, H. & Cryer, P.E. (1978) Exercise training and plasma catecholamines in patients with ischemic heart disease. *Am. J. Cardiol.* **42**, 372–376.

Cutler, J.A. & Furberg, C.D. (1985) Drug treatment trials in hypertension: a review. *Prev. Med.* **14**, 499–518.

DePlaen, J.F. & Detry, J.M. (1980) Hemodynamic effects of physical training in established arterial hypertension. *Acta Cardiol.* **35**, 179–188.

DeWood, M.A., Spores, J., Notske, R. *et al.* (1980) Prevalence of total coronary occlusion during the early hours of transmural myocardial infarction. *N. Engl. J. Med.* **303**, 897–902.

Dishman, R.K. (1985) Medical psychology in exercise and sport. *Med. Clin. North Am.* **69**, 123–143.

Donahue, R.P., Abbot, R.D., Reed, D.M. & Yano, K. (1988) Physical activity and coronary heart disease in middle-aged and elderly men: the Honolulu Heart Program. *Am. J. Public Health* **78**, 683–685.

Dufaux, B., Assmann, G. & Hollman, W. (1982) Plasma lipoproteins and physical activity: a review. *Int. J. Sports Med.* **3**, 123–126.

Duncan, J.J., Farr, J.E., Upton, S.J., Hagan, R.D., Oglesby, M.E. & Blair, S.N. (1985) The effects of aerobic exercise on plasma catecholamines and blood pressure in patients with mild essential hypertension. *J.A.M.A.* **254**, 2609–2613.

Dyken, M.L., Wolf, P.A., Barnett, H.J.M. *et al.* (1984) Risk factors in stroke: a statement for physicians by the Subcommittee on Risk Factors and Stroke of the Stroke Council. *Stroke* **15**, 1105–1111.

Ekelund, L.G., Haskell, W.L., Johnson, J.L., Whaley, F.S., Criqui, M.H. & Sheps, D.S. (1988) Physical fitness as a predictor of cardiovascular mortality in asymptomatic North American men. The Lipid Research Clinics Mortality Follow-up Study. *N. Engl. J. Med.* **319**, 1379–1384.

Epstein, L.H. & Wing, R.R. (1980) Aerobic exercise and weight. *Addict. Behav.* **5**, 371–378.

Erikssen, J. (1986) Physical fitness and coronary heart disease morbidity and mortality. A prospective study in apparently healthy, middle aged men. *Acta Med. Scand.* **711** (Suppl.), 189–192.

Folsom, A.R., Caspersen, C.J., Taylor, H.L. *et al.* (1985) Leisure time physical activity and its relationship to coronary risk factors in a population-based sample: The Minnesota Heart Survey. *Am. J. Epidemiol.* **121**, 570–579.

Garcia-Palmieri, M.R., Costas, R. Jr, Cruz-Vidal, M., Sorlie, P.D. & Havlik, R.J. (1982) Increased physical activity. A protective factor against heart attacks in

Puerto Rico. *Am. J. Cardiol.* **50**, 749–755.

Goldberg, L. & Elliot, D.L. (1987) The effect of exercise on lipid metabolism in men and women. *Sports Med.* **4**, 307–321.

Hagberg, J.M., Goldring, D., Ehsani, A.A. *et al.* (1983) Effect of exercise training on the blood pressure and hemodynamic features of hypertensive adolescents. *Am. J. Cardiol.* **52**, 763–768.

Hagberg, J.M., Montain, S.J., Martin, W.H. III & Ehsani, A.A. (1989) Effect of exercise training in 60- to 69-year-old persons with essential hypertension. *Am. J. Cardiol.* **64**, 348–353.

Harris, S.S., Caspersen, C.J., DeFriese, G.H. & Estes, E.H. Jr (1989) Physical activity counseling for healthy adults as a primary preventive intervention in the clinical setting. Report for the U.S. Preventive Services Task Force. *J.A.M.A.* **261**, 3588–3598.

Hartung, G.H., Foreyt, J.P., Mitchell, R.E., Vlasek, I. & Gotto, A.M. (1980) Relation of diet to high-density lipoprotein cholesterol in middle-aged marathon runners, joggers and inactive men. *N. Engl. J. Med.* **302**, 357–361.

Haskell, W.L. (1984) Exercise-induced changes in plasma lipids and lipoproteins. *Prev. Med.* **13**, 23–36.

Haskell, W.L. (1985) Physical activity and health: need to define the required stimulus. *Am. J. Cardiol.* **55**, 4D–9D.

Haskell, W.L., Montoye, H.J. & Orenstein, D. (1985) Physical activity and exercise to achieve health-related physical fitness components. *Public Health Rep.* **100**, 202–212.

Herbert, P.N., Bernier, D.N., Cullinane, E.M., Edelstein, L., Kantor, M.A. & Thompson, P.D. (1984) High density lipoprotein metabolism in runners and sedentary men. *J.A.M.A.* **252**, 1034–1037.

Herman, B., Schmitz, P.I.M., Leyten, A.C.M. *et al.* (1983) Multivariate logistic analysis of risk factors for stroke in Tilburg, the Netherlands. *Am. J. Epidemiol.* **118**, 514–525.

Hulley, S.B., Rosenman, R.H., Bawol, R.D. & Brand, R.J. (1980) Epidemiology as a guide to clinical decisions. The association between triglyceride and coronary heart disease. *N. Engl. J. Med.* **302**, 1383–1389.

Huttunen, J.K., Lansimies, E., Voutilainen, E. *et al.* (1979) Effect of moderate physical exercise on serum lipoproteins. A controlled clinical trial with special reference to serum high-density lipoproteins. *Circulation* **60**, 1220–1229.

Iverson, D.C., Fielding, J.E., Crow, R.S. & Christenson, G.M. (1985) The promotion of physical activity in the United States population: the status of programs in medical, worksite, community, and school settings. *Public Health Rep.* **100**, 212–224.

Kagan, A., Popper, J.S. & Rhoads, G.G. (1980) Factors related to stroke incidence in Hawaii Japanese men. The Honolulu Heart Study. *Stroke* **11**, 14–21.

Kannel, W.B., Belanger, A., D'Agostino, R. & Israel, I. (1986) Physical activity and physical demand on the job and risk of cardiovascular disease and death: The Framingham Study. *Am. Heart J.* **112**, 820–825.

Kannel, W.B. & Sorlie, P. (1979) Some health benefits of physical activity. The Framingham Study. *Arch. Intern. Med.* **139**, 857–861.

Kantor, M.A., Cullinane, E.M., Herbert, P.N. & Thompson, P.D. (1984) Acute increase in lipoprotein lipase following prolonged exercise. *Metabolism* **33**, 454–457.

Kemmer, F.W. & Berger, M. (1983) Exercise and diabetes mellitus: physical activity as part of daily life and its role in the treatment of diabetic patients. *Int. J. Sports Med.* **4**, 77–88.

Kiens, B., Jorgensen, I., Lewis, S. *et al.* (1980) Increased plasma HDL-cholesterol and apo A-I in sedentary middle-aged men after physical conditioning. *Eur. J. Clin. Invest.* **10**, 203–209.

Kramsch, D.M., Aspen, A.J., Abramowitz, B.M., Kreimendahl, T. & Hood, W.B. Jr (1981) Reduction of coronary atherosclerosis by moderate conditioning exercise in monkeys on an atherogenic diet. *N. Engl. J. Med.* **305**, 1483–1489.

Krotkiewski, M., Lonnroth, P., Mandroukas, K. *et al.* (1985) The effects of physical training on insulin secretion and effectiveness and on glucose metabolism in obesity and type 2 (non-insulin-dependent) diabetes mellitus. *Diabetologia* **28**, 881–890.

Kukkonen, K., Rauramaa, R., Voutilainen, E. & Lansimies, E. (1982) Physical training of middle-aged men with borderline hypertension. *Ann. Clin. Res.* **14**, 139–145.

Lapidus, L. & Bengtsson, C. (1986) Socioeconomic factors and physical activity in relation to cardiovascular disease and death: a 12-year follow-up of participants in a population study of women in Gothenburg, Sweden. *Br. Heart J.* **55**, 295–301.

LaPorte, R.E., Adams, L.L., Savage, D.D., Brenes, G., Dearwater, S. & Cook, T. (1984) The spectrum of physical activity, cardiovascular disease, and health: an epidemiologic perspective. *Am. J. Epidemiol.* **120**, 507–517.

LaRosa, J.C., Cleary, P., Muesing, R.A., Gorman, P., Hellerstein, H.K. & Naughton, J. (1982) Effect of long-term moderate physical exercise on plasma lipoproteins. The National Exercise and Heart Disease Project. *Arch. Intern. Med.* **142**, 2269–2274.

LeBlanc, J., Nadeau, A., Boulay, M. & Rousseau-Migneron, S. (1979) Effects of physical training and adiposity on glucose metabolism and ^{125}I-insulin binding. *J. Appl. Physiol.* **46**, 235–239.

Leon, A.S. (1983) Exercise and coronary heart disease. *Hosp. Med.* **19**, 38–57.

Leon, A.S., Connett, J., Jacobs, D.R. Jr & Rauramaa, R. (1987) Leisure-time physical activity levels and risk of coronary heart disease and death. The Multiple Risk Factor Intervention Trial. *J.A.M.A.* **258**, 2388–2395.

Lie, H., Mundal, R. & Erikssen, J. (1985) Coronary risk factors and incidence of coronary death in relation to physical fitness. Seven-year follow-up study of middle-aged and elderly men. *Eur. Heart J.* **6**, 147–157.

Lilienfeld, A.M. & Lilienfeld, D.W. (1980) *Foundations of Epidemiology*. Oxford University Press, New York.

Lipid Research Clinics Program (1984) The Lipid Research Clinics Coronary Primary Prevention Trial Results. I. Reduction in incidence of coronary heart disease. *J.A.M.A.* **251**, 351–364.

Lithell, H., Orlander, J., Schele, R., Sjodin, B. & Karlsson, J. (1979) Changes in lipoprotein-lipase activity and lipid stores in human skeletal muscle with prolonged heavy exercise. *Acta Physiol. Scand.* **107**, 257–261.

Lopez-S, A., Vial, R., Balart, L. & Arroyave, G. (1974) Effect of exercise and physical fitness on serum lipids and lipoproteins. *Atherosclerosis* **20**, 1–9.

Magnus, K., Matroos, A. & Strackee, J. (1979) Walking, cycling, or gardening, with or without seasonal interruption, in relation to acute coronary events. *Am. J. Epidemiol.* **110**, 724–733.

Manninen, V., Elo, M.O., Frick, M.H. *et al.* (1988) Lipid alterations and decline in the incidence of coronary heart disease in the Helsinki Heart Study. *J.A.M.A.* **260**, 641–651.

Martin, J.E. & Dubbert, P.M. (1982) Exercise applications and promotion in behavioral medicine: current issues and future directions. *J. Consult. Clin. Psychol.* **50**, 1004–1017.

Martin, J.E. & Dubbert, P.M. (1987) The role of exercise in preventing and moderating blood pressure elevation. *Bibl. Cardiol.* **41**, 120–142.

Maskin, C.S. (1986) Aerobic exercise training and cardiopulmonary disease. In: Weber, K.T. & Janicki, J.S. (eds) *Cardiopulmonary Exercise Training*, pp. 317–332. W.B. Saunders, Philadelphia.

Menotti, A. & Seccareccia, F. (1985) Physical activity at work and job responsibility as risk factors for fatal coronary heart disease and other causes of death. *J. Epidemiol. Comm. Health* **39**, 325–329.

Morris, J.N., Everitt, M.G., Pollard, R., Chave, S.P. &

Semmence, A.M. (1980) Vigorous exercise in leisure-time: protection against coronary heart disease. *Lancet* **ii**, 1207–1210.

Nakamura, N., Uzawa, H., Haeda, H. & Inomoto, T. (1983) Physical fitness, its contribution to serum high density lipoprotein. *Atherosclerosis* **48**, 173–183.

Neill, W.A. & Oxendine, J.M. (1979) Exercise can promote coronary collateral development without improving perfusion of ischemic myocardium. *Circulation* **60**, 1513–1519.

O'Connor, G.T., Buring, J.E., Yusuf, S. *et al.* (1989) An overview of randomized trials of rehabilitation with exercise after myocardial infarction. *Circulation* **80**, 234–244.

Paffenbarger, R.S. Jr & Hyde, R.T. (1984) Exercise in the prevention of coronary heart disease. *Prev. Med.* **13**, 3–22.

Paffenbarger, R.S. Jr, Hyde, R.T., Wing, A.L. & Hsieh, C.C. (1986) Physical activity, all-cause mortality, and longevity of college alumni. *N. Engl. J. Med.* **314**, 605–613.

Paffenbarger, R.S. Jr, Hyde, R.T., Wing, A.L. & Steinmetz, C.H. (1984) A natural history of athleticism and cardiovascular health. *J.A.M.A.* **252**, 491–495.

Paffenbarger, R.S. Jr, Laughlin, M.E., Gima, A.S. & Black, R.A. (1970) Work activity of longshoremen as related to death from coronary heart disease and stroke. *N. Engl. J. Med.* **282**, 1109–1114.

Paffenbarger, R.S. Jr, Wing, A.L., Hyde, R.T. & Jung, D.L. (1983) Physical activity and incidence of hypertension in college alumni. *Am. J. Epidemiol.* **117**, 245–257.

Pedersen, O., Beck-Nielsen, H. & Heding, L. (1980) Increased insulin receptors after exercise in patients with insulin-dependent diabetes mellitus. *N. Engl. J. Med.* **302**, 886–892.

Pomrehn, P.R., Wallace, R.B. & Burmeister, L.F. (1982) Ischemic heart disease mortality in Iowa farmers. The influence of life-style. *J.A.M.A.* **248**, 1073–1076.

Powell, K.E., Thompson, P.D., Caspersen, C.J. & Kendrick, J.S. (1987) Physical activity and the incidence of coronary heart disease. *Ann. Rev. Public Health* **8**, 253–287.

Rauramaa, R. (1984) Relationship of physical activity, glucose tolerance, and weight management. *Prev. Med.* **13**, 37–46.

Rauramaa, R., Salonen, J.T., Kukkonen-Harjula, K. *et al.* (1984) Effects of mild physical exercise on serum lipoproteins and metabolites of arachidonic acid: a controlled randomised trial in middle aged men. *Br. Med. J.* **288**, 603–606.

Rauramaa, R., Salonen, J.T., Seppanen, K. *et al.* (1986)

Inhibition of platelet aggregability by moderate-intensity physical exercise: a randomized clinical trial in overweight men. *Circulation* **74**, 939–944.

Raz, I., Rosenblit, H. & Kark, J.D. (1988) Effect of moderate exercise on serum lipids in young men with low high density lipoprotein cholesterol. *Arteriosclerosis* **8**, 245–251.

Richter, E.A. & Galbo, H. (1986) Diabetes, insulin and exercise. *Sports Med.* **3**, 275–288.

Ronnemaa, T., Mattila, K., Lehtonen, A. & Kallio, V. (1986) A controlled randomized study on the effect of long-term physical exercise on the metabolic control in type 2 diabetic patients. *Acta Med. Scand.* **220**, 219–224.

Salonen, J.T., Puska, P. & Tuomilehto, J. (1982) Physical activity and risk of myocardial infarction, cerebral stroke and death: a longitudinal study in Eastern Finland. *Am. J. Epidemiol.* **115**, 526–537.

Salonen, J.T., Slater, J.S., Tuomilehto, J. & Rauramaa, R. (1988) Leisure time and occupational physical activity: risk of death from ischemic heart disease. *Am. J. Epidemiol.* **127**, 87–94.

Schneider, S.H., Amorosa, L.F., Khachadurian, A.K. & Ruderman, N.B. (1984) Studies on the mechanism of improved glucose control during regular exercise in type 2 (non-insulin-dependent) diabetes. *Diabetologia* **26**, 355–360.

Scragg, R., Stewart, A., Jackson, R. & Beaglehole, R. (1987) Alcohol and exercise in myocardial infarction and sudden coronary death in men and women. *Am. J. Epidemiol.* **126**, 77–85.

Seals, D.R. & Hagberg, J.M. (1984) The effect of exercise training on human hypertension: a review. *Med. Sci. Sports Exerc.* **16**, 207–215.

Shephard, R.J. (1983) Employee health and fitness — state of the art. *Prev. Med.* **12**, 644–653.

Shephard, R.J. (1986) Exercise in coronary heart disease. *Sports Med.* **3**, 26–49.

Siscovick, D.S., Ekelund, L.G., Hyde. J.S., Johnson, J.L., Gordon, D.J. & LaRosa, J.C. (1988) Physical activity and coronary heart disease among asymptomatic hypercholesterolemic men. (The Lipid Research Clinics Coronary Primary Prevention Trial). *Am. J. Public Health* **78**, 1428–1431.

Siscovick, D.S., Weiss, N.S., Fletcher, R.H., Schoenbach, V.J. & Wagner, E.H. (1984) Habitual vigorous exercise and primary cardiac arrest: effect of other risk factors on the relationship. *J. Chron. Dis.* **37**, 625–631.

Siscovick, D.S., Weiss, N.S., Hallstrom, A.P., Inui, T.S. & Peterson, D.R. (1982) Physical activity and primary cardiac arrest. *J.A.M.A.* **248**, 3113–3117.

Slattery, M.L. & Jacobs, D.R. Jr (1988) Physical fitness and cardiovascular disease mortality. The U.S. Railroad Study. *Am. J. Epidemiol.* **127**, 571–580.

Slattery, M.L., Jacobs, D.R. Jr & Nichaman, M.Z.

(1989) Leisure time physical activity and coronary heart disease death. The US Railroad Study. *Circulation* **79**, 304–311.

Sobolski, J., Kornitzer, M., DeBacker, G. *et al.* (1987) Protection against ischemic heart disease in the Belgian Physical Fitness Study: physical fitness rather than physical activity? *Am. J. Epidemiol.* **125**, 601–610.

Soman, V.R., Koivisto, V.A., Deibert, D., Felig, P. & DeFronzo, R.A. (1979) Increased insulin sensitivity and insulin binding to monocytes after physical training. *N. Engl. J. Med.* **301**, 1200–1204.

Stamler, R., Stamler, J., Riedlinger, W.F., Algera, G. & Roberts, R.H. (1978) Weight and blood pressure. Findings in hypertension screening of 1 million Americans. *J.A.M.A.* **240**, 1607–1610.

Stephens, T., Jacobs, D.R. Jr & White, C.C. (1985) A descriptive epidemiology of leisure-time physical activity. *Public Health Rep.* **100**, 147–158.

Superko, H.R. & Haskell, W.H. (1987) The role of exercise training in the therapy of hyperlipoproteinemia. *Cardiol. Clin.* **5**, 285–310.

Taylor, C.B., Sallis, J.F. & Needle, R. (1985) The relation of physical activity and exercise to mental health. *Public Health Rep.* **100**, 195–202.

Thompson, P.D., Cullinane, E.M., Sady, S.P. *et al.* (1988) Modest changes in high-density lipoprotein concentration and metabolism with prolonged exercise training. *Circulation* **78**, 25–34.

Tipton, C.M. (1984) Exercise, training, and hypertension. *Exerc. Sport Sci. Rev.* **12**, 245–306.

US Department of Health and Human Services (1980) *Promoting Health/Preventing Disease: Objectives for the Nation.* Government Printing Office, Washington, D.C.

US Department of Health and Human Services (1991) *Healthy People 2000: National Health Promotion and Disease Prevention Objectives.* Government Printing Office, Washington, D.C.

US Preventive Services Task Force (1989) *Guide to Clinical Preventive Services, Report of the US Preventive Services Task Force.* US Department of Health and Human Services, Bethesda, Maryland.

Wilhelmsen, L., Bjure, J., Ekstrom-Jodal, B. *et al.* (1981) Nine year's follow-up of a maximal exercise test in a random population sample of middle-aged men. *Cardiology* **68** (Suppl. 2), 1–8.

Williams, R.S., Logue, E.E., Lewis, J.G. *et al.* (1980) Physical conditioning augments the fibrinolytic response to venous occlusion in healthy adults. *N. Engl. J. Med.* **302**, 987–991.

Wood, P.D., Haskell, W.L., Blair, S.N. *et al.* (1983) Increased exercise level and plasma lipoprotein concentrations: a one-year, randomized, controlled study in sedentary, middle-aged men. *Metabolism* **32**, 31–39.

Wood, P.D., Haskell, W., Klein, H., Lewis, S., Stein, M.P. & Farquhar, J.W. (1976) The distribution of plasma lipoproteins in middle aged male runners. *Metabolism* **25**, 1249–1257.

Wood, P.D., Stefanick, M.L., Dreon, D.M. *et al.* (1988) Changes in plasma lipids and lipoproteins in overweight men during weight loss through dieting as compared with exercise. *N. Engl. J. Med.* **319**, 1173–1179.

Chapter 40

Cardiac Problems in Endurance Sports

RICHARD ROST AND WILDOR HOLLMAN

Introduction

The heart of an endurance-trained athlete is of major cardiological interest from two, very different, viewpoints. First, endurance training of high intensity may stimulate cardiac adaptation in the form of 'athlete's heart', which doctors have long suspected as being a pathological phenomenon because of its extraordinary size and functional 'abnormalities', particularly the training bradycardia and some clinical signs such as abnormal electrocardiogram (ECG) patterns. Even if an athlete's heart is seen as healthy and very effective, it can sometimes be difficult to distinguish between physiological and pathological features.

Second, as in sedentary subjects, the heart of an athlete may dysfunction. Because of the large amount of work that has to be performed during training and competitions, slight cardiac conditions that may be of minor importance during everyday activity can result in serious cardiac disease and possibly even a fatal incident during a sports event.

The athlete's heart

Historical overview and evaluation

The athlete's heart is one of the oldest and most stimulating subjects for research in sports medicine. Credit for the first description of the athlete's heart belongs to Henschen (1899), who published two papers on the subject in the late 19th century. The recognition of athlete's heart and the development of modern, high-performance athletics are more than coincidental, since the first modern Olympic games were held in 1896. Only competitive sports lead to the development of athlete's heart, by virtue of the training that is required. Other physical activities, even occupation-related ones, do not have this effect, even though this has been claimed repeatedly. Henschen's concept that this is truly an 'athlete's heart' is valid.

Assessment of the athlete's heart has always been a scientific tug-of-war between those who view it as a physiologically adapted, extremely effective and healthy heart, and those who regard it as a sick heart or, at least, a heart on the borderline of the pathological.

Henschen (1899) arrived at his findings through simple physical diagnostic techniques. The size of the heart was determined through carefully performed percussion. When we consider the later, mistaken, interpretations of athlete's heart made by authors who had much more sophisticated tools at their command, it may be worthwhile quoting Henschen (1899):

> 'It follows from this, that skiing causes an enlargement of the heart, and that this enlarged heart can perform more work than the normal heart. There is therefore, a physiological enlargement of the heart, due to athletic activity: the athlete's heart.'

In spite of this ingenious interpretation many subsequent investigations considered athlete's heart as a pathological phenomenon. One of the most outstanding references can be found in the standard American cardiology textbook by Friedberg (1972). He made the statement that while the athlete's heart was formerly considered to be a physiological adaptation, it is today interpreted as a result of overexertion in a rheumatic, syphilitic or congenitally damaged heart.

All of these suspicions about the athlete's heart can be gathered together under the term athlete's heart syndrome. The frequent interpretation of the athlete's heart as a sick organ is readily understandable. Physiologists observe an enlargement of the heart in experimental animals as a result of overexertion. Many clinicians view the enlargement of the heart as an indication of incipient failure. For them, an increasing heart size is always a negative diagnostic sign. To this has to be added the fact that the enlarged athlete's heart is frequently accompanied by other changes, particularly ECG abnormalities. The false assumption that 'a large heart is a sick heart' is, when applied to the athlete's heart, based on a lack of recognition that in physiological experiments the adaptation factor is missing. In the athlete, enlargement of the heart also denotes an improvement in performance.

In isolated cases the above suspicions may be justified and exercise may aggravate a pre-existing pathological condition. But studies carried out over many years have substantiated the basic premise of Henschen (1899) that 'an enlarged heart is a good thing if it can perform more work over an extended period of time'.

When cardiac volume measured radiologically is compared with cardiac performance measured as maximal aerobic power ($\dot{V}_{O_2 max}$), Henschen's observations that the largest heart has the highest performance capacity, is substantiated (Fig. 40.1). This figure also demonstrates that the largest athlete's heart can be found in pure endurance sports and that athlete's heart is seen only in types of sport that have a substantial endurance component, such as soccer.

Functional aspects of athlete's heart: the training bradycardia

Among the functional aspects of athlete's heart, only bradycardia will be discussed here, because this phenomenon causes most clinical problems. The extremely low heart rate, which may slow down in some athletes to $20-30$ beats·min^{-1}, sometimes suggests to inexperienced investigators that a pacemaker might be needed in an otherwise healthy sportsperson.

However, in the endurance-trained athlete, an increased stroke volume can compensate without any difficulty for the decreased heart rate. Even high-performance athletes have no problems attributable to extreme bradycardia. The training bradycardia must therefore be considered a physiological response.

This still begs the clinical question as to whether the responsiveness of the heart to vagal tone may not be an additional pathogenic factor leading to a situation where a patient literally 'runs him/herself' into the need for an artificial pacemaker. Even though there is no evidence that training bradycardia can progress to the point where it produces a syncopal attack, there have been cases in which there was a high index of suspicion that the vagal effects of training contributed to organic or functional cardiac disturbances and therefore had to be considered as pathogenic.

This suspicion is demonstrated by a single case report. We studied a 46-year-old patient who had been running long distances for 5 years, who had five to six training sessions per week, and who ran the marathon distance in 3 h. It was known that he had had a slow heart rate since childhood and that his rate was further diminished to 30 beats·min^{-1} during periods of intensive training. The patient came to our attention when he complained of premature beats and dyspnoea, mostly at rest. In one of these episodes, when he had severe dyspnoea at night, his pulse rate was 30 beats·min^{-1}. The patient could barely walk, but under these conditions the symptoms were markedly de-

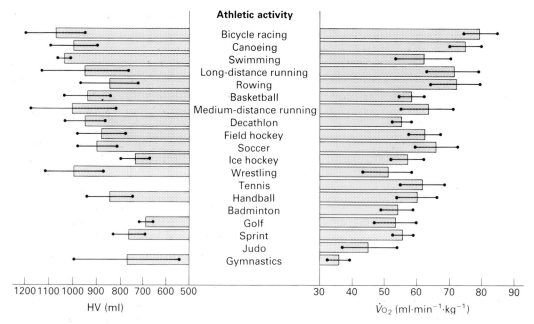

Fig. 40.1 Cardiac volumes (left) and maximal oxygen intake values (right) of the five best athletes from different athletic disciplines ever studied in the Cologne Institute for Cardiology and Sports Medicine. The largest hearts and oxygen intake values were seen in endurance athletes. The two variables were well correlated. From Heck, in Hollman & Hettinger (1976).

creased. He then stopped running completely and his pulse rate rose to 54 beats·min^{-1}. An intensive cardiac diagnostic work-up, including a His' bundle ECG, failed to reveal any cardiac pathology. The tentative diagnosis was one of isolated sinus node damage, with superimposed exercise-induced vagal sensitivity, resulting in a critical bradycardia.

Clinical aspects

Electrocardiographic findings

Experience obtained in a large outpatient, sports cardiology clinic has shown that the clinical problems associated with athlete's heart can be so dramatic that a colleague was moved to write a letter to the *Journal of the American Medical Association*, urging that routine ECGs should never be done in athletes, because the findings would cause more harm than good. On the basis of striking but unimportant ECG

abnormalities, athletes were advised to desist from any further athletic activity. These findings not infrequently also led to unnecessary and dangerous invasive diagnostic tests (Sheehan, 1973). This sarcastic letter underlines the need for physicians who treat athletes to become familiar with the peculiarities of the ECG in athlete's heart.

The most important ECG changes are briefly presented below. The reader interested in a more detailed discussion is referred to an earlier monograph (Rost & Hollman, 1980). No characteristic changes in the ECG are found only in athletes. However, a high incidence of variations can be observed in the athletic population.

Normal, physiological variants: These occur as a result of training and can lead to diagnostic difficulties if the physician is not aware of their incidence in athletes. *Physiological hypertrophy* may cause an increased Sokoloff–Lyon index (left ventricular hypertrophy) and/or an incomplete left bundle branch block (predominantly right ventricular hypertrophy). An increased vagal tone can lead to arrhythmias and functional conduction disturbances in addition to the training bradycardia. The arrhythmias are classified according to the location of the P wave. The *coronary sinus rhythm* shows an inverted P wave and a normal conduction time. In the *upper nodal rhythm* the conduction time is shortened. In a *middle nodal rhythm* there is no P wave. The *lower nodal rhythm* can be recognized by an inverted P wave, which falls after the ventricular complex. This phenomenon is found only very rarely in the athlete, and so is a *wandering pacemaker*, in which the impulse generation passes from the sinus node to the middle nodal rhythm.

The *simple atrioventricular (AV) dissociation*, which occurs frequently in athletes, is often mistakenly identified as a wandering pacemaker. The AV dissociation is characterized by a P wave, which is always upright, but which occurs at varying distances ahead of the ventricular complex. We are dealing here with the simplest form of an overlap between two pacemakers (simple para-arrhythmia), the sinus node and the AV node, which alternate in assuming control. In contrast to the AV node, the rate of the sinus node is significantly influenced by autonomic and respiratory effects. If the sinus wave is relatively late, the AV node will fire, and the P wave will fall just before the ventricular complex. This imitates the picture of a shortened conduction time, which, in fact, does not exist. Related to simple AV dissociation, but extremely rarely found in the athlete, is *interference dissociation*. It differs from simple AV dissociation by the appearance of a retrograde, protective block. The impulse originating in the AV node does not lead to retrograde atrial stimulation. Thus, the P wave is maintained and can 'wander' through the entire cardiac cycle. If it falls fairly late, it can again assume control. This picture, however, is usually reserved for pathological conditions, particularly digitalis intoxication. We have seen this phenomenon only very rarely in

the several thousand athletes whom we have studied.

Not uncommon, and yet always surprising to the physician unfamiliar with the athlete's ECG, is the appearance of a *ventricular escape rhythm* (Fig. 40.2). Such ECG tracings are frequently mistaken for an intermittent bundle branch block or for an intermittent Wolff–Parkinson–White syndrome. Such an error can be avoided by realizing that the widened ventricular complex is not preceded by a P wave. If such a ventricular escape rhythm is combined with simple AV dissociation, the picture of an apparent 'alternating axis deviation' can be seen, because of the fusion of atrial and ventricular beats. This is not uncommon in the athlete's heart ECG.

As far as functional conduction disturbances are concerned, prolongation of the conduction time (*first-degree AV block, second-degree Wenckebach-type AV block*) can occur in athletes. The prolongation of the conduction time is usually slight, and the PQ interval rarely exceeds 0.22 s. Significant first-degree AV blocks are extremely rare. While the Wenckebach periodicity is extremely rare in the untrained person, according to the literature, it appears in the ECG tracing of about 0.5–1% of athletes. By Holter monitoring the sleep ECG, we found a second-degree AV block in 10% of all athletes studied.

Although this was denied for a long time, even *third-degree heart blocks*, of a purely functional nature, can be seen in athletes. Venerando (1979) described two well-documented cases. We studied a female long-distance runner whose ECG showed periodic total AV dissociation (Fig. 40.3). Further study, including a His' bundle ECG, failed to show any organic cardiac disease.

The existence of a purely functional *sinoatrial block* in the athlete is usually denied in the literature. On the other hand, it is difficult to see why increased vagal tone should be unable to produce an AV block, but not a sinoatrial block. We have seen ECG changes in the trained person, which could be formally interpreted as

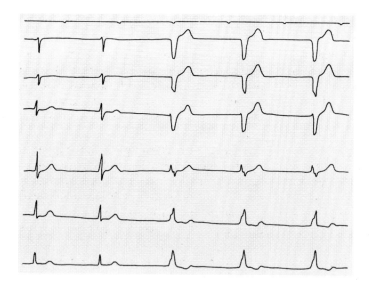

Fig. 40.2 Example of a ventricular escape rhythm in an athlete recorded from chest leads. The escape rhythm starts with the third beat.

sinoatrial blocks, even though it was difficult to decide in the individual case whether or not we were dealing with an extreme case of respiratory arrhythmia. If, however, such changes appear in conjunction with stress they cannot be interpreted as respiratory arrhythmia.

The functional nature of impulse-generating and conduction disturbances can be recognized by the fact that they disappear immediately during exercise. On the other hand, even functional impulse-generation disturbances may become clinically relevant if they are superimposed upon a damaged conduction system.

ECG changes due to physical conditioning which cannot be distinguished from pathological phenomena on the basis of their configuration: These can be seen primarily in the area of repolarization. ST-segment depression or elevation, and T-wave inversion, can be mistaken for epicardial injury as seen in pericarditis, or even for a myocardial infarction (Fig. 40.4). These changes are so striking and occur so frequently in athletes that they appear regularly in the literature. Only a brief discussion of these changes will be presented. Long-range studies by Venerando (1979) in 52 athletes who showed these changes failed to reveal the development of any pathological changes. On

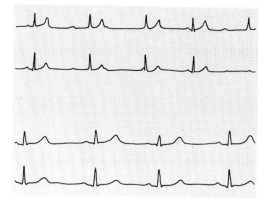

Fig. 40.3 Example of a functionally induced, third-degree atrioventricular disassociation in a female long-distance runner. This change occurred briefly in a switch from a Wenckebach periodicity. Under load, the block disappeared immediately (below). Standard leads I and II were used and the paper speed was 25 mm·s^{-1} (above) and 50 mm·s^{-1} (below).

the other hand, in the athletes studied by Maron *et al.* (1987), who died suddenly from a hypertrophic cardiomyopathy, there was one athlete who did show similar ECG changes.

On the basis of these facts it would be a mistake either to minimize or dramatize these ECG findings. They can occur in the trained heart without being based on any demonstrable pathology.

Naturally, careful cardiac surveillance and monitoring are essential. The athlete should be advised to abandon any significant conditioning stress or competitive activity until it can be assumed some months later that there is no organic heart disease present or in a stage of development.

ECG changes outside the physiological range: These cannot be discussed in detail here; all possible ECG changes may occur in the athlete. Only the most important problems that are likely to occur in the practice of sports cardiology will be mentioned. Even minor ECG changes, which would be ignored in the untrained person, may assume great importance under heavy stress. In sports cardiology apparently minor problems cause the greatest headaches for the physician. Usually there is no question that an athlete with a complete, organic AV block or a complete left bundle branch block should be forbidden to continue high endurance physical exercise. In contrast, a complete right bundle branch block is usually considered to be relatively harmless in the untrained person. Can this condition be tolerated in the endurance-conditioned athlete? If single premature beats are considered harmless, how many can be tolerated in athletes: 2, 5 or 20 per min?

According to a frequently held view, *premature contractions* occur more frequently in the athlete than in the untrained person, because of the increased resting vagal tone in the former. We found premature beats in only 0.6% of routine ECGs obtained from athletes. In 18-h Holter monitoring, the incidence was much higher. However, even with Holter monitoring the number of premature contractions in athletes was not higher than in untrained samples.

A particularly difficult problem is presented by the appearance of potentially dangerous *runs of premature beats* in apparently healthy endurance athletes. This problem is not specific to athletes: such findings can occasionally be seen in the untrained person without any demonstrable cardiac disease.

Paroxysmal tachycardia is usually considered to be relatively meaningless in young people without organic heart disease. How should it be viewed in the high-performance athlete, considering that under conditions of extreme acidosis even mild tachycardia may trigger ventricular fibrillation? For instance, some 400-m runners have an arterial blood pH of 6.8 after their race.

For this reason, high-performance athletes who are severely stressed during their athletic events should be forbidden to continue if they show such tachycardia. Unfortunately this can have serious economic repercussions, particularly for the professional athlete. In such instances it may be very difficult for the sports cardiologist to find the middle road between athletic, medical and economic considerations.

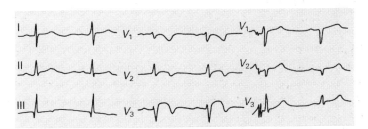

Fig. 40.4 Example of a significant repolarization disturbance in an athlete. The electrocardiogram was submitted to us by a general practitioner because of its peculiar configuration. The thorough cardiological work-up and a 10-year follow-up failed to reveal any cardiac pathology. The change consists of ST segment elevation and transiently inverted T waves, mostly in the V_2 and V_3 leads.

Even though medical considerations must be given absolute priority, the athlete should not suffer from medical 'overprotection'.

Paroxysmal tachycardias must be evaluated on the basis of frequency and configuration. If they are triggered relatively frequently by physical exercise, high-performance athletics should be forbidden. It would certainly be desirable to record the arrhythmia. Attacks are frequently triggered, at least to some extent, by sports-related physical exercise. Apparently some mechanical factors are involved, such as the physical agitation of the heart during certain athletic manoeuvres. Stress testing does not usually reproduce them. If they occur relatively frequently, an attempt should be made to record them by Holter monitoring. Very high frequencies and arrhythmias within the framework of the tachycardia, or a very frequent occurrence, should be sufficient cause to advise against further athletic activity.

Paroxysmal tachycardia plays a central role in the evaluation of Wolff−Parkinson−White (WPW) syndrome in athletes. This syndrome has a particular significance for the athlete's heart, for the following reasons:

1 The pre-excitation syndrome is considered to occur more frequently in the athlete than in the untrained person. According to our observations, WPW syndrome occurs in athletes slightly more frequently than in the average population. The average figures are, however, obtained from the general population. Since WPW syndrome is somewhat more frequent in young people, it is possible that the somewhat higher incidence in athletes is due to the fact that athletes belong to this subset of the population, and not to their level of physical conditioning.

2 WPW syndrome is frequently misread on the ECG tracing. Accordingly, the wrong diagnosis is frequently made in athletes with the syndrome. This happens particularly when the physician does not realize that in patients with WPW syndrome, stress ECGs frequently show false repolarization disturbances.

3 The frequent appearance of tachycardia in the athlete raises all the problems already discussed above.

Some authors in the literature occasionally mention WPW syndrome as the reason for forbidding high-performance athletics. We consider that these cases have an 'abnormality' of the ECG pattern only if there is no tachycardia, and no sign of organic heart disease. In these cases athletics can be continued. Conversely, fatal incidents during exercise in connection with paroxysmal tachycardia and WPW syndrome in athletes, were described in the same way as in patients with organic heart disease in combination with WPW.

There are many athletes, particularly professional athletes, who are well aware of the potential problems when they first notice the appearance of a tachycardia. For this reason they frequently deny its existence. If the appearance of tachycardia is known, its evaluation must take the above comments into serious consideration. In WPW syndrome, the tachycardia may present as an atrial fibrillation, leading to ventricular fibrillation if there is a 1 : 1 transmission. Younger athletes with WPW syndrome must be cautioned particularly, because serious attacks may only appear later. A 9- or 10-year-old child who shows WPW syndrome should avoid sports that require major effort. Such a youngster should choose activities such as 'play-sports', where the possibility of replacement during competition makes the appearance of tachycardia much less of a problem. If there is any doubt about the clinical assessment of WPW syndrome in an athlete, particularly if there is tachycardia and a rapid conduction in the Kent bundle which cannot be excluded by clinical means (for example, by a disappearance of the δ wave in stress testing), an invasive diagnosis by His' bundle ECG is recommended.

Among the conduction defects, a complete right bundle branch block is occasionally seen in athletes. In contrast to the incomplete right bundle branch block, this can never be considered a physiological variant. It appears to be a manifestation of a mild cardiac injury, such as a pericarditis in early childhood. Thus, forbidding all further athletic participation may not be indicated. Underlying pathology, particularly an atrial septal defect, must be excluded. A complete left bundle branch block is also always pathological and should be sufficient reason to advise against any further athletic activity that requires significant physical stress.

With regard to atrio-ventricular conduction disturbances, we wish to refer to the functional variants discussed above. A first-degree AV block, which disappears during exercise, should be considered physiological. If a similar block first appears under stress, it must be considered pathological. Among second-degree AV blocks, the Mobitz type II is always considered to be pathological, in contrast to the Wenckebach periodicity. Type II is characterized by a sudden failure of P-wave conduction without the typical 'accordion' effect of the Wenckebach cycle. The Mobitz pattern indicates infranodal damage. Holter monitoring reveals a 'Mobitz II-like' pattern in athletes as frequently as the Wenckebach pattern. However, the ECG differs from the true Mobitz II-type pattern: the abnormalities of rhythm disappears during physical exercise and a bundle block, which is more or less obligatory for Mobitz II, is never found. These differences should be understood to avoid improperly implanting a pacemaker into a healthy athlete.

A third-degree AV block of organic origin is obviously a contraindication for further high-performance athletics. It is nevertheless amazing how many reserve mechanisms the heart can exploit in the presence of a congenital AV block. We know of a high-performance soccer player who suffered from a total AV dissociation that was compensated for by a secondary supraventricular centre; during heavy exercise, this could generate a rate of 150 beats·min^{-1}.

Echocardiographic findings

Ultrasonography compensates for one of the significant shortcomings of routine radiography, i.e. the inability to distinguish between the chamber and wall of the heart. The echocardiogram makes it possible to investigate one of the old arguments about the athlete's heart — the distinction between dilatation and hypertrophy (Rost et al., 1972).

A new perspective on athlete's heart was introduced on echocardiographic grounds by Morganroth et al. (1975; Morganroth & Maron, 1977). They emphasized that there may be a particular form of cardiac adaptation in power athletes, although previously the athlete's heart was believed to belong entirely to the endurance-trained athlete. Morganroth et al. (1975) found a 'pure (concentric) hypertrophy' in power athletes, as contrasted with the 'pure dilatation' in the endurance athlete. Such a response model is understandable when one considers the different haemodynamic conditions that prevail in dynamic and isometric exercise. In the first case the volume-work is of primary importance, while in the second case the pressure-work is more important.

Yet, on purely theoretical grounds, the simple distinction made by Morganroth cannot be correct. It is contradicted by other findings, including our own. According to Laplace's law, an enlargement of the ventricular capacity must be accompanied by an increase in wall tension. A dilatation must therefore be accompanied by a thickening of the wall to compensate for the augmented work of the individual muscle fibres. The cardiac enlargement of the endurance-trained athlete is not pure dilatation but rather an eccentric hypertrophy (Fig. 40.5).

Our observations did not substantiate those of Morganroth et al. (1975) in 'static athletes' such as weightlifters (see Rost, 1987), even though we found individual weightlifters who had thickened cardiac walls; however, similar ECGs can also be found in the endurance-trained athletes.

Such differences must be attributed to differences in methodology. It is difficult to determine cardiac hypertrophy through 'single beam' measurement, as is attempted with the M-mode technique. All recent investigations, including our own, have confirmed that there is no sports-specific form of hypertrophy in static athletes. A clearly increased septal diameter in a weight-lifter of more than 12 mm therefore has to be considered abnormal.

Echocardiography has proved useful in sports cardiology, not only as an important tool in understanding the athlete's heart, but it has also opened up new diagnostic avenues. The athlete's heart comes to the physician's attention not only because of its size and abnormal ECG findings, but frequently also because of murmurs, which cannot always be classified as functional. In view of the heavy stress to which the athlete's heart is exposed, it is particularly important to perform a thorough diagnostic investigation. On the other hand, this diagnostic assessment should only rarely be invasive, since it rarely leads to surgical intervention. Generally, invasive investigations are not justified merely to reach a definitive decision concerning the continuation of athletic activities. The possibility of assessing valvular function through echocardiography is particularly significant. Modern techniques including Doppler echocardiography and colour imaging allow a perfect diagnosis of valvular as well as congenital cardiac conditions.

In addition, the introduction of ultrasonographic diagnostic techniques has popularized two cardiac diseases that can be considered as 'ultrasound specific'. These are hypertrophic cardiomyopathy and mitral valve prolapse. With regard to sports cardiology, two questions must be raised:

1 Since both of these conditions are seen primarily in young people, how often do they occur in athletes?

2 Can physical conditioning lead to the development of these conditions?

Roeske et al. (1976) pointed out that an asymmetrical septal hypertrophy could be found fairly frequently in athletes who had no apparent organic disease. He found that in 10% of athletes studied the relationship between the thickness of the septum and the posterior wall exceeded the permissible ratio of 1 : 1.3.

According to our experience, a value greater than 1 : 1.3 for the septum : posterior wall ratio is frequently due to a thin posterior wall. In cases of asymmetric septal hypertrophy observed by us, there was no instance of *hypertrophic cardiomyopathy*, or of a systolic anterior movement of the anterior mitral valve leaflet, or of decreased mobility of the septum.

In practice, then, septal thickening does occur in athletes, particularly in those who are engaged in the physically most demanding endurance sports. The meaning of these changes is still not clear. There is no convincing evidence to date that these changes can lead to a hypertrophic cardiomyopathy. It thus seems to be unjustified to forbid further athletic activity for such athletes. On the other hand, a careful cardiac evaluation is indicated, because, according to the findings of Maron et al. (1987), hypertrophic cardiomyopathy is among the most frequent causes of sudden death in apparently healthy athletes. If a clear diagnosis of pathological cardiac hypertrophy is made in an athletically active person, all forms of athletic activity that are known to cause further cardiac enlargement should be forbidden. These include all endurance and high-performance sports. Play-sports may be allowed to continue on the basis of individual assessment.

The discovery of a *mitral valve prolapse* frequently creates problems in a sports medicine clinic. We frequently see athletes who are symptom free, but in whom routine echocardiography has uncovered such a state of affairs. The question usually asked in this context is whether further participation in athletic activities should be forbidden. In resolving this question, the following points should be considered.

The incidence of mitral valve prolapse in healthy individuals is not well defined. It varies from 1% to 21% depending on the criteria set by the investigators. In our experience, pronounced mitral valve prolapse in an athlete is relatively rare.

The significance of mitral valve prolapse is unknown. There are at least two contradictory

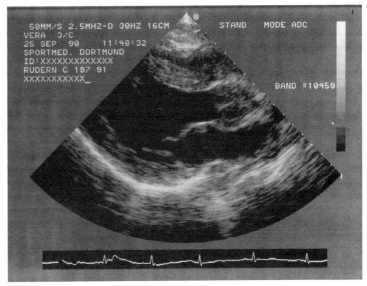

(a)

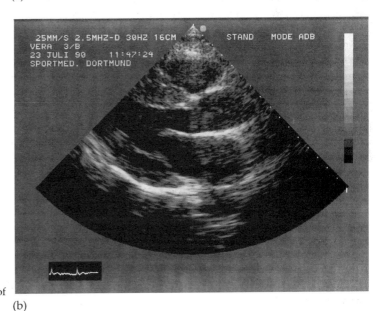

Fig. 40.5 Echocardiographic presentation of (a) a 'normal' athlete's heart, and (b) a clear concentric hypertrophy in the hypertrophic cardiomyopathy of an athlete.

(b)

theories regarding its origin. One theory claims that the phenomenon is purely valvular in nature and is due to a myxomatous change in the leaflets. The other theory claims that it is a functional myocardial disturbance, or is a peculiar form of cardiomyopathy. If the second hypothesis is correct, it would probably be a mistake to allow athletes with these findings to continue to participate in high-performance athletic activity.

However, when haemodynamic stress studies were performed in subjects with echocardiographically proven mitral valve prolapse, substantiated by auscultation, no disturbance in the pump function could be demonstrated. We therefore see no difficulty in allowing athletes to continue their activities if the prolapse is purely an incidental finding on echocardiography. The possibility of a significant associated arrhythmia must, however, be considered in mitral valve prolapse. No athletes should be allowed to continue high-performance athletics in the presence of an ultrasonographic diagnosis of prolapse, until the likelihood of arrhythmia has been excluded by stress ECG and Holter monitoring. To date no death has been attributed to this anomaly in top athletes. Maron *et al.* (1987) reported one athlete who died suddenly and had mitral prolapse. The cause of death, however, was questionable, since this same person had other cardiac pathologies, including a left-sided hypertrophy and dysplastic coronary arteries. When considering the possibility that training may contribute to the development of mitral valve prolapse, the theoretical possibility exists that after cessation of athletic activity and the regression of the physiological heart muscle hypertrophy, the valve leaflets become relatively too large and develop a tendency to prolapse. So far there is no evidence either for or against this hypothesis.

Fatal cardiac incidents during physical activity

Cardiac incidents are relatively rare in athletics. Nevertheless, the sudden death of a young apparently healthy athlete, or of an older, physically active person, while engaged in athletic activity, is a dramatic and devastating athletic incident. In such instances it is impossible to avoid the question whether the affected person might not be still alive if she or he had not engaged in athletics.

If a cardiac incident, for example sudden death or myocardial infarction, occurs during athletic activity, the question must be asked whether a causal relationship exists between physical activity and the cardiac incident. Since most people, including physicians, have a deep-seated need for explanations, such a

causal relationship is almost always assumed. But, on the other hand, because such incidents also occur at rest, it must be asked whether the cardiac incident occurred during athletic activity or because of athletic activity.

The following questions must be answered:
1 Does physical activity increase the risk of cardiac incidents?
2 If the answer to the first question is yes, is this true only for the already injured heart, or is the healthy heart also at risk?
3 Does the hypertrophy and increased vagal tone of the athlete's heart increase the risk at rest and/or during physical exercise?

Only epidemiological studies can find an answer to these questions. The frequency of sudden death in athletics varies considerably from report to report.

According to a statement from the German Athletic Association, the Sports Association Insurance Company reported 187 deaths in 1981 in connection with athletic activity. Sixty-two of these deaths were apparently due to trauma. The remaining 125 were listed as 'incidental deaths' and were thus considered to be more or less incidental to the athletic activity. If one assumes that the percentage of the general population that participates in athletics outside formal associations is approximately the same as the percentage that constitutes the membership of these associations, the total number of athletic-related deaths in former West Germany can be estimated to be 350–400 per year. Such estimates are naturally unsatisfactory, particularly when one considers that the health of those engaged in athletics outside of the sports associations is likely to be less satisfactory than those of the predominantly younger members of the associations.

A careful analysis of all sports-related deaths in the former German Federal Republic from 1966 to 1975, comprising a total of 124 cases, was reported by Munschek (1977). Twenty-eight of the cases were due to trauma, and 77 were due to organic pathology. Sixty-seven of the deaths were attributed to cardiac causes: 59 to coronary artery disease and eight to myocarditis.

The most important question is whether these were coincidental events that might have taken place at any time, anywhere, or whether physical activity increased the risk of sudden cardiac death. Moritz and Zamchek (1946) reviewed 40 000 autopsy records for the US Army between 1942 and 1946. In 98 sudden cardiac deaths, information was available about physical activity at the time of death. According to these statistics, the soldiers who died suddenly spent 33% of their time sleeping and 17% of their time in vigorous physical exercise. Fifteen per cent of the deaths occurred during sleep and 29% during major physical effort. These numbers suggest that in the presence of pre-existing heart disease, particularly coronary artery disease, physical activity is a possible trigger mechanism for sudden death.

The same conclusion can be drawn from more recent reports (Ragosta *et al.*, 1984; Siscovick *et al.*, 1984) showing an excess of deaths during physical activity. However, according to the results of Siscovick *et al.* (1984) the relative risk in trained subjects (5 : 1) is far lower than in untrained subjects (56 : 1). Additionally, if there is an increased risk *during* physical activity, sudden death in trained samples calculated for 24 h·day^{-1} is only 40% of that in the general population. In fact, sports increase health and lifespan; but if athletes are dying, they may die 'on the battle-field' (Pool, 1986).

It is not the type of sports that brings about the risk during physical activity, but the risk of the athletic population. Most fatal incidents occur in athletes who are considered to be healthy. Pool showed that in the Netherlands most people die while jogging. Among the 81 fatal incidents gathered by Ragosta *et al.* (1984), 19 occurred while playing golf. In Germany, according to Jung and Schäfer-Nolte (1982) a fairly high number of sudden deaths occurred while bowling. The common feature in all these types of sports is the fact that they are frequently performed by older people who have a high pre-existing risk of coronary heart disease. This observation is supported by the fact that sudden death during physical activity is a rare event in women, who have a low coronary risk.

These data lead to the conclusion that preventive sports medicine should seek to prevent sudden cardiac death and should particularly address men aged over 40 years. In these persons, the principal attention must be directed towards the early detection of coronary artery disease. In addition to routine clinical examination, they should also have a stress test. The resting ECG is normal in more than half of subjects with a documented coronary artery narrowing of 50% or more.

The picture of cardiac risk in the young athlete is considerably less clear, although coronary artery disease appears to be a primary cause of death. In the series of Munschek (1977), 16 of 39 athletes who died during athletic activity before their 30th birthday had coronary artery disease listed as the primary cause of death. Other important causes of death were myocarditis in six cases and aortic stenosis in only one case, even though aortic stenosis is frequently considered to be a major risk factor for sudden death. In three cases a viral infection and/or tonsillitis was held responsible for a fatal, toxic cardiovascular collapse. In a separate, second study, Munschek (1976) again emphasized the importance of myocarditis as a cause of death in the young athlete. He described 10 cases of sudden death in athletes aged between 16 and 35 years who died during physical activity from an inflammatory heart condition.

In this context it is interesting that the spectrum of the causes of death in young athletes is changing. This reflects less changes in the spectrum of disease than changes in pathological emphasis and pathological knowledge concerning the cardiomyopathies. It is surprising that Munschek (1977) did not list a single case of hypertrophic cardiomyopathy, a condition that was heavily emphasized by Maron *et al.* (1987). The widely discussed findings of Maron *et al.* proved first that the heart played an important role in the sudden death of young athletes. In a series of 29 young athletes who died suddenly, only one case had no cardiac pathology. Twenty-two of these athletes actually died during vigorous physical exercise. In 22 of the 29 cases, death was clearly due to cardiac causes, and in six this seemed very likely. Among the cases that were clearly attributable to cardiac causes, 14 could be explained on the basis of cardiac myopathy. Even though there were some clinical indications, the diagnosis was only rarely made before the cardiac death. Among the wrong diagnoses, the designation of 'athlete's heart' appears in some instances.

Among the dubious cardiac changes, which could not be clearly identified as a sufficient cause of death, there was one case of hypoplastic coronary arteries and five cases of idiopathic, left ventricular, concentric hypertrophy, which could not be definitely classified as an athletic cardiac hypertrophy. The other causes of death were listed as: arteriosclerotic heart disease, 3; aortic ruptures, 2; and anomalous left coronary arteries, 2. The classic lesions of aortic stenosis and myocarditis do not appear in this series. It must remain an open question as to whether the differences between Munschek's and Maron and coworkers' series are due to a difference in the groups studied (Munschek studied primarily average-calibre athletes, while Maron *et al.* (1987) studied high-performance, championship-calibre athletes), or to a difference in the pathological evaluation of the findings. In any case, the findings of Maron *et al.* should focus our attention on hypertrophic cardiomyopathy.

In summary, the following statements on sudden death during physical activity are supported by published data:

1 Sudden death during physical activity is a rare event, but not exceptional. An incidence of 10 cases per 10^6 population per year can be assumed.

2 There are some subsamples with a clearly increased risk: the relative risk of males is 10 times that of females. The same is true when old athletes are compared with young ones. Coronary risk factors increase the risk: there is a clear over-representation of smokers and hypertensive subjects.

3 In nearly all fatal incidents, pre-existing disease can be found, with 90% being of cardiovascular origin. There are very few incidents where necropsy cannot reveal the cause of death. In subjects aged over 30 years, 80% of cardiac death is related to a coronary heart disease. In younger athletes the most frequent reasons are myocarditis, hypertrophic abnormalities and aortic rupture in Marfan's syndrome. Rare reasons include valvular disease, particularly aortic stenosis, WPW syndrome, mitral valve prolapse, myocardial bridges, sarcoidosis, dilated cardiomyopathy and arrhythmogenesis of the right ventricle.

4 If there is a pre-existing cardiovascular condition, death can be triggered by physical exercise. Death during athletics therefore cannot be considered to be incidental.

5 Most cardiac incidents occur in sports that are preferred by older people, such as jogging, tennis, bowling, swimming or golf. This means that risk in sports is determined much more by pre-existing cardiac disease than by the type of activity. Therefore, in subjects with an increased cardiovascular risk, a careful medical preinvestigation, including stress testing, should be carried out.

6 There is no proof in the literature that athlete's heart *per se* involves an increased risk during sports. On the other hand, minor cardiac conditions that do not endanger the heart of sedentary subjects, such as slight myocarditis, may have fatal consequences in a competitive athlete. The athlete's heart therefore has to come under the careful supervision of a sports cardiologist.

References

Friedberg, C. (1972) *Erkrankungen des Herzens*, Deutsche Ausgabe, 2. Thieme Verlag, Stuttgart.

Henschen, S. (1899) Skilanglauf und Skiwettlauf. Eine medizinische Sport studie. *Mitt. med. Klin. Uppsala*, Jena.

Hollmann, W. & Hettinger, T. (1976) *Sportmedizin — Arbeits- und Trainings grundlagen*. Schattauer, Stuttgart.

Jung, K. & Schäfer-Nolte, W. (1982) Todesfälle im

Zusammenhang mit Sport. *Deutsche Z. Sportmed.* **33**, 6–11.

Maron, B., Epstein, S. & Roberts, W. (1987) Kardiale Risken im Leistungs sport. In: Rost, R. & Webering, F. (eds) *Kardiologie im Sport*, pp. 149–164. Deutscher Ärzteverlag, Köln.

Morganroth, J. & Maron, B. (1977) The athlete's heart syndrome. A new perspective. *Ann. N.Y. Acad. Sci.* **301**, 931–941.

Morganroth, J., Maron, B., Henry, W. & Epstein, S. (1975) Comparative left ventricular dimensions in trained athletes. *Ann. Intern. Med.* **82**, 521–524.

Moritz, A. & Zamchek, N. (1946) Sudden and unexpected death of young soldiers. *Arch. Path.* **42**, 459–494.

Munschek, H. (1976) Der plötzliche Tod beim Sport infolge Myokarditis. *Sportarzt Sportmed.* **27**, 201–210.

Munschek, H. (1977) Ursache des akuten Todes beim Sport in der Bundes republik Deutschland. *Sportarzt Sportmed.* **28**, 133–137.

Pool, J. (1986) Sudden death and sports. In: Fagard, R. & Bekaert, D. (eds) *Sports Cardiology*, pp. 223–227. Nijhoff, Dordrecht.

Ragosta, M., Crabtree, J., Sturner, W. & Thompson, P. (1984) Death during recreational exercise in the state of Rhode Island. *Med. Sci. Sports* **16**, 339–342.

Roeske, R., O'Rourke, R., Klein, H., Leopold, G. & Karlinger, J. (1976) Noninvasive evaluation of ventricular hypertrophy in professional athletes. *Circulation* **53**, 286–292.

Rost, R. (1987) *Athletics and the Heart.* Year Book Medical Publishers, Chicago.

Rost, R. & Hollmann, W. (1980) *Elektrokardiographie in der Sportmedizin.* Thieme Verlag, Stuttgart.

Rost, R., Schneider, K.W. & Stegmann, N. (1972) Vergleichende echokardiographische Untersuchungen am Herzen des Leistungssportlers und des Nichttrainierten. *Med. Welt.* **23**, 1088–1093.

Sheehan, G. (1973) Electrocardiography in athletes. *J.A.M.A.* **224**, 1296.

Siscovick, D., Weiss, N., Fletcher, P. & Lasky, T. (1984) The incidence of primary cardiac arrest during vigorous exercise. *N. Engl. J. Med.* **311**, 874–877.

Venerando, A. (1979) Electrocardiography in sports medicine. *Sports Med. Phys. Fitness* **19**, 107–128.

Chapter 41

Lung Fluid Movement

HUGH O'BRODOVICH

Introduction

Exercise is associated with an increase in cardiac output (and hence pulmonary blood flow) that is proportional to the work being performed. This fact, combined with the rare report of clinically evident pulmonary oedema and frequent reports of mild changes in lung function tests following exercise, has raised the question as to whether pulmonary oedema occurs during moderate to severe exercise. This chapter reviews how exercise affects the parameters determining fluid and solute movement in the lung.

Lung water and solute movement

In descriptive terms, the amount of fluid moving across a unit area of any membrane is equal to the product of the effective net *trans*vascular pressure gradient and the permeability of the membrane to that fluid (see Appendix). The total amount of fluid moving out of the entire lung's vasculature thus depends upon the amount of fluid movement per unit of membrane surface area and the total amount of perfused surface area. Even at rest, there is a continuous flow of fluid from the lung's vasculature into the interstitium of the lung. During many different physiological states (including exercise) and in pathophysiological conditions, this fluid movement will increase, but it is only when the increase exceeds the lung's clearance mechanisms that fluid accumulates within the lung. The fluid first accumulates in the lung's interstitium causing mild abnormalities in the distribution of inspired gases or blood flow. Significant abnormalities in gas exchange occur only when fluid floods into the alveolar spaces.

The lung has several protective mechanisms against the accumulation of excess fluid. First, the increase in fluid movement into the interstitium decreases the interstitial protein concentration by dilution and by increasing the protein's interstitial distribution volume. Both of these effects decrease the interstitial oncotic force. Second, under baseline conditions, the lung's interstitium has a very low compliance; thus trivial increases in the interstitial fluid volume increase the interstitial pressure from the normally negative to positive values. Both of these responses oppose the forces tending to an increase in fluid movement. Finally, the lung lymphatics can increase their flow rates at least 10-fold to aid in clearing the extra fluid escaping from the blood vessels. These phenomena are discussed elsewhere in greater detail (O'Brodovich & Albeda, 1991).

Exercise-induced changes in lung fluid movement

The physiological changes that develop during exercise under normal environmental conditions can alter several of the components that affect lung water and solute movement. Of greatest importance is the exercise-induced increase in pulmonary blood flow, which is associated with an increase in the perfused surface area (see Appendix). Experiments in animals and measurements of carbon monoxide diffusing capacity in humans suggest that the normal adult lung can undergo a 3–4-fold increase in perfused surface area (O'Brodovich & Coates, 1991). This is the likely reason why exercise of sufficient intensity to induce a three-fold increase of cardiac output is characterized by a linear relation between the augmentation of cardiac output and lung lymph flow (O'Brodovich & Coates, 1986). In addition to the cardiac output induced recruitment of additional pulmonary vascular surface area during exercise, there is, even at low and moderate levels of exercise, a small increase in the trans-vascular pressure of the fluid-exchanging vessels in the lung. This induces a further increase of transvascular fluid movement. There is evidence suggesting that a larger increase in transvascular pressure occurs during more intense short-term exercise (Newman *et al.*, 1988). There is likely to be little, if any, change in mean interstitial hydrostatic pressure during exercise, because the mean pleural pressure changes little in humans even during severe exercise; the increased ventilatory effort is characterized by equally large negative and positive pressure swings (Grimby *et al.*, 1971). In support of these predictions, animal experiments demonstrate little or no increase in lung lymph flow during eucapnoeic hyperventilation (O'Brodovich & Coates, 1991).

When exercise is performed under unusual environmental conditions (e.g., the hypoxic hypobaria of mountain climbing) or in patients with abnormalities of the cardiorespiratory system, the above exercise-induced changes in lung water and solute movement may have more dramatic effects (see below).

Lung water content during exercise

Direct measurements of lung water content

Does the exercise-induced increase in lung fluid movement result in clinically evident pulmon-ary oedema? For obvious reasons, there have not been any gravimetric measurements of lung water content in humans during or following exercise. However, Marshall *et al.* (1975) demonstrated that extravascular lung water content did not change in beagle dogs who had run at 10 km·h^{-1} for 20 min. There are rare reports of pulmonary oedema in humans who have performed severe prolonged exercise (for example, running a double marathon), and pulmonary oedema is not an uncommon complication of exercise at high altitudes. As discussed elsewhere (O'Brodovich & Coates, 1991), it is likely that other factors contribute to these reports of clinically evident gross pulmonary oedema.

Indirect assessment of lung water content

There are several indirect measurements that can be used to speculate whether or not interstitial or alveolar pulmonary oedema can occur during exercise. Regrettably, such measurements can only be consistent with, but not diagnostic of, pulmonary oedema.

Young healthy men undergoing relatively brief (15–30 min) maximal exercise tests do not develop abnormalities in either their chest radiographs or their radiographic lung density which would be consistent with pulmonary oedema (Gallagher *et al.*, 1988). Such measurements should detect a 25% increase in extravascular lung water content. Similarly, changes in pulmonary diffusing capacity for carbon monoxide following exercise are consistent with the changes in cardiac output, a finding that argues against the development of oedema with exercise (Miles *et al.*, 1986). In contrast, routine measurements of lung function have demonstrated small abnormalities in expiratory flow rates and/or lung volumes following exercise. As discussed elsewhere (O'Brodovich & Coates, 1991; Beck *et al.*, 1991), there are several potential explanations for the changes of lung function. These include technical difficulties in the actual measurement, an increase of thoracic blood volume, or small airway narrowing due to mechanical compression from interstitial oedema or to neurobronchomuscular reflex arcs.

More sophisticated techniques have also been used to assess lung water content indirectly during and after exercise. The exercise-induced changes in the volume 'seen' by the intravascular multiple indicator dilution technique have been attributed to an increase in the amount of perfused surface area rather than to an increase in total lung extravascular water content (Marshall *et al.*, 1971; Goresky *et al.*, 1975; Vaughan *et al.*, 1976). The multiple inert gas technique evaluates gas exchange, and although young fit men performing incremental maximal exercise tests do demonstrate a slight widening of the lung's ventilation/perfusion ratios, there are no regions of low ventilation/perfusion ratios or shunt (Wagner *et al.*, 1986; 1987). These data provide a strong argument against the development of interstitial or alveolar pulmonary oedema when fit young men perform short-term maximal exercise at sea level. In contrast, a group of highly trained and motivated young men who were chronically hypoxaemic during a time and altitude simulated ascent to the top of Mount Everest developed changes that were consistent with the development of interstitial pulmonary oedema (Wagner *et al.*, 1987). One might also argue that more prolonged severe exercise, as occurs in endurance competitions, might promote the development of pulmonary oedema. For example, there have been reports of pulmonary oedema during such events as a double marathon (O'Brodovich & Coates, 1991). It is, however, equally possible that significant concomitant fluid and electrolyte abnormalities may have produced pulmonary oedema by other mechanisms (e.g. neurogenic pulmonary oedema).

Clinical pulmonary oedema

Significant congenital or acquired diseases of the cardiopulmonary system would predispose an individual to the development of pulmonary oedema during exercise, although most of the potential causes are unlikely in a competitive athlete. An exhaustive list of such disorders is beyond the scope of this chapter. Rather, such conditions are best conceived in terms of the forces affecting transvascular fluid movement (Fig. 41.1). In the general population, the most common problem would be a disorder affecting left ventricular performance (for example, coronary artery disease); these would result in elevations of P_{mv} (pressure within the microvessel) as the left ventricle fails or increases its end-diastolic pressure in an attempt to increase cardiac output during exercise. A decrease in plasma albumin concentration resulting from inadequate or incomplete protein absorption, liver disease, or excessive protein losses (for example, nephrotic syndrome) would similarly

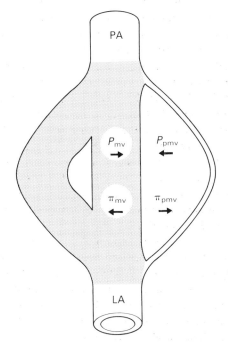

Fig. 41.1 A schematic diagram of the pulmonary circulation, with the perfused microvascular bed shown in stipple, and the direction that fluid moves in response to each of the forces indicated by the arrows. Unrecruited microvascular surface area is illustrated by the thin right-hand pathway. LA, left artery; PA, pulmonary artery. For other abbreviations, see Appendix.

promote increases in transvascular fluid flow. Finally, individuals who either have a congenitally absent lung, or have had significant amounts of lung tissue surgically removed would have less total vascular bed to recruit during exercise. If the vascular bed was fully recruited, then further increases in blood flow during exercise would promote greater increases in P_{mv}. Relevant to this last point, there is an increased incidence of high altitude pulmonary oedema in individuals with a congenitally absent lung.

Interstitial pulmonary oedema is 'clinically silent' as it produces only mild alterations in gas exchange and small changes in lung function. In contrast, alveolar oedema is heralded by marked dyspnoea, cyanosis and occasionally by the presence of frothy red-tinged oedema fluid. If alveolar oedema is suspected, supplemental oxygen is the most important medication to administer. If the patient is likely to be in left heart failure (for example, postmyocardial infarction), a semi-upright position and rotating medical phlebotomy are indicated to decrease P_{mv}. It is important, however, not to use such manoeuvres if the patient is suspected of being dehydrated and hypovolaemic, because a further reduction of circulating blood volume would have disastrous results.

Conclusion

There is irrefutable evidence that the amount of fluid leaving the pulmonary vasculature bed increases during exercise. In healthy individuals, the lung's normal protective mechanisms against oedema formation and the lymphatics' ability to clear excess fluid prevent the development of pulmonary oedema during relatively brief maximal exercise. However, under very unusual environmental conditions, or when there is a coexistent disease, prolonged exercise may contribute to oedema formation.

Acknowledgements

This research was supported by grants-in-aid from the Heart and Stroke Foundation of Ontario. Dr O'Brodovich is a Career Investigator of the Heart and Stroke Foundation of Ontario.

Appendix

In the 19th century, Starling discussed the forces that could influence the movement of fluid out of vessels (Starling, 1895–6). His observations were refined by subsequent investigators, who developed an equation that bears his name and provides us with an understanding of the factors that control water and solute movement across microvascular beds.

$$\dot{Q} = K_f (P_{mv} - P_{pmv}) - K_f \sigma (\pi_{mv} - \pi_{pmv})$$

Starling's equation is shown above; it states that the net movement of fluid ($\dot{Q}$) across a semipermeable membrane is influenced by:

1 The amount of vascular surface area available for fluid exchange and the permeability of that membrane to fluid (both are included in the K_f, permeability coefficient, term).

2 The net transmicrovascular hydrostatic pressure, which is the difference between the hydrostatic pressure within (P_{mv}) and immediately outside (P_{pmv}) the microvessel. P_{mv} is determined by the pulmonary arterial (P_{PA}) and left atrial (P_{LA}) pressures and by the distribution of the upstream and downstream resistances within the pulmonary circulation. P_{pmv} is likely close to zero in the middle of the alveolar capillary membrane, but is more negative around extra-alveolar vessels and is influenced by the pleural pressure.

3 The net transmicrovascular osmotic pressure which is the difference between the effective osmotic pressure within (π_{mv}) and immediately outside (π_{pmv}) the microvessel. The lung microvasculature is freely permeable to small ions and thus it is the protein concentration that influences π_{mv} and π_{pmv}. However, the reflection coefficient (σ) must also be included, since the microvessel is not completely impermeable to protein.

References

Beck, K.C., Babb, T.G., Staats, B.A. & Hyatt, R.E. (1991) Dynamics of breathing during exercise. In: Wasserman, K. & Whipp, B. (eds) *Pulmonary Physiology and Pathophysiology of Exercise*, pp. 67–92. Marcel Dekker, New York.

Gallagher, G.G., Huda, W., Rigby, M., Greenberg, D. & Younes, M. (1988) Lack of radiographic evidence of interstitial pulmonary edema after maximal exercise in normal subjects. *Am. Rev. Respir. Dis.* **137**, 474–476.

Goresky, C.A., Warnica, J.W., Burgess, J.H. & Nadeau, B.E. (1975) Effect of exercise on dilution estimates of extravascular lung water and on carbon monoxide diffusing capacity in normal lung. *Circ. Res.* **37**, 379–389.

Grimby, G., Saltin, B. & Wilhelmsen, L. (1971) Pulmonary flow-volume and pressure-volume relationship during submaximal and maximal exercise in young well trained man. *Bull. Phys. Pathol. Resp.* **7**, 157–168.

Marshall, B.E., Soma, L.R. & Neufeld, G.R. (1975) Lung water at rest and exercise in dogs. *J. Appl. Physiol.* **39**, 7–8.

Marshall, B.E., Teichner, R.L., Kallos, T., Sugarman, H.J., Wyche, M.Q. Jr & Tantum, K.R. (1971) Effects of posture and exercise on pulmonary extravascular water volume in man. *J. Appl. Physiol.* **31**, 375–379.

Miles, D.S., Enoch, A.D. & Grevey, S.C. (1986) Interpretation of changes in DL_{co} and pulmonary functions after running five miles. *Respir. Physiol.* **66**, 135–145.

Newman, J.H., Butka, J., Parker, R.E. & Roselli, R.J. (1988) Effect of progressive exercise on lung fluid balance in sheep. *J. Appl. Physiol.* **64**, 2125–2131,

O'Brodovich H. & Albelda S. (1991) Fluid and solute movement across the alveolar capillary membrane. In: Chernick, V. & Mellins, R.B. (eds) *Basic Mechanisms of Pediatric Respiratory Diseases: Cellular and Integrative*, pp. 188–202. B.C. Dekker, Philadelphia.

O'Brodovich, H. & Coates, G. (1986) Effect of isoproterenol or exercise on pulmonary lymph flow and hemodynamics. *J. Appl. Physiol.* **60**, 38–44.

O'Brodovich, H. & Coates, G. (1991) Lung water and solute movement during exercise. In: Wasserman, K. & Whipp, B. (eds) *Pulmonary Physiology and Pathophysiology of Exercise*, pp. 253–270. Marcel Dekker, New York.

Starling, E.H. (1895–6) On the absorption of fluids from the connective tissue spaces. *J. Physiol.* **19**, 312–326.

Wagner, P.D., Gale, G.E., Moon, R.E., Torre-Bueno, J.R., Stolp, B.W. & Saltzman, H.A. (1986) Pulmonary gas exchange in humans exercising at sea level and simulated altitude. *J. Appl. Physiol.* **61**, 260–270.

Wagner, P.D., Sutton, J.R., Reeves, J.T., Cymerman, A., Groves, B.M. & Malconian, M.K. (1987) Operation Everest II: pulmonary gas exchange during a simulated ascent of Mt. Everest. *J. Appl. Physiol.* **63**, 2348–2359.

Vaughan, T.R. Jr, DeMarino, E.M. & Staub, N.C. (1976) Indicator dilution lung water and capillary blood volume in prolonged heavy exercise in normal men. *Am. Rev. Respir. Dis.* **113**, 757–762.

Chapter 42

Hyperthermia, Hypothermia and Problems of Hydration

RICHARD L. HUGHSON

Introduction

Thermoregulatory problems that accompany endurance sports participation cannot be easily categorized because of the range of events, individual abilities and, especially, different climatic conditions. In this chapter, the health problems associated with thermoregulation are divided into three categories. Those individuals who are clearly hyperthermic or hypothermic are easily classified. On the other hand, it has recently become appreciated that a large number of cases of collapse are not associated with extremes of body temperature. This latter group does present with abnormal intra-vascular fluid volume regulation that might be either relatively hypovolaemic or hypervolaemic.

Classification of thermoregulatory disorders

Hyperthermic injuries

The classical description of heat injury breaks down into three primary categories. Heat cramps are often associated with prolonged and repeated loss of sodium (Na^+) in sweat without adequate replacement (Hubbard & Armstrong, 1989). Heat exhaustion is a common form of heat injury. It usually occurs as a conse-quence of a single bout, as opposed to repeated exercise. The major factor that differentiates between heat exhaustion and heat stroke is

impaired mental status in the latter (Taunton & McLean, 1986; Roberts, 1989), although some authors have indicated that achievement of an arbitrary rectal temperature of 40°C might also distinguish the two conditions from each other (Hubbard & Armstrong, 1989). In contrast with the heat exhaustion and heat stroke observed in non-athletic populations where failure of the sweating mechanism is common (Richards & Richards, 1986a), the heat injury seen during endurance exercise is often associated with continued sweating (Hughson et al., 1980; Richards & Richards, 1986a; Sutton, 1986).

Exertional collapse

A relatively new classification of thermal injury has been based on the observation of athletes collapsing at the finish line, or in the hours immediately after competition (Noakes, 1988; Roberts, 1989). Roberts (1989) suggested that exercise-associated collapse included hyper-thermic, normothermic and hypothermic sub-groupings. A useful description for athletes in the normothermic collapse category is hypo-natraemic (Noakes, 1988), because such indi-viduals show markedly reduced plasma sodium concentration.

Hypothermic injuries

The definition of hypothermia proposed by the International Union of Physiological Sciences is a core temperature below 35°C (Mills et al.,

1987). Roberts (1989) has classified mild, moderate and severe hypothermia following road racing as being associated with rectal temperatures below 36.1, 35.0, and 32.2°C respectively. As with hyperthermia, the level of central nervous system involvement increases with the severity of the condition. Given the fact that an athlete might have been exercising strenuously before hypothermic collapse, the presence of a body temperature below normal is a clear indicator of abnormal and excessive heat loss.

All thermal injuries associated with endurance exercise require direct measurement of rectal temperature to confirm the true status of the patient (Sutton, 1986; Taunton & McLean, 1986; Robertson, 1988; Roberts, 1989). The sensation of cold skin in victims of exertional heat stroke (Hughson et al., 1980), and especially the observation by Sutton (1986) of a collapsed runner who had an oral temperature of 35.5°C when the rectal temperature was 42°C, point quite clearly to the possibility of an incorrect diagnosis. One of the most famous cases of incomplete diagnosis was that of Alberto Salazar, who had an oral temperature of 31.1°C (88°F) at the end of the 1982 Boston marathon (Adner et al., 1988). It is not known whether he was hypothermic or hyperthermic. Disoriented and confused, he required 3 litres of intravenous fluid for rehydration.

Causes of hyperthermia in endurance exercise

There are a number of causes of hyperthermic injury during endurance exercise. These can be partitioned into factors related to the athlete, the competition, and the environment.

The athlete

The majority of élite runners are knowledgeable about the status of their bodies (Hughson et al., 1980). This means that they can gauge the rate of energy expenditure, so that the rise of body temperature that must occur with strenuous exercise is kept within safe limits. We studied élite and recreational runners, taking direct measurements of rectal and skin temperatures, while we monitored ambient conditions during simulated 8-km races (Hughson et al., 1983). An élite male runner completed 8 km in 25 min 11 s on a day when the wet bulb globe temperature (WBGT) index was 18°C. His mean skin temperature and rectal temperature were 33°C and 40°C respectively. On another day when the WBGT index was 28°C, this individual slowed his 8-km pace by 1 min 31 s, yet he still reached a rectal temperature of 40.2°C. Most athletes will slow their running pace on a warm day, thereby reducing the metabolic heat load and maintaining thermal balance. There are, however, exceptions to this when athletes perform in major national and international competitions. The result can be collapse, or near collapse.

Novice athletes are more susceptible to exertional heat injury than are experienced competitors (Hughson et al., 1980; Richards & Richards, 1986a). The former tend to be less well prepared in terms of both fitness and heat acclimatization (Hughson et al., 1980). They are also less aware of their personal level of exertion, and because they expect that running in a competitive event will be associated with a certain level of 'pain', they persevere through symptoms that should have caused them to stop or slow their pace.

Heat-intolerant individuals have a greater risk of hyperthermic heat injury (Hughson et al., 1980). The cause of the impaired thermoregulation is not yet understood (Armstrong et al., 1988; Epstein, 1990).

The competition

Most cases of exertional hyperthermic injury occur in relatively short distance events (Hughson et al., 1980; Noakes, 1988). The most thoroughly documented series of competitions where exertional heat injury has been a major problem is the Sydney Sun 'City-to-Surf' 14-km run (Sutton et al., 1972; Richards & Richards, 1986a; Sutton, 1986). In 1971, 29 of 1600 runners, or 1.8%, collapsed from exertional heat injury. Years of experience and careful medical planning reduced the incidence to less than 0.2% of 144 950 starters between 1978 and 1984 (Richards & Richards, 1986a). Likewise, the majority of heat injuries in North America have occurred during 10-km road races (Hughson *et al.*, 1980; Hughson, 1986). As noted above, most of these heat injuries have been in novice competitors.

While there can be many causes of exertional heat injury, the most important is the relationship between the rate of heat production and the rate of heat loss. At some point, the thermal load simply exceeds the body's capacity to lose heat (Hughson *et al.*, 1980; Hughson, 1986; Noakes, 1988; Robertson, 1988). If a 65-kg runner covers a 10-km race in a moderate time of 48 min, the total body metabolic heat production rate is approximately 725 W (Hughson, 1986). A solar radiation load of 275 W might be added to this, for a total of 1000 W. Sweat rate can reach $1-2$ $l \cdot h^{-1}$, with about 50% of this evaporating (Hughson, 1986). Therefore, the rate of heat loss from sweat amounts to approximately $350-700$ W. For thermal balance to occur, additional heat must be lost by the athlete through convection, conduction, radiation, or some combination of these factors. As the environmental temperature rises, the ability of these mechanisms to maintain body temperature within a healthy range may be severely challenged.

The metabolic load of the runner is directly related to running velocity. Fast runners are potentially at greater risk, but the capabilities of the thermoregulatory system are enhanced in physically fit individuals (Harrison, 1985), so that the increase in rectal temperature during exercise is usually related more closely to the relative work rate (percentage of maximal oxygen intake) than to the absolute work rate (Åstrand & Rodahl, 1985).

The environment

There is a general relationship between the environmental heat load and the incidence of exertional heat injury (Richards & Richards, 1986a). However, rectal temperatures as high as 43°C have sometimes been observed even under moderate conditions (Sutton, 1986). Recognition of the strain placed on the thermoregulatory system by adverse environmental conditions has led various authors and organizations to suggest guidelines for conducting endurance events in the heat (see below). Unfortunately, these guidelines are often ignored by event organizers, even when holding major international games. A case in point was the 1988 World Junior Track and Field Championships in Sudbury, Ontario.

The organizers of the World Junior Championships were asked by their medical team to schedule competitions at a time that would prevent excessive environmental heat load. Rather, they chose to assume that cool weather would prevail. When it did not (temperatures reached daytime highs of over 30°C), it was necessary to make last-minute decisions to move some competitions to cooler periods of the day. Well-planned medical services that included prominent display of colour-coded temperature warning flags (Hughson *et al.*, 1983; American College of Sports Medicine, 1985) and appropriate monitoring and treatment of injured athletes prevented any serious complications. When scheduling also includes television contracts, there is a danger that the safety of athletes may be sacrificed to other obligations.

In endurance events that last for several hours, it is unusual for athletes to show signs of hyperthermic heat injury. The reason for this is believed to be the relatively slower pace of the athletes in long endurance events (Noakes, 1988). There are documented cases of both hyperthermic and hypothermic injuries occurring in the same series of marathon races (Roberts, 1989). Several events are conducted in extreme environmental conditions. The Hawaii Ironman Triathlon stands out as an event that is demanding on the capabilities of the body's thermoregulatory system (O'Toole *et al.*, 1989).

Here, it is important for the athlete to monitor fluid and electrolyte intake and rate of energy expenditure carefully in order to avoid serious heat injury.

Collapse without extremes of body temperature in endurance athletes

Endurance athletes quite commonly collapse at or near the finish line. The majority of affected individuals have rectal temperatures in the normal range of 36.1–39.4°C (Roberts, 1989). The causes of collapse could be related to energy supply, to fluid volume regulation (hypovolaemia), or to serum electrolyte concentration (hyponatremia) (Richards & Richards, 1986a; Taunton & McLean, 1986; Noakes, 1988; Robertson, 1988; Roberts, 1989).

Energy supply and collapse

In a 10-km, or similar short duration, endurance event, it is unlikely that the supply of metabolic substrate will become rate limiting. However, for events that last 2 h or longer, this can be a major limiting factor. Hypoglycaemia occurs in a small percentage of athletes who compete in long-duration endurance events (Robertson, 1988; O'Toole et al., 1989). Muscle glycogen stores are depleted, as are liver glycogen stores (Åstrand & Rodahl, 1985). When the liver glycogen is no longer sufficient to sustain blood glucose, hypoglycaemia can lead to signs of central nervous system dysfunction (Robertson, 1988). In ultraendurance competitions, athletes must ingest carbohydrate to supplement the body's stores (Noakes, 1988; Robertson, 1988; O'Toole et al., 1989). In a triathlon, a recommended feeding pattern includes some solid food during the cycling portion of the event (O'Toole et al., 1989), while in running events, food intake is normally restricted to drinks containing carbohydrate (Lamb & Brodowicz, 1986; Murray, 1987).

Hypovolaemic collapse

Sweat rates can range from 1 to > 2 l·h^{-1} during strenuous exercise in a warm or hot environment (Nadel, 1983; Hughson, 1986). This leads to a reduction in total blood volume. Exercise performance is impaired if the blood volume is reduced by 3% or more (Harrison, 1985). Attempts to maintain thermal equilibrium probably involve peripheral vasodilatation, further decreasing the effective total blood volume. However, the muscle pump continues to return blood to the heart, albeit at a reduced rate. As long as the athlete continues the activity, blood pressure remains adequate for cerebral perfusion. Immediately on crossing the finish line, the action of the muscle pump is removed; the sympathetic vasoconstrictor response is usually not invoked rapidly enough, so that venous return declines, postural hypotension develops, and the oxygen supply of the brain becomes inadequate. Noakes and coworkers (Noakes, 1988; Noakes et al., 1988) have suggested that postural hypotension is the major cause of collapse in ultraendurance athletes. The most severely affected are those who are undertrained and not heat acclimatized (Noakes, 1988).

Hypovolaemic collapse is a consequence of the body's attempts to thermoregulate during strenuous exercise. The balance of body fluids and electrolytes needs to be considered carefully when analysing the reasons for collapse, and the appropriate therapy (Sutton, 1986; Noakes, 1988; Noakes et al., 1988; Laird, 1989).

Hyponatraemia, dehydration and overhydration

Homoeostatic mechanisms maintain the concentration of sodium between 136 and 143 mmol·l^{-1} over a wide range of sweat rates and fluid losses during exercise of several hours duration (Costill et al., 1976; Harrison, 1985). However, ultraendurance competitors may develop serum sodium concentrations as low as 112 mmol·l^{-1} (Nelson et al., 1986; Noakes, 1988). Hyponatraemia may be associated with central nervous system dysfunction, including altered mental status and seizures, and pulmonary oedema (Nelson *et al.*, 1986). There is currently no consensus concerning either the cause or the extent of hyponatraemia with endurance exercise.

Hiller and Laird (1986) have suggested that hyponatraemia is a consequence of losing large quantities of fluid and sodium with sweating. However, sweat is hypotonic relative to plasma (Costill *et al.*, 1976; Harrison, 1985). Acutely, sodium ion concentration ($[Na^+]$) increases as more fluid is lost than electrolytes (Röcker *et al.*, 1989). For shorter endurance competitions, hyponatraemia is not a problem, because both fluid loss and fluid intake are relatively small. Hyponatraemia has been observed with ultraendurance competitions (Noakes, 1988; Laird, 1989) and marathons (Nelson *et al.*, 1986; Robertson, 1988). Hiller and Laird (1986) attribute this to a replacement of hypotonic sweat by fluids that are even more hypotonic, such as plain water. Hiller (1989) advocates programmed drinking.

Noakes (Noakes, 1988; Noakes *et al.*, 1985; 1988) suggests that the problem is not so much consumption of water, or an electrolyte replacement drink, as excessive water replacement. Based on the loss of body mass, it has been suggested that runners should consume large volumes of fluid (American College of Sports Medicine, 1985). However (Noakes, 1988; Noakes *et al.*, 1988), a significant portion of the lost fluid came from water that had been stored with muscle glycogen. This water did not need to be replaced. Neither did water from oxidation of foodstuffs.

Let us assume that a 70-kg male exercises for 6 h at a power output equivalent to 2.0 $l \cdot min^{-1}$ (89.2 $mmol \cdot min^{-1}$) oxygen uptake ($\dot{V}O_2$). Other assumptions are: sweat rate 1 $l \cdot h^{-1}$; sweat sodium concentration 50 $mmol \cdot l^{-1}$; metabolic respiratory quotient 0.85; metabolic consumption of 1 mol of oxygen during carbohydrate metabolism produces 1 mol of water; consumption of 1 mol of oxygen during fat metabolism produces 0.65 mol of water; initial muscle glycogen concentration of 20 $g \cdot kg^{-1}$ distributed over 15 kg of muscle mass; and 80% of this

glycogen is used in a progressive manner over the 6 h.

For a respiratory quotient of 0.85, 50% of the energy would be derived from carbohydrate and 50% from fat. Per hour, metabolic production of water would be:

$$\text{Total } \dot{V}O_2 = 89.2 \text{ mmol} \cdot min^{-1} \times 60$$
$$= 5352 \text{ mmol} \cdot h^{-1}$$
$$H_2O \text{ from carbohydrate } 5352 \times 0.5 \times 1$$
$$= 2676 \text{ mmol } H_2O \cdot h^{-1}$$
$$H_2O \text{ from fat } 5352 \times 0.5 \times 0.65$$
$$= 1739 \text{ mmol } H_2O \cdot h^{-1}$$
$$\text{Total } H_2O \text{ from metabolism } = 4415 \text{ mmol} \cdot h^{-1}$$
$$= 79.5 \text{ g} \cdot h^{-1}$$

Likewise, one can calculate the water released from glycogen metabolism.

$$\text{Total glycogen in muscle } = 20 \text{ g} \cdot kg^{-1} \times 15 \text{ kg}$$
$$= 300 \text{ g}$$
$$\text{Glycogen used in 6 h } = 300 \times 0.80 = 240 \text{ g}$$
$$\text{Total water released } = 240 \text{ g} \times 3 \text{ g } H_2O \cdot g^{-1}$$
$$= 720 \text{ g}$$
$$\text{Water per hour } = 720/6 = 120 \text{ g} \cdot h^{-1}$$

The sum of water obtained from metabolism plus glycogen breakdown is 20% of hourly sweat production, equivalent to 1.2 litres of the total sweat secretion of 6 litres over the 6-h period.

To take these numbers further, the effects on sodium concentrations can be examined (Table 42.1). The normal low concentration of intracellular Na^+ is contained in a relatively large volume of fluid, so that 12% of total Na^+ is in this compartment. Interstitial fluid contains some 65% and the plasma compartment some 23% of the total body Na^+. Table 42.1 illustrates the uniform distribution of an expanded or a reduced total body water volume of 1.2 litres. This example has used the observations of Costill *et al.* (1976) as a reference point. This is, 10% of fluid is drawn from plasma, 60% from interstitial fluid, and 30% from intracellular fluid. The 1.2-litre volume is selected because it is the water volume that should not need to be replaced, according to the above calculations. The effects on $[Na^+]$ are relatively small. The

Table 42.1 Effects of changes in body water and sodium on body compartment volume and sodium concentration ([Na$^+$]).

	Body compartment		
	Intracellular	Interstitial	Plasma*
Normal total volume (litres)	28	10.5	3.5
+1.2 litres expanded volume (litres)[†]	28.4	11.2	3.6
−1.2 litres reduced volume (litres)[†]	27.6	9.8	3.4
Normal total Na$^+$ (mmol)	280	1522.5	535.5
[Na$^+$] normal volume (mmol·l^{-1})	10	145	153 (142)
[Na$^+$] expanded volume (mmol·l^{-1})	9.8	136	149 (138)
[Na$^+$] reduced volume (mmol·l^{-1})	10.1	155	158 (147)
With Na$^+$ loss of 50 mmol·l^{-1} for 6 h			
Total Na$^+$ (mmol)[‡]	244	1327	467
[Na$^+$] normal volume (mmol·l^{-1})	8.7	126	133 (124)
[Na$^+$] expanded volume (mmol·l^{-1})	8.6	118	130 (120)
[Na$^+$] reduced volume (mmol·l^{-1})	8.8	135	137 (127)

* Plasma values are expressed in litres of plasma water, except for values in parentheses (which represent total plasma).
† Redistribution based on data from Costill *et al.* (1976).
‡ Assumes proportional loss from each compartment.

normal total plasma [Na$^+$] of 142 mmol·l^{-1} is increased or decreased 4−5 mmol·l^{-1} by a 1.2-litre change in 42 litres of body water.

An individual who sweats at a rate of 1 l·h^{-1} for 6 h, with a sweat [Na$^+$] of 50 mmol·l^{-1} would lose a total of 300 mmol Na$^+$. If this loss was distributed equally between body compartments, then the total Na$^+$ would change as shown in Table 42.1. Given the smaller total Na$^+$, the [Na$^+$] in each of the body compartments would be reduced, no matter what fluid replacement schedule was followed. In each case, hyponatraemia (plasma [Na$^+$] < 136 mmol·l^{-1}) would result. Only if the 300 mmol Na$^+$ loss was accompanied by a reduced water replacement could [Na$^+$] fall into the normal range. However, there would then be a severe dehydration.

Before reaching any conclusions from this theoretical examination of body water and sodium loss, it is appropriate to consider some of its limitations. A very important simplification was the assumed distribution of water loss between the different compartments (Costill *et al.*, 1976; Harrison, 1985). Respiratory

water loss is important, but it has been ignored. The sweat rate and the sweat sodium concentration would probably vary with the duration of exercise, hydration state, environmental conditions, chronic body Na$^+$ balance, state of training and acclimatization (Nadel, 1983; Harrison, 1985; Hargreaves *et al.*, 1989). Both the 1 l·h^{-1} sweat rate and the 50 mmol·l^{-1} [Na$^+$] of sweat are probably at the upper limit of likely findings for ultradistance competitors for two reasons. The pace is generally slow enough that sweat rates are low, and the sweat becomes more dilute in trained, acclimatized athletes. Noakes (Noakes, 1988; Noakes *et al.*, 1988) suggested that fluid requirements probably would not exceed 500 ml·h^{-1}.

One conclusion from the current calculations is that water from metabolism and glycogen utilization can contribute significantly to fluid needs. In this example, for every litre of water lost during exercise, only 800 ml needed to be replaced. If the sweat rate is high for long periods of time, and if sweat [Na$^+$] is moderately high, then Na$^+$ depletion can also become important. The final conclusion is that both

Noakes (1988) and Hiller (1989) could be correct. Noakes has recognized that, especially in slower participants, the loss of plasma volume is less than simple changes in body mass would indicate. Water intoxication is a real possibility in athletes who are given too much time to consume water. On the other hand, it is possible to lose large quantities of sodium. In this example, the loss of 300 mmol Na^+ represents 12.8% of the total body Na^+ pool; thus, if exercise continues for as long as 6 h, Na^+ should be replaced during exercise.

Causes of hypothermic injury in endurance athletes

Running events

Rectal temperatures were recorded in 100 athletes treated for collapse during and after the Twin Cities Marathon; 16 cases were hypothermic (Roberts, 1989). Maughan and colleagues found a number of hypothermic athletes at the conclusion of the Aberdeen and Dundee marathons (Maughan, 1985; Maughan et al., 1985). Rectal temperatures were inversely related to running times over the last half of the marathon (Maughan, 1985).

The metabolic rate is markedly elevated during an endurance competition. Because of this, thermoregulatory processes are invoked in an attempt to maintain body temperature. In the latter part of a race, fatigue due to substrate depletion, dehydration or some other factor might cause the competitor to slow down. With a reduction in the rate of heat production, yet continued heat loss, the body temperature can start to fall (Taunton & McLean, 1986), particularly if the weather is cool or cold and there is rain (Sutton, 1987).

Swimming events

Dulac and colleagues (1987) reported the metabolic and hormonal responses of male and female swimmers to a 32-km swim in 18.5°C water. Rectal temperatures in finishers were 35.5°C for men and 36°C for women. Of 10 non-finishers, seven had to withdraw from the competition within 3 h because of marked hypothermia. All of these individuals had computed body fat percentages of less than 10%. Clearly, insulation and the maintenance of metabolic heat production are important to the prevention of hypothermia in these individuals.

Triathlon competitions frequently involve swimming, but the distance is normally no greater than 4 km (O'Toole et al., 1989). Several competitions are held with water temperatures near 20°C; large drop-out rates are reported (Hiller, 1989). The use of wet suits has been recommended (Hiller, 1989) Cold water also increases the oxygen cost of swimming, and maximal oxygen intake is reduced (Pendergast, 1988). A reduction of cardiac output contributes to the reduction in maximal exercise capacity. Differences in cooling responses between men and women may be related to brain thermoregulatory processes (Graham, 1988).

Other factors influencing thermoregulation

Age, sex and fitness

The incidence of heat injury is similar in males and females (in our observations of a 10-km road race, 1.3% and 1.2% for female and male participants, respectively; Hughson et al., 1980). When females are compared with males of similar fitness, they show similar thermoregulatory responses (Davies, 1979). There are apparently differences in thermoregulatory mechanisms, but the net effect is similar (Harrison, 1985).

Female thermoregulation is influenced by the menstrual phase. Stephenson and Kolka (1988) found a lower plasma volume in the luteal phase, a time when plasma progesterone, aldosterone and renin activity are elevated. Four of five subjects were unable to complete a passive heat exposure during the luteal phase. When exercising in the heat, the plasma volume decreased more rapidly during the follicular phase, so that there were no phase-related differences of plasma volume during exercise in the heat.

While the cold responses of females may differ from those of males (Graham, 1988), in a long-distance swim the ability to regulate body temperature is related to the percentage of body fat in both males and females (Dulac *et al.*, 1987).

In general, young and old individuals have greater difficulty dealing with thermal stress (Bar-Or, 1980; Kenney & Gisolfi, 1986; Kenney & Hodgson, 1987). A disproportionate number of the casualties of heat injury in 10 km road races are young males and females (Hughson *et al.*, 1980). The sweat rate of young people tends to be less than that of mature individuals (Bar-Or, 1980). In cold water, children lose heat more rapidly because of their relatively high surface area to mass ratio (Bar-Or, 1980).

Older individuals can tolerate exercise in the heat if they are fit (Kenney & Gisolfi, 1986). There are generally no differences of heat tolerance between middle-aged and young persons when they undergo the same acclimatization schedule (Pandolf *et al.*, 1988). Some researchers have suggested, though, that there are differences between old and young subjects matched for fitness (Kenney & Hodgson, 1987).

Medications and health status

During exercise with β-blockade the skin is cool and clammy (Freund *et al.*, 1987), suggesting a reduction of skin blood flow and transfer of heat to the skin. Freund *et al.* (1987) observed a smaller forearm blood flow and lower skin temperatures during exercise with propranolol β-blockade, but there was no unusual elevation in rectal temperature. In contrast, Pescatello *et al.* (1987) found that the oesophageal temperature during exercise was increased by β-blockade with propranolol. In agreement with Freund *et al.*, Pescatello *et al.* found a reduction in forearm blood flow for any given oesophageal temperature, reducing convective heat

transfer to the skin. However, there remains some uncertainty about the effect of β-blockade on core temperatures during exercise in the heat.

Fever increases susceptibility to exertional heat injury. In some of the earliest guidelines for the prevention of heat injury during fun runs, Sutton *et al.* (1972) indicated that athletes should not take part if they had recently developed a fever. Illness adversely affects total body water and sodium stores. Armstrong *et al.* (1988) point to the role of bacterial or viral infections in altering intestinal electrolyte absorption and thus reducing heat tolerance.

Individual susceptibility to heat injury has been noted. Genetic factors may possibly be involved (Armstrong *et al.*, 1990; Epstein, 1990) and individuals who have suffered previous exertional heat injury tolerate heat poorly (Armstrong *et al.*, 1990).

Type of exercise

Runners are probably most at risk of hyperthermic heat injury. Unlike cycling, where the increased relative air velocity can contribute to both convective and evaporative heat loss, runners often experience an effective 'zero' wind velocity (Hughson *et al.*, 1983). Runners also have more difficulty than cyclists in consuming fluids during competition.

Paraplegics are now becoming more involved in endurance activities. In such individuals oesophageal temperature rises more rapidly than rectal temperature (Gass *et al.*, 1988). This presumably reflects a different pattern of return of blood from the active muscle mass than is seen during leg exercise. Paraplegic athletes encounter a greater relative wind velocity for cooling, and they have easy access to fluids during exercise. However, the high power output and heat-generating capacity of some paraplegic athletes, together with disturbances of sympathetic nerve function in high-level lesions, warrant a further consideration of their cardiovascular and thermoregulatory problems.

Treatment of thermal injuries

Primary prevention of hyperthermia

Without doubt, the best treatment is prevention. This has been the basis for the guidelines published by Sutton *et al.* (1972), Hughson (1980), the American College of Sports Medicine (1985) and many others. With regard to shorter (5–20 km) endurance runs, even maximally activated thermoregulatory mechanisms may be unable to cope with metabolic heat production under certain climatic conditions. For this reason, it has been recommended that competitive schedules avoid the hottest parts of the day, and potentially hot times of the year (Hughson, 1980; American College of Sports Medicine, 1985). In addition, athletes can be warned about the environmental heat load on any given day by a colour-coded system based on the WBGT index (Hughson *et al.*, 1983; American College of Sports Medicine, 1985).

The race course preparation is also important in prevention of injuries. Adequate supplies of water must be provided at the start and at frequent intervals (3 km) along the race course. The necessary medical support is described by several authors (American College of Sports Medicine, 1985; Richards & Richards, 1986b).

Perhaps the most important component of prevention is the education of competitors. Because most injuries occur in novice runners (Hughson *et al.*, 1980), it is necessary to teach these individuals that heat stroke can kill otherwise healthy runners (Richards & Richards, 1986b; Robertson, 1988). Adequate training and heat acclimatization are required. On hot days, competitors must slow down to avoid heat injury. They should be encouraged to drink about 250 ml water every 3 km. Water consumption *per se* probably does not prevent heat injury (Hughson *et al.*, 1980), but it encourages competitors to monitor their health status. Runners must be told to question their condition, and to slow down or stop if any of the following warning signs are observed: clumsiness, stumbling, excessive sweating, cessation

of sweating, headache, nausea, dizziness, apathy, or gradual loss of consciousness (Hughson, 1980; American College of Sports Medicine, 1985).

In races of 42 km or longer, hyperthermia may be a problem, although the rate of metabolic heat production is usually not high enough to cause difficulties in itself. The athlete becomes susceptible to hyperthermia only when dehydration compounds the effects of heat production and a hot environment. An adequate intake of water and/or electrolyte solution is required to prevent hyperthermia. Guidance to athletes is presently complicated by uncertainty regarding the physiology of water and salt loss in long endurance events (Noakes *et al.*, 1988; Hiller, 1989). For some races, a fluid intake of 500 ml·h^{-1} may be adequate (Noakes, 1988). However, in the author's experience, a marathon in a hot environment may stimulate sweat rates in excess of 2.5 l·h^{-1}. Here, a larger volume of water and some electrolyte replacement is required. Hiller (1989) has suggested that competitors in ultra-triathlons replace fluids at a sufficient rate to counter the loss of body weight, and that approximately 1 g·h^{-1} of Na$^+$ be replaced in events of over 4 h duration. The potential for water intoxication (Noakes, 1988; Noakes *et al.*, 1988) remains real, and only a portion of sweat loss must be replaced to maintain body fluid volume. As sweat rate declines, the proportion requiring replacement is probably reduced.

Treatment of hyperthermia

There were earlier problems in the treatment of hyperthermia, because race organizers were unaware of the potential for heat injury (Hughson *et al.*, 1980). Now, extensive guidelines leave no excuse for inadequate preparation. The incidence of heat injuries in fun runs has apparently declined from over 1% (Hughson *et al.*, 1980; Richards & Richards, 1986a) to 0.2% or less (Richards & Richards, 1986a) with the institution of appropriate primary and secondary care. In the Hawaii

Ironman Triathlon, the incidence of hyper-thermia was only two of 1275 competitors (Laird, 1989). Hyperthermia is less common in long and ultra-long distance events; here the problem is with hydration and/or electrolytes (see below).

Two critical indicators of the severity of heat injury are direct measurement of rectal temperature and observation of mental status. Athletes who have marked central nervous system disturbances and a grossly elevated rectal temperature, typically but not invariably over 41°C, should be treated aggressively to lower body temperature. Even athletes who are relatively lucid should be treated for marked hyperthermia (Richards & Richards, 1986a). Hyperthermic injuries are potentially cases of thermoregulatory failure in which the body continues to generate large amounts of heat while shutting down normal heat loss mechanisms. Many victims of heat stroke have cool, clammy skin in spite of core temperatures in excess of 41°C. Skin blood flow should be elevated by massage to try to release body heat.

Treatment should include a rapid reduction of body temperature to 38–39°C (Richards & Richards, 1986a; Taunton & McLean, 1986). This is accomplished by application of cold towels over the neck, axillary and femoral vessels or by spraying with cool water. Most authors do not recommend immersion in ice baths (Nash, 1985), but some do (Nash, 1985; Costrini, 1990). Intravenous therapy is appropriate in severe cases. Transport from the onsite medical centre to a hospital is required if there is difficulty in lowering the rectal temperature.

Primary prevention of collapse

Athletes who collapse usually present with rectal temperatures in the range of 36.1–39.4°C (Roberts, 1989). The main cause is hypotension with or without hypovolaemia (Noakes, 1988; Robertson, 1988; Roberts, 1989).

The majority of cases of collapse are seen at the finish line, but some occur in the latter stages of the race. In long and ultralong events,

hypoglycaemia may be a cause. Prevention of hypoglycaemia depends upon competitor education. Recommendation should include a high carbohydrate diet before competition, consumption of a carbohydrate-containing liquid during competition, and selection of an appropriate pace so that glycogen stores are not depleted.

Most collapse victims are not hypoglycaemic, but are apparently hypovolaemic (Taunton & McLean, 1986; Noakes, 1988). Hypovolaemia is prevented by ensuring adequate access to fluids on the race course. Instructions concerning fluid requirements are not easy to give. In cool environments, about 500 ml·h^{-1} may be adequate (Noakes, 1988), but in warm or hot environments, 1 l·h^{-1}, or more, may be required (Hiller, 1989). The limiting factor here is the maximal rate of fluid uptake from the gut (Lamb & Brodowicz, 1986). The ideal volume is always somewhat less than the total sweat loss because of metabolic water production.

The electrolyte content of the fluid depends upon the total sweat loss. If this exceeds about 4 litres, then consumption of sodium chloride (about 1 g·h^{-1} (Hiller, 1989)) is recommended.

Treatment of collapse

The first step is to identify the cause. Rectal temperature is measured immediately, to rule out hyperthermic or hypothermic injury. At the Hawaii Ironman Triathlon, plasma electrolytes are also determined immediately (Laird, 1989). In marathon distance runs, hypovolaemia can probably be countered by oral consumption of fluids in the recovery area (Taunton & McLean, 1986). In longer races, it is essential to determine plasma electrolyte concentrations as part of the evaluation. Treatment is complex, and a consensus has not yet been reached. One approach is to treat athletes who collapse as victims of hypovolaemia and hyponatraemia (Laird, 1989). However, Noakes (1988) found that the most severely hyponatraemic patient in the Commrades Marathon responded well to diuretic therapy, showing the need for further study of this problem.

Primary prevention of hypothermia

Hypothermia can develop in competitors who run slowly, or who slow markedly in the latter stages of a road race; in cool, damp conditions; in swimmers and triathletes competing in cool water; in hikers and mountain-climbers; and in winter sports enthusiasts such as cross-country skiers. In most cases, proper selection of clothing can go a long way to prevent hypothermia. Signs of hypothermic injury include shivering, disorientation and muscular weakness (Taunton & McLean, 1986; Mills *et al.*, 1987).

Specific guidelines have been established for some sports to help prevent hypothermia. In running events, a WBGT index of less than 10°C indicates a high risk for hypothermia (American College of Sports Medicine, 1985). Cross-country skiing associations have established temperature guidelines, largely to prevent frostbite. For example, the Canadian Cross Country Ski Association has specified −20°C for races of 15 km or less, and −18°C for races over 15 km as critical temperatures for the postponement or cancellation of events (unpublished guidelines, 1990).

Treatment of hypothermia

Hypothermia induced by exercising in wet, cool conditions is best treated by removal of wet clothing, drying of the skin and wrapping the victims in wool blankets (Roberts, 1989). The treatment room must be kept warm. Possible dehydration must be assessed, because the affected individuals are often hypovolaemic (Bohn, 1987; Mills *et al.*, 1987). The technique of rewarming depends on the severity of the hypothermia. Simply maintaining the mildly hypothermic individual in blankets may be adequate. In more severe cases, it may be necessary to warm and humidify the inspired air, or to infuse warm saline (Bohn, 1987).

Conclusion

Endurance exercise places great demands on the body for the elimination of heat. The environment interacts with metabolic heat production in such a way that, under most circumstances, thermoregulatory balance is achieved. However, in certain environments, heat accumulates and hyperthermic injury can result. In contrast, excessive heat loss can give rise to hypothermic injury. Because of the wide range of environments and of individual responses, a careful diagnosis is needed before treatment is initiated. Rectal temperature must be measured. If plasma electrolyte disturbances are expected (ultraendurance events), then plasma mineral concentrations should also be measured.

Collapse can occur without extremes of body temperature. Postural hypotension is the most common cause. This could be a consequence of dehydration-induced hypovolaemia. Again, anticipation of the possible causes of collapse will aid in treatment.

The best treatment for all thermal problems is primary prevention (Hughson, 1980). The environmental heat stress can be minimized by selecting appropriate competitive conditions and making adequate plans according to published guidelines (American College of Sports Medicine, 1985). The heat stress on a particular day can be indicated to participants by the use of the WBGT index scale (Hughson *et al.*, 1983; American College of Sports Medicine, 1985). Finally, the athlete should be taught about the need for appropriate training, acclimatization and clothing to handle extreme environments.

References

Adner, M.M., Scarlet, J.J., Casey, J., Robison, W. & Jones, B.H. (1988) The Boston marathon medical care team: ten years of experience. *Phys. Sportsmed.* **16**, 99–105.

American College of Sports Medicine (1985) Position statement on the prevention of thermal injuries during distance running. *Med. Sci. Sports* **16**, ix–xiv.

Armstrong, L.E., Hubbard, R.W., Szlyk, P.C., Sils, I.V. & Kraemer, W.J. (1988) Heat intolerance, heat exhaustion monitored: a case report. *Aviat. Space Environ. Med.* **59**, 262–266.

Armstrong, L.E., Luca, J.P. De & Hubbard, R.W. (1990) Time course of recovery and heat acclimation ability of prior exertional heatstroke patients. *Med. Sci. Sports Exerc.* **22**, 36–48.

Åstrand, P.-O. & Rodahl, K. (1985) *Textbook of Work Physiology*. McGraw-Hill, New York.

Bar-Or, O. (1980) Climate and the exercising child — a review. *Int. J. Sports Med.* **1**, 53–65.

Bohn, D.J. (1987) Treatment of hypothermia: in the hospital. In: Sutton, J.R., Houston, C.S. & Coates, G. (eds) *Hypoxia and Cold*, pp. 286–305. Praeger Publishers, New York.

Costill, D.L., Cote, R. & Fink, W. (1976) Muscle water and electrolytes following varied levels of dehydration in man. *J. Appl. Physiol.* **40**, 6–11.

Costrini, A. (1990) Emergency treatment of exertional heatstroke and comparison of whole body cooling technique. *Med. Sci. Sports Exerc.* **22**, 15–18.

Davies, C.T.M. (1979) Thermoregulation during exercise in relation to sex and age. *Eur. J. Appl. Physiol.* **42**, 71–79.

Dulac, S., Quirion, A., DeCarufel, D. *et al.* (1987) Metabolic and hormonal responses to long-distance swimming in cold water. *Int. J. Sports Med.* **8**, 352–356.

Epstein, Y. (1990) Heat intolerance: predisposing factor or residual injury. *Med. Sci. Sports Exerc.* **22**, 29–35.

Freund, B.J., Joyner, M.J., Jilka, S.M. *et al.* (1987) Thermoregulation during prolonged exercise in heat: alterations with β-adrenergic blockade. *J. Appl. Physiol.* **63**, 930–936.

Gass, G.C., Camp, E.M., Nadel, E.R., Gwinn, T.H. & Engel, P. (1988) Rectal and rectal vs esophageal temperatures in paraplegic men during prolonged exercise. *J. Appl. Physiol.* **64**, 2265–2271.

Graham, T.E. (1988) Thermal, metabolic, and cardiovascular changes in men and women during cold stress. *Med. Sci. Sports Exerc.* **20**, S185–S192.

Hargreaves, M., Morgan, T.O., Snow, R. & Guerin, M. (1989) Exercise tolerance in the heat on low and normal salt intakes. *Clin. Sci.* **76**, 553–557.

Harrison, M.H. (1985) Effects of thermal stress and exercise on blood volume in humans. *Physiol. Rev.* **65**, 149–209.

Hiller, W.D.B. (1989) Dehydration and hyponatremia during triathlons. *Med. Sci. Sports Exerc.* **21**, S219–S221.

Hiller, W.D.B. & Laird, R.H. (1986) Hyponatremia and ultramarathons. *J.A.M.A.* **256**, 213.

Hubbard, R.W. & Armstrong, L.E. (1989) Hyperthermia: new thoughts on an old problem. *Phys.*

Sportsmed. **17**, 97–113.

Hughson, R.L. (1980) Primary prevention of heat stroke in Canadian long-distance runs (editorial). *Can. Med. Assoc. J.* **112**, 1115–1116.

Hughson, R.L. (1986) Heat stroke in Northern climates. In: Sutton, J.R. & Brock, R.M. (eds) *Sports Medicine for the Mature Athlete*, pp. 145–149. Benchmark Press, Indianapolis.

Hughson, R.L., Green, H.J., Houston, M.E., Thomson, J.A., MacLean, D.R. & Sutton, J.R. (1980) Heat injuries in Canadian mass participation runs. *Can. Med. Assoc. J.* **122**, 1141–1144.

Hughson, R.L., Staudt, L. & Mackie, J. (1983) Monitoring road racing in the heat. *Phys. Sportsmed.* **11**, 94–105.

Kenney, M.J. & Gisolfi, C.V. (1986) Thermal regulation: effects of exercise and age. In: Sutton, J.R. & Brock, R.M. (eds) *Sports Medicine for the Mature Athlete*, pp. 133–143. Benchmark Press, Indianapolis.

Kenney, W.L. & Hodgson, J.L. (1987) Heat tolerance, thermoregulation and ageing. *Sports Med.* **4**, 446–456.

Laird, R.H. (1989) Medical care at ultraendurance triathlons. *Med. Sci. Sports Exerc.* **21**, S222–S225.

Lamb, D.R. & Brodowicz, G.R. (1986) Optimal use of fluids of varying formulations to minimise exercise-induced disturbances in homeostasis. *Sports Med.* **3**, 247–274.

Maughan, R.J. (1985) Thermoregulation in marathon competition at low ambient temperature. *Int. J. Sports Med.* **6**, 15–19.

Maughan, R.J., Leiper, J.B. & Thompson, J. (1985) Rectal temperature after marathon running. *Br. J. Sports Med.* **19**, 192–195.

Mills, W.J., Hackett, P.H., Schoene, R.B., Roach, R. & Mills, W., III (1987) Treatment of hypothermia: in the field. In: Sutton, J.R., Houston, C.S. & Coates, G. (eds) *Hypoxia and Cold*, pp. 271–285. Praeger Publishers, New York.

Murray, R. (1987) The effects of consuming carbohydrate–electrolyte beverages on gastric emptying and fluid absorption during and following exercise. *Sports Med.* **4**, 322–351.

Nadel, E.R. (1983) Factors affecting the regulation of body temperature during exercise. *J. Thermal Biol.* **8**, 165–169.

Nash, H.L. (1985) Treating thermal injury: disagreement heats up. *Phys. Sportsmed.* **13**, 134–144.

Nelson, P.B., Robinson, A.G., Kapoor, W. & Rinaldo, J. (1986) Hyponatremia in a marathoner. *Phys. Sportsmed.* **16**, 78–87.

Noakes, T.D. (1988) Why endurance athletes collapse. *Phys. Sporstmed.* **16**, 24–26.

Noakes, T.D., Adams, B.A., Myburgh, K.H., Greeff, C., Lotz, T. & Nathan, M. (1988) The danger of an inadequate water intake during prolonged exercise. *Eur. J. Appl. Physiol.* **57**, 210–219.

Noakes, T.D., Goodwin, N. & Rayner, B.L. (1985) Water intoxication: a possible complication during endurance exercise. *Med. Sci. Sports Exerc.* **17**, 370–375.

O'Toole, M.L., Douglas, P.S. & Hiller, W.D.B. (1989) Applied physiology of a triathlon. *Sports Med.* **8**, 201–225.

Pandolf, K.B., Cadarette, B.S., Sawka, M.N., Young, A.J., Francesconi, R.P. & Gonzalez, R.R. (1988) Thermoregulatory responses of middle-aged and young men during dry-heat acclimation. *J. Appl. Physiol.* **65**, 65–71.

Pendergast, D.R. (1988) The effect of body cooling on oxygen transport during exercise. *Med. Sci. Sports Exerc.* **20**, S171–S176.

Pescatello, L.S., Mack, G.W., Leach, C.N. Jr & Nadel, E.R. (1987) Effect of β-adrenergic blockade on thermoregulation during exercise. *J. Appl. Physiol.* **62**, 1448–1452.

Richards, R. & Richards, D. (1986a) Prevention of exercise-induced heat stroke. In: Sutton, J.R. & Brock, R.M. (eds) *Sports Medicine for the Mature Athlete*, pp. 151–166. Benchmark Press, Indianapolis.

Richards, R. & Richards, D. (1986b) Providing medical care in fun runs and marathons in Australasia. In: Sutton, J.R. & Brock, R.M. (eds) *Sports Medicine for the Mature Athlete*, pp. 167–180. Benchmark Press, Indianapolis.

Roberts, W.O. (1989) Exercise-associated collapse in endurance events: a classification system. *Phys. Sportsmed.* **5**, 49–55.

Robertson, J.W. (1988) Medical problems in mass participation runs. Recommendations. *Sports Med.* **6**, 261–270.

Röcker, L., Kirsch, K.A., Heyduck, B. & Altenkirch, H.-U. (1989) Influence of prolonged physical exercise on plasma volume, plasma proteins, electrolytes, and fluid-regulating hormones. *Int. J. Sports Med.* **10**, 270–274.

Stephenson, L.A. & Kolka, M.A. (1988) Plasma volume during heat stress and exercise in women. *Eur. J. Appl. Physiol.* **57**, 373–381.

Sutton, J.R. (1986) Thermal problems in Masters athletes. In: Sutton, J.R. & Brock, R.M. (eds) *Sports Medicine for the Mature Athlete*, pp. 125–131. Benchmark Press, Indianapolis.

Sutton, J.R. (1987) Hypothermia in joggers and marathon runners. In: Sutton, J.R., Houston, C.S. & Coates, G. (eds) *Hypoxia and Cold*, pp. 257–263. Praeger Publishers, New York.

Sutton, J.R., Coleman, M.J., Millar, A.P., Lazarus, L. & Russo, P. (1972) The medical problems of mass participation in athletic competition. The 'City-to-Surf' race. *Med. J. Aust.* **2**, 127–133.

Taunton, J.E. & McLean, R.S. (1986) Road racing medical management. In: Sutton, J.R. & Brock, R.M. (eds) *Sports Medicine for the Mature Athlete*, pp. 205–212. Benchmark Press, Indianapolis.

Chapter 43

Problems of High Altitude

ROY J. SHEPHARD

Introduction

The performance and safety of competitors at high altitudes is modified relative to that observed under sea-level conditions because of decreases in gravitational acceleration, wind resistance and temperature, a potential local accumulation of air pollutants, high levels of radiation, and above all a low partial pressure of inspired oxygen. The impact of these factors upon performance and health is likely to be greatest during endurance events, because the successful and safe completion of such activities depends largely upon an adequate delivery of oxygen to the active tissues (see Chapter 3).

Sports physicians have expressed some concern about the potential risk of endurance competitions at altitudes of 2000–3000 m (Jokl & Jokl, 1968; Shephard, 1974), with the Fédération Internationale de Médecine Sportive (FIMS, Melbourne Meeting, 1974) urging extreme caution above 2290 m, and avoidance of competition above 3050 m. The practising sports physician should be prepared to advise the competitor on likely acute changes of performance (Goddard, 1967; Margaria, 1967; Jokl & Jokl, 1968), an optimum acclimatization schedule (Goddard, 1967) and any possible residual benefits from altitude training, real or simulated (Richardson, 1974). Treatment may also be required both for pre-existing conditions aggravated by altitude exposure, and for specific pathologies such as mountain sickness, pulmonary, cerebral and retinal oedema (Jokl & Jokl, 1968; Shephard, 1974; Fletcher et al., 1985; Hachett & Hornbein, 1989).

Physical environment

Gravity: The acceleration due to gravity diminishes by about 0.3 cm·s^{-1} for every 1000 m of altitude. At 2000–3000 m, there is thus a measurable but unimportant benefit to competitors ($<$0.1%), most obvious when cycling or running uphill; in practical terms, a much larger effect would result from a latitudinal change, for instance if the site of competition were moved from the equator to near the north pole ($>$0.5%).

Wind resistance: Wind resistance accounts for a substantial component of the work performed by some classes of endurance athlete (see Chapter 15). Such resistance is due largely to turbulent airflow over the body surface, and it is thus proportional to $\frac{1}{2} (Apv^2)$, where A is the projected area of the competitor and any associated equipment, p is the density of the atmosphere, and v is the relative velocity of air movement. Density decreases in exponential fashion as the altitude increases, by 20% at 1850 m, 26% at 2500 m, and 31% at 3000 m.

At sea level, wind resistance accounts for about 11% of the energy that an athlete expends in running 5000 m. The decrease of atmospheric density at 3000 m thus has the potential to boost a distance runner's performance by some

3.4%. The work performed against turbulence (resistive force × distance) is proportional to the third power of relative velocity, and in a racing cyclist it accounts for some 90% of the total energy expended, so that his or her advantage is about 28% when competing at 3000 m.

Temperature: The ambient temperature drops by about 2°C for each 300 m of altitude. Wind velocities also tend to be greater at high and exposed sites, while a diminution of ground haze increases solar radiation (see below). In general, the loss of body heat (see Chapter 16) thus proceeds more readily at altitude than at sea level. The likelihood of heat stress is reduced at tropical latitudes, and the chances of hypothermia are increased at greater latitudes. There may be interactions between hypoxia and cold stress (Sutton *et al.*, 1987).

Air pollution: Petrol-driven vehicles operate less efficiently as altitude is increased, and narrow mountain valleys may encourage the local accumulation of pollutants. The problems encountered when competing in a polluted environment (see Chapter 44) are thus likely to be exacerbated at altitude. From the viewpoint of endurance, an adverse interaction between carbon monoxide exposure and altitude is particularly likely (Shephard, 1983; Horvath *et al.*, 1988).

Radiation: Direct ultraviolet radiation (at a wavelength of 295 nm) increases by as much as 35% for an ascent of 1000 m, but because the atmosphere is less hazy there is a decrease in scattered radiation. At an altitude of 4000 m, the ultraviolet irradiation at 400 nm is increased by 147%, but that at 300 nm is increased by 250% (Heath & Williams, 1989).

Cosmic radiation also increases rapidly at altitudes above 1000 m (Heath & Williams, 1989), and at 3000 m there is a threefold increase in the anticipated sea-level exposure of about 24 mrad·year^{-1} (0.24 mGY·year^{-1}).

Oxygen partial pressure: The partial pressure of oxygen decreases exponentially, in parallel with the decrease of atmospheric density. Thus, unit volume of air at ambient pressure contains some 31% less oxygen at 3000 m than at sea level. Experience in Mexico City (stadium altitude about 2240 m, 24% reduction of oxygen pressure) has shown that the effects of hypoxia outweigh the benefits attributable to gravity, wind resistance and temperature, so that the times for endurance events of 5000 and 10 000 m are some 8% poorer than at sea level.

Acute effects

At a moderate altitude such as Mexico City, the acute effects upon the resting state and the body's responses to light exercise are quite small. The normal, sigmoid shape of the oxygen dissociation curve is in itself an important defence mechanism against hypoxia (Ernsting & Shephard, 1951), and until the athlete has reached an altitude of 1500–2000 m, the resting arterial oxygen saturation remains near normal despite any reduction of alveolar oxygen pressure. On the other hand, during maximal aerobic exercise the arterial oxygen saturation of an endurance competitor with a large maximal cardiac output may be less well protected (Tucker *et al.*, 1984). Often a small increase of the respiratory minute volume suffices to restore the normal sea-level arterial oxygen saturation, and thus the oxygen transported per unit volume of cardiac output while at altitude. If this is not the case, a moderate tachycardia restores oxygen transport at the expense of some diminution of the cardiac reserve (Shephard, 1974). As acid–base balance is adjusted to the new altitude, a greater hyperventilation becomes possible, and the tachycardia diminishes. The loss of plasma and tissue bicarbonate affects fluid balances, and perhaps as a consequence of this there is a progressive decrease of stroke volume over the first few weeks at altitude, particularly in unfit subjects. The maximal cardiac output and thus the maximal oxygen intake are depressed yet more, since there is also a decrease of maximal heart rate, possible effects from an increase of blood viscosity, and at higher altitudes direct effects of oxygen lack on myocardial contractility (Ferretti *et al.*, 1990).

The pulmonary arterial pressure is increased, by 18% at rest and 30% during submaximal exercise at 2370 m (Sime *et al.*, 1974; Lockhart & Saiag, 1981). This response may increase perfusion of the upper parts of the lungs, and thus allow a better matching of ventilation and perfusion, with advantages for alveolar gas exchange.

Acclimatization

If an athlete remains at high altitude, the body makes physiological and biochemical adjustments that restore endurance performance towards sea-level values. Athletes who took 8.5% longer to complete a distance run on arrival in Mexico City were running only 5.7% slower by the 29th day at this altitude (Heath & Williams, 1989).

In addition to the reduction of blood and tissue bicarbonate content already noted, acclimatization leads to increased haemoglobin levels, any early decrement of blood volume is made good, and the activity of various tissue enzymes is increased. Choice of an appropriate acclimatization schedule is based upon the anticipated rates of these various responses.

The bicarbonate content of the cerebral fluid is reduced within a few hours of moving to altitude, and parallel adjustments of blood and tissue buffers develop over the following week. As a result, the endurance competitor can hyperventilate slightly without developing intermittent ventilation and other signs of carbon dioxide lack. The immediate consequence is that the oxygen content of the arterial blood rises, and perhaps a fifth of the lost capacity to transport oxygen is restored. However, hyperventilation is a mixed blessing to an endurance competitor, because it increases the oxygen consumed by the respiratory muscles to the point where this factor may limit per-

formance. There have been suggestions that the carotid bodies of the well-trained endurance competitor show a decreased sensitivity to oxygen lack. In theory, the decrease of tissue buffering should also reduce the athlete's tolerance of lactate accumulation, so that prolonged exercise above the anaerobic threshold would become more fatiguing. Certainly, the measurements of lactate used by some laboratories become much more difficult to interpret at altitude (McLellan *et al.*, 1988).

An increase in the haemoglobin content of unit volume of blood tends to restore the arterial oxygen content in the face of the reduced partial pressure of oxygen in the alveoli. Immediate increases in red cell count and haemoglobin concentration are due to haemoconcentration, but an increase of haemopoiesis leads to a true increase in total red cell mass over several months of exercise at high altitudes (Boutellier *et al.*, 1990). Stimulation of erythropoiesis decreases the average age of the red cells, and thus increases their $2-3$ diphosphoglycerate (DPG) levels, with a rightward shift of the oxygen dissociation curve (Mairbäurl *et al.*, 1986); the reduced oxygen affinity of the haemoglobin presumably helps oxygen delivery in the tissues. At extreme altitudes, a very large increase of red cell count may increase the blood viscosity to such an extent as to limit maximal cardiac output (Buick *et al.*, 1982) and increase the risk of intravascular clotting.

The team physician should check both the haemoglobin concentration and the serum iron levels of competitors while they are at sea level, because plasma volume expansion, fads of diet, poor iron absorption, losses in sweat, depressed red cell formation, haemorrhage and intravascular haemolysis can all predispose the endurance athlete to the unnecessary handicap of an initial anaemia or latent iron deficit. If measurements are made after a competitor has moved to high altitude, it must be remembered that 'normal' values should then be higher than at sea level (Tufts *et al.*, 1985).

Other reported tissue adaptations to high altitude include an increase in the myoglobin content of the muscles, and an augmentation of activity in the various enzyme systems; these responses develop over 1–2 weeks. At the altitudes encountered by mountaineers, there may also be a negative nitrogen balance (Guilland & Klepping, 1985), with a loss of protein from the myofibrils (Hoppeler *et al.*, 1990), but no change in the capillary network, making capillary oxygen more readily available to the muscle mitochondria.

Acclimatization must strike a reasonable balance between useful respiratory adaptations and the disadvantage of a cumulative fluid loss. At altitudes below 2250 m, respiratory gains seem to outweigh any circulatory losses, at least for the person who is training hard, and where practicable most authorities recommend a 3–4-week period of acclimatization. During this time, the athlete must be guarded against unfamiliar microorganisms, the psychological problems of living in an unfamiliar environment, and the practical risks of interrupting a well-established training plan. At 3000 m, the cumulative loss of plasma fluid can no longer be ignored, and it may be wise for the athlete to compete within 72 h of reaching altitude. Opportunity is thereby allowed for recuperation from the journey, adjustments of cerebrospinal bicarbonate levels, and recovery from any immediate mountain sickness, but competition is completed before there has been time for a serious decrease of maximum cardiac output. The main disadvantage of permitting only a short pre-event stay at altitude is that the athlete has little chance to learn the peculiarities of the course or an appropriate competitive pace. An early precontest site visit is thus desirable.

The high-altitude native has a clear advantage over the sea-level resident when endurance competitions are conducted at great heights. The high-altitude native experiences less early mountain sickness, and a smaller decrease of oxygen transport (Maresh *et al.*, 1983). In the 1968 Mexico City Olympic Games, the first five places in the 10 000-m event were taken by those who were either native to high altitude,

or who had lived at high altitude for long periods (Heath & Williams, 1989). Such individuals also have some advantage when endurance competitions are conducted at sea level; specific characteristics include a high haemoglobin concentration and (at least in some populations) a limited response of the carotid body chemoreceptors to oxygen lack (Hackett *et al.*, 1980; Milledge, 1986). The latter feature reduces the likelihood of hyperventilation, excessive carbon dioxide washout and intermittent breathing during vigorous effort. Moreover, diversion of the available oxygen supply to the chest muscles is reduced.

High-altitude training camps

Because sea-level residents ultimately adapt well to endurance competition at moderate altitudes, and there is some evidence that high-altitude natives have a persistent advantage at a sea-level venue, there has been considerable discussion of the desirability of training endurance competitors at high altitudes. Where this tactic has been adopted, the physiological objective has been to time the return to sea level so that the altitude polycythaemia is preserved, but body buffers have been restored to their sea-level values. Red cell production is severely depressed immediately after return to sea level, and if the altitude exposure has been extreme, the suppression of haemopoiesis can be such that a temporary anaemia develops (Heath & Williams, 1989). There remains a theoretical possibility of gaining some advantage of oxygen transport 4–20 days following altitude exposure, but this must be set against such practical disadvantages as the likely curtailment of training and the learning of an incorrect pace while at altitude. If athletes are in peak condition before a mountain sojourn, the net result of a period at an altitude camp seems no change or even a small deterioration in maximal oxygen intake and times for endurance competition (Shephard, 1974; Adams *et al.*, 1975; Jackson & Sharkey, 1988; Terrados *et al.*, 1988). Most teams are now disillusioned about altitude training, except where competition is planned at altitude and a long period of residence is possible at an agreeable training site.

A few authors have experimented with hypoxic training at sea level, for instance putting cyclists on ergometers in a decompression chamber, or having competitors rebreathe through long tubes during practice periods (D'Urzo et al., 1986; notice that the latter technique also induces a marked hypercarbia). Any physiological benefits from such artificial forms of acclimatization have again been slight, and the impact of such tactics upon performance has generally been offset by the disruption of normal training.

Altitude pathologies

Mountain sickness

The liability to mountain sickness shows much interindividual variability (Forster, 1984), and the condition can be quite difficult to diagnose, as the symptoms are non-specific. Complaints include a headache that becomes progressively more severe, insomnia, irritability and a variety of gastrointestinal disturbances. There is an increase of extracellular fluid, with a risk of progression to cerebral oedema (Ravenhill, 1913), pulmonary oedema (Hackett & Hornbein, 1988), generalized oedema (Malconian & Rock, 1988) and (particularly in severe cases) retinal haemorrhages (Frayser et al., 1970; Sutton, 1990). The volume and composition of the intestinal secretions is also modified. All of these changes seem secondary to hyperventilation, disturbances of acid−base balance, and associated fluid shifts.

During moderate recreational activity, the threshold altitude for the development of mountain sickness seems to be 2000−3000 m (Montgomery et al., 1989). The heavy training schedule of the international endurance athlete may increase the risk, with a potential for the appearance of symptoms at a somewhat lower altitude. However, at the altitudes relevant to most types of competition, the disorder usually

lasts only 2−3 days, and most patients respond well to conservative treatment. Training schedules should be lightened temporarily, little activity being taken on the first day. Symptomatic therapy can be given for headache and sleeplessness, although an excess of sedatives may worsen the condition by depressing the athlete's respiration during sleep. Carbonic anhydrase-inhibiting diuretics such as acetazolamide (250 mg four times daily) are quite popular with mountaineers who must face more severe altitudes for longer periods, and there have been claims that in such situations the administration of acetazolamide conserves muscle mass with gains of performance (Bradwell & Coote, 1987). However, at the moderate altitudes of typical international competitions, carbonic anhydrase inhibitors are best avoided if possible. Although symptoms are undoubtedly relieved, the course of natural acclimatization is slowed, and the resultant fluid loss may further aggravate the deterioration of performance associated with acid−base disturbances and a shrinking plasma volume (Hackett et al., 1985; Stager et al., 1990). Dexamethasone may be considered for severe cases (Ferrazzini et al., 1987).

Cerebral oedema is a medical emergency that usually presents as an exacerbation of acute mountain sickness. A severe headache may be accompanied by hallucinations, incoherence, weakness and ataxia, progressing to loss of consciousness and even a stroke (Clarke, 1988). Treatment includes betamethasone (4 mg intravenously, immediately and every 4 h), acetazolamide (250 mg immediately and every 8 h), provision of an airway, oxygen, and general care as for any unconscious patient.

Chronic mountain sickness is most unlikely at 2000−3000 m. If symptoms persist, they may reflect a compounding of the original episode with an intercurrent gastrointestinal infection, irrational fears of altitude, discouragement from poor track times, and a progressive loss of physical condition due to the interruption of training schedules.

Pulmonary oedema

An intense pulmonary oedema is a medical emergency that occasionally develops within 9–36 h of reaching altitude. There is a substantial leakage of high molecular weight proteins, erythrocytes, macrophages and various enzymes into the alveolar spaces (Schoene et al., 1986). Among recreational athletes, the threshold altitude for pulmonary oedema seems about 2500 m, but because unusually vigorous exercise is a precipitant, endurance competitors could conceivably encounter this disorder at lower elevations. Circumstances predisposing to the onset of pulmonary oedema include recent respiratory infection, pulmonary venous constriction (secondary to oxygen lack), peripheral vasoconstriction (secondary to hyperventilation), an increase of total blood volume, and pulmonary hypertension (exacerbated by previous residence at altitude). The syndrome is most commonly encountered in competitors with past experience of altitude; typically, they initiate vigorous training without allowing adequate time for the body to readapt to the low partial pressure of oxygen.

The classical patient presents with an acute dyspnoea, a phlegm that is bloodstained, watery and sometimes frothy, noisy breathing, chest discomfort, a cough (initially dry, but becoming wet), nausea, vomiting, and a cold, clammy skin. There are the usual physical signs of alveolar exudate (including poor air entry, dullness to percussion, râles, and cyanosis), tachycardia, an increased pulmonary second sound, and usually a low-grade fever. The electrocardiogram shows evidence of right ventricular strain, and intense pulmonary vascular congestion with coarse parahilar mottling is seen in chest radiographs (Fig. 43.1).

If neglected, pulmonary oedema can prove fatal. Prompt diagnosis is thus vital. However, there is usually a good response to bed rest, oxygen at high flow rates (6–8 l·min⁻¹), frusemide (40 mg intravenously, immediately and every 6 h), acetazolamide (250 mg immediately, and repeated every 8 h) and antibiotics (to counter secondary infection). Morphia was once administered, but is not now recommended because it leads to a further depression of ventilation (Heath & Williams, 1989).

General medical conditions

At moderate altitudes, problems of oxygen transport can often be accommodated by the simple expedient of moving a little more slowly

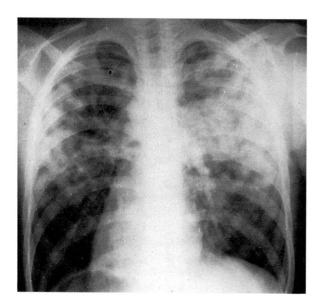

Fig. 43.1 Pulmonary oedema is one of the most serious adverse responses to high altitude and the accompanying hypoxic conditions. Radiograph courtesy of Altitude Research Division, US Air Force Research Institute of Environmental Medicine.

than at sea level. However, the athlete who attempts to sustain a normal pace inevitably increases the risk of developing general medical conditions, including myocardial infarction and cardiac arrest. Even slight reductions of the arterial oxygen saturation increase the likelihood that exercise will induce cardiac arrhythmias and manifestations of cerebral hypoxia such as central scotomata, impairment of colour vision, and disturbances of coordination. The hazards remain small for a young, healthy, medically screened athlete who is competing at moderate altitudes, but must be kept in mind, particularly in events that involve Masters' competitors. There have been disturbing reports of permanent brain damage in habitual explorers of higher altitudes (Hornbein *et al.*, 1989).

Black athletes should be checked for sickle cell disease, since several deaths from splenic rupture have occurred at altitudes of around 2500 m. Athletes of other ethnic groups are not totally exempt from risk of splenic rupture, and the condition should be suspected in anyone who suddenly develops upper left quadrant abdominal pain (Lane & Githens, 1985).

The cold, dry air and the likelihood of increased ozone concentrations make the vulnerable contestant more liable to exercise-induced bronchospasm.

Ultraviolet radiation is greater at altitude than at sea level (see above), and exposure is likely to be longer because the air is cooler. Particularly when such radiation is reflected from snow, it can cause not only sunburn, but also temporary blindness. Barrier creams and dark glasses with side-protectors (Brandt & Malla, 1982) should be used as necessary.

Conclusions

Both the practical experience of high-altitude endurance competitions and the theoretical considerations presented above support the FIMS position that problems attributable to altitude are unlikely below 2300 m. Between 2300 and 3000 m, there is an increasing chance that the more vulnerable members of a team could develop mountain sickness, pulmonary oedema and other medical problems such as cardiac arrhythmias and cerebral hypoxia. On present knowledge, the likelihood of occasional incidents above 3000 m seems sufficient to justify both the categoric prohibition of major competitions, and the urging of caution upon recreational skiers and mountain climbers.

References

Adams, W.C., Bernauer, E.M., Dill, D.B. & Bomar, J.B. (1975) Effects of equivalent sea-level and altitude training on $V_{O_2 max}$ and running performance. *J. Appl. Physiol.* **39**, 262–266.

Boutellier, U., Dériaz, O., diPrampero, P. & Cerretelli, P.V. (1990) Aerobic performance at altitude: effects of acclimatization and haematocrit with reference to training. *Int. J. Sports Med.* **11**, S21–S26.

Bradwell, A.R. & Coote, J.H. (1987) Expedition to the Himalayas. *Postgrad. Med. J.* **63**, 165–167.

Brandt, F. & Malla, O.K. (1982) Eye problems at high altitudes. In: Brendel, W. & Zink, R.A. (eds) *High Altitude Physiology and Medicine*, pp. 212–214. Springer-Verlag, New York.

Buick, F.J., Gledhill, N., Froese, A.B. & Spriet, L.L. (1982) Red cell mass and aerobic performance at sea level. In: Sutton, J.R., Jones, N.L. & Houston, C.S. (eds) *Hypoxia: Man at Altitude*, pp. 43–50. Thième-Stratton, New York.

Clarke, C. (1988) High altitude cerebral oedema. *Int. J. Sports Med.* **19**, 170–174.

D'Urzo, A.D., Liu, F.L.W. & Rebuck, A.S. (1986) Influence of supplemental oxygen on the physiological response to the P_{O_2} aerobic exerciser. *Med. Sci. Sports Exerc.* **18**, 211–215.

Ernsting, J. & Shephard, R.J. (1951) Respiratory adaptations in congenital heart disease. *J. Physiol.* **112**, 332–343.

Ferrazzini, G., Maggiorini, M., Kriemler, S., Bärtsch, P. & Oelz, O. (1987) Successful treatment of acute mountain sickness with dexamethasone. *Br. Med. J.* **294**, 1380–1382.

Ferretti, G., Boutellier, U., Pendergast, D.R. *et al.* (1990) IV. Oxygen transport system before and after exposure to chronic hypoxia. *Int. J. Sports Med.* **11**, S15–S21.

Fletcher, R.F., Wright, A.D., Jones, G.T. & Bradwell, A.R. (1985) The clinical assessment of acute mountain sickness. *Q. J. Med.* **54**, 91–100.

Forster, P. (1984) Reproducibility of individual response to exposure to high altitude. *Br. Med. J.* **289**, 1269.

Frayser, R., Houston, C.S., Bryan, A.C., Rennie, I.D. & Gray, G. (1970) Retinal hemorrhage at high altitude. *N. Engl. J. Med.* **282**, 1183–1184.

Goddard, R.F. (ed.) (1967) *The Effects of Altitude on Physical Performance*. Athletic Institute, Chicago.

Guilland, J.C. & Klepping, J. (1985) Nutritional alterations at high altitude in man. *Eur. J. Appl. Physiol.* **54**, 517–523.

Hackett, P.H. & Hornbein, T. (1988) Disorders of high altitude. In: Murray, J.F. & Nadel, J.A. (eds) *Textbook of Respiratory Medicine*, pp. 1646–1663. W.B. Saunders, Philadelphia.

Hackett, P.H., Reeves, J.T., Reeves, C.D., Grover, R.F. & Rennie, D. (1980) Control of breathing in Sherpas at low and high altitude. *J. Appl. Physiol.* **49**, 374–379.

Hackett, P.H., Schoene, R.B., Winslow, R.M., Peters, R.M. & West, J.B. (1985) Acetaezolamide and exercise in sojourners to 6300 meters – a preliminary study. *Med. Sci. Sports Exerc.* **17**, 593–597.

Heath, D. & Williams, D.R. (1989) *High Altitude Medicine and Pathology*. Butterworths, London.

Hoppeler, H., Kleinert, E., Schlegel, C. *et al.* (1990) II. Morphological adaptations of human skeletal muscle to chronic hypoxia. *Int. J. Sports Med.* **11**, S3.

Hornbein, T.F., Townes, B.B., Schoene, R.B., Sutton, J.R. & Houston, C.S. (1989) The cost to the central nervous system of climbing to extremely high altitudes. *N. Engl. J. Med.* **321**, 1714–1719.

Horvath, S.M., Bedi, J.F., Wagner, J.A. & Agnew, J. (1988) Maximum aerobic capacity at several ambient concentrations of CO at several altitudes. *J. Appl. Physiol.* **65**, 2696–2708.

Jackson, C.G.R. & Sharkey, B.J. (1988) Altitude, training and human performance. *Sports Med.* **6**, 279–284.

Jokl, E. & Jokl, P. (1968) *Exercise and Altitude*. University Park Press, Baltimore.

Lane, P.A. & Githens, J.H. (1985) Splenic syndrome at mountain altitudes in sickle cell trait: its occurrence in non-black persons. *J.A.M.A.* **253**, 2251–2254.

Lockhart, A. & Saiag, B. (1981) Altitude and the human pulmonary circulation. *Clin. Sci.* **60**, 599–605.

McLellan, T., Jacobs, I. & Lewis, W. (1988) Acute altitude exposure and altered acid–base states. I. Effects on the exercise ventilation and blood lactate responses. *Eur. J. Appl. Physiol.* **57**, 435–444.

Mairbäurl, H., Schobersberger, W., Humperler, E., Hasibeler, W., Fischer, W. & Raas, E. (1986) Beneficial effects of exercising at moderate altitude on red cell oxygen transport and on exercise performance. *Pflügers Arch.* **406**, 594–599.

Malconian, M.K. & Rock, P.B. (1988) Medical problems related to altitude. In: Pandolf, K.B., Sawka, M.N. & Gonzalez, R.F. (eds) *Human Performance Physiology and Environmental Medicine at Terrestrial Extremes*, pp. 545–563. Benchmark Press, Indianapolis.

Maresh, C.M., Noble, B.J., Robertson, K.L. & Sime, W.E. (1983) Maximal exercise during hypobaric hypoxia (447 Torr) in moderate altitude natives. *Med. Sci. Sports Exerc.* **15**, 360–365.

Margaria, R. (ed.) (1967) *Exercise at Altitude*. Excerpta Medica Foundation, Amsterdam.

Milledge, J.S. (1986) The ventilatory response to hypoxia: how much is good for a mountaineer? *Postgrad. Med. J.* **63**, 169–172.

Montgomery, A.B., Mills, J. & Luce, J.M. (1989) Incidence of acute mountain sickness at intermediate altitude. *J.A.M.A.* **261**, 732–734.

Ravenhill, T.H. (1913) Some experiences of acute mountain sickness in the Andes. *J. Trop. Med. Hyg.* **20**, 313–320.

Richardson, R.G. (ed.) (1974) Altitude training. *Br. J. Sports Med.* **8**, 1–63.

Schoene, R.B., Hackett, P.H., Henderson, W.R. *et al.* (1986) High altitude pulmonary edema. Characteristics of lung lavage fluid. *J.A.M.A.* **256**, 63–69.

Shephard, R.J. (1974) Altitude training camps. *Br. J. Sports Med.* **8**, 38–45.

Shephard, R.J. (1983) *Carbon Monoxide: The Silent Killer*. C.C. Thomas, Springfield, Illinois.

Sime, F., Penaloza, D., Ruiz, L., Gonzalez, N., Covarrubias, E. & Postigo, R. (1974) Hypoxaemia, pulmonary hypertension and low cardiac output in newcomers to low altitude. *J. Appl. Physiol.* **36**, 561–565.

Stager, J.M., Tucker, A., Cordain, L., Engebretsen, B.J., Brechue, W.F. & Matulich, C.C. (1990) Normoxic and acute hypoxic exercise tolerance in man following acetazolamide. *Med. Sci. Sports Exerc.* **22**, 178–184.

Sutton, J.R. (1990) Exercise at high altitudes. In: Torg, J., Welsh, P. & Shephard, R.J. (eds) *Current Therapy in Sports Medicine 2*, pp. 155–158. B.C. Decker, Toronto.

Sutton, J.R., Houston, C.S. & Coates, G. (eds) (1987) *Hypoxia and Cold*. Praeger, New York.

Terrados, N., Melichna, J., Sylvén, J., Jannson, E. & Kaijser, L. (1988) Effects of training at simulated altitude on performance and muscle metabolic capacity in competitive road cyclists. *Eur. J. Appl. Physiol.* **57**, 203–209.

Tucker, A., Stager, J.M. & Cordain, L. (1984) Arterial O_2 saturation and maximum O_2 consumption in moderate-altitude runners exposed to sea level and 3050 m. *J.A.M.A.* **252**, 2867–2871.

Tufts, D.A., Haas, J.D., Beard, J.L. & Spielvogel, H. (1985) Distribution of hemoglobin and functional consequences of anemia in adult males at high altitude. *Am. J. Clin. Nutr.* **42**, 1–11.

Chapter 44

Ambient Air Pollution and Endurance Performance

LAWRENCE J. FOLINSBEE

Introduction

Among the environmental concerns that élite endurance athletes may consider in their quest for optimal performance is the quality of the large quantities of air that they must breathe during heavy exercise. Many major athletic events are conducted within the environs of heavily populated urban areas, where air pollutants such as ozone (O_3), carbon monoxide (CO), sulphur dioxide (SO_2), nitrogen dioxide (NO_2), and acid aerosols may be present at unacceptably high levels. Depending on personal exposure history and individual physiological or disease factors which may alter responsiveness, high pollution levels may have an impact on performance or present a health risk. In addition to the immediate potential impact of air pollutants on performance, the athlete should consider the possible long-term effects of training for years in areas dominated by poor air quality. Indoor air may be an additional source of inhaled toxic substances.

Exposure to air pollutants

Endurance athletes constitute a group at special risk from exposure to air pollutants because of the large amount of time they spend training in polluted ambient air. Physiological responses to air pollutants are influenced by the amount inhaled and subsequently deposited in or delivered to various target organs. The major factors determining the dose received are the concentration of the pollutant, the duration of exposure, and the volume of air inhaled (i.e. the respiratory minute volume). Other factors such as chemical reactions (modifying or neutralizing the air pollutant) or an accumulation of the substance within the body may modify the 'dose'. Because respiratory minute volume increases proportionately with the intensity of exercise, the potential effects of air pollutants on athletic performance should be considered in the context not only of pollutant concentrations, but also of the intensity and duration of activity of the athletes concerned. If the pulmonary health effects of air pollutants occur at low pollutant levels or after short exposure periods, they are almost invariably associated with moderate or heavy exercise.

Ozone

Ozone is a major urban air pollutant produced by the action of sunlight on vehicular and industrial emissions. Ozone has marked effects on lung function and impairs exercise performance at levels known to exist in ambient air. Concentrations of ozone in urban areas depend upon the interaction of meteorological factors with the quantity of internal combustion engine exhaust emissions, pollution transport, and the industrial and community output of ozone precursors such as nitrogen oxides and hydrocarbons. A study of high-school cross-country runners in Los Angeles indicated that increased ambient ozone concentrations might impair athletic performance. Controlled laboratory studies (Folinsbee & Raven, 1984; Gong et al. 1986; Adams, 1987) have demonstrated reductions in peak oxygen consumption or endurance time, or failure to complete prescribed exercise as a result of ozone exposure. The reduction in exercise performance was accompanied by pronounced respiratory symptoms, including cough and pain on deep inspiration, a more rapid and shallow breathing pattern during exercise, and a substantial decrease in spirometric measurements of lung function. The exercise performance of trained athletes has been impaired after 1 h of moderately heavy exercise at ozone concentrations as low as 0.18 parts per million (p.p.m.). (All ozone concentrations have been referenced to equivalent levels using the current US Environmental Protection Agency (USEPA) ultraviolet measurement standard.) Such levels are frequently exceeded in cities such as Los Angeles, Athens and Mexico City. Higher ozone concentrations are reached much less frequently, but the effects on exercise performance and lung function are more pronounced (Table 44.1).

Exercise performance can be limited by large increases in ventilatory resistive or elastic work. However, the increase in airways resistance caused by ozone exposure is small, and lung compliance is not significantly altered, so that the reduction in exercise performance cannot be attributed to increased ventilatory work. There is no evidence that ozone alters cardiac output or maximal heart rate. Because ozone is oedemagenic, impaired diffusion of oxygen across the alveolocapillary membrane could result from ozone exposure. However, relative to breathing clean air, 0.18 p.p.m. ozone caused no alterations in arterial oxygen saturation in highly trained runners who were susceptible to mild exercised-induced hypoxaemia. Thus none of the major physiological systems responsible for oxygen delivery during exercise appears to be compromised by ozone exposure. Adams (1987) recently reviewed the effects of prior ozone exposure on exercise performance, and concluded that ozone-induced decrements

of performance are probably not due to impaired oxygen diffusion, transport or delivery.

Nevertheless, if athletes are exposed to ozone before performance of maximum exercise tests, their performance decreases. Exercise after ozone exposure is typically accompanied by rapid shallow breathing. Ozone exposure also causes significant respiratory symptoms, most notably cough and discomfort, when taking a deep breath. Anecdotally, individuals have reported consciously modifying their breathing pattern to avoid the discomfort that is associated with large tidal volumes. Furthermore, athletes have indicated that they would be unable to perform maximally under conditions inducing such symptoms (Folinsbee & Raven, 1984; Adams, 1987). With the respiratory minute volumes typical of endurance training or competition in highly trained athletes ($70-120$ l·min^{-1}), ozone-induced symptomatic discomfort sufficient to limit exercise performance develops after $45-75$ min of exposure to ozone concentrations of around 0.18 p.p.m. As with other responses induced by ozone, there is considerable interindividual variability in the severity of symptoms; some individuals are sufficiently incapacitated to limit performance, whereas others may be unaffected.

Exposures to ozone levels as low as 0.12 p.p.m. for $1-2$ h can cause a significant reduction of lung function. The magnitude of the impairment is a function of the inhaled dose, as shown in Fig. 44.1. Increased ozone concentration, respiratory minute volume, or duration of exposure/exercise all exacerbate the loss of pulmonary function. Prolonged exposure (6.5 h) to levels as low as 80 parts per billion (p.p.b.) (common in many cities) can impair lung function (Folinsbee et al., 1988; Horstman et al., 1990), although the effect on exercise performance is uncertain. In addition to these changes in lung function, ozone also induces a hyper-responsiveness to bronchoactive drugs such as methacholine or histamine, and it may cause an athlete to become more responsive to aeroallergens. Furthermore, ozone causes an increased epithelial perme-

Table 44.1 Effects of ozone exposure on exercise performance. See Adams (1987) for details of references.

Reference	Ozone concentration (p.p.m.)	Exposure time (min)	Exercise ventilation ($l \cdot min^{-1}$)	Effects on peak $\dot{V}O_2$, endurance time, breathing pattern, lung function, etc.	Subjects
Gong et al. (1986)	0.12	60	89	Reduced (−6%) FEV_1, no change in breathing pattern, peak $\dot{V}O_2$, or endurance time	17 élite cyclists
	0.20	60	89	Reduced (−22%) FEV_1, decreased V_T, increased f_R, reduced (−30%) endurance time, reduced (−16%) peak $\dot{V}O_2$, cough and chest tightness, 5 out of 16 failed to complete 60 min at 0.20 p.p.m. ozone	
Folinsbee et al. (1986)	0.18	55−85	75−85% peak $\dot{V}O_2$	Reduced FEV_1, reduced V_T, reduced (−7%) endurance time, cough and chest discomfort after ozone exposure	Trained runners
Schelegle & Adams (1986)	0.12	30 30	55 120	1 out of 10 failed to complete last 30 min	10 highly trained cyclists
	0.18	30 30	55 120	5 out of 10 failed to complete last 30 min, reduced (−26%) endurance time at 120 $l \cdot min^{-1}$, reduced (−6%) FEV_1	
	0.24	30 30	55 120	7 out of 10 failed to complete last 30 min, reduced (−34%) endurance time at 120 $l \cdot min^{-1}$, reduced (−11%) FEV_1	
Adams & Schelegle (1983)	0.20	30 30	52 100	4 out of 10 felt they could not compete maximally under these conditions, cough and shortness of breath in 7 out of 10, reduced (−6%) FEV_1	10 trained distance runners
	0.35	30 30	52 100	4 out of 10 failed to complete at 100 $l \cdot mm^{-1}$, 9 out of 10 felt they could not compete maximally under these conditions, cough and shortness of breath in 9 out of 10, reduced (−21%) FEV_1	
Folinsbee et al. (1984)	0.21	60	90	No reduction in endurance time, reduced (−15%) FEV_1, chest discomfort and cough, 3 out of 5 competitive cyclists felt ozone would affect their performance adversely	7 trained cyclists
Foxcroft & Adams (1986)	0.35	60	60	Reduced (−6%) peak $\dot{V}O_2$, reduced (−17%) endurance time in peak $\dot{V}O_2$ test, reduced (−23%) FEV_1, reduced V_T, 5 out of 8 could not perform maximally after ozone exposure	8 trained men

FEV_1, forced expiratory volume in 1 s; V_T tidal volume; f_R, respiratory frequency.

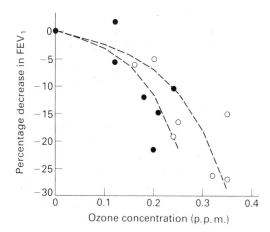

Fig. 44.1 Percentage decrease in lung function (forced expiratory volume in 1 s, FEV$_1$) after 1 h of continuous exercise exposure to 0.12–0.35 p.p.m. ozone. Response curves have been estimated for two exercise intensities, based on respiratory minute volumes of 60–70 l·min^{-1} (○) and 80–100 l·min^{-1} (●). Data from Avol *et al.*, 1984; Folinsbee *et al.*, 1984, 1986; Foxcroft *et al.*, 1986; Gong *et al.*, 1986; Horstman *et al.*, 1986; Schelegle *et al.*, 1986; and Brookes *et al.*, 1989; all are cited in Adams (1987).

ability and inflammation of the airways, presumably subsequent to damage to the airway epithelium.

Much of the recovery from ozone-induced lung function and respiratory symptom responses occurs within a few hours, although some minimal dysfunction may persist for up to 24 h. Respiratory discomfort and cough also persist for several hours after exposure, and indeed inflammatory responses have been observed as late as 18 h after exposure. If an individual is exposed to high concentrations (0.25–0.50 p.p.m.) of ozone on two consecutive days, the degree of pulmonary function impairment is generally larger on the second day.

Repeated exposures to ozone, whether in the laboratory or from seasonal exposure to the urban environment, is associated with a diminished responsiveness to ozone. Los Angeles residents who experience frequent exposure to ozone, especially during the summer months, experience fewer symptoms and less impairment of lung function from ozone in the autumn than in the spring (Linn *et al.*, 1988). Anec-

dotally, athletes training in the Los Angeles area experience more discomfort and performance impairment in the spring (the start of the smog season) than in the summer or autumn (during or after the smog season). Thus, effects on symptoms, lung function and exercise performance seem to be diminished by repeated exposure to ozone. However, the diminished acute responsiveness does not eliminate concerns regarding chronic effects of exposure.

The effects of ozone on spirometry and respiratory symptoms are at least partially blocked by the cyclo-oxygenase inhibitor indomethacin (and presumably also by aspirin and ibuprofen). However, there is no compelling evidence that dietary supplementation with vitamins C or E will alter the effects of ozone in humans.

Chronic effects of exposure to air pollution

Lung function declines with age; among other changes, vital capacity is decreased and residual volume increases. The decline in function is clearly accelerated by habitual cigarette smoking and there is some suggestion that chronic exposure to air pollution may also accelerate such changes. Thus, athletes who train in polluted ambient air on a routine basis should be concerned about the potential long-term effects of the polluted environment upon their lungs. The absence of symptoms and the normality of the immediate ventilatory response to exercise does not guarantee the absence of adverse chronic lung responses. Subtle cellular 'remodelling', including changes in the thickness of airway epithelial cells, an increased turnover and deposition of collagen, and repetitive bouts of airway inflammation may all contribute to lung 'ageing'. Studies (Detels *et al.*, 1987) comparing high oxidant pollution areas with low pollution areas of the Los Angeles basin suggest that the decline in lung function is more rapid for residents of high ozone areas, although habitual outdoor exercisers have not been specifically studied in this regard. Nevertheless, whenever possible, athletes should avoid endurance training during that part of the day when ozone levels are elevated, typically midday to late afternoon during the summer months. The most desirable training time with regard to ozone levels (usually early morning) will vary from city to city, depending upon the urban air dynamics (for example, ozone precursor emissions, climate, and the long-range transport of pollutants).

Sulphur dioxide

Sulphur dioxide is an ubiquitous air pollutant; it is emitted primarily from stationary fuel combustion sources (for example, power plants), but it is also produced by smelters, refineries and other industries. Sulphur dioxide emissions are primarily involved in the formation of acid aerosols and acid rain. Neither sulphur dioxide nor acid aerosols reach ambient levels that have a significant effect on lung function or exercise performance in normal healthy individuals.

However, sulphur dioxide causes bronchoconstriction in asthmatics. (In the context of this chapter, individuals with clinically defined, exercise-induced bronchoconstriction have been considered as 'asthmatics' even though they may not have been specifically diagnosed as such.) The proportion of athletes with asthma may be as high as 10–12%. Many such individuals require chronic or pre-exercise medication to prevent or ameliorate the onset of exercise-induced bronchoconstriction, which can be exacerbated by cold and/or dry air. These factors must be considered when assessing the potential impact of sulphur dioxide on asthmatic athletes (Horstman & Folinsbee, 1989).

Brief periods of 2–5 min exposure to sulphur dioxide levels as low as 0.40 p.p.m. will induce bronchoconstriction, wheezing and chest tightness, of sufficient magnitude to require the use of medication in some asthmatics. Concurrent exposure to cold and/or dry air can clearly exacerbate the effects of sulphur dioxide in moderately exercising asthmatics. Increased

respiratory minute volume associated with high intensity exercise may also worsen the effects of sulphur dioxide exposure, although the interaction of exercise and sulphur dioxide exposure does not appear to be simply additive. The degree of bronchoconstriction induced by exercise in asthmatics will vary with the intensity of exercise, the temperature and dryness of the air, and the current severity of the disease. With exercise levels that induce a moderate degree of exercise-induced bronchoconstriction (a doubling or tripling of airway resistance), sulphur dioxide exposure causes additional bronchoconstriction. However, if a substantial level of bronchoconstriction is induced by a bout of heavy submaximal exercise in cold air, it is not clear that the symptoms or bronchoconstriction would be quantitatively worsened by the addition of sulphur dioxide exposure. The maximum changes in forced expiratory volume (FEV_1) and airway resistance observed with sulphur dioxide exposure are similar to those observed with other non-immunological stimuli such as exercise or voluntary eucapnic hyperpnoea with cold–dry air.

A considerable quantity of inhaled sulphur dioxide can be removed in the supraglottic upper airway, the nose being a more efficient scrubber of sulphur dioxide than the mouth. During resting breathing, little, if any, sulphur dioxide reaches the trachea in nose-breathing individuals. Increased mouth breathing during heavy exercise tends to increase sulphur dioxide delivery to the lower airway, and hence increases the bronchoconstrictive response. Many asthmatics have congestive allergic rhinitis which, because of increased nasal resistance, may prompt initiation of mouth breathing at a lower exercise levels.

Exercise under cold–dry winter conditions in combination with sulphur dioxide exposure is the condition of greatest concern for the asthmatic athlete. Sulphur dioxide breathing in combination with cold–dry air causes markedly greater increases in airway resistance than sulphur dioxide breathed at room temperature or under warm humid conditions.

It is well established that breathing cool, dry air during exercise markedly enhances exercise-induced bronchoconstriction. Both airway evaporative cooling and evaporative drying of airway surface fluids (both leading to changes in osmolarity) appear to play a role in inducing a response. Drying of the upper (supraglottic) airways and a consequent reduction in the capacity to absorb sulphur dioxide may also lead to an increased penetration of sulphur dioxide to the intrathoracic airway sites where bronchoconstriction is induced.

Common asthma medications (approved by the International Olympic Committee) such as sodium cromoglycate and β_2-sympathomimetics (salbutamol, terbutaline) inhibit the effects of sulphur dioxide on airway resistance in a dose-dependent manner. Sulphur dioxide-induced bronchoconstriction is often self-limiting, and recovery is usually spontaneous in individuals with mild asthma. Recovery generally occurs within 30–60 min. Subsequent sulphur dioxide exposures within about 3 h are typically associated with lessened symptoms and functional effects. Therefore, the effects of sulphur dioxide on performance could be diminished by modest sulphur dioxide-induced bronchoconstriction during precompetition warm-up. Any 'refractory period' persists for less than 6 h. However, the use of approved medication to prevent exercised-induced bronchoconstriction seems a more sensible and effective prophylactic approach. In some asthmatics, sulphur dioxide may induce sufficient wheezing and chest discomfort that discontinuation of exercise and treatment with inhaled bronchodilators is necessary. The effects of repeated ambient sulphur dioxide exposure on the long-term severity of asthma has yet to be studied adequately.

Acid aerosols

In the atmosphere, sulphur oxides, mainly sulphur dioxide, can be converted to aerosols of sulphuric acid (and hence to acid rain). At currently encountered ambient levels, there is no reason to suspect that acid aerosols will have any impact on performance, even in asthmatics (who are considerably more responsive to inhaled acids than non-asthmatics).

Nitrogen dioxide

Nitrogen dioxide is one of the precursors of ambient ozone, and as such is present in varying amounts in oxidant atmospheres. Even at the highest ambient levels, nitrogen dioxide causes no known acute effects in normal healthy adults. However, there is some suggestion that quite low levels of nitrogen dioxide (0.2–0.5 p.p.m.) may cause an increase of airway responsiveness in asthmatics. If this is true, then exposure of asthmatic athletes to ambient air containing a combination of nitrogen dioxide and sulphur dioxide or nitrogen dioxide and ozone, could result in greater changes in lung function than with exposure to either sulphur dioxide or ozone alone.

Carbon monoxide

Carbon monoxide (CO) is a commonly occurring air pollutant which can have a substantial effect on human performance by reducing maximal oxygen intake (Horvath, 1981; Folinsbee & Raven, 1984). Carbon monoxide binds reversibly with haemoglobin to form carboxyhaemoglobin (COHb). The sites on the haemoglobin molecule occupied by carbon monoxide can no longer transport oxygen to the tissues; a COHb level of 5% translates to a 5% loss in oxygen-carrying capacity. The presence of increased COHb levels also causes a shift in the haemoglobin–oxygen dissociation curve that interferes with the unloading of oxygen at the tissue level.

Carbon monoxide exposure occurs in urban areas (especially close to roadways), in smoke-filled rooms, and in poorly ventilated areas contaminated by combustion sources (for example, parking garages and traffic tunnels). Although carbon monoxide is also produced endogenously by the degradation of haemo-globin, COHb levels are normally less than 1% in non-smokers.

Because of the high affinity of carbon mono-xide for haemoglobin, the clearance of carbon monoxide from the blood is slow, with a half-time of 2–4 h. Carbon dioxide can accumulate in the blood as a result of prolonged exposure to low concentrations or brief exposure to high concentrations of the gas. For example, an hour of training in heavy traffic (40–50 p.p.m. carbon monoxide) could raise COHb levels to above 5%. Once COHb is elevated, exposure to rela-tively low levels of carbon monoxide (25 p.p.m.) will slow the subsequent clearance of carbon monoxide from the blood. Thus exposure to carbon monoxide sources should be avoided for an extended period before endurance competition.

A 10% increase in COHb results in an ap-proximate 10% decrease in maximal oxygen intake in non-smokers at sea level. Although the relationship between exercise performance decrements and COHb levels is essentially linear (Fig. 44.2), no statistically significant ef-fects on exercise performance have been ob-served below about 4% COHb. Carbon monoxide reduces peak $\dot{V}_{O_2}$ primarily by reducing the oxygen-carrying capacity of the blood: maximal cardiac output is not appreci-ably altered. Although significant reductions in peak $\dot{V}_{O_2}$ occur, moderate submaximal exercise performance (30–60% of maximum) is not impaired below COHb levels of 15%, because a compensatory increase in cardiac output main-tains tissue oxygen delivery. However, as the exercise intensity is increased to the levels sustained in endurance events (75–95% of maximum), the cardiovascular system be-comes unable to compensate for the reduced oxygen-carrying capacity.

Both altitude exposure and carbon monoxide have the potential to produce tissue hypoxia, at altitude because of a decreased saturation of haemoglobin due to a reduced partial pressure of inspired oxygen, and in carbon monoxide exposure by blocking the oxygen transport sites

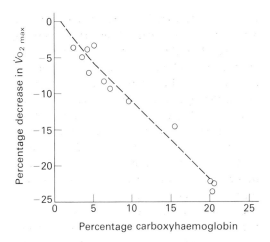

Fig. 44.2 Effect of increased carboxyhaemoglobin (COHb) level on $\dot{V}_{O_2\,max}$ in healthy men. The dashed line is the linear regression from 5% to 20% COHb; the line was adjusted below 5% COHb to intersect the abscissa at 0.7% COHb, the mean resting level of COHb in unexposed non-smokers. Data from Ekblom *et al.*, 1972; Horvath *et al.*, 1975; Pirnay *et al.*, 1971; Vogel *et al*, 1972a; 1972b; and Raven *et al.*, 1974; all are cited in Folinsbee & Raven (1984). Additional data from Weisser *et al.* (1979) and Horvath *et al.* (1988).

on the haemoglobin molecule. However, in moderate altitude residents, the reductions in peak $\dot{V}_{O_2}$ after carbon monoxide exposure are similar to those seen at sea level, provided that COHb levels are below 6%. At moderate alti-tudes and with moderate increases to COHb, altitude and carbon monoxide appear to cause reductions in peak $\dot{V}_{O_2}$ by independent and non-additive mechanisms. However, at higher altitudes and/or higher carbon monoxide levels, hypoxiasensitive tissues may be affected by a combined response to carbon monoxide and altitude. Such effects may have influenced the outcome of past mountaineering and polar expeditions (Folinsbee, 1990a; 1990b).

Summary

Three major air pollutants are of concern for endurance athletes: ozone, carbon monoxide and, for asthmatics, sulphur dioxide. Exposure to high levels of vehicle exhaust fumes or other sources of carbon monoxide should be avoided for at least 4 h before competition, to prevent any potential reduction in $\dot{V}o_2$ max. Asthmatic athletes should also avoid training near sources of sulphur dioxide, because even brief exposures to this gas may cause bronchoconstriction, wheezing and chest discomfort; such individuals should use an approved prophylactic bronchodilator medication to avoid impairment of performance. Ozone exposure may impair the performance of healthy individuals, especially in longer duration events such as running or cycling road races. Symptoms that limit performance may be reduced by several days of training in an oxidant-polluted area before competition. Anti-inflammatory medication may also be beneficial to the ozone-exposed competitor, although recommended doses have not been established. Although the long-term consequences of repeatedly exercising in polluted air are not yet clearly established, the prudent athlete will avoid routine training under such conditions.

References

Adams, W.C. (1987) Effects of ozone exposure at ambient air pollution episode levels on exercise performance. *Sports Med.* **4**, 395−424.

Brookes, J., Adams, W.C. & Schelegle, E.S. (1989) 0.35 ppm O_3 exposure induces hyperresponsiveness on 24-h re-exposure to 0.20 ppm O_3. *J. Appl. Physiol.* **66**, 2756−2762.

Detels, R., Tashkin, D.P., Sayre, J.W. *et al.* (1987) Lung function changes associated with chronic exposure to photochemical oxidants — a cohort study among never smokers. *Chest* **92**, 594−603.

Folinsbee, L.J., (1990a) Discussion: exercise and the environment. In: Bouchard, C., Shephard, R.J., Stephens, T., Sutton, J.R. & McPherson, B.D. (eds) *Exercise, Fitness, and Health*, pp. 179−183. Human Kinetics, Champaign, Illinois.

Folinsbee, L.J. (1990b) Human clinical studies of sulfur dioxide. Human clinical studies of acid aerosols. Human clinical studies of ozone and other photochemical oxidants. Human clinical studies of nitrogen oxides. In: *National Acid Precipitation Assessment Program. Direct Health Effects of Air Pollutants Associated with Acid Precursor Emissions.* State of the Science/Technology Reports, Vol. 22, Washington, D.C. (in press).

Folinsbee, L.J., McDonnell, W.F. & Horstman, D.H. (1988) Pulmonary function and symptom responses after 6.6 hour exposure to 0.12 p.p.m. ozone with moderate exercise. *JAPCA* **38**, 28−35.

Folinsbee, L.J. & Raven, P.B. (1984) Exercise and air pollution. *J. Sports Sci.* **2**, 57−75.

Gong, H., Bradley, P.W., Simmons, M.S. & Tashkin, D.P. (1986) Impaired exercise performance and pulmonary function in elite cyclists during low-level ozone exposure in a hot environment. *Am. Rev. Respir. Dis.* **134**, 726−733.

Horstman, D.H. & Folinsbee, L.J. (1989) Sulfur dioxide-induced bronchoconstriction in asthmatics exposed for short durations under controlled conditions: a selected review. In: Utell, M.J. & Frank, R. (eds) *Susceptibility to Inhaled Pollutants*, pp. 195−206. ASTM Publication No. STP 1024. American Society for Testing and Materials, Philadelphia.

Horstman, D.H., Folinsbee, L.J., Ives, P.J., Abdul-Salaam, S. & McDonnell, W.F. (1990) Ozone concentration and pulmonary response relationships for 6.6-hour exposures with 5 hours of moderate exercise to 0.08, 0.10 and 0.12 ppm. *Am. Rev. Resp. Dis.* **142**, 1158−1163.

Horvath, S.M., Agnew, J.W., Wagner, J.A. & Bedi, J.F. (1988) *Maximal Aerobic Capacity at Several Ambient Concentrations of Carbon Monoxide at Several Altitudes.* Research Report No. 21. Health Effects Institute, Cambridge, Massachusetts.

Horvath, S.M. (1981) Impact of air quality in exercise performance. *Exerc. Sport Sci. Rev.* **9**, 265−296.

Linn, W., Avol, E., Shamoo, D. *et al.* (1988) Repeated laboratory ozone exposures of volunteer Los Angeles residents: an apparent seasonal variation in response. *Toxicol. Ind. Health* **4**, 505−520.

Weiser, P.C., Cropp, G.J.A., Morill, C.G., Kurt, T.L. & Dickey, D.W. (1979) *Low Level Carbon Monoxide Exposure and Work Capacity at 1600 meters.* U.S. Environmental Protection Agency Report EPA-600-1-79-037, pp. 1−24. Research Triangle Park, North Carolina.

Chapter 45

Effects of Endurance Exercise on the Immune Response

DAVID C. NIEMAN AND SANDRA L. NEHLSEN-CANNARELLA

Introduction

The immune system is comprised of two functional divisions: the innate, which acts as a first line of defence against infectious agents, and the adaptive, which, when activated, produces a specific reaction and immunological memory to each infectious agent (Male & Roitt, 1989).

The innate immune system is comprised of cells (natural killer (NK) cells and phagocytes including neutrophils, eosinophils, basophils, monocytes and macrophages) and soluble factors (acute phase proteins, complement, lysozyme and interferons). The adaptive immune system is also comprised of cells (B and T lymphocytes) and soluble factors (immuno-globulins). Significant populations of cells found in these two systems and of interest in exercise physiology are listed in Table 45.1.

Intense endurance exercise is associated with significant sympathoadrenal and corticosteroid alterations. These systems also respond to other forms of stress, and have important effects on the immune response. This chapter will summarize the immune system changes that accompany endurance exercise, their probable mechanisms, and their clinical significance. Studies utilizing exercise protocols of less than 30 min duration are not included. Several reviews of research employing maximal and short submaximal exercise protocols are available (Simon, 1984; Mackinnon & Tomasi, 1986;

Table 45.1 Characterization of major monoclonal antibodies to human lymphocyte subpopulations by cell surface structures. From Lydyard & Grossi (1989).

Cell type	Antigen cluster designation	Antibody	Normal circulating concentrations of lymphocytes (%) (mean ± s.d.)
T cells	CD5	Anti-Leu-1	72 ± 7
T cytotoxic/ suppressor cells	CD8	Anti-Leu-2a	28 ± 8
T helper/inducer cells	CD4	Anti-Leu-3a	45 ± 10
B cells	CD19	Anti-Leu-12	10 ± 5
Fc IgG receptor on NK cells and neutrophils	CD16	Anti-Leu-11a Anti-Leu-11b Anti-Leu-11c	15 ± 7
NK cells, cytotoxic T cell subsets	CD56	Anti-Leu-19	15 ± 6

Keast *et al.*, 1988; McCarthy & Dale, 1988; Mackinnon, 1989; Nieman *et al.*, 1989b).

Effects of endurance exercise on the immune system

Cells of the innate immune system

The studies summarized in Table 45.2 and Fig. 45.1 demonstrate that acute endurance exercise, especially marathon running, is associated with a significant and pronounced leucocytosis. The magnitude of the response is related to the intensity and duration of the exercise bout (for review, see McCarthy & Dale, 1988). The increase in total leucocytes is accompanied by a strong increase in granulocytes, but only a mild increase in total lymphocytes. The granulocytosis occurs primarily because of a marked increase in neutrophils, which represent over 90% of the circulating granulocytes (Dickson *et al.*, 1982). Eosinophils tend to decrease following endurance exercise, while basophils show little or no change (McCarthy & Dale, 1988; Nieman *et al.*, 1989a). Most researchers have reported that circulating monocytes also increase strongly (Dickson *et al.*, 1982; Davidson *et al.*, 1987; Nieman *et al.*, 1989a).

The total granulocyte pool is composed of circulating and marginated pools, both of approximately equal size. The marginated pool consists of granulocytes adhering to the endothelium of veins in areas of sluggish circulation or sequestered within sinusoidal circulations, as in the spleen and liver. Several factors may explain the exercise-induced increase in circulating granulocytes: (i) significant demargination, resulting from increased blood flow and a rise in plasma catecholamines; (ii) splenic contraction; (iii) reduction in postexercise plasma volume; and (iv) cortisol-induced release of granulocytes from the bone marrow.

Both catecholamine infusion and exercise-induced increased blood flow cause neutrophils to be released from the lungs, which is a major site of the large marginated pool of neutrophils (Muir *et al.*, 1984; Foster *et al.*, 1986). The spleen, which is also a major site, appears to contribute few leucocytes to the circulation in response to exercise (McCarthy & Dale, 1988). Plasma volume changes during endurance exercise are modest in most cases; values decrease about 6.5% if subjects drink no water while running a marathon under moderate environmental conditions (Davidson *et al.*, 1987), and not at all if subjects drink approximately 1 litre every hour of exercise (Nieman *et al.*, 1989a). Thus

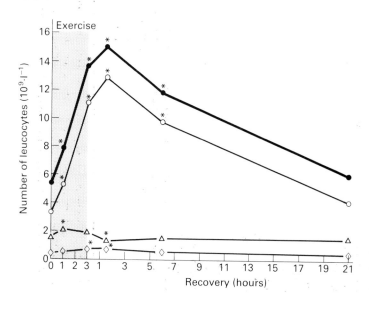

Fig. 45.1 Changes in total leucocyte count and leucocyte subset counts at rest, exercise, and throughout 21 h of recovery. Ten trained marathon runners ran for 3 h at 70% $\dot{V}o_{2\,max}$ in a laboratory setting. Repeated measures ANOVA showed significant within-subjects effects for each variable. *, $p < 0.05$, significant change from baseline value. ●, Total leucocytes; ○, granulocytes; △, lymphocytes; ◇, monocytes. From Nieman *et al.* (1989a).

Table 45.2 Review of the literature on endurance exercise and acute immune system changes. Data are expressed as the percentage change in mean circulating numbers of cells (before and 0–30 min after exercise).

	Davidson et al. (1987)	Dickson et al. (1982)	Eskola et al. (1978)	Gmünder et al. (1988)	Hanson & Flaherty (1981)	Moorthy & Zimmerman (1978)	Nieman et al. (1989a); Berk et al. (1990)	Oshida et al. (1988)	Pedersen et al. (1988); Tvede et al. (1989)	Wells et al. (1982)
No. of subjects	90	18	8	7	6	11	10	11	6–16	10
Subject description	Trained	Trained	Trained	Trained	Trained	Trained	Trained	5 Untrained 6 Trained	Untrained	Trained
Mode of exercise	Running	Running	Running	Running	Running	Running	Running	Cycling	Cycling	Running
Distance or time	42.2 km	56 km	42.2 km	42.2 km	12.8 km	32.4 km	37.2 km	2 h	60 min	42.2 km
Total leucocytes	265*	175*	174*	184*	33 (n.s.)	226*	154*	Increased*	73*	Increased*
Granulocytes	434*	262*		349*	29 (n.s.)	375*	236*	Increased*	52*	Increased*
Monocytes	150*	222*				−11% (n.s.)	67*			
Lymphocytes	25*	−26*	n.c.	n.c.	24 (n.s.)	38*	19 (n.s.)	Increased*	125*	Increased (n.s.)
Lymphocyte function[+]	−26*		Decreased	−30–99*		n.c.		Decreased*		
B cells				Decreased*	25 (n.s.)	85*	17*	n.c.	62*	
T cells				n.c.	24 (n.s.)	29 (n.s.)	6 (n.s.)	Increased	58*	
T helper				n.c.			7 (n.s.)	n.c.	40*	
T suppressor				n.c.			16 (n.s.)	Increased*	51*	
NK cells (CD16)							42 (n.s.)		369*	
NK cell activity (25:1 or 50:1 E:T)							10 (n.s.)		56*	15 (n.s.)
Cortisol			93%	Increased*		135*	59*		25*	
Adrenaline				Increased*			156*		689*	
Noradrenaline				Increased*			102*		1450*	
Other information	Plasma volume decreased 6.5%	Band cells increased sharply	Antibody formation to tetanus toxoid unimpaired	T helper cells rose after 2 days of recovery	Activity of K lymphocytes increased for 24 h	Rise in cortisol correlated with rise in WBC	NK cell activity depressed 24% at 1.5 h of recovery	Trained and untrained did not differ	All values normal by 24 h but not at 2 h of recovery	Total WBC count increased at 8 h of recovery; normal by 24 h

* $p < 0.05$ (significant change in postexercise value in comparison with baseline). n.s., non-significant change (percentage change included in table for comparison); n.c., no change; blank space denotes that no information was available for that particular variable. Note: The terms 'decreased' or 'increased' are used when the percentage change could not be determined owing to the use of graphs rather than tables in the published article. E:T, effector:target cells; NK, natural killer; WBC, white blood cells. [+] Mitogen stimulation.

haemoconcentration cannot account for the 236–434% increase in granulocytes that occurs following marathon running events (Table 45.2). Circulating numbers of band cells (immature neutrophils from the bone marrow) increase strongly following endurance exercise, their release being promoted by the presence of cortisol (Moorthy & Zimmerman, 1978; Dickson et al., 1982; MaCarthy & Dale, 1988). In a study by Nieman et al. (unpublished data; 1989a), the number of band cells increased from $0.1 \times 10^9 \cdot l^{-1}$ to $1.8 \times 10^9 \cdot l^{-1}$ (1700% increase) after 6 h of recovery from 3 h of intense running, the final count representing approximately 20% of the total circulating granulocytes.

NK cells, first discovered in the early 1970s, are unique in that they express spontaneous cytolytic activity against a variety of tumour and virus-infected cells (Male & Roitt, 1989). Unlike T lymphocytes, NK cells do not require the involvement of major histocompatibility antigens to initiate cytotoxicity. NK cells account for about 15% of mononuclear cells in the peripheral blood; they respond rapidly to foreign materials, and initially control them until the antigen-specific immune system begins to respond. Interest in NK cells and their activity has grown, because they represent a major first-line defence system against viral infection. NK activity is decreased in a number of conditions associated with reduced immuno-surveillance (Mackinnon, 1989).

Nearly all studies to date have measured the acute effect of short-term submaximal or graded maximal exercise on NK cell activity and numbers (Brahmi et al., 1985; Deuster et al., 1988; Pedersen et al., 1988; Fiatarone et al., 1989). This type of physical activity is associated with a considerable increase in NK cell number and activity immediately following exercise. Few researchers have reported changes in NK cell number and activity following long endurance exercise (Mackinnon et al., 1988; Berk et al., 1990) or endurance training. Pedersen et al. (1989) have reported increased levels of NK cell activity at rest in trained vs. untrained males.

In randomized controlled studies with both animal and human models, 6–15 weeks of moderate exercise training has been associated with a considerable increase in resting NK cell activity (Fernandez et al., 1985; Nieman et al., 1990b).

Berk et al. (1990) found a significant 30.7% decrease in total NK activity in marathoners 1.5 h following a 3-h run; this was negatively correlated with the elevation of cortisol concentration 5 min after exercise (Table 45.3). In agreement with these findings, other researchers have shown that cortisol inhibits NK activity (Gatti et al., 1987). Prostaglandins released by monocytes may also decrease NK cell activity (Pedersen et al., 1988). The decrease in NK activity was coincident with a 50% decrease in lymphocytes bearing the surface antigen CD16 (see Table 45.1 for an explanation of antigen cluster designations). No change occurred, however, in the number of lymphocytes bearing the surface antigen CD56. No increase in NK activity was seen immediately following the 3-h run, which contrasts with findings in short-term submaximal or graded maximal exercise.

Mackinnon et al. (1988) have reported similar findings. Seven competitive cyclists rode cycle ergometers for 2 h at approximately 75% $\dot{V}o_{2\,max}$. NK activity was not elevated immediately following exercise. Although total NK activity decreased 24% by 1 h of recovery, this was accompanied by a 50% decrease in the percentage of lymphocytes exhibiting the CD16 antigen. When adjusted to a 'per CD16 cell' basis, an absolute increase of 40% in cytotoxic activity was described.

Adjusting for the decrease in number of lymphocytes exhibiting the CD16 antigen alone may lead to inappropriate conclusions as to the effect of exercise on NK activity. The antigen CD56 may be more specific in identifying the most effective lymphocyte subpopulation with NK activity. Table 45.3 suggests that the decrease in NK cell activity following long endurance exercise is not due to a redistribution of blood lymphocytes with the antigen CD56 to

Table 45.3 Lymphocyte count, spontaneous blastogenesis ratio, natural killer (NK) cells and NK activity before, during and after a 3-h treadmill run. From Berk *et al.* (1990) and Nieman *et al.* (1989a).

Variable	Baseline	Exercise (1-h exercise)	Recovery 1 (5-min post)	Recovery 2 (1.5-h post)	Recovery 3 (6-h post)	Recovery 4 (21-h post)	F-ratio	p-value
Lymphocyte count ($10^9 \cdot l^{-1}$)	1.61 ± 0.09	$2.09 \pm 0.24^*$	1.88 ± 0.16	$1.31 \pm 0.09^*$	1.48 ± 0.11	1.49 ± 0.09	5.8	<0.001
Spontaneous blastogenesis ratio	1.19 ± 0.13	1.42 ± 0.15	1.29 ± 0.14	$1.98 \pm 0.31^*$	1.70 ± 0.29	$1.86 \pm 0.19^\dagger$	4.5	0.002
NK activity (%) (25:1 E:T)	56.1 ± 3.4	65.0 ± 4.5	61.6 ± 3.4	$38.9 \pm 5.1^*$	46.3 ± 3.4	48.9 ± 4.4	6.4	<0.001
NK cell count (CD16) ($10^9 \cdot l^{-1}$)	0.24 ± 0.03	0.35 ± 0.06	0.34 ± 0.07	$0.12 \pm 0.02^\ddagger$	$0.13 \pm 0.02^\ddagger$	$0.15 \pm 0.02^\ddagger$	12.3	0.008
NK cells, cytotoxic T cell subsets (CD56) ($10^9 \cdot l^{-1}$)	0.14 ± 0.03	$0.22 \pm 0.05^*$	$0.30 \pm 0.08^*$	0.17 ± 0.03	0.10 ± 0.02	0.18 ± 0.03	13.0	0.007

Values are mean ± s.e.m.; F-ratio and p-value represent within-subject effects, repeated measures ANOVA.
E:T, effector:target cells. * $p < 0.05$, † $p < 0.01$, ‡ $p < 0.001$, contrast with baseline.

peripheral tissues. Rather, a suppression in the activity of circulating NK cells and cytotoxic T cell subsets appears to occur within 1.5 h following endurance exercise, and these changes may persist for several hours. Pedersen *et al.* (1988) have also concluded that the decrease in NK activity 2 h after 60 min of intense cycling is not due to a decrease in the size of the NK cell circulating pool.

Some types of NK cells, specifically those bearing the CD16 antigen, appear to leave the circulation following long endurance exercise. This redistribution may be promoted by cortisol, with NK cells redirected to lymphoid tissues to assist in non-specific immune responses to antigens introduced during the exercise bout. Some NK cells may travel to areas of damaged muscle cells. Muscle cell injury occurs following marathon running. Stauber *et al.* (1988) have reported that NK cells are present in the injured tissue and may assist in the process of repair.

Soluble factors of the innate immune system

Severe exertion or heavy exercise training is associated with muscle cell damage and local inflammation (Armstrong, 1986). Indicators of muscle cell leakage and of haemolysis remain elevated in the plasma for up to 7 days following a marathon race (Lijnen *et al.*, 1988). The acute phase reaction (1–4 days after the event) is similar to that seen during a septic or aseptic inflammatory response (Liesen *et al.*, 1977; Dufaux *et al.*, 1984; Taylor *et al.*, 1987), with an accompanying elevation of C-reactive protein (CRP). CRP can activate the complement system and initiate the cell-damaging and inflammatory reactions necessary for resolution and repair processes. Other plasma enzyme systems are also important in mediating the inflammatory response and the resolution of tissue damage.

The tissue macrophage activity of athletes is increased following endurance running (Fehr *et al.*, 1989). The degenerative changes that occur in the muscles following long endurance exercise are accompanied by an invasion of macrophages and other cells of the immune system which assist in the regeneration process (Michna, 1988). Macrophages have surface receptors which allow them to react non-specifically to a variety of substances, a process enhanced by the presence of opsonins (primarily complement and antibody). Complement is a complex of humoral factors that can augment non-specific immunity (Male & Roitt, 1989). The precise mechanism by which autologous tissue products may become coated with opsonins and be engulfed by macrophages and neutrophils is still undetermined (Dufaux & Order, 1989b).

Hanson and Flaherty (1981) reported that resting levels of serum complement C3 and C4 were not significantly altered in six trained males 10 min after running 12.8 km at training pace (70–75% of $\dot{V}o_{2\,max}$). However, Nieman *et al.* (unpublished data; 1989a) showed that serum complement C3 levels exhibited significant within-subject effects over time in 10 marathoners who ran for 3 h at marathon race pace (Fig. 45.2). Serum complement C3 and C4 levels reached their lowest points at 1.5 h of recovery (down 11.2% and 9.8%, respectively, vs. baseline), slowly rising to baseline levels by 21 h of recovery. Dufaux and Order (1989a) have provided evidence for complement activation after 2.5 h of running. Together, these data suggest that serum complement may contribute to extravascular pools during recovery from marathon running, assisting macrophages in the resolution and repair process of injured muscle cells.

Complement C3 and C4 levels are significantly lower in marathoners vs. age-matched, sedentary controls during rest, graded maximal exercise, and at 45 min of recovery (Nieman *et al.*, 1989c). The possibility exists that repeated long distance running may overload the liver's ability to produce adequate levels of complement to amplify the non-specific immune response toward muscle cell inflammation.

Interferons comprise a group of proteins that

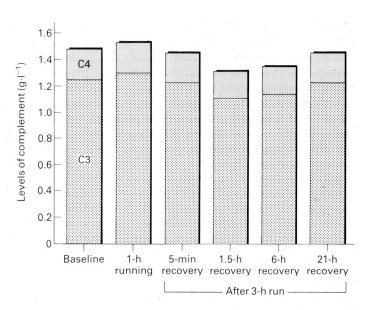

Fig. 45.2 Changes in complement C3 and C4 (same subjects and study as described in Fig. 45.1). C3 and C4 tended to show within-subject effects over time, using repeated measures ANOVA [$F(5, 35) = 2.38$, $p = 0.05$], [$F(5, 45) = 2.78$, $p = 0.14$] respectively, despite no change in plasma volume [$F(5, 45) = 0.50$, $p = 0.78$]. C3 and C4 tended to decrease during recovery, reaching their lowest points at 1.5 h of recovery (11.2% and 9.8% vs. baseline), rising slowly to baseline levels by 21 h of recovery.

are important in viral infections. One group of interferons is produced in cells which have become virally infected; another type is released by certain activated T cells (Male & Roitt, 1989). Interferons induce a state of antiviral resistance in uninfected tissue cells, and are produced very early in infection, representing a first line of resistance against many viruses. Plasma α-interferon activity is significantly increased following 1 h of cycling at 70% $\dot{V}o_{2\,max}$ (Viti *et al.*, 1985). The proteins and enzymes released by injured muscle and connective tissues may potentiate the production of α-interferon.

Cells of the adaptive immune system

In response to acute endurance exercise, the number of circulating lymphocytes increases moderately (Moorthy & Zimmerman, 1978; Davidson *et al.*, 1987; Oshida *et al.*, 1988) or remains unchanged (Eskola *et al.*, 1978; Gmünder *et al.*, 1988) (see Table 45.2). Dickson *et al.* (1982) reported a 26% decrease in lymphocyte count after a 56-km run. However, blood samples in this study were collected 30 min following exercise, in contrast to the 0–10 min adopted by the other researchers listed (see list

in Table 45.2). The timing of blood sampling is very important, because lymphocytes leave the circulation rapidly during recovery (see below).

Pedersen *et al.* (1988) and Tvede *et al.* (1989) reported an unusually strong lymphocytosis (125%) immediately after 60 min of cycling at 75% $\dot{V}o_{2\,max}$ in untrained male medical students (Table 45.2). These results are similar to those of others who have utilized graded maximal or short-term submaximal exercise protocols. Immediately following such exercise, a transient mild leucocytosis but strong lymphocytosis (usually 60–130%) is seen (Hedfors *et al.*, 1983; Landmann *et al.*, 1984; Deuster *et al.*, 1988; Lewicki *et al.*, 1988). Thus intense cycling for 1 h may result in immune system changes that are more similar to short-term submaximal and maximal exercise than to prolonged endurance exercise. Alternatively, immune system changes may differ depending on the mode of exercise. Data from Oshida *et al.* (1988) showed that 2 h of cycling resulted in a stronger lymphocytosis (about 60%) than occurs during distance running (see Table 45.2). Data from Nieman *et al.* (1989a) suggest that a significant but moderate lymphocytosis (31%) occurs during the first hour of endurance running, a much smaller response than reported by Pedersen *et al.* (1988) and Tvede *et al.* (1989) after 1 h of cycling.

Catecholamines rise early during endurance exercise. They are associated with a mild leucocytosis but a strong and rapid lymphocytosis; the lymphocytes are probably being supplied by several storage sites and walls of high endothelial venules (Crary *et al.*, 1983). Cortisol, which is increased by 59–135% (see Table 45.2) following exhaustive endurance exercise, induces a leucocytosis while inhibiting the entry of lymphocytes into the circulation and facilitating their egress to peripheral tissues (Yu *et al.*, 1977; Robertson *et al.*, 1981; McCarthy & Dale, 1988; Nieman *et al.*, 1989a). Immediately after prolonged endurance running, the effects of cortisol may predominate, an event that may explain the strong leucocytosis, but the mild or absent lymphocytosis.

Several researchers have reported that from 30 min to 3 h following long endurance exercise, a significant lymphocytopaenia is observed (Dickson *et al.*, 1982; Davidson *et al.*, 1987; Pedersen *et al.*, 1988; Nieman *et al.*, 1989a; Tvede *et al.*, 1989). The decrease in lymphocyte count is moderate (about 20–25%), and short lived, with counts returning to normal after 6 h of recovery (Nieman *et al.*, 1989a). Cortisol which stays elevated for at least 1.5 h following prolonged endurance exercise (Nieman *et al.*, 1989a) may reduce circulating lymophocytes by redirecting them to peripheral tissues (Cupps & Fauci, 1982). Data from Stauber *et al.* (1988) and Michna (1988) suggest that lymphocytes invade injured muscle cell areas to aid in the process of repair. Lymphocytes may also sequester in lymphoid and other peripheral tissue areas to improve their likelihood of being exposed to antigen-presenting cells (macrophages, dendritic cells, Langerhans' cells, fibroblasts) that process various antigens introduced into the body during an exercise bout.

Few researchers have reported changes in lymphocyte subpopulations following acute endurance exercise (see Table 45.2). Immediately after endurance running, little or no change is seen in circulating T and NK cell counts, but there is a moderate increase in B cells (Moorthy & Zimmerman, 1978; Hanson & Flaherty, 1981; Gmünder *et al.*, 1988; Nieman *et al.*, 1989a). This is in contrast to the situation immediately after endurance cycling, when large increases are seen in T cytotoxic/suppressor cells and NK cells (Oshida *et al.*, 1988; Pedersen *et al.*, 1988; Tvede *et al.*, 1989).

Figure 45.3 suggests that during the first several hours following intensive endurance running, the decline in circulating lymphocytes is best explained by concomitant decreases in T cytotoxic/suppressor cells and NK cells (Nieman *et al.*, 1989a). Both of these types of cells are involved in cell-mediated cytotoxicity, possessing the ability to lyse target cells (usually virus-infected autologous cells). Macrophages, which also play a central role in cell-mediated immunity, are more active in the connective tissue of athletes following an intense 15-km run (Fehr *et al.*, 1989). The activity of plasma interleukin-1 (Cannon *et al.*, 1986) and interferon (Viti *et al.*, 1985) also increases significantly following acute endurance exercise. Interleukin-1 is produced by many cell types to help activate T cells, NK cells and macrophages. Interferon is produced by activated T cells and NK cells, and plays a critical role in the antigen-presenting function of macrophages and dendritic cells (Feldmann & Male, 1989). Together, these results suggest that cell-mediated immunity is increased in the peripheral tissues of athletes following acute endurance exercise. Proteins and enzymes released by injured muscle and connective tissues may play a role in stimulating the increased cell-mediated immune activity.

An increased ratio of helper to suppressor T cells (H:S ratio) is important in predicting a favourable immune response. There are significant decreases in the H:S ratio immediately after graded maximal or short-term submaximal exercise (Hedfors *et al.*, 1983; Landmann *et al.*, 1984; Brahmi *et al.*, 1985; Lewicki *et al.*, 1988) and after 1–2 h of endurance cycling (Oshida *et al.*, 1988; Pedersen *et al.*, 1988), but the H:S ratio is unchanged following endurance

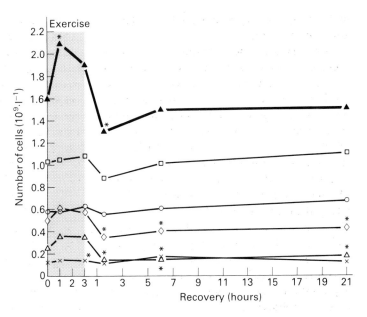

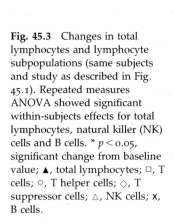

Fig. 45.3 Changes in total lymphocytes and lymphocyte subpopulations (same subjects and study as described in Fig. 45.1). Repeated measures ANOVA showed significant within-subjects effects for total lymphocytes, natural killer (NK) cells and B cells. * $p < 0.05$, significant change from baseline value; ▲, total lymphocytes; □, T cells; ○, T helper cells; ◇, T suppressor cells; △, NK cells; ×, B cells.

running (Gmünder *et al.*, 1988; Nieman *et al.*, 1989a). The H:S ratio tends to be elevated during recovery (up to 24 h) from all forms of exercise (Brahmi *et al.*, 1985; Pedersen *et al.*, 1988; Nieman *et al.*, 1989a). Following endurance running, the increase in H:S ratio appears to be brought about by a significant decrease in the number of suppressor T cells (see Fig. 45.3), perhaps induced by elevated cortisol levels.

Lymphocyte responsiveness to mitogen stimulation is decreased immediately after both short-term exercise (Robertson *et al.*, 1981; Hedfors *et al.*, 1983; Brahmi *et al.*, 1985) and prolonged endurance exercise (Eskola *et al.*, 1978; Gmünder *et al.*, 1988; Oshida *et al.*, 1988; Mahan & Young, 1989; Tvede *et al.*, 1989; but not Moorthy & Zimmerman, 1978) (see Table 45.2). The decrease in lymphocyte transformation lasts for several hours following exhaustive endurance exercise (Eskola *et al.*, 1978). In animals, endurance training is also associated with a significant decrease in mitogen-induced lymphocyte proliferation (Hoffman-Goetz *et al.*, 1986; Pahlavani *et al.*, 1988). The mechanism by which acute and chronic endurance exercise leads to a reduction in lymphocyte plastogenesis may involve both

a suppression by macrophage-secreted prostaglandin E_2 and increased activity of T suppressor cells (Mahan & Young, 1989). Each of these researchers measured lymphocyte function using mitogen stimulation (either phytohaemagglutinin or concanavalin A) which is an in vitro procedure. Mitogen stimulation of lymphocytes in vitro is believed to mimic events that occur after antigen stimulation of lymphocytes in vivo.

Spontaneous blastogenesis (SB) activity is also utilized to detect specific and non-specific in vivo lymphocyte activation by alloantigens, mitogens, cytokines, hormones or neuropeptides. SB activity is assayed by incubating blood lymphocytes with tritiated thymidine in tissue culture. The quantity of radionucleotide uptake is directly correlated with the level of activation. SB ratios are calculated by dividing the experimental counts per minute by a standard. Table 45.3 summarizes changes in the SB ratio in a group of 10 marathoners who ran for 3 h at 70% $\dot{V}o_{2\,max}$ (Nieman *et al.*, 1989a). In contrast with results from studies using mitogen stimulation, spontaneous in vivo lymphocyte activation was increased during recovery, with no change experienced immediately following exercise. Further research is needed to delineate differences between mitogen stimulation and SB, and to assign clinical significance to these results.

Few researchers have measured the effect of prolonged endurance exercise training on either resting immune system values or the changes induced by short-term exercise. Changes in immune system values in response to 2 h of cycling at 60% $\dot{V}_{O_2 max}$ vary little between untrained and trained individuals (Oshida *et al.*, 1988). Figure 45.4 compares immune system changes in six marathon runners vs. six untrained, age-matched control subjects in response to a graded maximal exercise test (Balke protocol) (Nieman *et al.*, 1989c; unpublished data). Changes in total leucocytes, lymphocytes, T cells and B cells were remarkably

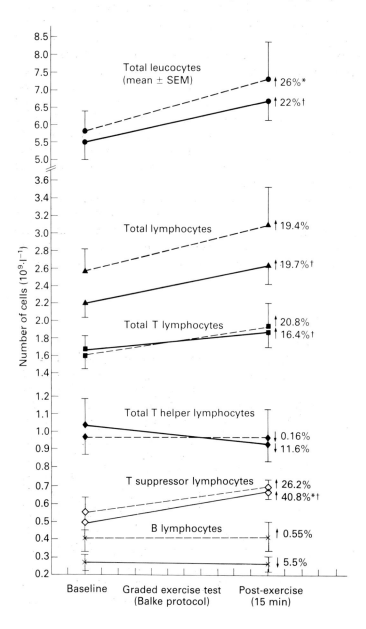

Fig. 45.4 Changes in total leucocytes, lymphocytes and lymphocyte subpopulations in six athletes (——) and six non-athletes (− − −) in response to a maximal graded exercise test using the Balke protocol. Blood samples were collected 10 min before exercise and 15 min after maximal exertion. * $p < 0.05$, significant change from baseline value within the group; † $p < 0.05$, significant change from baseline for both groups combined. ●, Total leucocytes; ▲, total lymphocytes; ■, total T lymphocytes; ◆, total T helper lymphocytes; ◇, total T suppressor lymphocytes; x, total B lymphocytes.

similar between the two groups, as reported by others (Brahmi *et al.*, 1985; Deuster *et al.*, 1988). The decrease in T helper cells tended to be greater in the athletes (37% decrease in the H:S ratio in contrast to 21% for the non-athletes). NK cells increased by about 120% in both groups. Changes in immunoglobulins, β-endorphin, cortisol, adrenocorticotrophic hormone and catecholamines were the same for both groups (Nieman *et al.*, 1989c). The resting values for total leucocytes and lymphocytes tended to be somewhat lower in the athletes, as reported by other researchers (Green *et al.*, 1981; Davidson *et al.*, 1987; Deuster *et al.*, 1988; McCarthy & Dale, 1988).

Soluble factors of the adaptive immune system

Relatively few authors have described exercise-induced changes in serum and salivary immunoglobulin levels (Table 45.4). Hanson and Flaherty (1981) studied serum immunoglobulins in six male runners who ran 13 km at 72% $\dot{V}o_{2\,max}$. Values did not rise significantly above baseline levels at 10 min postexercise. However, IgM did rise by 34%, and was still elevated by 29% the next morning, although these changes were not statistically significant. Changes in plasma volume were not reported.

Changes in serum immunoglobulins were measured in 10 experienced marathoners who exercised for 3 h at marathon race pace (Nieman & Nehlsen-Cannarella, 1991). Blood samples were collected at baseline, after 1 h of exercise, and after 5 min, 1.5 h, 6 h, and 21 h of recovery (Fig. 45.5). IgM ($p = 0.09$) and IgG ($p = 0.07$), but not IgA ($p = 0.28$) tended to show within-subject effects over time despite the absence of change in plasma volume. IgG tended to decrease during recovery, reaching its lowest point (7.6% below baseline) at 1.5 h of recovery, before rising slowly to baseline by 21 h of recovery. Mean serum IgA values followed a similar pattern, but variance between subjects was greater. IgM rose by 7.2% during exercise, returning to baseline levels throughout recovery.

Israel *et al.* (1982) have reported changes in serum immunoglobulins in athletes running 45 or 75 km at high intensity (Table 45.4). Serum immunoglobins were decreased 10–28% by 24 h of recovery, stayed low for an additional

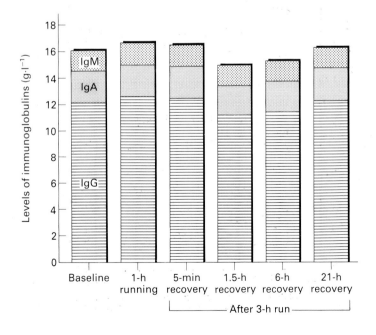

Fig. 45.5 Changes in serum immunoglobulins (same subjects and study as described in Fig. 45.1). IgG and IgM tended to show within-subject effects over time, using repeated measures ANOVA [$F(5, 45) = 4.18$, $p = 0.07$], [($F(5, 35) = 2.07$, $p = 0.09$]. IgG tended to decrease during recovery, reaching its lowest point at 1.5 h of recovery (down 7.6% vs. baseline). IgM rose 7.2% ($p < 0.05$) during exercise and then fell to baseline levels throughout recovery.

Table 45.4 Literature summary of percentage changes of serum immunoglobulin (Ig) in response to submaximal exercise.

Reference	No. of subjects	Mode of exercise	Change in plasma volume	Workload/distance	% change Ig (before vs. within 15-min postexercise)			% change Ig (before vs. 18–25-h postexercise)		
					IgM	IgG	IgA	IgM	IgG	IgA
<40-km exertion										
Hanson & Flaherty (1981)	6	Running		12.8 km, 72% $\dot{V}O_{2\,max}$	34	2	2	29	−1	−5
Nieman & Nehlsen-Cannarella (1991)	10	Running	n.c.	37.2 km, 70% $\dot{V}O_{2\,max}$	5	3	0.4	1	1	2
>40-km exertion										
Israel et al. (1982)	10	Running		45 km	−28	−1	−21*	−24	−18*	−20
Israel et al. (1982)	10	Running		75 km	−20	−4	−17	−10	−22*	−28
Poortmans & Haralambie (1979)	7	Running	n.c.	100 km		7*	1		−4	−12

* $p < 0.05$.

n.c., no reported change; blank space denotes that no information was available.

24 h, and then rose slowly to baseline levels by the fourth day of recovery. Poortmans and Haralambie (1979) reported a significant 7% increase in IgG in 11 male runners 15 min after completing a 100-km run, despite the absence of change in mean plasma volume. After 18−25 h of recovery, serum IgG and IgA levels were still 4% and 12%, respectively, below baseline levels. IgM was not measured. These data suggest that intense ultramarathon exertion may be associated with a greater and more prolonged depression of serum immunoglobulins than those seen over shorter distances. IgA and IgG, immunoglobulins commonly found in airway and alveolar space secretions, may diffuse from the serum in response to microbial agents and antigens introduced into the airways during the exercise bout. In addition, natural (IgM) autoantibodies may assist macrophages in disposal of muscle cell breakdown products (Nieman & Nehlsen-Cannarella, 1991).

Tomasi et al. (1982) reported that resting salivary IgA levels were lower in élite cross-country skiers than in age-matched controls, and that IgA levels decreased further after 2−3 h of exhaustive ski competition. In a follow-up study, eight well-trained male competitive bicyclists exercised on a cycle ergometer for 2 h at 70−75% $\dot{V}o_{2\,max}$ (Mackinnon et al., 1987). In contrast to the first study, resting salivary IgA levels were no different from those found in untrained controls. However, the skiers were studied in New York during the winter and the cyclers during the summer in New Mexico. Thus, factors other than exercise training may have affected resting salivary IgA levels. Immediately after the 2 h of ergometer exercise, salivary but not nasal lavage fluid IgA decreased by an average of 65%, values returning to baseline levels at 1−24 h following exercise. Serum IgM, IgG, IgA and serum antibody titres to specific antigens were unchanged after exercise. In addition, the in vitro production of IgG and IgA by pokeweed mitogen-stimulated peripheral blood lymphocytes was unaltered following exercise.

Other researchers have also investigated the ability of B lymphocytes to produce antibodies following exertion. Eskola et al. (1978) reported that four well-trained runners who were vaccinated with tetanus toxoid 30 min after a marathon race showed a normal 14-day antibody production. This occurred despite a decrease in T lymphocyte transformation which persisted for several hours following the marathon event. Although activated T cells are important in helping B cells develop into immunoglobulin-secreting plasma cells, the transient nature of the decrease in T lymphocyte transformation following prolonged endurance exercise may mean that the longer-term in vivo antibody response is unaltered.

Cross-sectional studies suggest that resting serum immunoglobulin levels are similar in athletes and non-athletes, especially when adjusted for differences in plasma volume (Röcker et al., 1976; Nieman & Nehlsen-Cannarella, 1991). However, some élite athletes may develop low concentrations of serum and secretory immunoglobulins during the competitive season, with a possible increased risk of infection (von Weiss et al., 1985; Ricken & Kindermann, 1986). Muscular injections of immunoglobulins are useful in reducing the duration but not the incidence of infections in such individuals. Moderate exercise training (45 min of brisk walking, five sessions per week for 15 weeks), on the other hand, has been associated with a net 20% increase in serum immunoglobulins, a change that was inversely correlated with total acute upper respiratory tract symptom days (Nehlsen-Cannarella et al., 1991). These data suggest that while the combined psychosocial−physiological stress of competitive exercise training may be associated with depressed serum immunoglobulin levels in some élite athletes, moderate exercise training slightly improves serum immunoglobulin levels, with a lessened risk of infection. However, such data require confirmation, using more exacting methodologies.

Clinical significance

Much attention has recently been focused on stress, both physical and psychological, as a potent suppressor of the immune system (Graham *et al.*, 1986; Landmann *et al.*, 1984; Mackinnon & Tomasi, 1986). Athletes training for long endurance events, such as the marathon, experience repeated cycles of physical stress which can be accompanied by mental stress. Anecdotal reports from coaches have reflected a concern over an increased incidence of infectious episodes in their competitive endurance athletes (Jokl, 1974). Many athletes, however, feel that their training programmes promote resistance to upper respiratory tract infections. Nieman *et al.* (1989a) administered a questionnaire to 10 experienced marathon runners; nine out of 10 felt that their training programme during the previous 5 years had helped them to reduce the number of upper respiratory tract infections while one felt that the incidence was increased. However, seven of the 10 marathoners felt that following marathon race events, their risk of upper respiratory tract infections was increased, while three felt that their risk was the same as normal.

The influence of exercise training on resistance to infection has been investigated using animal models since the turn of the century. Cannon and Kluger (1984) concluded that moderate exercise before infection may increase resistance to infection, but that exhaustive exercise after contracting an infection may be detrimental. Nieman *et al.* (1990b), in a randomized controlled study of adult females, showed that moderate exercise training (five 45-min brisk walking sessions per week for 15 weeks) was associated with a 50% reduction in the duration of infectious episodes.

Several epidemiological reports have suggested that athletes engaging in marathon type events and/or very heavy training are at increased risk of acute respiratory infections (Jokl, 1974; Peters & Bateman, 1983; Linde, 1987; Nieman *et al.*, 1990a). In 2311 runners training for ≥97 vs. <32 km per week, the odds ratio for

upper respiratory tract infection (URI) during a 2-month period prior to the Los Angeles Marathon (LAM) was 2.0 (95% confidence interval, 1.2–3.4) (Nieman *et al.*, 1990a). Of the 1828 LAM participants without URI during the week before the race, 236 (12.9%) reported URI during the week following the LAM vs. three of 134 (2.2%) similarly experienced runners who did not participate (odds ratio = 5.9, 95% confidence interval, 1.9–18.8).

Changes in many immune system factors could be involved, but the evidence to date does not give strong support for immunosuppression following heavy exercise training or prolonged endurance events. Although serum and salivary immunoglobulins may be low in élite athletes during the competitive season, data to link these low levels of immunoglobulins to an increased risk of acute respiratory infection are unconvincing (Israel *et al.*, 1982).

Following long endurance exercise, the total number of circulating granulocytes remains significantly elevated for more than 6–12 h of recovery (Wells *et al.*, 1982; Lijnen *et al.*, 1988; Nieman *et al.*, 1989a) (see Fig. 45.1). The clinical significance is open to conjecture, but nonspecific immunity may be enhanced (McCarthy & Dale, 1988).

The postendurance exercise lymphocytopaenia probably does not last for more than 5–6 h. However, several lymphocyte subpopulation changes, primarily decreases in T cytotoxic/suppressor and NK cells, may persist for more than 21 h of recovery (see Fig. 45.3), and as a consequence cell-mediated immunity in the peripheral tissues of athletes may be increased following endurance exercise (Michna, 1988; Fehr *et al.*, 1989). Although NK activity is depressed in the circulatory compartment of the body following endurance exercise, no one has yet measured NK cell activity in peripheral lymphoid and tissue areas during recovery from such exercise. The decrease in circulatory NK activity is transitory, and Pedersen *et al.* (1989) have reported that resting NK activity in male racing cyclists is significantly greater than in sedentary controls.

There is an interesting similarity between the metabolic and immunological responses to prolonged endurance exercise and to an infectious challenge (Cannon & Kluger, 1983; Lewis et al., 1986; Schaefer et al., 1987). In both conditions, the number of circulating leucocytes increases, lymphocytopaenia occurs (especially T cells), with cells trafficking to peripheral tissues; the lymphocyte responses to phytohaemagglutinin and concanavalin A decrease, body core temperature rises, plasma levels of acute-phase proteins increase, and degranulation of neutrophils develops. These similarities suggest that endurance exercise leads to an activation of immunity. Because endurance exercise is associated with muscle cell damage and an increased intake of potential pathogens through augmented ventilation, it is logical that in preparation for such a challenge, the immune system should receive a signal from the neuroendocrine network that activates the immune system.

Why, then, do epidemiological data and clinical experience point toward an increased risk of URI in some athletes? The mass of evidence favours the view that psychosocial variables play an important role in impairing immunological competence; changes include reduced NK activity, low levels of circulating and secretory antibodies, and suppressed mitogenic responses to phytohaemagglutinin (Jemmott & Locke, 1984; Brahmi et al., 1985; Mackinnon & Tomasi, 1986; Kronfol & House, 1989). The net effect of combined psychological and physiological stress from unusually heavy endurance exercise, especially during times of competition, may lead to suppression or down-regulation of the immune system.

The increased susceptibility of some endurance athletes to infections may be better explained by exercise-induced deficiencies of innate immunity than by alterations in adaptive immunity. Athletes tend to have low serum complement levels (Nieman et al., 1989c), decreased phagocytic function (Petrova et al., 1983; Lewicki et al., 1987), and lowered serum

CRP (Dufaux et al., 1984). In addition, the acute decrease in NK cell activity following prolonged exercise may provide a brief interval of vulnerability (Berk et al., 1990). Thus heavy endurance exercise may weaken first-line defence mechanisms, increasing the risk of URI. More information is needed to correlate actual changes in immune system parameters following long endurance exercise with episodes of URI.

References

Armstrong, R.B. (1986) Muscle damage and endurance events. *Sports Med.* **3**, 370–381.

Berk, L.S., Nieman, D.C., Youngberg, W.S. et al. (1990) The effect of long endurance running on natural killer cells in marathoners. *Med. Sci. Sports Exerc.* **22**, 207–212.

Brahmi, Z., Thomas, J.E., Park, M. & Dowdeswell, I.R.G. (1985) The effect of acute exercise on natural killer cell activity of trained and sedentary human subjects. *J. Clin. Immunol.* **5**, 321–328.

Cannon, J.G., Evans, W.J., Hughes, V.A., Meredith, C.N. & Dinarello, C.A. (1986) Physiological mechanisms contributing to increased interleukin-1 secretion. *J. Appl. Physiol.* **61**, 1869–1874.

Cannon, J.G. & Kluger, M.J. (1983) Endogenous pyrogen activity in human plasma after exercise. *Science* **220**, 617–619.

Cannon, J.G. & Kluger, J.J. (1984) Exercise enhances survival rate in mice infected with *Salmonella typhimurium* (41830). *Proc. Soc. Exp. Biol. Med.* **175**, 518–521.

Crary, B., Hauser, S.L., Borysenko, M. et al. (1983) Epinephrine-induced changes in the distribution of lymphocyte subsets in peripheral blood of humans. *J. Immunol.* **131**, 1178–1181.

Cupps, T.R. & Fauci, A.S. (1982) Corticosteroid-mediated immunoregulation in man. *Immunol. Rev.* **65**, 133–155.

Davidson, R.J.L., Robertson, J.D., Galea, G. & Maughan, R.J. (1987) Hematological changes associated with marathon running. *Int. J. Sports Med.* **8**, 19–25.

Deuster, P.A., Curiale, A.M., Cowan, M.L. & Finkelman, F.D. (1988) Exercise-induced changes in populations of peripheral blood mononuclear cells. *Med. Sci. Sports Exerc.* **20**, 276–280.

Dickson, D.N., Wilkinson, R.L. & Noakes, T.D. (1982) Effects of ultra-marathon training and racing on hematologic parameters and serum ferritin levels in well-trained athletes. *Int. J. Sports Med.* **3**, 111–117.

Dufaux, B. & Order, U. (1989a) Complement activation after prolonged exercise. *Clin. Chim. Acta* 179, 45–49.

Dufaux, B. & Order, U. (1989b) Plasma elastase-alpha₁-antitrypsin, neopterin, tumor necrosis factor, and soluble interleukin-2 receptor after prolonged exercise. *Int. J. Sports Med.* 10, 434–438.

Dufaux, B., Order, U., Geyer, H. & Hollman, W. (1984) C-reactive protein serum concentrations in well-trained athletes. *Int. J. Sports Med.* 5, 102–106.

Eskola, J., Ruuskanen, O., Soppi, E. *et al.* (1978) Effect of sport stress on lymphocyte transformation and antibody formation. *Clin. Exp. Immunol.* 32, 339–345.

Fehr, H.G., Lötzerich, H. & Michna, H. (1989) Human macrophage function and physical exercise: phagocytic and histochemical studies. *Eur. J. Appl. Physiol.* 58, 613–617.

Feldmann, M. & Male, D. (1989) Cell cooperation in the immune response. In: Roitt, I.M., Brostoff J., Male, D.K. (eds) *Immunology*, 2nd edn, pp. 8.1– 8.12. Gower Medical Publishing, New York.

Fernandez, G., Jeng, G. & Baker, D. (1985) Effect of exercise during middle age on immune function in mice maintained on a normal and/or restricted calorie intake. *Fed. Proc.* 44, 767.

Fiatarone, M.A., Morely, J.E., Bloom, E.T., Benton, D., Solomon, G.F. & Makinodan, T. (1989) The effect of exercise on natural killer cell activity in young and old subjects. *J. Gerontol.* 44, M37–M45.

Foster, N.K., Martyn, J.B., Rangno, R.E., Hogg, J.C. & Pardy, R.L. (1986) Leukocytosis of exercise: role of cardiac output and catecholamines. *J. Appl. Physiol.* 61, 2218–2223.

Gatti, G., Cavallo, R., Sartori, M.L. *et al.* (1987) Inhibition by cortisol of human natural killer (NK) cell activity. *J. Steroid Biochem.* 26, 49–58.

Gmünder, F.K., Lorenzi, G., Bechler, B. *et al.* (1988) Effect of long-term physical exercise on lymphocyte reactivity: similarity to spaceflight reactions. *Aviat. Space Environ. Med.* 59, 146–151.

Graham, N.M.H., Douglas, R.M. & Ryan, P. (1986) Stress and acute respiratory infection. *Am. J. Epidemiol.* 124, 389–401.

Green, R.L., Kaplan, S.S., Rabin, B.S., Stanitski, C.L. & Zdziarski, U. (1981) Immune function in marathon runners. *Ann. Allergy* 47, 73–75.

Hanson, P.G. & Flaherty, D.K. (1981) Immunological responses to training in conditioned runners. *Clin. Sci.* 60, 225–228.

Hedfors, E., Holm, G., Ivansen, M. & Wahren, J. (1983) Physiological variation of blood lymphocyte reactivity: T-cell subsets, immunoglobulin production, and mixed-lymphocyte reactivity. *Clin. Immunol. Immunopathol.* 27, 9–14.

Hoffman-Goetz, L., Keir, R., Thorne, R., Houston, M.E. & Young, C. (1986) Chronic exercise stress in mice depresses splenic T lymphocyte mitogenesis *in vitro*. *Clin. Exp. Immunol.* 66, 551–557.

Israel, S., Buhl, B., Krause, M. & Neumann, G. (1982) Die Konzentration der Immunoglobuline A, G und M im Serum bei Trainierten und Untrainierten sowie nach verschiedenen sportlichen Ausdauerleistungen. *Mediz. Sport* 22, 225–231.

Jemmott, J.B. & Locke S.E. (1984) Psychosocial factors, immunologic mediation, and human susceptibility to infectious diseases: How much do we know? *Psychol. Bull.* 95, 78–108.

Jokl, E. (1974) The immunological status of athletes. *J. Sports Med.* 14, 165–192.

Keast, D., Cameron, K. & Morton, A.R. (1988) Exercise and the immune response. *Sports Med.* 5, 248–267.

Kronfol, Z. & House, J.D. (1989) Lymphocyte mitogenesis, immunoglobulin and complement levels in depressed patients and normal controls. *Acta Psychiatr. Scand.* 80, 142–147.

Landmann, R.M.A., Müller, F.B., Perini, Ch., Wesp, M., Erne, P. & Bühler, F.R. (1984) Changes in immunoregulatory cells induced by psychological and physical stress: relationship to plasma catecholamines. *Clin. Exp. Immunol.* 58, 127–135.

Lewicki, R., Tchórzewski, H., Denys, A., Kowalska, M. & Golinska, A. (1987) Effect of physical exercise on some parameters of immunity in conditioned sportsmen. *Int. J. Sports Med.* 8, 309–314.

Lewicki, R., Tchórzewski, H., Majewska, E., Nowak, Z. & Baj, Z. (1988) Effect of maximal physical exercise on T-lymphocyte subpopulations and on interleukin 1 (IL 1) and interleukin 2 (IL 2) production in vitro. *Int. J. Sports Med.* 9, 114–117.

Lewis, D.E., Gilbert, B.E. & Knight, V. (1986) Influenza virus infection induces functional alterations in peripheral blood lymphocytes. *J. Immunol.* 137, 3777–3781.

Liesen, H., Dufaux, B. & Hollmann, W. (1977) Modifications of serum glycoproteins in the days following a prolonged physical exercise and the influence of physical training. *Eur. J. Appl. Physiol.* 37, 243–254.

Lijnen, P., Hespel, P., Fagard, R. *et al.* (1988) Indicators of cell breakdown in plasma of men during and after a marathon race. *Int. J. Sports Med.* 9, 108–113.

Linde, F. (1987) Running and upper respiratory tract infections. *Scand. J. Sports Sci.* 9, 21–23.

Lydyard, O. & Grossi, C. (1989) Cells involved in the immune response. In: Roitt, I.M. Brostoff, J. & Male, D.K. (eds) *Immunology*, 2nd edn, pp. 2.2–2.17. Gower Medical Publishing, New York.

McCarthy, D.A. & Dale, M.M. (1988) The leukocytosis of exercise: a review and model. *Sports Med.* 6, 333–63.

Mackinnon, L.T. (1989) Exercise and natural killer cells: what is the relationship? *Sports Med.* **7**, 141–149.

Mackinnon, L.T., Chick, T.W., van As, A. & Tomasi, T.B. (1988) Effects of prolonged intense exercise on natural killer cell number and function. In: Dotson, C.O. & Humphrey, J.H. (eds) *Exercise Physiology: Current Selected Research*, pp. 77–89. AMS Press, New York.

Mackinnon, L.T., Chick, T.W., van As, A. & Tomasi, T.B. (1987) The effect of exercise on secretory and natural immunity. *Adv. Exp. Med. Biol.* **216A**, 869–876.

Mackinnon, L.T. & Tomasi, T.B. (1986) Immunology of exercise. *Ann. Sports Med.* **3**, 1–4.

Mahan, M.P. & Young, M.R. (1989) Immune parameters of untrained or exercise-trained rats after exhaustive exercise. *J. Appl. Physiol.* **66**, 282–287.

Male, D. & Roitt, I. (1989) Adaptive and innate immunity. In: Roitt, I.M., Brostoff, J. & Male, D.K. (eds) *Immunology*, 2nd edn, pp. 1.1–1.9. Gower Medical Publishing, New York.

Michna, H. (1988) The human macrophage system: activity and functional morphology. *Bibl. Anat.* **31**, 1–84.

Moorthy, A.V. & Zimmerman, S.W. (1978) Human leukocyte response to an endurance race. *Eur. J. Appl. Physiol.* **38**, 271–276.

Muir, A.L., Cruz, M., Martin, B.A., Thommasen, H., Belzberg, A. & Hogg, J.C. (1984) Leukocyte kinetics in the human lung: role of exercise and catecholamines. *J. Appl. Physiol.* **57**, 711–719.

Nehlsen-Cannarella, S.L., Nieman, D.C., Balk-Lamberton, A.J. *et al.* (1990) The effects of moderate exercise training on immune response. *Med. Sci. Sports Exerc.* **23**, 64–70.

Nieman, D.C., Berk, L.S., Simpson-Westerberg, M. *et al.* (1989a) Effects of long endurance running on immune system parameters and lymphocyte function in experienced marathoners. *Int. J. Sports Med.* **10**, 317–323.

Nieman, D.C., Johansen, L.M. & Lee, J.W. (1989b) Infectious episodes in runners before and after a roadrace. *J. Sports Med.* **29**, 289–296.

Nieman, D.C., Johansen, L.M., Lee, J.W. & Arabatzis, K. (1990a) Infectious episodes in runners before and after the Los Angeles Marathon. *J. Sports Med. Phys. Fitness* **30**, 316–328.

Nieman, D.C. & Nehlsen-Cannarella, S.L. (1991) The effects of acute and chronic exercise on immunoglobulins. *Sports Med.* **11**, 182–201.

Nieman, D.C., Nehlsen-Cannarella, S.L., Markoff, P.A. *et al.* (1990b) The effects of moderate exercise training on natural killer cells and acute upper respiratory tract infections. *Int. J. Sports Med.* **11**, 467–473.

Nieman, D.C., Tan, S.A., Lee, J.W. & Berk, L.S. (1989c) Complement and immunoglobulin levels in athletes and sedentary controls. *Int. J. Sports Med.* **10**, 124–128.

Oshida, Y., Yamanouchi, K., Hayamizu, S. & Sato, Y. (1988) Effect of acute physical exercise on lymphocyte subpopulations in trained and untrained subjects. *Int. J. Sports Med.* **9**, 137–140.

Pahlavani, M.A., Cheung, T.H., Chesky, J.A. & Richardson, A. (1988) Influence of exercise on the immune function of rats of various ages. *J. Appl. Physiol.* **64**, 1997–2001.

Pedersen, B.K., Tvede, N., Christensen, L.D., Klarlund, K., Kragbak, S. & Halkjr-Kristensen, J. (1989) Natural killer cell activity in peripheral blood of highly trained and untrained persons. *Int. J. Sports Med.* **10**, 129–131.

Pedersen, B.K., Tvede, N., Hansen, F.R. *et al.* (1988) Modulation of natural killer cell activity in peripheral blood by physical exercise. *Scand. J. Immunol.* **27**, 673–678.

Peters, E.M. & Bateman, E.D. (1983) Respiratory tract infections: an epidemiological survey. *S. Afr. Med. J.* **64**, 582–584.

Petrova, I.V., Kuz'min, S.N., Kurshakova, T.S., Suzdail'nitskii, R.S. & Pershin, B.B. (1983) Neutrophil phagocytic activity and the humoral factors of general and local immunity under intensive physical loading. *Zh. Mikrobiol. Epidemiol. Immunobiol.* **12**, 53–57.

Poortmans, J.R. & Haralambie, G. (1979) Biochemical changes in a 100 km run: proteins in serum and urine. *Eur. J. Appl. Physiol.* **40**, 245–254.

Ricken, K.H. & Kindermann, W. (1986) Behandlungsmöglichkeiten der Infektanfälligkeit des Leistungssportlers. *Dtsch Zeit. Sportsmediz.* **37**, 146–150.

Robertson, A.J., Ramesar, K.C.R.B., Potts, R.C. *et al.* (1981) The effect of strenuous physical exercise on circulating blood lymphocytes and serum cortisol levels. *Clin. Lab. Immunol.* **5**, 53–57.

Röcker, L., Kirsch, K.A. & Stoboy, H. (1976) Plasma volume, albumin and globulin concentrations and their intravascular masses. A comparative study in endurance athletes and sedentary subjects. *Eur. J. Appl. Physiol.* **36**, 57–64.

Schaefer, R.M., Kokot. K., Heidland, A. & Plass, R. (1987) Jogger's leukocytes. *N. Engl. J. Med.* **316**, 223–224.

Simon, H.B. (1984) The immunology of exercise. *J.A.M.A.* **252**, 2735–2738.

Stauber, W.T., Fritz, V.K., Vogelbach, D.W. & Dahlmann, B. (1988) Characterization of muscles injured by forced lengthening. I. Cellular infiltrates. *Med. Sci. Sports Exerc.* **20**, 345–353.

Taylor, C., Rogers, G., Goodman, *et al.* (1987) Hematologic, iron-related, and acute-phase protein responses to sustained strenuous exercise. *J. Appl. Physiol.* **62**, 464–469.

Tomasi, T.B., Trudeau, F.B., Czerwinski, D. & Erredge, S. (1982) Immune parameters in athletes before and after strenuous exercise. *J. Clin. Immunol.* **2**, 173–178.

Tvede, N., Pedersen, B.K., Hansen, F.R. *et al.* (1989) Effect of physical exercise on blood mononuclear cell subpopulations and in vitro proliferative responses. *Scand. J. Immunol.* **29**, 383–389.

Viti, A., Muscettola, M., Paulesu, L., Bocci, V. & Almi A. (1985) Effect of exercise on plasma interferon levels. *J. Appl. Physiol.* **59**, 426–428.

Weiss, M. von, Fuhrmansky, J., Lulay, R. & Weicker, H. (1985) Häufigkeit und Ursache von Immunoglobulin-Mangel bei Sportlern. *Dtsch. Zeit. Sportmediz.* **36**, 146–153.

Wells, C.L., Stern, J.R. & Hecht, L.H. (1982) Hematological changes following a marathon race in male and female runners. *Eur. J. Appl. Physiol.* **48**, 41–49.

Yu, D.T.Y., Clements, P.J. & Pearson, C.M. (1977) Effect of corticosteroids on exercise-induced lymphocytes. *Clin. Exp. Immunol.* **28**, 326–331.

Chapter 46

Overuse Syndromes

R. PETER WELSH AND LINDA J. WOODHOUSE

Introduction

The overuse syndromes include a pot pourri of maladies that afflict endurance athletes of all ages, no matter what the type of activity or the level of competition. Loosely defined, they include not only tendinitis and bursitis resulting from chronic overload and overuse but also chronic muscle strains, joint overload syndromes, stress fractures and compartment syndromes.

The common feature of these diverse conditions is that they result from repetitive load and use. The loads may not necessarily be excessive, but repetition results in a state which has come to be defined loosely as an inflammation. In reality, there is little clinical evidence of acute inflammation in many of these conditions. Injuries occur when activity is sustained at a level that exceeds the body's adaptive ability. Problems are often precipitated by a sudden increase in training frequency, intensity or duration and/or change in mode of exercise. The resultant effects include pain, inhibited function and impaired performance. Management should focus mainly on prevention, with the most important aspect being adequate physical preparation of the athlete. If an overuse injury develops, it is also crucial to continue training to maintain cardiovascular fitness. Although the mode of exercise may need adaptation to reduce direct loading of the injured tissues, the training regimen should remain as specific as possible in terms of the muscle groups and the energy systems involved.

The focus of this section will be on management of the specific soft tissue injury. From a rehabilitative perspective this includes a programme aimed at attaining a high degree of flexibility concomitant with balanced strength around the involved joint. The training programme must be designed to avoid chronic overload or fatigue. Once established, such conditions can be pernicious to deal with and may lead to a permanent impairment of performance.

Overuse syndromes include such diverse conditions as supraspinatus tendinitis, tennis elbow, shin splints and Achilles tendinitis. They also include chronic muscle strains, bursitis and compartment syndromes. The one common denominator is tissue fatigue from overuse. The forces are not necessarily pathological in themselves, but the repetitive nature of the activity results in a physiological incapacity to deal with the demands placed upon the body.

Individual endurance sports lead to characteristic problems. Thus the swimmer is prone to the shoulder impingement syndrome, while the runner will develop Achilles tendinitis and shin splints. A simple classification is shown in Tables 46.1 and 46.2.

Table 46.1 Classification of overuse syndromes.

Muscle−tendon or tendon−bone junction
   syndromes
Tenosynovitis and bursitis states
Chronic joint overload
Stress fractures
Muscle overload conditions
Muscle compartment syndromes

The genesis of overuse syndromes: pathophysiology

Muscle−tendon and tendon−bone junction syndromes

The prototypical example of an overuse syndrome involving the bone−tendon junction is Achilles tendinitis. The muscle tendon complex of the heel is not just a force-generating and transmission system but a shock-absorbing mechanism as well. Force is generated concentrically by the calf muscle and is transmitted via the tendon to the calcaneum, controlling push-off and propelling the whole body upward or forward. Similarly, when landing on the foot, loads must be transmitted from distal to proximal through the Achilles tendon to the shock absorption provided by eccentric muscle contraction.

Repetitive loading leads to Achilles tendinitis. This may have three foci:

1 At the muscle−tendon junction, where there is diffusion of force from the tendon to the muscle or vice versa.

2 In the substance of the Achilles tendon; approximately 2 cm above its insertion into the tubercle of the os calcis, there is a dysvascular zone where a 'watershed' occurs between the blood supply that percolates down from the muscle and a second source of blood supply flowing up from the os calcis (Schatzker & Branemark, 1967). When the muscle contracts and the tendon is taut, the blood supply to this region is interrupted; for example, the concentric contraction of push-off reduces blood flow to this zone from both muscle and tendon

sources. Repetitive interruption of blood flow renders this zone of the tendon susceptible to degeneration or breakdown.

3 Bone−tendon junction overload. At the transition from tendon to bone, there is another site of 'stress concentration' as the relatively flexible tendon makes attachment to the much more rigid bone (Welsh et al., 1971). Tendon degeneration and microfracture are prevalent at this site.

Analogous features have been observed in association with lateral and medial epicondylitis of the elbow. At the bone−tendon junction and in the tendon itself degenerative features are seen, with microfracture, granulation tissue formation and attempts at repair. In a histological review of 50 specimens from patients undergoing tendon release for chronic epicondylitis, fibrinoid degeneration was present in 26%, with fibrovascular hyperplasia present in another 28%. There were areas of focal necrosis or granular calcification in 24%, and evidence of partial rupture of the tendon fibre in 42% of the specimens (Welsh et al., 1988).

In the shoulder, the common overuse syndrome has taken a new name — the shoulder impingement syndrome. This is not a diagnosis, but is rather a descriptive term, denoting a clinical picture of pain in the shoulder associated with repetitive overhead activity. There is an associated pathology of rotator cuff tendinitis and a concomitant reactive bursitis in the adjacent subacromial bursa. The pathophysiological features of Achilles tendinitis are also, to some extent, evident around the shoulder:

1 Extrinsic compression of the supraspinatus tendon by the subacromial arch, acromion, acromial ligament and outer edge of the clavicle during overhead activity produces a reaction in the tendon and bursa (Neer & Welsh, 1977).

2 The blood supply to the supraspinatus tendon enters from the lesser tuberosity attachment, and from the body of the supraspinatus (Rathbun & Macnab, 1970).

3 At the tendon attachment to the tuberosity, there is a concentration of stress, leading to a breakdown of tendon structure.

Table 46.2 Classification of overuse syndromes by region of body.

Region	Syndrome	Region	Syndrome
Spine	Facet joint strain	Lower extremity	
	Discogenic back pain	Hip	Bursitis
			Ischial
Pelvis	Ischial tendinitis		Trochanteric
	Iliac apophysitis		Gluteal
			Tendinitis
Upper extremity			Adductor
Shoulder	Impingement syndrome		Psoas
	Supraspinatus tendinitis		Ischial
	Subacromial bursitis		Stress fracture of femoral neck
	Biceps tenosynovitis	Knee	Tendinitis
	Rotator cuff tear		Infrapatellar
	Joint overload		Osgood−Schlatter
	Recurrent subluxation		apophysitis
	Dead arm syndrome		Bursitis
	Thoracic outlet syndrome		Pes anserine
Elbow	Epicondylitis		Iliotibial syndrome
	Medial (golfer's elbow)		Prepatellar
	Lateral (tennis elbow)		Patellar overload syndrome
	Biceps tendinitis		Chondromalacia patellae
	Olecranon impaction syndrome		Fat pad compression
	Posterior interosseous nerve		Stress fractures
	entrapment		Femoral condyle
Wrist	De Quervain's tenosynovitis		Tibial plateau
	Extensor carpi ulnaris	Leg	Tendinitis
	tenosynovitis		Shin splints
	Carpal tunnel syndrome with		Stress fractures of tibia
	flexor tenosynovitis		Compartment syndromes
			Anterior and posterior
			Anterolateral
		Ankle and foot	Tendinitis
			Achilles tendon
			Plantar fasciitis
			Tenosynovitis
			Peroneal tendon
			Tibialis anterior
			Apophysitis
			Sever's disease
			Stress fractures
			Metatarsals and fibula

Tenosynovitis and bursitis

Whenever a tendon runs in a confined space or is retained by a retinaculum, it is protected by a gliding layer of tenosynovium, a sensitive and vascular membrane that is subject to in-flammation. Irritation can occur through in-creased pressure or tightness in the space, or by repetitive use at a level exceeding normal tolerances. The result is a tenosynovitis, seen for example around the ankle, on the inside (where the tendons of tibialis posterior pass beneath the medial retinaculum) or on the outer side (where the peroneal tendons are constrained by the peroneal retinaculum).

Similarly in the shoulder, part of the impingement syndrome is a bursal reaction to: (a) extrinsic compression within the subacromial space; and (b) intrinsic changes within the tendon.

Reactive changes include: (i) inflammation; (ii) repair; and (iii) scarring and thickening, clinically presenting as a bursitis of the shoulder.

Other types of bursitis develop similarly where tendons move over bony prominences; the synovium normally forms a protective layer, but if it becomes irritated by 'overuse', reactive changes occur as in the shoulder bursa. Potential sites include the greater trochanter of the hip and around the knee — on the inside (pes anserine bursitis), the outside (beneath the iliotibial tract), and the front (prepatellar area).

Joint overload syndromes

Any joint that is subjected to abnormal loads, abnormal ranges of excursion or abnormal levels of activity is prone to a reactive synovitis. Such a reaction from the joint lining is not necessarily associated with any damage to the joint structure, and is not a precursor of arthritis or an indication of other significant joint derangement.

The synovial lining responds to 'overuse' with a reactive effusion and a reactive thickening of the membrane itself, with an inflammatory response which in most instances is reversible once the provocative activity is discontinued.

The knee joint is most commonly affected; patellofemoral pain made up over 60% of the problems seen in a sports knee clinic in Toronto. The genesis of the patellofemoral syndrome is multifactorial; it includes periarticular tendinitis, bursitis, fat pad impingement, plical band syndrome and chondromalacia patellae. Three factors should be considered if there is overload: (i) the structure and mechanics of the

joint itself; (ii) complication of intrinsic joint forces by muscle tightness and lack of flexibility; and (iii) the extrinsic load.

The facet overload syndrome in the lumbar or cervical spine is another prime example of joint overload where structural alignment, force mechanics and loading, as well as intrinsic forces, must be considered in the genesis of the complaint.

Bone overload syndromes

Bone, like other structural materials, is subject to chronic mechanical fatigue and on occasion failure. Unlike inanimate materials, it is capable of remodelling, thus reducing the likelihood of fatigue or stress fractures.

The femoral neck is subject to forces equivalent to two to five times body mass, depending on the activity undertaken, and it is thus vulnerable to stress fractures. Typically, a fissure-like crack develops tangential to the long axis of the bone. Repair is stimulated locally and the fracture may become manifest as an area of periosteal reaction, with the crack itself scarcely visible on radiographs. Common sites of stress fractures include the neck of the femur, the shaft of the tibia, the distal fibula, and the shaft of a metatarsal (with the second or fifth metatarsal being most commonly involved). On occasion, stress fractures may also be seen in the tibial or femoral condyles.

Muscle overload syndromes

Muscle tissue is quite plastic and is rarely the weakest link in the kinetic chain. Overuse injuries usually involve microtears within the connective tissue (tendon or fascia). The site of injury is usually the musculotendinous junction. Adhesions altering resistance and range of motion, pain or swelling contributing to neural inhibition, or overtraining of the agonist relative to the antagonist muscle group may alter forces about the joint and predispose to injury. Internal rotators that are overdeveloped with respect to external rotators, bilaterally in swimmers and in the dominant arm of water-polo players, are not uncommon examples. The ability to develop high torques through concentric contractions of strong internal rotators places a tremendous eccentric load on the external rotators and posterior rotator cuff muscles to decelerate the limb. If these latter muscle groups are weaker, or if fatigue, pain, or swelling alters their normal pattern of recruitment, the joint complex may be predisposed to injury. In the absence of an equal and opposite decelerating force from the external rotators, the humerus can glide anteriorly and superiorly, predisposing the shoulder to an anterior labrum tear or impingement syndrome. Thus, it is essential that one considers the range of motion, force—velocity relationship, type of muscle contraction and fibre type of the muscle groups involved in the activity.

Muscle compartment syndromes

All muscles are contained within a fascial sheath, which may impair the efficiency of function by restricting either blood inflow or the drainage of metabolites (Amendola & Rorabeck, 1989). Problems may arise from one of the following:
1 Interference with the arterial supply, as in the gastrocnemius/soleus arch syndrome.
2 Obstruction of venous outflow from similar pressure.
3 Build-up of intracompartmental pressures due to: (a) hypertrophy of the muscle within the compartment; (b) constraint by the fascial envelope; or (c) fluid accumulation within the compartment.

Pain develops with the build-up of pressure and the restricted efflux of metabolites.

Obstruction occurs most commonly in the anterior or peroneal compartments of the leg. It can also occur from obstruction of the vascular supply to the calf, as previously noted. In the forearm, the extensor compartment, and on rare occasions the forearm musculature, can be affected. In these instances, though, the com-

partment syndromes are usually associated with trauma rather than chronic use.

Management of overuse syndromes

Clinical features

Overuse syndromes usually present in an insidious manner, from repetitive activity, although there may occasionally have been an acute strain or definable injury. Obviously located at a bone—tendon junction or tendo-muscular interface, the tendinitis—bursitis group will present with pain, but often little other than some tenderness is evident on examination. There is not a lot of reactive swelling; fluid accumulation occurs only in the joint overload, while there may be some reactive thickening of the tendon sheath in the tenosynovitis group.

The chronicity of the complaint makes management difficult. The impact on an athlete's career can be very severe; of 50 athletes from the University of Toronto involved in the track programme, 56% of those afflicted with Achilles tendinitis of over 6 months' duration never again competed successfully at an élite level, while 9% had to give up athletic participation because of persistent symptoms (Welsh & Clodman, 1980).

Prevention

The best form of management is prevention. Training sessions must be graduated and monitored to guard against fatigue. Fatigue leads to other imbalances and strain, imposing loads on structures that are less protected than they would normally be, leading to the development of an overuse syndrome.

Basic cardiorespiratory fitness, strengthening and flexibility drills are essential aspects of prevention for the endurance athlete. The training conditions must also be considered; repeated running on hard roads may predispose to chronic overuse states.

Modification of activity

Once the overuse state develops, activity must be modified. Continuation of the provocative activity causes further aggravation of the lesion and chronicity which may be extremely hard to resolve (Clancy, 1974).

Avoidance of the provocative activity does not mean cessation of all activity. Cardiorespiratory fitness and sport-specific skills must be maintained, but activity that evokes significant symptoms must be strictly limited. Thus the runner with Achilles tendinitis must reduce running on uneven terrain or a hard road surface. Cycling, swimming, walking or rowing are alternative activities that will maintain endurance fitness while the condition slowly resolves. For the swimmer with supraspinatus tendinitis or an impingement syndrome of the shoulder, a change in stroke or technique may be required. On other occasions, emphasis can be put on leg work, while the upper body is exercised by a weight programme that emphasizes activity outside the impingement range and strengthens the external rotators (Penny & Welsh, 1981).

Muscle strengthening and balancing

Many overuse syndromes arise because activity is pursued at an intensity which overdevelops one particular muscle group, creating a relative imbalance of strength about the joint. The swimmer or waterpolo player, for example, may develop a chronic overload syndrome because the internal rotator group is overdeveloped, while the external rotators and accessory muscles of the shoulder girdle are less well emphasized. Similarly, patellar overload is greatly benefited by a programme that strengthens the hip flexors, hip abductors and hamstring muscles rather than the quadriceps.

Flexibility

The muscle system must be rendered as flexible as possible in order to reduce strain and stress at the bone–tendon or tendon–muscle junction, as well as reducing loads on the bones and joints themselves. A flexibility programme is thus essential, both to enhance performance and to prevent or treat injury.

Role of physical treatment

Objectives are to relieve pain and to see that injured joints are fully mobilized, that the muscles acting around those joints are strengthened to optimal levels, and that full flexibility is restored.

While there is no difference in oxygen cost or electrical activity between concentric and eccentric contractions, the maximum absolute weight that can be lowered eccentrically exceeds that which can be lifted concentrically. The difference is that the passive elements or series elastic components that contribute to eccentric force generation are not metabolically or electrically active. Thus, concentric contractions stress only muscle tissue, while eccentric contractions stress both muscle and connective tissue. The injury sustained is commonly a partial rupture or microruptures at the musculotendinous junction. Overuse injuries of the patellar tendon ('jumper's knee'), Achilles tendinitis or medial ('tennis elbow') and lateral epicondylitis ('golfer's elbow') are commonly the result of cumulative trauma from repetitive eccentric loading.

Conservative physiotherapeutic treatment may include a combination of ice and ultrasound or other modalities to reduce the local inflammatory reaction. While a period of rest may indeed alleviate symptoms, such treatment offers little long-term benefit and may predispose to reinjury. The absence of stress on bone, muscle and connective tissue has deleterious, rather than neutral, effects.

Successful rehabilitation requires thorough evaluation to identify factor(s) contributing to the injury. A comprehensive programme is then developed to overload the affected tissue and elicit adaptation of bone, muscle and connective tissue. Information is elicited on any previous related injuries, the mechanism of injury, and a detailed profile of mode, intensity, frequency and duration of training. Often a change in training has precipitated symptoms.

Objective evaluation includes a static and a dynamic component. The latter recreates the sequence of isometric, concentric and/or eccentric contractions that occur when performing the activity in question, in order to identify the injured tissue. The example of an overhand throw (e.g. baseball pitcher) will be used to illustrate how characterization of the soft tissue injury can be augmented through delineation of the position, type and velocity of muscle contraction eliciting the symptoms. This information not only assists with differential diagnosis but forms the basis for functional physical rehabilitation of the soft tissue injury.

The overhand throw comprises a well-integrated series of coordinated movements, commencing from the foot, through the lower extremity, pelvis, trunk, shoulder, elbow and wrist. The end-result is a whipping motion of the upper extremity and release of the ball at speeds up to 160 km·h^{-1}.

While success in attaining high-speed controlled delivery of the ball depends on precise timing and coordination of movement of all body parts, the focus here will be on shoulder movement. The shoulder is one of the most mobile joints in the human body. The surrounding musculature (particularly the rotator cuff muscles) plays a crucial role in stabilizing the humerus into a shallow acetabulum. The overhand throw requires elevation of the humerus and proximal stabilization at the glenohumeral and scapulothoracic joints. The overhead position of the arm and stabilizing isometric muscle contractions further compromise blood flow in a region already suffering from a relatively poor blood supply (the supraspinatus). Isometric contractions start to occlude blood flow at about 20% of maximal voluntary contraction (MVC) and result in complete occlusion at about 60% MVC (Royce, 1958; Ahlborg et al., 1972; Karlsson & Ollander, 1972). Given the relatively small muscle mass

involved, stabilizing the arm in an overhead position requires contraction at a relatively high percentage of MVC. This contributes to delayed removal of local fatiguing metabolites. While the reduced blood flow is short lived during a single throw, the cumulative effects of repeated throwing and early fatigue may affect the normal neuromuscular function of this muscle–joint complex.

Motion can be broken down into three phases during the overhead throw. There is a winding or cocking phase, the delivery and follow-through. During the wind-up phase the glenohumeral joint attains a position of approximately 90° abduction, 30° horizontal abduction and maximal external rotation. This occurs at slow to moderate velocity and results in maximal stretch of the anterior structures at the glenohumeral joint and internal rotators of the humerus. In terms of the supporting musculature, the posterior deltoid retracts the humerus, assisted by the supraspinatus, infraspinatus and teres minor, which also contract to stabilize the head of the humerus. A burst of concentric and isometric contractions, respectively, from these muscles accelerates the limb towards a posterior, externally rotated position. A timely eccentric contraction of the subscapularis and internal rotators (pectoralis major and latissimus dorsi) decelerates the movement of the humerus before the limb reaches a position of full external rotation. This movement results in 'preloading' of the horizontal adductors and internal rotators. During this phase, muscles around the scapula act as synergists, firing to stabilize the scapula, thereby providing a solid base on which movements of the humerus occur.

The phasic bursts of muscle activity during the delivery phase are similar to those during the wind-up, except that different muscle groups are firing. The humerus is rapidly accelerated into horizontal adduction, through concentric contraction of the anterior muscles (pectoralis major and latissimus dorsi) as the triceps contracts concentrically to extend the elbow from 90° to 25° or so. The head of the humerus glides anteriorly and superiorly, stressing the anterior superior aspect of the labrum, as extremely high torques are produced. This places tremendous strain on the rotator cuff muscles (to stabilize the head of the humerus) and on the scapular stabilizers (to continue providing a stable base of support). Weakness of the posterior rotator cuff may contribute to an anterior labrum tear. The relative amount of pronation/supination of the forearm and wrist controls the type of pitch that is tossed. After the ball has been released, the posterior muscles of the rotator cuff must contract eccentrically at high velocity to decelerate the limb. The biceps muscles must also contract eccentrically to decelerate elbow extension.

The force−velocity relationship is also important to consider. According to Hill's model (Hill, 1938), as the velocity of a muscle contraction increases, the maximal force generated concentrically decreases, while the reverse is true with eccentric contractions. Clinically, there has been a tremendous rise in the use of isokinetic devices which allow for control of velocity during concentric and eccentric loading. This allows in vivo examination of the torque−velocity relationship. While the relationship described by Hill has been demonstrated for lower extremity movement patterns, the same has not held true for the upper extremity, particularly the shoulder complex, where torque tends to plateau with increasing velocity up to speeds of 400° per second (the maximum velocity presently available on clinical isokinetic devices).

Following injury, it is important to delineate whether adaptation should be effected in the active contractile tissue or the passive connective tissue (series elastic component), using concentric and eccentric muscle contractions, respectively.

To effect change in muscular strength, it is important to load muscle tissue with a high resistance, above 85% of MVC and a small number of repetitions (8−10 per set) for three sets per session (for reviews see Ahta, 1981; Sale & McDougall, 1981). Training muscle to

improve local muscle endurance requires submaximal loading of the tissue with forces between 50% and 85% MVC, making a greater number of repetitions (20−30 repetitions) or continuing for a time of 30−60 s. Alternation is recommended between agonist and antagonist muscle groups, undertaking successive exercises on alternate days (that is, three to four times per week). Others prefer daily workouts, alternating daily between upper and lower extremity work.

Three different modes of training are used to develop muscular strength or local muscular endurance. The first is *isometric contractions* with no change in muscle length. Such training is angle-specific with approximately a 20° window, i.e. benefit is seen at the training angle ± 20° (Gardner, 1963; Lindh, 1979; Knapik et al., 1983). The second is *isotonic contractions*, where velocity is uncontrolled, resistance varies with joint angle, and the external load is constant. This type of training may include contractions that are either concentric or eccentric. The difficulty with eccentric loading, when using this mode, is that maximal loading is limited by the maximum load that can be lifted concentrically.

The third is the *isokinetic mode*, where velocity is held constant and resistance is accommodating. Devices designed to evaluate isokinetic muscle strength and endurance have become common place in rehabilitation departments over the past decade. Most active systems can be used to measure isometric, isotonic and isokinetic strength in both the concentric and eccentric modes. These devices monitor position, angular velocity (degrees per second) and torque (Newton-metres). The advantage of isokinetic exercise is that the type of contraction, angular velocity, torque and range of motion can be preselected. This is a particular advantage with respect to eccentric loading. Some devices allow controlled loading of the tissue relative to the immediately preceding concentric contraction.

Regardless of the training mode that is selected, improvement in force or torque generation within the first 3 weeks reflects mostly neural adaptation (Sale, 1987). This is particularly true of eccentric loading. Muscular adaptation usually takes 3–6 weeks, while connective tissue adaptation takes much longer. Animal models suggest that adaptation of collagen tissue to physical stress becomes significant only after 12 months or so (Woo *et al.*, 1982). Eccentric loading at more than 85% of maximum force may result in muscle injury (delayed onset muscle soreness, DOMS). Thus, eccentric loading needs to commence at between 50% and 85% MVC, with a slower progressive increase in resistance than when training concentrically (McCully & Faulkner, 1986; Friden *et al.*, 1988). There is a high incidence of recurrence of overuse tendinitis injuries, in part because improvement in neural recruitment and muscle adaptation occur before strengthening of connective tissue; thus, increased resistance places relatively more stress on the tissue that is slowest to adapt. A programme of prolonged submaximal eccentric loading is required to elicit connective tissue adaptation in the treatment of overuse tendinitis.

Functional activities bridge the gap between rehabilitation of the physical components and full return to sport. While isokinetic devices offer a safe, controlled method of loading soft tissue, the joint movement is restricted to a single axis of rotation. Athletic performance, however, involves well-coordinated movement about multiple axes of rotation. That is the justification for training internal and external rotation of the shoulder at $400°·s^{-1}$ while a baseball pitcher's arm travels at much higher velocities. Hence a graduated return to sport is necessary to enable the muscle strength and endurance gains to be integrated in a functional manner.

Role of assistive devices

In addition to physical treatment, simple assistive devices may be of considerable benefit in both prevention of and rehabilitation from overuse syndromes. Orthoses for the runner can modify footwear, reduce loads and balance forces that are imposing undue stress or strain on the musculoskeletal system (Bull, 1989).

Athletes predisposed to shin splints, Achilles tendinitis or tenosynovitis around the ankle may benefit from orthotic devices. Likewise, the tennis player with chronic epicondylitis of the elbow will benefit from a stress-relieving support around the forearm muscles just below the elbow. Such devices may be used in rehabilitation, but there is limited place for them on a continuing basis.

Role of the physician: medication

Oral non-steroidal anti-inflammatory drugs

The non-steroidal anti-inflammatory drugs (NSAIDs) are of some benefit for acute strains and inflammatory states but probably do not have a major place in the continuing management of chronic overuse syndromes (Hodge, 1989).

While the conditions are often loosely described as associated with chronic inflammation, there is scant histological evidence of a true inflammatory reaction; rather, degenerative features have been observed. The rationale for the use of NSAIDs is thus limited, although they do have an analgesic effect.

Non-steroidal drugs may be used acutely, often with good effect. Under these circumstances, they are best prescribed at maximum dose for 10–14 days. If no benefit is noted in the first 3 days, then there is likely to be little benefit from their continuation.

While glucocorticoids have been used on occasion, there are few confirmed data on their efficacy; and their long-term use should be actively discouraged because of extreme side-effects.

Injection of corticosteroids

Glucocorticoid injections have an important place in the management of some overuse states. Although these are powerful agents, their exact mode of action is still open to debate, and certain principles should be followed when recommending their administration. In particular, steroid injections can harm normal tissues. This is evidenced by the depigmentation of skin at the site of an extravasated injection, particularly in black athletes. Dissolution of subcutaneous fat tissue also occurs at an injection site. Intra-articular injection can damage normal articular cartilage by breaking down the mucopolysaccharide and collagen components of this tissue. Direct intratendinous injection has a similar adverse effect on tendon structure, leading to tissue breakdown and degeneration which in certain sites, for example the patellar tendon or the Achilles tendon, may predispose to tendon rupture.

Therefore, direct bone–tendon junction injections are to be avoided, except perhaps in moderate dose in specific non-clinical sites such as the epicondyle of the elbow in golfer's elbow or tennis elbow.

Tendon sheath injections, in contrast, are very effective; but the injection should be peritendinous rather than intratendinous, and it should be made into the tenosynovial sleeve rather than the surrounding tissue, for example when treating tibialis posterior tenosynovitis of the ankle or De Quervain's tenosynovitis of the wrist.

Intrabursal injections are similarly to be made into the bursal space and not into the tendon or muscle. For example, the injections around the shoulder should be into the subacromial space, not into the supraspinatus tendon or some other locally tender focus.

Intra-articular injections should be made only when there is significant reactive synovitis with an effusion. Other sources of joint derangement should already be ruled out, and a 'dry' joint should never be injected.

If steroid injections are used, then the question arises as to how many and how often. The answer seems self-evident. If one injection does not work, why try two or three? If one injection does work, why would one need another?

There is no reason for multiple injections in most instances, although there is a legitimate place for repeated use of these agents should the condition relapse some months later. If benefit was earlier derived from injection, another injection can be tried. However, a limit should be set. If the condition proves refractory, then a maximum of three injections should be given at any one site.

Surgical treatment

In certain chronic overuse states, the condition may become refractory; there is then a limited yet well-defined role for surgical treatment, as outlined below:

1 *Bone–tendon junction syndromes*: tendon release, excision of degenerate tissue and, on occasion, drilling of the underlying bone to enhance revascularization and to encourage regrowth of healthy tissue may be appropriate treatments, for example of lateral epicondylitis and infrapatellar tendinitis.

2 *Tenosynovitis*: release of a tight compartment space may be needed, for example in De Quervain's tenosynovitis or parallel tenosynovitis of the ankle.

3 *Joint overload conditions*: arthroscopic review of such lesions enables a direct visualization of the interior of the joint. Thus, any internal derangement can be ruled out. A light debridement of the irritated synovium and redundant fat pad with lavage may greatly alleviate the situation.

4 *Bone overload syndromes*: stress fractures generally heal uneventfully, but certain fractures require particularly careful attention. Fracture of the femoral neck has to be very carefully protected.

5 *Muscle compartment syndromes*: myofascial release may be required to decompress a tense compartment in the lower extremity, as with the anterior compartment syndrome.

Conclusion

Overuse syndromes collectively account for the vast majority of chronic musculoskeletal problems affecting the endurance athlete. Such conditions are not to be treated lightly. They are serious afflictions which require diligent attention from the athlete, the trainer, the coach and the therapist as well as the medical team if morbidity is to be reduced and the athlete is to achieve optimal performance.

References

Ahlborg, B., Bergstrom, J., Ekelund, L.G. *et al.* (1972) Muscle metabolism during isometric exercise performed at constant force. *J. Appl. Physiol.* **33**(2), 224−228.

Ahta, J. (1981) Strengthening muscle. *Exerc. Sport Sci. Rev.* **9**, 1−73.

Amendola, A. & Rorabeck, C.H. (1989) Chronic exertional compartment syndrome. In: Torg, J., Welsh, P. & Shephard, R.J. (eds) *Current Therapy in Sports Medicine*, Vol. 2, pp. 250−253. B.C. Decker, Philadelphia.

Bull, C.R. (1989) Orthotic devices: indications. In: Torg, J., Welsh, P. & Shephard, R.J. (eds) *Current Therapy in Sports Medicine*, Vol. 2, pp. 217−220. B.C. Decker, Philadelphia.

Clancy, W.G. (1974) Lower extremity injuries in the jogger and distance runner. *Phys. Sports Med.* **2**, 46.

Friden, J., Serger, J. & Ekblom, B. (1988) Sublethal fiber injuries after high tension anaerobic exercise. *Eur. J. Appl. Physiol.* **57**, 360−368.

Gardner, G.W. (1963) Specificity of strength changes of the exercised and non-exercised limb following isometric training. *Res. Q.* **34**, 98−101.

Hill, A.B. (1938) The heat of shortening and the dynamic constants of muscle. *Proc. R. Soc. Lond. [Biol.]* **126**, 136−195.

Hodge, N.A. (1989) Athletic injuries and the use of medication. In: Torg, Welsh & Shephard (eds) *Current Therapy in Sports Medicine − 2.* pp. 178−182.

Karlsson, J. & Ollander, B. (1972) Muscle metabolites with exhaustive static exercise of different duration. *Acta Physiol. Scand.* **86**, 309−314.

Knapik, J.J., Mawdsley, R.H. & Ramos, N.U. (1983) Angular specificity and test mode specificity of isometric and isokinetic strength training. *J. Orthop. Sports Phys. Ther.* **5**, 58−65.

Lindh, M. (1979) Increase of muscle strength from isometric quadriceps exercise at different knee angles. *Scand. J. Rehab. Med.* **11**, 33−36.

McCully, K.K. & Faulkner, J.A. (1986) Characteristics of lengthening contractions associated with injury to skeletal muscle fibres. *J. Appl. Physiol.* **61**(1), 293−299.

Neer, C.S. & Welsh, R.P. (1977) The sports injured shoulder. *Orthop. Clin. North Am.* **8**, 583−591.

Penny, J.N. & Welsh, R.P. (1981) Shoulder impingement syndromes in athletes and their surgical management. *Am. J. Sports Med.* **9**, 11−15.

Rathbun, J. & Macnab, I. (1970) The microvascular pattern of the rotator cuff. *J. Bone Joint Surg.* **52B**, 540−553.

Royce, J. (1958) Isometric fatigue curves in human muscle with normal and occluded circulation. *Res. Q.* **29**, 204−212.

Sale, D.G. (1987) Influence of exercise and training on motor unit activation. *Exerc. Sport Sci. Rev.* **15**, 95−151.

Sale, D.G. & McDougall, D. (1981) Specificity in strength training: a review for the coach and athlete. *Can. J. Appl. Sports Sci.* **6**, 87−92.

Schatzker, J. & Branemark P.I. (1967) Intravital observations on the microvascular anatomy and microcirculation of the tendon. *Acta Orthop. Scand.* **126** (Suppl.), 3−23.

Welsh, R.P. & Clodman, J. (1980) Clinical survey of Achilles tendinitis in athletes. *Can. Med. Assoc. J.* **122**, 193−194.

Welsh, R.P., Doman, A. & Barrie, H.J. (1988) *A Clinical Histological Review of Tennis Elbow.* American Shoulder and Elbow Surgeons Annual Meeting, October 1988, Santa Fe, New Mexico.

Welsh, R.P., Macnab, I. & Riley, V. (1971) Biomechanical studies of rabbit tendon. *Clin. Orthop.* **81**, 171−177.

Woo, S.L.Y., Gomez, M.A., Woo Y.-K. & Akeson, W.H. (1982) Mechanical properties of tendons and ligaments. II. The relationship between immobilization and exercise on tissue remodelling. *Biorheology* **19**, 397−408.

Chapter 47

Other Health Benefits of Physical Activity

ROY J. SHEPHARD

Introduction

Discussions of sports participation and health have tended to focus rather narrowly upon the potential of endurance activity to reduce the number of fatal heart attacks, with a resultant extension of longevity. While the importance of such gains should not be minimized, it is also worth emphasizing that the product of lifespan and life quality is of more concern to most people than a mere extension of life (Shephard, 1982b). Personal justifications of involvement in a prolonged training programme are thus made more commonly in terms of 'feeling better' than in the anticipation of a prolongation of lifespan. For the athlete, such perceptions are shaped by personal and social gains associated with participation in competitive events.

In addition to a favourable influence upon the incidence of ischaemic heart disease, hypertension and obesity, a regular programme of moderate endurance exercise is likely to improve perceived health, to extend the period of independence and self-care as a senior citizen, to enhance respiratory and musculoskeletal function, to decrease the incidence of hormonal disorders and neoplasms, to boost immune function and to enhance various aspects of psychological function (Shephard, 1985). Regular exercise may also have a favourable impact upon certain aspects of personal lifestyle (Shephard, 1989), with potential improvements in future health. However, there is relatively little information on the optimum intensity, frequency and duration of exercise needed to achieve such gains; in general, the competitive athlete may realize additional benefits relative to the recreational exerciser because of more vigorous participation, but in some instances the amount of training demanded by international competition may exceed the personal optimum, with adverse consequences for both immediate and long-term health.

Perceived health

Every person lives on a biological continuum that extends from a state of complete physical, mental and social health to overt illness (Herzlich, 1973; Fig. 47.1). Perceptions of health on a given day, the impact of such perceptions upon competitive performance, and the likelihood that an athlete will seek medical services all depend on his or her current location along this continuum.

Because international athletes are under extreme pressure to produce outstanding performances, some competitors show a marked impairment of function and make strident demands for medical services if their perceived health suffers even a small displacement in the direction of clinical illness. On the other hand, the improvement of mood-state that accompanies regular bouts of moderate endurance exercise tends to displace personal perceptions of health in a positive direction. One biochemical factor that contributes to an en-

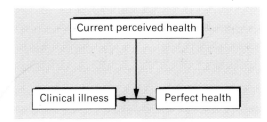

Fig. 47.1 Diagram illustrating the concept of perceived health. An individual lies at some point on a continuum extending from perfect health to clinical illness. The location on this continuum influences the likelihood of symptoms and the demand for medical services. Appropriate amounts of exercise or success in competition, by elevating mood-state, may displace perceived health to the right; conversely, if the demands of the coach exceed the capacity of the individual or the rewards of training seem disappointing, perceived health may be displaced to the left.

hanced mood-state is the secretion of β-endorphins; this response is associated with prolonged endurance activity (the distance runner's 'high'; Harber & Sutton, 1984), and thus may be greater in the international athlete than in the recreational exerciser. Both personal satisfaction (a sense of 'self-actualization') and the praise of significant others (such as the coach or team-mates) may further enhance perceived health in the successful competitor, but if a prolonged season of preparation has been pursued to the point of over-training, diminishing performance and physical injuries, the perceived health of the athlete may deteriorate.

The average perceived health of a population has considerable practical importance in terms of controlling medical expenditure, since the majority of physician consultations reflect a worsening of perceived health rather than the development of some specific organic disease. Controlled studies of the general population have now documented that regular involvement in a moderate endurance training programme reduces the demands for both physician and hospital services, with parallel reductions in absenteeism from work and the purchase of non-prescribed medications

(Shephard, 1986a). It would be difficult to conduct analogous studies on top-level athletes, for even if it were shown that international competitors made less than average overall demands for medical services, this advantage could have developed because particularly healthy individuals elected to participate in high-level competition, rather than through a specific effect of endurance training upon perceived health. There is indeed some suggestion that over-training is associated with a higher than normal level of consultations for minor medical complaints (T.J. Verde, unpublished data).

Prolongation of independence

The typical senior citizen spends about 10 years with some limitation of daily activity, and a final year of life when a relative or an institution must provide almost total support (Health & Welfare, Canada, 1982). There are many reasons for such dependency, sociological, psychological and medical. In some instances, there is a clinical catastrophe — a sudden stroke, or the onset of blindness. Often, the prime cause is physiological: oxygen transport, muscular strength or flexibility have declined to a level where the individual has insufficient residual function to sustain independent living. However, much also depends on motivation, and some highly motivated senior citizens are able to continue living alone despite severe physical handicaps (Shephard, 1987).

The potential for physiological limitation may conveniently be illustrated with reference to the age-related decline of maximal oxygen intake, since regular endurance training has a particularly important impact upon the magnitude of this variable. Many of the lighter tasks of daily living require three or four times the resting level of energy expenditure (3−4 METS, equivalent to an oxygen consumption of 11−14 ml·kg·min^{-1}), and independence is likely to be limited by severe fatigue if the sustainable oxygen transport cannot satisfy this minimum requirement. The average person finds difficulty in deploying their full maximal oxygen intake for more than a few minutes. It is possible to sustain about 70% of the maximum value over an hour of vigorous exercise, but fatigue develops over an 8-h day, if energy demands exceed 40% of maximum.

Comparisons between endurance athletes and the general population do not suggest that continued participation in endurance sports slows the intrinsic rate of ageing of oxygen transport; the loss amounts to about 5 ml·kg^{-1}·min^{-1} for every 10 years of adult life in both athletes and their sedentary peers (Kavanagh *et al.*, 1989). On the other hand, at any given age an appropriately graded programme of endurance training can increase a person's maximal oxygen intake by up to 10 ml·kg^{-1}·min^{-1}, equivalent to a rejuvenation of 20 years in terms of this particular variable (Sidney & Shephard, 1978; Fig. 47.2). The status of the endurance athlete at any given age is further enhanced by initial selection. Thus, in terms of oxygen transport, the endurance competitor should have the functional resources to live independently for many more years than a sedentary person. In the age range where the capacity for independent living is likely to be a practical issue (80 years and above), the impact of endurance training upon overall longevity is

no more than a few months (Paffenbarger *et al.*, 1986; Pekkanen et al., 1987); the net effect of sports participation is thus to increase the likelihood that a person will remain in good functional health until close to the time of death. Retrospective questioning of the institutionalized elderly has offered some confirmation of this hypothesis, showing that those who are currently unable to care for themselves had a low level of physical activity at the age of 50 years (Shephard & Montelpare, 1988).

Similar arguments may be advanced with regard to the loss of function in other body systems. For example, the independence of an elderly person may be threatened by an inability to lift the body mass from a chair or a toilet seat, or the loss of flexibility in a major joint may make it impossible to dress without assistance. Again, there is good evidence that an appropriate pattern of regular physical exercise can sustain the fucntion of an active person in a way that offers the equivalent of 10−20 years of rejuvenation. The competitor who has participated in an event demanding muscular endurance may show a major functional advantage in terms of absolute strength, but this can be offset by a bulky frame. A large lean body mass can lead to a relatively low peak oxygen transport per unit of body mass,

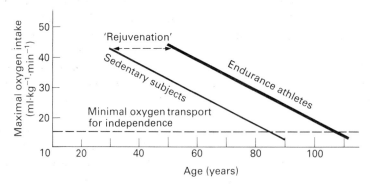

Fig. 47.2 The influence of regular endurance training upon the ageing of maximal oxygen intake. The rate of loss of oxygen transport is about 5 ml·kg^{-1}·min^{-1} for each 10 years of adult life in both the athletes and their sedentary peers, but regular training can enhance oxygen transport by 10 ml·kg^{-1}·min^{-1}, equivalent to a rejuvenation of 20 years with respect to this particular variable. Initial selection further enhances the status of the competitive athlete at any given age.

and thus a poor cardiovascular endurance; the overall impact of muscle-strengthening activity upon the age of dependency thus remains unknown.

Any advantage of flexibility in an endurance competitor tends to be quite localized. Thus, if there have been no injuries or dislocations, a person with very flexible shoulder joints may continue to sustain an outstanding performance in a specific swimming event to an advanced age.

Respiratory function

Many athletes — particularly swimmers and contestants in events that use the chest muscles — have a very large vital capacity. This arises in part from athletic selection, but also in part from a specific, training-induced strengthening of the thoracic muscles. Since oxygen transport is limited by the cardio-vascular system rather than by respiratory function, enhanced development of the chest normally has no great significance for health, even in extreme old age (when oxygen tran-sport may be limiting functional capacity). On the other hand, if the individual has the mis-fortune to contract a chronic respiratory disease such as tuberculosis, the added lung capacity may ultimately have considerable importance in reducing the extent of disability.

In many people, a substantial part of the decrease in vital capacity and other aspects of lung function that occurs over adult life is at-tributable to cigarette smoking with resultant chronic bronchitis and obstructive lung dis-ease. Probably because endurance exercise en-courages a life-long abstinence from cigarettes, the average age-related decrease of lung func-tion tends to be smaller in athletes than in the general population.

Endurance exercise has been advocated as a useful form of therapy in various forms of chronic respiratory disease such as asthma, cystic fibrosis and chronic obstructive lung dis-ease. Swimming may be helpful for asthmatics partly because it teaches breathing control, and partly because it offers activity in a humid atmosphere; the latter loosens mucus and re-duces the probability of exercise-induced bronchospasm relative to other forms of physi-cal activity. Some asthmatic patients have reached the highest levels of international competition in swimming events.

There is no evidence that the development of either cardiovascular or muscular endurance can restore damaged lung tissue, and while the symptoms of chronic chest disease may be alleviated by a progressive exercise programme, respiratory function is not normally enhanced. The mechanisms of benefit in such patients seem to be: (i) an increase in the mechanical ef-ficiency of physical activity, reducing the oxy-gen demands of both limb and chest muscles; (ii) a strengthening of the limb muscles, facili-tating their perfusion; this reduces the pro-duction of anaerobic metabolites, and thus curbs the respiratory minute volume associ-ated with a given intensity of effort; (iii) the postural drainage and encouragement of ex-pectoration associated with vigorous body movements; and (iv) psychological factors (including a breaking of the vicious cycle of dyspnoea, fear of exercise, muscular weakness and greater dyspnoea (Shephard, 1976).

Musculoskeletal factors

For a while, experts in preventive medicine recommended that middle-aged adults should develop cardiovascular endurance, but they categorically rejected forms of exercise that were designed to strengthen the skeletal muscles. The two arguments advanced against the de-velopment of muscular strength were that the added body mass increased the cardiac work rate, and that heavy isotonic or isometric straining might in itself precipitate a heart attack. Those who followed such advice liter-ally, concentrating all of their conditioning efforts upon endurance events such as distance running, sometimes showed a weakening of muscles elsewhere in the body that had not been used during competitive performance.

Certainly, the athlete who has developed a large lean body mass must perform more work when displacing the body, but if the limb muscles have been strengthened by appropriate muscular training, the necessary body movements may be accomplished with a lesser rise of blood pressure than in a weaker individual. Since blood pressure is in turn the main determinant of cardiac work rate, the loading of the heart may also be smaller in a well-muscled subject than in a person whose muscles have been weakened by an exclusive focus upon cardiovascular training. Muscle loss is particularly likely to occur if an athlete is worried about becoming too fat or failing to make a desired weight category; gymnasts and ballet dancers are especially vulnerable groups.

The blood pressure rises progressively during either a sustained isometric contraction or a rapidly repeated series of heavy isotonic efforts (Fig. 47.3). However, muscles can be strengthened by quite brief contractions, with extended rest intervals, and this pattern of training is to be preferred for older competitors.

Muscle training programmes increase the strength of tendons and ligaments (Fig. 47.4) so that more force is required to rupture them or to tear them from their ligaments (Tipton et al., 1975). On the other hand, if a ligament or joint capsule has been repeatedly damaged by athletic trauma, it may become more vulnerable to reinjury. The effects upon articular cartilage follow a similar pattern. The immediate effect of endurance activity is to decrease the water content of the cartilage and thus its thickness, but with repeated bouts of such exercise, there is an increase in its thickness and resistance to compression, reducing the danger of tears and subsequent osteoarthritis. On the other hand, either over-training or repeated local trauma may increase the vulnerability to osteoarthritis. Retrospective studies of runners do not suggest an unusually high incidence of osteoarthritis of the knees or hips (Lane et al., 1986; Eichner, 1989; Pascale & Grana, 1989), and in older individuals who have developed either osteoarthritis or rheumatoid arthritis an increase of habitual physical activity often has a beneficial effect upon function (Ike et al., 1989), in part because it corrects muscular weakness associated with overprotection of the patient, and in part because the patient's tolerance of discomfort is increased.

The influence of endurance training upon

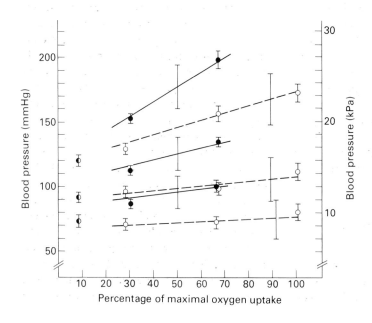

Fig. 47.3 Rise of arterial systolic, mean and diastolic pressure in response to selected intensities of endurance work performed with the arms (●——●) or the legs (○– – –○). Data obtained by femoral artery catheterization. ◐, At rest. From Åstrand & Rodahl (1986), with permission.

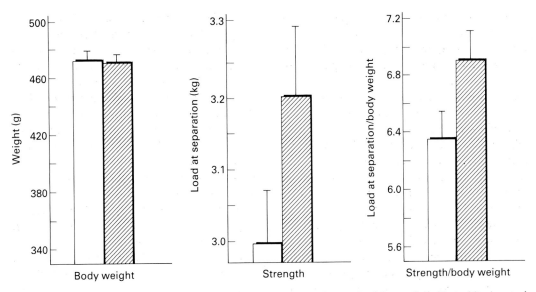

Fig. 47.4   The influence of endurance training upon the junctional strength of the medial collateral ligament of rats. Diet of untrained animals restricted so that animals had equal body mass in untrained group (□) and trained group (▨). From Tipton *et al.* (1975), with permission.

bone density (Table 47.1) depends in part upon the volume of training, and in part upon nutritional status; other important variables include dietary calcium and hormonal balance. Moderate, recreational training clearly increases the density of weight-bearing bones (Bailey & McCulloch, 1990), and there may also be a local strengthening of bone architecture (for example, in the playing arm of tennis competitors). But if conditioning is pursued to the point that sex hormone levels are reduced, there can be a reduction of bone density (Drinkwater *et al.*, 1986). Some recent studies suggest that the effects of over-training are reversed once normal sex hormone levels are restored, and the need for specific calcium and hormonal supplements remains the subject of debate.

Metabolic factors and the incidence of hormonal disorders

Obesity was classically attributed to overeating, but more recent observations have shown that regular endurance exercise contributes in many ways to the avoidance of obesity. In particular: (i) the greater self-esteem of an athlete avoids the need to seek consolation of snacks and energy-rich 'treats'; pride is also developed in maintaining a neat body form, and this tendency is reinforced by the advice of the coach; and (ii) large amounts of energy are consumed, both by the performance of prolonged endurance exercise and by the subsequent stimulation of metabolism. If a fat-rich diet is consumed (as is commonly the case for groups such as football players), it may be less easy to overeat, and a smaller percentage of the ingested energy is absorbed; however, many endurance competitors prefer a carbohydrate-rich diet, because they are repeatedly seeking to boost their muscle glycogen stores. On the other hand, the proportion of fat that is metabolized is higher in those classes of athletes who operate for long periods at intensities below the anaerobic threshold, and who pursue individual bouts of exercise to significant glycogen depletion. Some male long-distance runners carry as little as 5% body fat, compared with 20–25% in a sedentary young man. The

Table 47.1 Cross-sectional studies showing influence of sports participation on bone mass. For details of references see primary source, Schoutens et al. (1989), with permission.

Reference	No. of subjects/type of exercise	Sex/mean age (years) of subjects (range) [SD]	Bone studied (technique)*	Results
Tennis players				
Huddlestone et al. (1980)	35 senior tennis players	M (70–84)	Radius (SPA)	Playing side + 11%
Jones et al. (1977)	44 professional tennis players / 23 professional tennis players	M/27 (18–50) / F/24 (14–34)	Humerus, 11 cm proximal to distal end (X-ray); cortical thickness	Playing side + 34.9% (M); + 28.4% (F)
Montoye (1980)	61 senior tennis players	M/64 [4.4]	Hand-wrist and hand (X-ray) Radius, ulna, humerus (SPA)	Bone width and mineral content greater in dominant limb
Physical activity				
Aloia et al. (1978)	30 marathon runners; 16 controls	M/42 (30–60) [7.7]	Total body calcium (NAA); radius, distal (SPA)	Total body calcium + 11% in marathon runners; radius no difference
Brewer et al. (1983)	42 with history of running > 2 years; 38 physically inactive	F/39 (30–49) [5.8] premenopausal	Phalanx 5th finger, os calcis (X-ray). Radius, distal + midshaft (SPA)	Bone mineral in marathon runners greater in finger and midshaft radius; equal in distal radius; less in os calcis
Cann et al. (1984)	11 amenorrhoeic athletes; 16 premature ovarian failure; 50 controls	F/41.6 (16–49)	Lumbar spine (CT); radius, distal one third (SPA)	Amenorrhoeic athletes (vs. controls): spinal trabecular bone − 24%; radial cortical bone not significantly low

Drinkwater et al. (1984)	25 marathon runners: 11 amenorrheic (67 km·week⁻¹); 14 cyclic (40 km·week⁻¹)	F/25 [4.5]	Lumbar spine (DPA); radius, 2 sites (SPA)	Bone density L1–L4: cyclic > amenorrhoeic; radius no difference
Laval-Jeantet et al. (1984)	136; 5 grades of physical activity	F/90 aged 28–40; 17 aged 41 to menopause; 27 menopausal	Vertebra L3 (CT)	Activity level influences vertebral density (especially level 4)
Marcus et al. (1985)	17 marathon runners (less than 3 h), >65 km·week⁻¹; no oestrogen therapy: 11 secondary amenorrhoea; 6 regular menses	F (20–29)	Lumbar spine (CT); radius (SPA)	Mineral density lumbar spine: menstruating athletes > amenorrhoeic runners. Mineral density radius normal in both groups
Nilsson & Westlin (1971)	9 top rank athletes; 55 athletes; 24 controls exercising; 15 controls	M/22	Femur, distal end (SPA)	Bone density top rank > athletes > controls exercising > controls. Weightlifters + throwers + runners > soccer players + swimmers
Stillman et al. (1986)	19 low activity (mean age 51.5 years); 36 moderate activity (age 53.2 years); 28 high activity (age 43.1 years; no patient > 60 years)	F (30–85)	Radius; distal one third (SPA)	Bone mineral/bone width adjusted for age and menstrual status: high activity > moderate > low

* Technique for bone mass measurement: CT, computed tomography; DPA, double photon absorptiometry; NAA, neutron activation analysis; SPA, single photon absorptiometry.

adverse health consequences of a substantial (20–25 kg) accumulation of body fat have been well documented by actuarial statistics; there is an increased risk of diabetes, circulatory diseases, pneumonia and influenza, digestive diseases and renal diseases (Society of Actuaries, 1959). The impact of smaller accumulations of fat is less clear, in part because smokers tend to have a below-average body mass, and in part because a low body mass in the general population may reflect a lack of lean tissue rather than an optimization of body fat content.

Endurance exercise has favourable effects upon the blood lipid profile. Regular endurance training has little impact upon total blood cholesterol levels, particularly if body mass is held constant, because the body can: (i) alter the amounts of cholesterol excreted via the bile and reabsorbed from the intestines; and (ii) the liver is capable of synthesizing substantial quantities of cholesterol from the normal building blocks of metabolism (acetoacetyl coenzyme A (CoA) and acetyl CoA). However, the prolonged running associated with marathon training can increase serum concentrations of the useful, scavenging high density lipoprotein (HDL) fraction of cholesterol (particularly the HDL_2 subfraction and the associated apoprotein A-I), while decreasing the concentration of the undesirable low density lipoprotein (LDL) fraction and speeding the clearance of chylomicrons from the circulation (Haskell, 1984). These changes seem to be related to an increase of lipoprotein lipase (LPL) and lecithin cholesterol acyltransferase (LCAT) activity, with a greater breakdown of triglycerides in endurance competitors; a decrease of body mass may also be involved, since LDL-cholesterol is particularly low in very lean long-distance runners.

It has been widely suggested that regular endurance exercise is helpful to the diabetic patient. In the young adult, it is not clearly established that an increase of physical activity will help the course of the disease. It is quite possible for those with mild diabetes to participate in vigorous endurance sport, but care must be taken to ensure that an accelerated uptake of insulin and increased carbohydrate usage does not provoke a hypoglycaemic crisis during bouts of physical activity. The main value of exercise for the young diabetic contestant is in reducing the likelihood of late complications (particularly ischaemic heart disease). In the older person who is affected by maturity-onset diabetes, renewed involvement in regular endurance sport can lower resting blood sugar and increase insulin sensitivity, reducing the need for insulin injections and in some cases eliminating the need for insulin treatment (Holm & Krotkiewski, 1985). However, it does not seem to normalize the glucose tolerance curve.

Neoplasms

There has been much discussion about the possible impact of sports participation upon the risk of developing a neoplasm (Shephard, 1986b). Divergent conclusions have reflected the wide range of potential neoplasms and the differing categories of athlete that have been investigated.

In some specific situations, the athlete may be at increased risk of malignancy. Swimmers, dinghy sailors and other contestants in water sports may have a high exposure to ultraviolet radiation, and thus an above-average risk of skin tumours. Likewise, athletes who have required repeated radiographs because of recurrent injuries may develop neoplasms attributable to local X-irradiation. On the other hand, the endurance competitor is at a lower risk of several types of tumour because of life-long abstinence from cigarettes.

The end-result for most competitors is that the overall risk of malignancy does not differ greatly from that anticipated in the general population. One particular item that has been consistently documented is an association between endurance activity and a reduced incidence of colonic cancers. This could reflect differing dietary preferences in an active person, but the main explanation is probably an increase of gastrointestinal motility associated with endurance exercise (the 'runner's trots'). As a consequence of the increased gastrointestinal motility, toxic materials remain in the large intestine for a shorter time period than would be likely in a sedentary individual. One study of female endurance competitors has also demonstrated a low incidence of breast and uterine cancers; this has been attributed to the reduced blood levels of oestrogens associated with prolonged endurance training.

Immune function

The acute effect of endurance activity is a suppression of immune function, with (at least theoretically) an increased vulnerability to both infections and neoplasms. However, repeated bouts of endurance training reduce the vulnerability of the individual to a given intensity of exercise, so that the immune system of a well-trained athlete may be superior to that of a sedentary person. The potential gains from endurance training can be negated if the individual is perceiving the demands of either training or competition as stressful. Over-training also appears to be associated with a depression of immune function.

Psychological function

The potential of sports involvement to improve mood-state has already been noted. There may be an increase of self-esteem, related to (i) the approval of significant others (the coach, team-mates or spectators), or (ii) the satisfaction of personal goals (self-actualization). Such influences seem more likely to operate in team than in individual sports. At the same time, bouts of prolonged vigorous exercise tend to increase the level of cerebral arousal through both an increase of proprioceptive stimulation and an increased output of catecholamines. Finally, prolonged exercise may increase the output of

β-endorphins (the 'runner's high'), with a positive influence upon mood-state (Harber & Sutton, 1984).

There have been reports suggesting that regular physical activity improves the intellectual performance of young children and slows the deterioration of neural function in seniors. In young children, the enhanced academic performance has been linked to an increase of body awareness, including a more accurate perception of body dimensions, a better appreciation of the vertical, and more accurate finger recognition, in accord with the classical French concept of a linkage between motor development and intellectual attainment (Shephard, 1982a). The optimal pattern of sport has yet to be delineated, but if the French hypothesis is well founded, greater gains of academic performance might be anticipated in forms of sport that required highly skilled movements, rather than the repetitive movements typical of many endurance activities.

In older adults, it has been speculated that exercise may help cerebral performance by periodically raising the systemic blood pressure and thus increasing the perfusion of the brain. If this hypothesis is true, the greatest response might be anticipated from sports demanding vigorous muscular straining. However, elderly subjects have shown gains in response to cardiovascular endurance-type activities, so that the true explanation of the findings may be an increase of arousal, a greater awareness of the surrounding environment, or even an increased interest in life associated with membership of a sports club, rather than an improvement of cerebral perfusion (Dustman *et al.*, 1984).

Personal lifestyle

It seems likely that involvement in endurance sport would have a beneficial influence upon various aspects of personal lifestyle, such as diet, the consumption of cigarettes, alcohol and other drugs, sleep patterns and other variables (Shephard, 1989). In practice, the overall impact upon the lifestyle and thus the risk of future disease is surprisingly small.

Some studies have suggested that athletes have an increased tendency to die violent deaths; this has been attributed to their leadership in war, their quest for vertiginous stimulation, and their willingness to take risks when driving a vehicle (Polednak, 1978).

In the USA, there have also been suggestions that former 'major letter'-winners are more likely to be overweight, heavy smokers, and heavy consumers of alcohol than their non-competitive peers by the time that they reach middle-age (Montoye et al., 1956). This reflects the social nature of many of the 'major-letter' sports, and the relatively short period of active participation. In contrast, Scandinavian studies of cross-country skiers have shown continued vigorous participation to an advanced age, with relatively few members of this group becoming addicted to cigarettes; apparently as a consequence of the favourable lifestyle, the cross-country skiers were found to live several years longer than their sedentary counterparts (Fig. 47.5, Table 47.2; Karvonen et al., 1974). Masters' athletes (mainly swimmers and distance runners) are also rarely current smokers, although the cessation of smoking in members of this group often antedates involvement in sport; smoking withdrawal and sport involvement seem to be expressions of an inherent above-average interest in health (Kavanagh et al., 1989).

Conclusion

Involvement in endurance sport induces changes in various body systems that intuitively seem to have a positive value for health, supplementing the well-accepted gains of cardiovascular condition. However, the dose–response relationship is non-linear, and in many instances a careful watch must be kept to avoid excessive training; this not only negates the anticipated gains, but can also have a negative effect upon overall health.

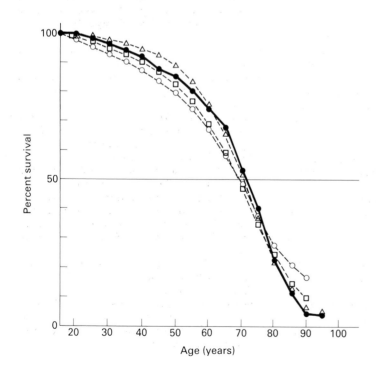

Fig. 47.5 Survival of Finnish male cross-country ski champions (●) (median year of death 1947) compared with three cohorts of the general Finnish male population. ○, 1931–35; □, 1946–50; △, 1956–60. From Karvonen et al. (1974), with permission.

Table 47.2 Numbers of Finnish male cross-country skiers surviving at various ages compared with three cohorts of the general Finnish population. Compare with Fig. 47.5. From Karvonen *et al.* (1974), with permission.

Age (years)	Skiers	Total male population 1931−35	1946−50	1956−60
15−19	1000	1000	1000	1000
20−24	1000	981	988	995
25−29	982	953	967	987
30−34	963	928	946	976
35−39	945	901	925	964
40−44	917	871	901	946
45−49	872	836	870	923
50−54	847	793	826	887
55−59	800	738	765	832
60−64	738	666	685	753
65−69	672	578	583	646
70−74	527	478	465	515
75−79	397	372	341	368
80−84	224	273	238	228
85−89	113	203	144	120
90−94	38	164	100	63
95−99	38	−	−	43

References

Åstrand, P.-O. & Rodahl, K. (1986) *Textbook of Work Physiology*, 3rd edn. McGraw Hill, New York.

Bailey, D.A. & McCulloch, R.G. (1990) Bone tissue and physical activity. *Can. J. Sport Sci.* **15**, 229−239.

Drinkwater, B., Nilson, K., Ott, S. & Chestnut, C.H. (1986) Bone mineral density after resumption of menses in amenorrheic athletes. *J.A.M.A.* **256**, 380−382.

Dustman, R.E., Ruhling, R.O., Russell, E.M. *et al.* (1984) Aerobic exercise and improved neuropsychological function of older individuals. *Neurobiol. Aging* **5**, 35−42.

Eichner, E.R. (1989) Does running cause osteoarthritis? An epidemiological perspective. *Phys. Sportsmed.* **17**(3), 147−154.

Harber, V.J. & Sutton, J.O. (1984) Endorphins and exercise. *Sports Med.* **1**, 154−171.

Haskell, W.L. (1984) The influence of exercise on the concentration of triglyceride and cholesterol in plasma. *Exerc. Sport Sci. Rev.* **12**, 205−244.

Health & Welfare, Canada (1982) *Canada Health Survey*. Health & Welfare, Ottawa.

Herzlich, C. (1973) *Health and Illness*. Academic Press, London.

Holm, G.A.L. & Krotkiewski, M.J. (1985) Exercise in the treatment of diabetes mellitus. In: Welsh, P. & Shephard, R.J. (eds) *Current Therapy in Sports Medicine*, pp. 105−108. B.C. Decker, Burlington, Ontario.

Ike, R.W., Lampman, R.M. & Castor, C.W. (1989) Arthritis and aerobic exercise: a review. *Phys. Sportsmed.* **17**(2), 128−139.

Karvonen, M.J., Klemola, H., Virkajarvi, J. & Kekkonen, A. (1974) Longevity of endurance skiers. *Med. Sci. Sports* **6**, 49−51.

Kavanagh, T., Mertens, D. & Shephard, R.J. (1989) Health and aging of Masters athletes. *Clin. Sports Med.* **1**, 72−88.

Lane, N.E., Bloch, D.A., Jones, N.H. *et al.* (1986) Long-distance running, bone density and osteoarthritis. *J.A.M.A.* **255**, 1147−1151.

Montoye, H.J., van Huss, W.D., Olson, H., Hudec, A. & Mahoney, E. (1956) Study of longevity and morbidity of college athletes. *J.A.M.A.* **162**, 1132−1134.

Paffenbarger, R.S., Hyde, R.T., Wing, A.L. & Hsieh, C.C. (1986) Physical activity, all-cause mortality and longevity of college alumni. *N. Engl. J. Med.* **314**, 605−613.

Pascale, M. & Grana, W.A. (1989) Does running cause osteo-arthritis? An orthopedic perspective. *Phys. Sportsmed.* **17**(3), 156−166.

Pekkanen, J., Marti, B., Nissinen, A., Tuomilehto, J., Punsar, S. & Karvonen, M.J. (1987) Reduction of premature mortality by high physical activity: a 20-year follow-up of middle-aged Finnish men. *Lancet* **i**, 1473−1477.

Polednak, A.P. (1978) *The Longevity of Athletes*. C.C. Thomas, Springfield, Illinois.

Schoutens, A., Laurent, E. & Poortmans, J.R. (1989) Effects of inactivity and exercise on bone. *Sports Med.* **7**, 71−81.

Shephard, R.J. (1976) Exercise and chronic obstructive lung disease. *Exerc. Sport Sci. Rev.* **4**, 263−296.

Shephard, R.J. (1982a) *Physical Activity and Growth*. Year Book Publishers, Chicago.

Shephard, R.J. (1982b) Are we asking the right questions? *J. Cardiac Rehabil.* **2**, 21−26.

Shephard, R.J. (1985) The value of physical fitness in preventive medicine. In: Evered, D. & Whelan, J. (eds) *The Value of Preventive Medicine*, pp. 164−182. CIBA Foundation Symposium Pitman, London.

Shephard, R.J. (1986a) *The Economic Benefits of Enhanced Fitness*. Human Kinetics Publishers, Champaign, Illinois.

Shephard, R.J. (1986b) Exercise and malignancy. *Sports Med.* **3**, 235−241.

Shephard, R.J. (1987) *Physical Activity and Aging*. Croom Helm, London.

Shephard, R.J. (1989) Exercise and lifestyle change. *Br. J. Sports Med.* **23**, 11–21.

Shephard, R.J. & Montelpare, W. (1988) Geriatric benefits of exercise as an adult. *J. Gerontol.* **43**, M86–M90.

Sidney, K.H. & Shephard, R.J. (1978) Frequency and intensity of exercise training for elderly subjects. *Med. Sci. Sports* **10**, 125–131.

Society of Actuaries (1959) *Build and Blood Pressure Study*. Society of Actuaries, Chicago.

Tipton, C.M., Matthes, R.D., Maynard, J.A. & Carey, R.A. (1975) The influence of physical activity on ligaments and tendons. *Med. Sci. Sports* **7**, 165–175.

PART 7

SPECIFIC ISSUES IN INDIVIDUAL SPORTS

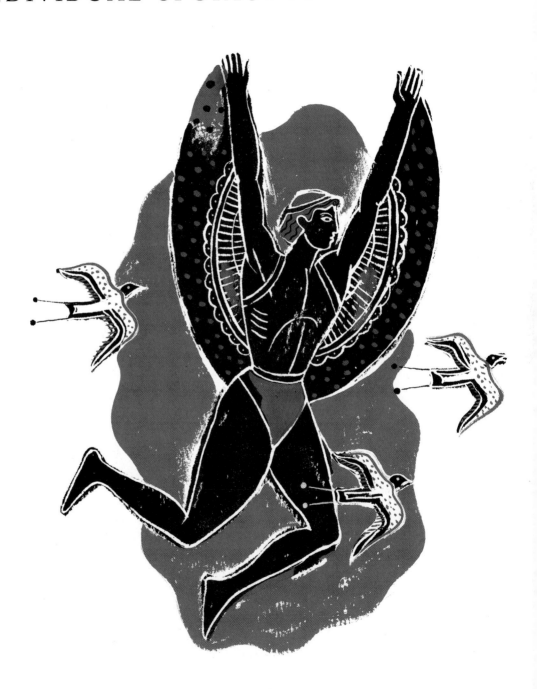

Chapter 48

Swimming as an Endurance Sport

LENNART GULLSTRAND

Introduction

Swimming is in many ways a peculiar sport. From a physiological point of view, one of the most striking aspects of competitive swimming is that it is dominated by anaerobic events (Table 48.1; Houston, 1978; Maglischo, 1982; Troup, 1984), while practice for most distances is still dominated by aerobic workouts. This is supported by the fact that 10 out of a total of 13 events for both sexes in international competitions are swum at distances taking less than about 2 min. When all 4×100-m and 4×200-m relays are included, the number of anaerobic events is increased even further.

During 1986, the 50-m freestyle was added to the international programme for both men and women. By analogy with track and field, this event is similar in duration to the running distance of 200 m.

That swimming during training is dominated by aerobic exercises can be seen by the high values of maximal oxygen intake measured for swimmers (Holmér, 1979). In a review table with other sports we find female and male swimmers with values of 3.5 and 5.5 $l \cdot min^{-1}$, respectively, in the top third of athletes from endurance sports such as long-distance running, cross-country skiing, and orienteering. Similar figures have repeatedly been measured for Swedish national team swimmers since the early 1960s (Åstrand & Rodahl, 1986).

Table 48.1 Relative contribution of anaerobic and aerobic metabolism in international swim distances.

Race distance (m)	Approximate time* (min : s)	Anaerobic metabolism									Aerobic metabolism (%)		
		ATP–PCr (alactic) (%)			HLa (lactic) (%)			Total (%)					
		M	T	H	M	T	H	M	T	H	M	T	H
50	0:23	78	98	—	20	2	—	98	100	—	2	—	—
100	0:50	25	80	—	65	15	—	90	95	80	10	5	20
200	1:50	10	30	—	65	65	—	75	95	60	25	5	40
400	3:50	7	20	—	40	55	—	47	75	40	53	25	60
800	7:50	5	—	—	30	—	—	35	—	17	65	—	83
1500	15:00	3	10	—	20	20	—	23	30	10	77	70	90

* Male élite swimmers.
ATP, adenosine triphosphate; PCr, phosphocreatine; HLa, lactic acid; M, Maglischo (1982); T, Troup (1984); H, Houston (1978).

Comparison with maximal oxygen intake expressed in $ml\cdot kg^{-1}\cdot min^{-1}$ is in this case not justified because the static lifting force influences the body. Extra body fat has only a minor negative effect on performance in water compared with dry land.

A superficial analysis of the training performed by élite swimmers allows us to understand their large aerobic power. It is usual to swim between eight and 12 workouts per week with a distance of 4000–12000 m (60–120 min) per workout. Strangely enough, the character of the training is similar for long periods regardless of the distance being trained for.

To draw up a training plan based on a physiological competition profile, as in Table 48.1, is unrealistic for most swimmers competing over 50, 100 and 200 m. A 100-m and 200-m swimmer cannot, for example, stand workouts in which 80–90% is at an anaerobic intensity, especially since 65% of this training is calculated to be of a lactic acid nature, with the remaining part being aerobic. Nevertheless, there has been a certain change in the training design over the past 10 years. More and more anaerobic sessions are seen in a 100-m swimmer's training, as well as more frequent periods of both active and passive rest (Gullstrand, 1985; 1986a; 1986b).

One of the reasons for the dominance of aerobic training is probably that swimming is very much an 'arm and upper body sport'. All leg-dependent athletes on land have special training for the lower extremities plus the daily stimulation of walking and standing. A swimmer while not actually swimming receives virtually no training of the upper body, and especially not of the 'proper' arm muscles. Perhaps this is one of the reasons for the distance and time the swimmer has to undertake to be successful, regardless of short or long distance performance. Compared with a runner, a swimmer could reduce the workout time if she or he could swim to and from school, work or a training session. In such a fantasy situation the 100-m swimmer would probably do better with a training based on the competitive profile mentioned above.

The fact that the arms and upper body must be well trained locally can be seen from longitudinal oxygen intake measurements for the Olympic champion Gunnar Larsson from 1970 to 1975 (Fig. 48.1). The top values in swimming were recorded when he was a double gold medal winner at the 1972 Olympics. Between the major competitions his maximal oxygen intake was reduced when swimming, while for running it remained unchanged. The conclusion can be drawn that treadmill testing does not mirror swimming performance.

It was mentioned above that maximal oxygen intake of swimmers should not be expressed in $ml\cdot kg^{-1}\cdot min^{-1}$. Litres per minute is a better measure, but is by itself incomplete when expressing endurance in swimming.

A better way is probably to calculate the

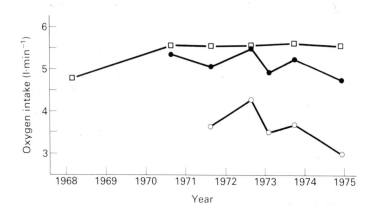

Fig. 48.1 Oxygen intake during maximal swimming and running for World and Olympic medal swimmer Gunnar Larsson over a period of 8 years. □, Running; ●, front crawl (whole stroke); ○, front crawl (arms only). From Åstrand & Rodahl (1986).

oxygen intake in $l \cdot min^{-1} \cdot kg^{-1}$ *body weight in water* because that is where the athlete is performing. Hydrostatic weight is measured with the swimmer completely submerged after a maximal exhalation. This way of expressing swimming endurance includes some of the swimmer's sinking force, which is crucial for the water resistance the swimmer has to overcome to attain certain swim speeds.

Using this method, we can see from Table 48.2 that female swimmer A has a higher oxygen intake per kg body weight in water than female swimmer B, even though swimmer B has higher values expressed both in $l \cdot min^{-1}$ and $ml \cdot kg^{-1} \cdot min^{-1}$ based on dry land weight.

Swimmer A had better race results for long-distance events than swimmer B, but both were national champions at long distances. A similar comparison can be made between female swimmers C and D, who also look more or less favourable depending on whether the oxygen intake is based on land or underwater weight. D had a maximum of more than $12~ml \cdot kg^{-1} \cdot min^{-1}$ higher than C on dry land, but C had a higher oxygen intake when weight in water is used. However, these women competed at 100 and 200 m, where maximal aerobic power plays only a minor role. The swimmers thus had similar competitive times.

Other findings also illustrate the problem of correlating high oxygen intake values with swim endurance. Earlier longitudinal studies on top swimmers showed that they could beat national records for 400-m distances during championships, with approximately 15% lower oxygen intake values compared with their corresponding measurements during the pre-season months (Gullstrand & Holmér, 1983). Less remarkably, the maximal oxygen intake values for 100 and 200-m swimmers usually decline at the time of championships compared with 'hard work periods'. The dominating anaerobic energy delivery at these distances could explain the decline (L. Gullstrand, unpublished data).

Heart rate and lactate tests

The linear relationship between heart rate and work rate is one of the cornerstones of Åstrand's cycle ergometer test for predicting maximal oxygen intake. In the past, Treffene (1978) in swimming and Conconi *et al.* (1982) in other sports have used this correlation to construct sport-specific tests.

The heart rate (oxygen intake)/performance line is shifted rightwards with improved endurance capacity, which means, for example, that given swim speeds can be performed at a lower heart rate. The linear part of the lactate performance curve similarly undergoes a shift to the right.

Conconi's test additionally identifies a so-called heart rate deflection point (HR_d), where the heart rate no longer increases linearly with work rate, but does so at a reduced rate.

Approximately 600 tests on Swedish national team swimmers have indicated that when swimming, the HR_d point does not coincide with the start of the rise in blood lactate con-

Table 48.2 Comparison of maximal oxygen intake calculated using dry land weight and hydrostatic weight in female subjects A−D. The measurements were made in a swimming flume. From Gullstrand (1988).

Race distances (m)	Subject	$\dot{V}O_{2\,max}$ ($l \cdot min^{-1}$)	Mass (kg)	Test value ($ml \cdot kg^{-1} \cdot min^{-1}$)	Hydrostatic weight (kg)	Test value in water ($l \cdot kg^{-1} \cdot min^{-1}$)
400, 800 &	A	2.8	57.3	48.9	1.3	2.2
1500	B	3.6	61.8	58.3	2.9	1.2
100 & 200	C	2.8	74.3	37.7	2.2	1.3
	D	3.4	67.6	50.3	3.0	1.1

centration in the stepwise manner that Conconi imputes to runners. In a 10 × 100-m increased speed swim test with simultaneous measurements of heart rate and blood lactate, the HR_d occurred at higher speeds. In Fig. 48.2, showing an example of one world-class swimmer, it can be seen that HR_d correlates better with what other investigators call maximal lactate steady state, at about the 4 mmol·l^{-1} level.

This finding, together with the linear heart rate performance finding, could be useful when evaluating and monitoring endurance training in swimmers.

Lactate testing

In recent years the worldwide use of lactate tests in swimming has become very popular. Different kinds of lactate performance curves and threshold tests based on 'micro' blood samples have been constructed after various swim performances. The aims of these tests are to evaluate training, prescribe optimal loading during training, predict race results, and detect talent.

These methods are particularly applicable to swimming because the pool offers relatively constant conditions over time, and because swimming is a 'cyclic sport', with an even pace as one of the most important considerations during races and in training.

Mader's two-point test is one of the most well-known threshold tests (Mader et al., 1976). However, it has been criticized for the use of a fixed 4 mmol·l^{-1} point to describe the aerobic–anaerobic threshold and optimal training load. Heck et al. (1985) and others have pointed out that this threshold is individual and can occur below as well as above 4 mmol·l^{-1} (see Stegmann et al., 1983, Olbrecht et al., 1985).

The aerobic–anaerobic threshold is defined as the work rate at which the maximal balance is found between production and elimination of lactate. This has also been called the maximal lactate steady state (Heck et al., 1985). From 1977 to 1982 Swedish national team swimmers were frequently tested with a battery of tests. The first year included the two-point test described by Mader et al. (1976), but certain problems led to a more training-related test (L. Gullstrand, unpublished results). One hundred metres were swum from eight to 10 times with increased effort, starting at a low speed and ending with a maximal effort. With this design, the time reduction per repetition was about 2 s. Microsamples of blood were taken from the earlobe after each 100-m swim. The resulting lactate performance curve includes lactate concentration during aerobically dominated metabolism, the individual aerobic–anaerobic transition, and lactate levels during anaerobically dominated metabolism

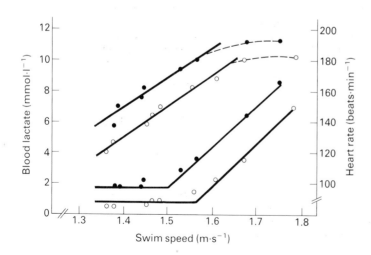

Fig. 48.2 Blood lactate and heart rate values at 8–10 × 100-m freestyle for one world-class 200-m swimmer. Values shown as open circles are from an extensive and aerobically dominated period of training. Black circles denote values obtained after a 3-week period of increased training for speed and anaerobic qualities with less distance training. The dashed lines indicate heart rates beyond the deflection point (see text). From Gullstrand (1988).

(Fig. 48.2). All parts of the curve could be of interest for evaluation and training, as swimming during training is traditionally carried out over the whole 'metabolic scale'.

By using a standardized treatment of the lactate performance curve (Fig. 48.2), the base lactate level, the speed at aerobic—anaerobic transition, and the increase in (and maximal) lactate concentration can be compared during different periods of training. An indication of the true maximal anaerobic metabolism can probably be found only after maximal effort races during important competitions or during simulated races where the swimmers are highly motivated (L. Gullstrand, unpublished results). Measurement of maximal anaerobic power is probably impossible because the actual energy demand cannot be predicted.

The lactate performance profile showed typical variations at several points depending on whether the tests were conducted during hard training periods or in direct connection with championships (Table 48.3). The Swedish national team swimmers from whom the data were derived had different specializations with regard to both distance and technique. However, very rarely has anyone broken the general pattern by showing a lower base level, higher transition speed or lower maximal lactate concentration when hard training periods have been compared with tests connected with important races.

Lower base level of lactate at aerobically dominated speeds and a lower maximal lactate value after the final 10th 100-m repetition during hard training could be seen as an effect resulting from metabolic adaptation to the type of training that was conducted. Extended periods of interval training and the covering of long distances more or less automatically lead to aerobically dominated training.

During the weeks of physiological tapering leading up to competition, the total amount of training is usually reduced gradually and more competition-speed oriented training is introduced. The elevated maximal lactate—and elevated base—levels that can be seen in Table 48.3 are thus logical.

The significant decrease in transition speed noticed at the 10 × 100-m test at the time for competition, especially for the 400−1500-m swimmers, should be considered when evaluating swimmers during tapering training. The reason for this is that mid- to long-distance races are swum in this specific speed zone. Therefore, one would want swimmers' tran-

Table 48.3 Comparison of mean values from four well-defined parts of the lactate performance curve obtained during extensive training and at the time of competition. Values are from 8 to 10 × 100-m freestyle stroke (see also Fig. 48.2). From Gullstrand (1988).

	Base level $(mmol \cdot l^{-1})$	Transition speed $(m \cdot s^{-1})$	Slope $(y = a + bx)$	HLa_{max} $(mmol \cdot l^{-1})$
Men ($n = 11$)				
Preparation training	1.3	1.550	39.8	7.3
Competition	1.7	1.532	44.6	9.2
p-value	0.01	n.s.	n.s.	0.01
Women ($n = 11$)				
Preparation training	1.2	1.425	51.1	7.0
Competition	1.7	1.402	50.8	8.7
p-value	0.001	0.01	n.s.	0.05

HLa_{max}, maximal blood lactate concentration; n.s., not significant.

sition speeds to increase, and definitely not to decline. This discussion should probably also include 200-m swimmers.

Specific methods of endurance training

Without doubt, the most frequently practised swim training method is the interval method. To develop aerobic power and capacity, extended series of laps with relatively short resting intervals of 10–30 s are often performed. The total distance of the series can range from 1000 to 5000 m, sometimes even more, and is usually divided into distances of from 50 to 800 m. The series can be 'straight', which means that the same distance is repeated throughout, or it can consist of mixed distances.

The rest periods between laps and swim strokes are also mixed. Every coach and swimmer has a set-up of their own, and their inventive capacity is enormous. Often the top athlete group consists of 15–20 swimmers using a very limited space in the pool. Therefore, the swimmers are usually organized to swim in a 'loop' in the lanes. In these cases, the straight series are the easiest to control for both swimmers and coaches, with regard to speed, heart rate and rest intervals.

Less frequently used are long-distance swimming of 2000–3000 m, or maximal distance over a given time of 20–50 min. These series are mostly swum with the whole stroke to create the greatest possible load on the cardiovascular system (see more about endurance training at the end of this chapter).

A study of top-level swimmers by Huber *et al.* (1978) revealed less discrepancy in heart rate between series of whole stroke, pulling and kicking (170, 160 and 150 beats·min^{-1}, respectively) than might be expected. The differences were even less among regional swimmers (175, 175 and 170 beats·min^{-1}). These findings indicate that the muscle mass engaged during kicking and pulling is large enough to result in a good central stimulation of the cardiovascular system.

Risks in endurance training

There are several risks with the extensive training regarded as necessary for top-level swimmers to attain a high level of swimming endurance. One is that a major portion of the training does not correspond well with the metabolic competition profile described in Table 48.1.

Planned endurance training is frequently executed at too high an intensity and results in substantial lactate accumulation, which in top-level swimming often leads to what is known as over-training. The swimmer feels very weak and cannot reproduce normal training speeds. It can take days or even weeks of easy swimming or rest for the swimmer to recover to 'normal' capacity.

Madsen (1982/83) emphasized the need for controlled intensity training to obtain the desired effect. The control method he recommended was frequent measurement of blood lactate concentration.

Too low a training intensity is often the result of extensive workouts that primarily stimulate aerobic metabolism. One reason for this is that stored glycogen will have had time to be only partially restored (Costill, 1985). In this case fat becomes the dominant energy source during training. Poor training results and tiredness during the third day of a two-workouts-per-day training camp are classical and are caused by emptied or partially emptied glycogen stores.

This theory is supported by the lower base lactate level in the lactate performance curve. Lower values of RQ (respiratory quotient) for a given submaximal oxygen intake are also found during endurance training compared with competition periods. Some of these negative metabolic effects can be eliminated by more effective scheduling of training. In this connection, the importance of good nutrition must be emphasized. According to several investigations, athletic nutrition can be improved a great deal.

Another risk associated with low-speed, extensive training is found at the neuromuscular level. During low-speed training, swimming movements are accomplished with low limb speed. Several investigators have shown that low-speed training gives good results for the practised limb speed, but a doubtful transfer of the training effect to higher limb speeds. On the other hand, high-speed movements give good effects at both high and low speeds (Lesmes et al., 1978).

Other researchers mostly agree with these findings, but some narrow the training effect of fast-movement training to fast limb movements (Caiosso et al., 1981; Kanehisa & Miyashita, 1983). The stroke frequency of a good 100-m freestyle swimmer repeating 100-m swims in training at a speed of 60–70 s corresponds to 30–38 arm cycles per min (one cycle is one left and one right arm stroke). At a maximal swim speed of 50 s over a 100-m distance, the frequency of the same swimmer will be roughly 66 cycles per min (Craig et al., 1979). The difference between training and race movement

speeds is approximately 50%. Because much endurance training for good male 100-m swimmers today is swum at a speed of 60–70 s, it can be concluded that there is a substantial difference between the movement speed in training and competitions.

One way of solving both the metabolic and the neuromuscular problems can be found in 15:15 training, which is a way of including a large number of repetitions during 15-s exercise at race pace and 15-s rest. The first study in this area was published in 1960 and was performed on runners (Christensen et al., 1960). In recent years the same design has been used for good swimmers (Gullstrand & Lawrence, 1987). In Fig. 48.3 the acute effect on blood lactate levels and heart rate can be seen during and after 40×25-m freestyle with an average speed corresponding to race pace at 100 m. The relatively low lactate level of 3 mmol·l^{-1} and high mean heart rate of 179 beats·min^{-1} indicate a low level of anaerobic work and a high aerobic loading.

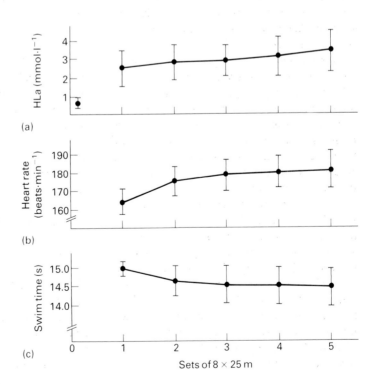

Fig. 48.3 Mean values of (a) blood lactate (HLa), (b) heart rate and (c) swim time for five sets of 8×25-m swim efforts at 100-m race pace ($n = 9$). From Gullstrand & Lawrence (1987).

After a 100-m maximal swim the mean lactate concentration was 7.1 mmol·l^{-1} and heart rate was 191 beats·min^{-1}. The 40×25-m freestyle with a 15:15 design resulted in 43% of maximal lactate and 93% of maximal heart rate.

In conclusion, this study shows the advantages of 'intermittent training': swimming a good deal at race pace; reaching a high aerobic load; and swimming with a low anaerobic lactic stress.

Tapering and endurance

It is not yet fully understood how the tapering phase affects factors related to swim endurance. The problem seems to be how to become rested and 'superadapted' for the competition without losing endurance quality during the tapering phase. Few investigations have been carried out in this area, although the physiological changes seen in well-trained endurance athletes after the cessation of training have been described (Houston et al., 1979; Costill et al., 1985).

In comparison with maximal oxygen intake, endurance is reduced more quickly with detraining and inactivity. The reason is the reduction of oxidative enzyme activity. This activity is reduced by 50% after a week of inactivity (Henriksson & Reitman, 1977). Houston and coworkers (1979) demonstrated a 4% decrease in maximal oxygen intake, 24% lower SDH (succinate dehydrogenase) activity, and a 25% reduction in endurance during a 15–18-min run in a group of highly trained runners after a training interruption of 15 days. Costill et al. (1985) studied the phosphorylase and phosphofructokinase activity of top-level swimmers during a 4-week period of no training, but did not find any significant change in these variables. As the investigation was carried out after a tapering and competition phase, reasons were given for believing that the swimmers had already started to reduce their enzyme activity during the tapering phase. They probably also competed with a reduced endurance capacity. These swimmers trained for 5 months, with 6 days of training per week

and an average swimming distance of 10 900 m per day.

In another study, eight female national team swimmers were followed over a 6-week tapering period (L. Gullstrand, unpublished data). Maximal oxygen intake was significantly reduced, from 3.5 to 3.2 l·min^{-1}, in the 6-week period.

Lactate performance testing in connection with the $8-10 \times 100$-m protocol was carried out every week and aerobic–anaerobic transition speeds had significantly reduced, for 2.4 s per 100 m between measurements undertaken 3 weeks before and they 1 day after the championships. The results indicated that the group using a traditional tapering pattern had reduced their performances in both types of endurance test.

The female swimmers had specialized for 100 and 200-m distances and they performed well as a group at the meet. A reduced endurance is not so important at these distances. On the other hand, the swimming times might have been better with higher maximal oxygen intake and lactate threshold values.

Conclusion

Endurance training in top-level swimming is very important for both short- and long-distance swimmers. In fact, many world class short-distance swimmers were also highly ranked when competing over 400–1500 m when they were younger. Whether this results from a necessary and natural development of better performance over shorter distances or from a failure to identify sprinting talent is unclear.

The trend over the past few years has been to adapt swim training more and more to the physiological profile of the distances competed at. This should not be regarded as a way of short-cutting the work necessary to become a top-level swimmer, but more as a trial of more effective training.

To make swim training more effective, sophisticated methods of testing can be used such as measuring blood lactate concentrations, although any one test method alone probably should not be relied on. Several physiological qualities need to be considered, and a battery of relevant tests is desirable.

For endurance, maximal oxygen intake or heart rate measurements will be suitable for evaluation of the central capacity, while lactate performance tests will say more about the peripheral capacity.

Föhrenbach et al. (1984) divided the lactate performance curve into five intensity zones and attributed to each zone a major training effect. Absaliamow (1984) constructed a table with lactate and heart rate values for each training zone. This way of classifying training has major advantages for the understanding, monitoring and evaluation of training for swimming. It is important to understand that these recommendations must be adapted for each individual swimmer.

The Soviet coach Koshkin (1984) demonstrated how both frequent heart rate and lactate measurement were a part of Vladimir Salnikov's training (Fig. 48.4). During one period, all training was controlled by heart rate. As a world record-holder for the longest distance in swimming (1500 m), Salnikov may be seen as one of the leading representatives of endurance and endurance training in swimming. However, we do not know whether his performance would have been still better if his training had been modified.

Acknowledgements

The author's results in this paper originate from investigations undertaken at the Department of Physiology III, Karolinska Institute, Stockholm, Sweden with grants from the Swedish Swimming Federation and at the Department of Human Movement and Recreation Studies at the University of Western Australial, Perth, Australia.

References

Absaliamow, T. (1984) Controlling the training of top level swimmers. In: Cramer, J.L. (ed.) How to Develop Olympic Level Swimmers, pp. 14–21. International Sport Media, Finland.
Åstrand, P.-O. & Rodahl, K (1986) Textbook of Work Physiology, 3rd edn. McGraw Hill, New York.
Caiosso, V.J., Perrine, J.J. & Edgerton, W.R. (1981)

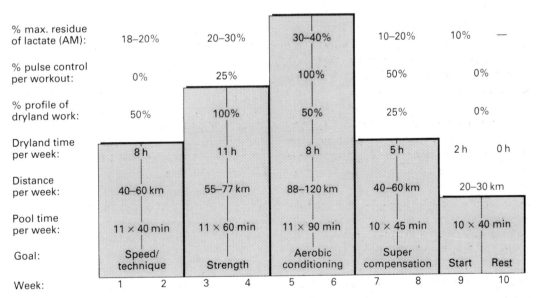

Fig. 48.4 Coach Koshkin's basic training pattern for 1500-m swimmer Salnikov and other Soviet top swimmers. The pattern is repeated five times a year in 10-week cycles. From Koshkin (1984).

Training induced alterations of the *in-vivo* force–velocity relationship of human muscle. *J. Appl. Physiol.* **51**(3), 750–754.

Christensen, E.H., Hedman, R. & Saltin, B. (1960) Intermittent and continuous running. *Acta Physiol. Scand.* **50**, 269–286.

Conconi, F., Ferrari, M., Liglio, P., Drogetti, P. & Codeca, L. (1982) Determination of the anaerobic threshold by a non invasive field test in runners. *J. Appl. Physiol.* **52**(4), 869–873.

Costill, D.L. (1985) Carbohydrate nutrition before, during and after exercise. *Fed. Proc.* **44**, 364–368.

Costill, D.L., Fink, W.J., Hargreaves, M., King, D.S., Tomas, R. & Fielding, R. (1985) Metabolic characteristics of skeletal muscle during detraining from competitive swimming. *Med. Sci. Sports Exerc.* **17**, 339–343.

Craig, A.B., Boomer, W.L. & Gibbons, J.F. (1979) Use of stroke, distance per stroke and velocity relationships during training for competitive swimming. In: Terauds, J. & Bedingfield, E.W. (eds) *Swimming III*, pp. 263–272. University Park Press, Baltimore.

Föhrenbach, R., Liesen, H., Mader, A., Heck, H., Vellage, E. & Hollmann, W. (1984) Wettkampf-und Trainingssteuerung von Marathonläuferinnen undläufern mittels leistungsdiagnostischer Felduntersuchungen. (Competition and training monitoring of female and male marathon runners by means of performance diagnostic field tests.) In: Heck, H., Hess, G. & Mader, A. (eds) *Comparative Study of Different Lactate Threshold Concepts*. Special issue, German Journal of Sports Medicine, Vol. 36, Nos 1 and 2.

Gullstrand, L. (1985) Soviet swimming: analysis, planning and research. *Simsport* **1**, 36–37 (in Swedish).

Gullstrand, L. (1986a) Periodization in training swimmers. In: Quinlan, P. (ed.) *Swim 86 Yearbook*, pp. 45–48. Australian Swimming Incorporated and Swimming Coaches Association, Mt Gravatt.

Gullstrand, L. (1986b) Physiological aspects of tapering swimmers. In: Quinlan, P. (ed.) *Swim 86 Yearbook*, pp. 39–43. Australian Swimming Incorporated and Swimming Coaches Association, Mt Gravatt.

Gullstrand, L. (1988) Swimming. In: Forsberg, A. & Saltin, B. (eds) *Konditionsträning*, pp. 280–291. Idrottens Forskningsråd, Sveriges Riksidrottsförbund (in Swedish).

Gullstrand, L. & Holmér, I. (1983) Physiological characteristics of champion swimmers during a five year follow-up period. In: Hollander, P. & de Groot, G. (eds) *Biomechanics and Medicine in Swimming*, pp. 258–262. Human Kinetics, Champaign, Illinois.

Gullstrand, L. & Lawrence, S. (1987) Heart rate and blood lactate response to short intermittent work at race pace in highly trained swimmers. *Aust. J. Sci. Med. Sport* **19**(1), 10–14.

Heck, H., Mader, A., Hess, G., Mucke, S., Muller, R. & Hollmann, W. (1985) Justification of the 4-mmol/l lactate threshold. *Int. J. Sports Med.* **6**, 117–130.

Henriksson, J. & Reitman, S. (1977) Time course of changes in human skeletal muscle succinate dehydrogenase and cytochrome oxidase activities and maximal oxygen uptake with physical activity and inactivity. *Acta Physiol. Scand.* **99**, 91–97.

Holmér, I. (1979) Physiology of swimming man. *Exerc. Sport Sci. Rev.* **7**, 87–123.

Houston, M.E. (1978) Metabolic responses to exercise with special reference to training and competition in swimming. In: Eriksson, B. & Furberg, B. (eds) *Swimming Medicine IV*, pp. 207–232. University Park Press, Baltimore.

Houston, M.E., Bentzen, H. & Larsen, H. (1979) Interrelationships between skeletal muscle adaptations and performance as studied by detraining and retraining. *Acta Physiol. Scand.* **105**, 163–170.

Huber, G., Keul, J., Kindermann, W. & Stocklasa, L. (1978) Herzfrequenzen, Lactatspiegel und pH-Wert bei verschiedenen Trainingsformen im Kraulschwimmen. (Heart rate, lactate level and pH value at different training regimes in swimming.) *Dtsch. Z. Sportmedizin* **X**, 282–291.

Kanehisa, H. & Miyashita, M. (1983) Specificity of velocity in strength training. *Eur. J. Appl. Physiol.* **52**, 104–106.

Koshkin, I. (1984) The training program that developed Salnikov. In: Cramer, J.L. (ed.) *How to Develop Olympic Level Swimmers*, pp. 107–116. International Sport Media, Finland.

Lesmes, G.R., Costill, D.L., Coyle, E.F. & Frick, W.J. (1978) Muscle strength and power changes during maximal isometric training. *Med. Sci. Sports* **10**(4), 266–269.

Mader, A., Heck, H. & Hollmann, W. (1976) Evaluation of lactic acid anaerobic energy contribution by determination of post exercise lactic acid concentration of capillary blood in middle distance runners and swimmers. In: Landry, F. & Orban, W. (eds) *Exercise Physiology*, pp. 187–199. Symposia Specialists Incorporated, Florida.

Madsen, Ö. (1982/83) Aerobic training: not so fast there. *Swimming Technique* **19**(3), 17–19.

Maglischo, E. (1982) *Swimming Faster*. Chico: Mayfield Publishing Company, Palo Alto.

Olbrecht, J., Madsen, Ö., Liesen, H. & Hollmann, W. (1985) Relationship between swimming velocity and lactic acid concentration during continuous and intermittent training exercises. *Int. J. Sports Med.* **6**(2), 74–77.

Stegmann, H., Weiler, B. & Kindermann, W. (1983) Vergleich verschiedener anaerober Schwellen-konzepte bei Sportlern unterschiedlicher Sportarten. (Comparison of different anaerobic threshold concepts for athletes representing various sports events.) In: Heck, H., Hollmann, W., Liesen, H. & Rost, R. (eds) *Sport, Leistung und Gesundheit*, pp. 163–167. Deutsche Ärzte Verlag, Cologne.

Treffene, R. (1978) Swimming performance test. A method of training and performance fine selection. Aust. J. Sports Med. **10**, 33–38.

Troup, J. (1984) Energy systems and training considerations. *J. Swimming Res.* **1**, 13–16.

Chapter 49

The Energetics of Running

PIETRO E. DI PRAMPERO

Introduction

The energetics of running (and indeed of many other forms of locomotion on land or in water) can be described appropriately, provided that the energy cost is known. This is defined as the amount of energy required to transport the subject's body over one unit distance. According to SI units the energy cost of running, which will here be given the symbol C_r, ought to be expressed in $kJ \cdot km^{-1}$, or in $J \cdot m^{-1}$; however, it is often convenient to express C_r in $kcal \cdot km^{-1}$ or in ml of oxygen per metre of distance. The above units can be converted into one another, considering that 1 litre of oxygen consumed in the body yields 5.0 kcal or 20.9 kJ (strictly true only when the respiratory quotient equals 0.96).

The energy expenditure per unit of time, or metabolic power output ($\dot{E}_r$), is given by the product of the energy cost multiplied by the running speed (v):

$$\dot{E}_r = C_r\, v \tag{1}$$

where, if C_r is expressed in $J \cdot m^{-1}$ and v in $m \cdot s^{-1}$, $\dot{E}_r$ is in watts. (To obtain $\dot{E}_r$ in terms of oxygen consumption, it is often convenient to express C_r in eqn. 1 in ml oxygen per metre of distance and v in $m \cdot min^{-1}$.) Rearranging eqn. 1 and applying it to maximal conditions:

$$v_{max} = \dot{E}_{r\,max}\, C_r^{-1} \tag{2}$$

where $\dot{E}_{r\,max}$ is the subject's maximal metabolic power during running, irrespective of the sources (aerobic and/or anaerobic) providing the energy for muscle contraction.

Equation 2 shows that the maximal running speed is set by the maximal metabolic power of the subject and by the energy cost of transport. Thus, for any given subject, v_{max} can be calculated provided that these two variables are known. However, $\dot{E}_{r\,max}$ is a function of the effort duration and C_r depends on the speed of progression.

This article is devoted to a discussion of: (i) the effects of the speed of progression on the energy cost of running; and (ii) the duration of the effort on $\dot{E}_{r\,max}$. It will then become possible (iii) to predict performances both in track and endurance running. Finally, (iv) a few paragraphs are devoted to a general discussion of the approach briefly described above.

Metabolic power requirement in running

The energy cost of level running at constant speed is the sum of the energy spent against air resistance and against non-aerodynamic forces. This last is essentially independent of the speed, whereas the former increases with the square of the speed (for a review on this and related matters see di Prampero, 1986). When the energy spent to accelerate the body from zero to the speed v is taken into account, the overall energy cost of track running from a still start can be described by:

$$C_r = C_{r\,NA} + k'\, v^2 + 0.5\, Mv^2\, \eta^{-1}\, d^{-1} \tag{3}$$

where $C_{r\,NA}$ is the energy cost per unit distance against non-aerodynamic forces, k' is the proportionality constant relating energy cost to air resistance and speed squared, M is the mass of the subject, d is the distance covered, and η is the efficiency of transformation of metabolic into kinetic energy. This last can be assumed to be 0.25, since in the initial acceleration phase no recovery of elastic energy takes place (Cavagna et al., 1971) and the overall efficiency of exercise must therefore approach the efficiency of muscular contraction. On the basis of published data (see di Prampero, 1986), for a subject with a body mass of 70 kg and a height of 175 cm, eqn. 3 becomes:

$$C_r = 270 + 0.72\, v^2 + 140\, v^2\, d^{-1} \qquad (3')$$

where C_r is given in kJ·km^{-1}, or J·m^{-1}, v in m·s^{-1} and d in m. It can be calculated from this equation that the kinetic energy term plays an appreciable role in the shortest distances, amounting to about 8% of the total for 400 m covered at world record speed; for longer distances it decreases progressively, to attain 0.2% for 10 000 m.

In eqn. 3', the energy expended against air resistance was calculated on the basis of the value of k' (0.72) applying at sea level conditions and 20°C. However, the energy expenditure against the wind (∂) is directly proportional to the air density, itself a function of barometric pressure (PB) and temperature (T):

$$\partial = \partial_0\, PB\, 760^{-1}\, 273\, T^{-1} \qquad (4)$$

where ∂_0 is the density of dry air at 760 torr and 273°K (1.29 kg·m^{-3}). Therefore, for conditions appreciably different from those specified above, k' must be appropriately corrected using eqn. 4.

The energy requirement per unit of time ($\dot{E}_r$ = metabolic power output) for running at speed v in the absence of wind (i.e. when ground and air speed are equal), is given by the product $C_r\, v$ (eqn. 1). Hence, from eqn. 3':

$$\dot{E}_r = C_r\, v = 270\, v + 0.72\, v^3 + 140\, v^3\, d^{-1} \qquad (5)$$

or, setting $v = d/t$:

$$\dot{E}_r = 270\, d\, t^{-1} + 0.72\, d^3\, t^{-3} + 140\, d^2\, t^{-3} \qquad (6)$$

For any given track event d is constant and known. Equation 6 therefore allows calculation of the metabolic power requirement as a function of the time employed to cover the distance in question. This has been done in Fig. 49.1 where the three steeper curves represent $\dot{E}_r$ during 800, 1000 and 1500-m track running for performance times extending below and above the corresponding world records.

This section has been devoted exclusively to track running, because this is the main object of this chapter. With the appropriate modifications, however, the above analysis can be applied to any other form of locomotion whose energy cost per unit distance as a function of speed is known.

Maximal metabolic power

The maximal power a given subject can maintain at a constant level throughout the effort is

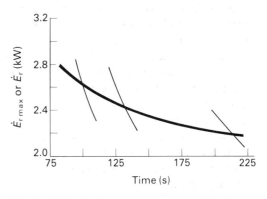

Fig. 49.1 Metabolic power requirement in track running ($\dot{E}_r$, kW, thin lines) to cover the 800, 1000 or 1500-m distance from a still start in the time indicated for a 70-kg, 175-cm subject at sea level, 20°C, in the absence of wind (see eqn. 6). The maximal metabolic power that an élite athlete of the same body build can develop as a function of the duration of effort ($\dot{E}_{r\,max}$, kW, thick line) is also indicated on the same time axis (see eqn. 8). Individual theoretical record times over the three distances are given by the abscissa value at which the $\dot{E}_{r\,max}$ function crosses the appropriate $\dot{E}_r$ curve. See text for details and references and Table 49.1 for the actual numerical values.

a decreasing function of the exhaustion time and, as shown by Scherrer and Monod (1960), this decrease can be approximated by a hyperbola. Wilkie (1980) has analysed the relationship between external power in cycling ($\dot{w}_{max}$) and duration of the exercise to exhaustion between 40 s and 10 min; longer durations were excluded because of the difficulty of assessing the exhaustion time precisely. The relationship between $\dot{w}_{max}$ (kW) and exhaustion time (t_e, s) is described by Wilkie (1980):

$$\dot{w}_{max} = A\, t_e^{-1} + B - B\, k^{-1}\, (1 - e^{-kt_e})\, t_e^{-1} \quad (7)$$

where A is the amount of mechanical work that can be derived from maximal utilization of the anaerobic (lactic + alactic) sources, i.e. from lactate production and high energy phosphate depletion; B is the mechanical power sustainable on the basis of $\dot{V}_{O_2\,max}$ alone; and $k = 0.1$ s^{-1} is the time constant with which $\dot{V}_{O_2\,max}$ is attained at the onset of exercise. The third term in eqn. 7 reflects the fact that $\dot{V}_{O_2\,max}$ cannot be instantaneously reached at the onset of exercise: it is rather small and decreases in relative importance with increasing t_e, from 11% of w_{max} at 40 s, to 1.5% at 10 min. A and B in eqn. 7 depend on the athletic characteristics of the subject; in Wilkie's case, $A = 16$ kJ and $B = 0.273$ kW.

On the basis of Wilkie's analysis, it seems reasonable to describe the relationship between maximal metabolic power in running ($\dot{E}_{r\,max}$) and exhaustion time in similar terms:

$$\dot{E}_{r\,max} = AnS\, t_e^{-1} + MAP - MAP\, k^{-1}$$
$$(1 - e^{-kt_e})\, t_e^{-1} \quad (8)$$

where AnS is the maximal amount of energy released by anaerobic (lactic + alactic) sources, MAP is the subject's maximal aerobic power, and k has the same value and meaning as in eqn. 7. If this is so, $\dot{E}_{r\,max}$ can be calculated as a function of t_e, assigning to AnS and MAP the values applicable to the subject in question. This has been done in Fig. 49.1 where the continuous thick curve represents $\dot{E}_{r\,max}$ for an élite athlete (70 kg, 175 cm) assuming $MAP = 1.8$ kW (corresponding to a $\dot{V}_{O_2\,max}$ of

74 ml·kg^{-1}·min^{-1} above resting) and $AnS = 100$ kJ (68 ml oxygen·kg^{-1}), this last being a reasonable estimate of the amount of energy released by complete utilization of lactic and alactic anaerobic stores in a top athlete (di Prampero, 1981). In summary, $\dot{E}_{r\,max}$ can be calculated for any given value of t_e, provided that the maximal aerobic power and the maximal anaerobic capacity of the subject are known.

The performance

Track running

As discussed above: (i) the metabolic power requirement in running ($\dot{E}_r$) for a given distance is a decreasing function of the time of performance; and (ii) the maximal metabolic power ($\dot{E}_{r\,max}$) for a given subject is a decreasing function of the duration of effort to exhaustion. $\dot{E}_r$ for three distances and $\dot{E}_{r\,max}$ for a hypothetical élite athlete are shown in Fig. 49.1. It can be seen from this figure that, for a given distance and a given set of t_e values, $\dot{E}_{r\,max}$ is below the metabolic power requirement in running ($\dot{E}_r$). Hence, this set of times over this distance will forever be unattainable by the (hypothetical) athlete in question. For longer t_e values, $\dot{E}_{r\,max}$ is higher than $\dot{E}_r$. Hence our hypothetical athlete could have covered the distance at stake in a shorter time, his record time being given by the abscissa value at which the two functions cross.

In summary, this type of analysis allows calculation of the theoretical record time for any given subject and any given type of locomotion provided that: (i) the relationship between energy cost and speed, and (ii) the maximal aerobic power and anaerobic capacity of the subject are known. An additional requirement is that the performance time be such as to allow complete utilization of anaerobic stores (i.e. ≥ 90 s) and is shorter than about 30 min. For longer performances, eqn. 8 is not appropriate, because $\dot{V}_{O_2\,max}$, and hence MAP, cannot be maintained at the 100% level for longer than about 30 min (Lacour & Flandrois, 1977).

The calculations summarized in Fig. 49.1 for the 800, 1000 and 1500-m events have been repeated for other track events. The results, reported in Table 49.1, show that theoretical and actual records are essentially equal ($\pm 2\%$) for track running events from 800 to 10 000 m.

Endurance running

As shown in eqn. 8, with increasing t_e the contribution of the anaerobic sources to the overall energy expenditure becomes progressively smaller; it amounts to about 5% of the total for $t_e = 15$ min and is reduced to about 2.5% for $t_e = 30$ min. Therefore, in endurance running, the only relevant term in eqn. 8 is the metabolic power that the subject can develop on the basis of $\dot{V}o_{2\,max}$ alone (MAP in eqn. 8).

However, $\dot{V}o_{2\,max}$ cannot be maintained indefinitely. Indeed, according to di Prampero et al. (1986), the maximal fraction of $\dot{V}o_{2\,max}$ that can be maintained at a constant level in endurance running (F) decreases with the duration of effort (t_e, min), as described by:

$$F = 0.905 - 0.91 \ 10^{-3} \ t_e \qquad (9)$$

($r = 0.60$, $n = 36$). This equation applies to well-trained amateur male subjects for t_e between 80 and 240 min and is close to that described by Saltin (1973) for cycle ergometric exercise over a similar range of exhaustion times.

It follows that for long-distance running such as the semimarathon (21.1 km) or the marathon (42.195 km), eqn. 8 reduces to:

$$\dot{E}_{r\,max} = F \ MAP = F \ \dot{V}o_{2\,max} \qquad (10)$$

Under these conditions, and substituting eqn. 10 into eqn. 2:

$$v_{max} = F \ \dot{V}o_{2\,max} \ C_r^{-1} \qquad (11)$$

where F is the maximal fraction of $\dot{V}o_{2\,max}$ that can be maintained throughout the duration of the effort in question (see eqn. 9).

The theoretical performances predicted on the basis of eqn. 11 were calculated by di Prampero et al. (1986) for 36 male amateur runners taking part in a marathon or semimarathon. F was estimated from eqn. 9 on the basis of the individual times of performance,

Table 49.1 1987 world records and predicted record times for indicated distances. Ratios of calculated to predicted values are also given.

Distance (km)	World record 1987 (s)	World record predicted* (s)	Ratio of predicted to actual record
0.8	101.73 (1:41.73)	100.40	0.987
1.0	132.18 (2:12.18)	132.40	1.002
1.5	209.46 (3:29.46)	213.60	1.020
3.0	452.10 (7:32.10)	459.70	1.017
5.0	778.39 (12:58.39)	789.00	1.014
10.0	1633.81 (27:13.81)	1614.20	0.988

* Predicted records were calculated from eqns 6 and 8, assuming a maximal aerobic power of 1.8 kW (corresponding to a $\dot{V}o_{2\,max}$ of 74 ml·kg^{-1}·min^{-1} above resting) and a maximal anaerobic capacity of 100 kJ (68 ml oxygen·kg^{-1}) in a 70-kg, 175-cm élite male athlete. For further details see text and Fig. 49.1.

while $\dot{V}_{O_2\,max}$ and C_r were determined during treadmill running. The ratio of predicted to actual speed was not significantly different from unity (Table 49.2).

However, according to Péronnet and Thibault (1989) in élite athletes, F decreases exponentially with effort duration, as described by:

$$F = 1.00 - 0.050 \ln(0.14\, t_e) \qquad (12)$$

and by:

$$F = 1.00 - 0.056 \ln(0.14\, t_e) \qquad (12')$$

for females and males, respectively (Péronnet & Thibault, 1989). Thus, for values of t_e from 80 to 240 min (the range over which eqn. 9 was obtained), the F values applicable to amateur runners are from 3.2% to 11.6% lower than those for élite athletes (see also Davies, 1981).

The theoretical performances for 21 100 m, 30 000 m and marathon events, calculated from eqns 11 and 12 on the basis of the same values of maximal anaerobic capacity and maximal aerobic power used for Table 49.1, are also reported in Table 49.2, together with the 1987 world records for the same events. This table shows that the agreement between theoretical and actual performances, even if quite satisfactory, is not as good for long distance as for shorter distances (see Table 49.1).

General discussion

In the preceding sections, maximal individual performances in running were calculated on the basis of the ratio between the maximal metabolic power of the subject ($\dot{E}_{r\,max}$) and the metabolic power requirement in running ($\dot{E}_r$).

$\dot{E}_{r\,max}$ was obtained from the relationship between maximal mechanical power in cycling and the time to exhaustion, established by setting the power output at a constant level and pedalling until exhaustion (eqn. 7; Wilkie, 1980). Whereas this strategy may not be appropriate for winning a race, it does seem to be the best method to set a record. Indeed, it has been shown on theoretical grounds (Keller, 1973) that to establish a record performance in running: (i) the power output must be held constant throughout at the maximal value appropriate to a given duration of effort. This implies that (ii) the duration of performance must coincide with the time to exhaustion. The performance times, as calculated in this study, meet the above requirements. Hence it seems legitimate to assume them to represent the theoretical individual record times.

Because of the acceleration phase at the onset of running, the average speed underestimates the final value. The calculated metabolic power

Table 49.2 1987 world records, predicted record times and ratios of predicted to actual values for the three indicated long-distance events. Ratios of predicted to actual values obtained for a group of 36 male amateur runners are also given.

Distance (km)	World record 1987 (s)	World record predicted* (s)	Ratio of predicted to actual record
21.100	3655.0 (1:00:55.0)	3847.6	1.053
30.000	5358.8 (1:28:18.8)	5608.9	1.047
42.195	7632.0 (2:07:12.0)	8063.1	1.056
21.100			$0.980 \pm 0.070 (\text{s.d.})^\dagger$
42.195			$0.974 \pm 0.084 (\text{s.d.})^\dagger$

* Predicted records were calculated from eqns 11 and 12 assuming $\dot{V}_{O_2\,max} = 74$ ml·kg^{-1}·min^{-1} above resting; † not significantly different from 1.00; $n = 24$ for the semimarathon and $n = 12$ for the marathon. From di Prampero et al. (1986).

requirement is also underestimated, since $\dot{E}_r$ was obtained on the basis of the average speed and eqns 5 and 6 contain terms increasing with the cube of the speed. However, for the distances reported in this study, the differences between $\dot{E}_r$ values calculated on the basis of average or final speeds are negligible.

The validity of the predictions depends on the accuracy with which the numerator and denominator of the relevant equations (eqns 2 and 11) are assessed. The calculations reported in Table 49.3 show that a 5% change in the estimated anaerobic energy stores (AnS) leads to a difference of the predicted performance decreasing from 1.3% to 0.1% as the distance is increased from 800 to 10000 m. On the contrary, the effect of the same 5% change in the estimated $\dot{V}_{O_2\,max}$ is much larger and increases with distance, from 2.4% for the 800-m to 3.9% for the 10000-m distance. Finally, the effects of a 5% change in the estimated energy cost of running (C_r) are close to 4% throughout. For exhaustion times extending beyond 30 min, the term F of eqn. 11 plays a role whose relative importance is equal to that of MAP. Moreover,

in this time range, and independently of the precise shape of the function relating F to exhaustion time (see eqns 9 and 12), the scatter of measurement becomes rather large; for example, in the case of the experiments from which eqn. 9 was obtained (di Prampero et al., 1986), F ranged from 0.72 to 0.88 for $t_e = 100$ min. Other things being equal, this is equivalent to a variation of marathon performance from 140 to 171 min — a large margin indeed.

A similar line of reasoning to that pursued to calculate the effects of the variability of the different terms appearing in eqns 2 and 11 on the estimated running performance can be used to estimate the importance of the relevant variables in establishing the performance itself. It can thus be shown that for distances up to 5000 m, the most important variable is C_r, followed by MAP and finally by AnS. For the 10000-m event or beyond, the relative importance of AnS becomes vanishingly small and MAP and C_r become about equally important. For even longer distances, F must be taken into account on equal terms with MAP and C_r. It should also be pointed out that C_r is affected by the type of

Table 49.3 Predicted percentage decrease in record times in the indicated events when maximal aerobic power (MAP), maximal anaerobic capacity (AnS) or energy cost of running (C_r) are changed by 5%. The last column gives predicted changes in record times when all three variables are changed.

Distance (km)	MAP 100 AnS 100 C_r 100	MAP 100 AnS 100 C_r 95	MAP 100 AnS 105 C_r 100	MAP 105 AnS 100 C_r 100	MAP 105 AnS 105 C_r 95
0.8	100 (100.4)	96.3 (96.7)	98.3 (98.7)	97.2 (97.6)	92.0 (92.4)
1.0	100 (132.4)	96.3 (127.4)	98.6 (130.6)	97.0 (128.4)	92.1 (121.0)
1.5	100 (213.6)	96.3 (205.6)	99.1 (211.7)	96.6 (206.4)	92.1 (196.8)
3.0	100 (459.7)	96.3 (442.7)	99.6 (457.9)	96.3 (442.9)	92.3 (424.5)
5.0	100 (789.0)	96.3 (760.0)	99.8 (787.4)	96.2 (759.2)	92.4 (729.2)
10.0	100 (1614.2)	96.3 (1553.9)	99.9 (1612.0)	96.1 (1550.6)	92.4 (1491.7)

100%: $MAP = 1.8$ kW (corresponding to a $\dot{V}_{O_2\,max}$ of 74 ml·kg^{-1}·min^{-1} above resting; $AnS = 100$ kJ (68 ml oxygen·kg^{-1}); $C_r = 0.185$ ml oxygen·kg^{-1}·m^{-1} (3.87 J·kg^{-1}·m^{-1}) in a 70-kg, 175-cm élite male athlete. Absolute record times are given in parentheses. For calculations see text (eqns 6 & 8) and Fig. 49.1.

terrain, by its slope (a fact that should not be forgotten when dealing with marathon running) and by fatigue. This last factor plays only a minor role, at least up to the distance of the marathon (i.e. a 0.12% increase of C_r per km of distance; Brueckner et al., 1991).

The approach presented in this chapter was originally proposed by di Prampero (1984; 1985; 1986; 1989). More recently it was further elaborated by Péronnet and Thibault (1989). The latter model yields very good predictions of actual records from 60 m to the marathon and has been extrapolated to predict 'ultimate' performances. Its main differences, in comparison with the model presented above, are the following: (i) the assumption of larger values of both maximal aerobic power and maximal anaerobic capacity ($79.7\,\text{ml}\cdot\text{kg}^{-1}\cdot\text{min}^{-1}$ for $\dot{V}_{O_2\,max}$ above resting and $79.3\,\text{ml oxygen}\cdot\text{kg}^{-1}$, respectively, compared with values of 74 and 68 in the approach described here); (ii) the assumption that $\dot{V}_{O_2\,max}$, and hence MAP, cannot be maintained at the 100% level beyond the seventh minute of exercise, see eqn. 12 (30th minute in this model); (iii) the assumption that at the onset of exercise the rate of aerobic metabolism increases with a time constant of 30 s (10 s in this model); the assumption that the amount of energy available from the anaerobic stores: (iv) increases with a time constant of 20 s up to the seventh minute of effort, and (v) for longer distances decreases exponentially, being reduced to about 66% of the total for a duration of 30 min. Taken together, these two last assumptions imply that the entirety of AnS is available only for exercises lasting between about 120 and 420 s.

Assumption (iv) is crucial for predicting sprint running performances. It was not needed in the model presented in this chapter, which was limited to distances equal to or longer than 800 m (100 s). Assumption (v) does not introduce great differences between the two models, since the contribution of the anaerobic energy stores becomes a progressively smaller fraction of the overall energy expenditure with increasing duration of effort (about 5% of the

total for a performance time of 15 min, see eqn. 8). The other differences between the two models, (i)–(iii) above, must cancel out since they both fit the world records curve amazingly well, at least between 800 and 10 000 m.

Both models, however, suffer from the drawback of utilizing the same set of values for the maximal aerobic power and anaerobic capacity of sprinters, middle-distance and long-distance runners. In order to gain further insight into this type of problem, comparison between actual and theoretical performances should be made on the basis of individually measured data, rather than on estimates of an 'ideal' athlete, as was necessarily the case here.

Conclusions

The agreement between theoretical and actual performances emerging from the above discussion and calculations is remarkably good. Its degree of precision depends essentially on the accuracy with which we can assess the individual values of the energy cost of running, maximal anaerobic capacity, maximal aerobic power and the fraction of the last variable that can be sustained throughout the duration of the effort. This seems to provide sound proof that our knowledge of the energetics of muscular exercise, on the one hand, and of human locomotion, on the other, are satisfactory.

The conclusions derived above have an obvious practical use in sports physiology. They have also a more general value, however, in providing us with a clearer understanding of the basic mechanisms underlying human motion.

Summary

In running, the relationship between the metabolic power requirement ($\dot{E}_r$) and speed is known. Hence, the value of $\dot{E}_r$ necessary to cover a given distance can be calculated as a function of the performance time. In addition, the maximal metabolic power ($\dot{E}_{r\,max}$) that a subject can maintain at constant level is a known function of (i) his or her maximal aerobic power; (ii) his or her maximal anaerobic capacity; and (iii) the effort duration to exhaustion. Thus, both $\dot{E}_r$ (for a given distance) and $\dot{E}_{r\,max}$ (for a given subject) can be calculated as a function of time (performance time for $\dot{E}_r$, exhaustion time for $\dot{E}_{r\,max}$). For a given set of times, $\dot{E}_{r\,max}$ is lower than $\dot{E}_r$. Hence, this set of performance times will be unattainable by the subject in question. For longer times, $\dot{E}_{r\,max}$ is higher than $\dot{E}_r$. Hence the runner could have covered the distance at stake in a shorter time, his or her individual record time being given by the time for which $\dot{E}_{r\,max} = \dot{E}_r$. Theoretical records in track running (800–10 000 m) and long-distance running (21.1, 30 and 41.195 km) have been calculated for a hypothetical subject with the metabolic characteristics of a top athlete, and compared with actual records. The two sets of data are essentially equal ($\pm2\%$) for track running, whereas actual records are underestimated by about 5% for long-distance running. In spite of these discrepancies, it is concluded that present knowledge of the energetics of muscular exercise and of human locomotion is remarkably good.

References

Brueckner, J.C., Atchou, G., Capelli, C. *et al.* (1991) The energy cost of running increases with the distance covered. *Eur. J. Appl. Physiol.* (in press).

Cavagna, G.A., Komarek, L. & Mazzoleni, S. (1971) The mechanics of sprint running. *J. Physiol. (Lond.)* **217**, 709–721.

Davies, C.T.M. (1981) Physiology of ultra-long distance running. In: di Prampero, P.E. & Poortmans, J.R. (eds) *Physiological Chemistry of Exercise and Training*, Med. Sport, Vol. 13, pp. 77–84. Karger, Basel.

di Prampero, P.E. (1981) Energetics of muscular exercise. *Rev. Physiol. Biochem. Pharmacol.* **89**, 144–222.

di Prampero, P.E. (1984) I record del mondo di corsa piana. *Riv. Cult. Sportiva* **3**, 3–7.

di Prampero, P.E. (1985) *La Locomozione Umana su Terra, in Acqua, in Aria. Fatti e Teorie.* Edi-Ermes, Milan.

di Prampero, P.E. (1986) The energy cost of human locomotion on land and in water. *Int. J. Sports Med.* **7**, 55–72.

di Prampero, P.E. (1989) Energetics of world records in human locomotion. In: Wieser, W. & Gnaiger, E. (eds) *Energy Transformations in Cells and Organisms*, pp. 248–253. G. Thième, Stuttgart.

di Prampero, P.E., Atchou, G., Brueckner, J.C. & Moia, C. (1986) The energetics of endurance running. *Eur J. Appl. Physiol.* **55**, 259–266.

Keller, J.B. (1973) A theory of competitive running. *Phys. Today* **26**, 43–47.

Lacour, J.R. & Flandrois, R. (1977) Le rôle du métabolisme aérobie dans l'exercice intense de longue durée. *J. Physiol. (Paris)* **73**, 89–130.

Péronnet, F. & Thibault, G. (1989) Mathematical analysis of running performances and world running records. *J. Appl. Physiol.* **67**, 453–465.

Saltin, B. (1973) Oxygen transport by the circulatory system during exercise in man. In: Keul, J. (ed.) *Limiting Factors of Physical Performance*, pp. 235–252. G. Thième, Stuttgart.

Scherrer, J. & Monod, H. (1960) Le travail musculaire local et la fatigue chez l'homme. *J. Physiol. (Paris)* **52**, 419–501.

Wilkie, D.R. (1980) Equations describing power input by humans as a function of duration of exercise. In: Cerretelli, P. & Whipp, B.J. (eds) *Exercise Bioenergetics and Gas Exchange*, pp. 75–80. Elsevier/North Holland, Amsterdam.

Chapter 50

Canoeing

ANTONIO DAL MONTE, PIERO FACCINI AND ROBERTO COLLI

Introduction

Canoeing was invented for both necessity and pleasure. Canoes were the first objects built for moving on rivers and lakes. Three characteristics differentiate the canoe from other crafts:

1 The person, seated or on their knees, looks in the direction in which they are heading.

2 The propelling element is a paddle without a fixed support on the boat, held free in the hands of the paddler.

3 The canoe is a craft with a pointed stem and stern. These particular characteristics permit a great mobility and manageability.

Around 1745, as we can tell from a report written by some Russian hunters, Europeans knew about this particular type of boat, used by Eskimos from Greenland. About 100 years later, the Scot John McGregor designed and built a canoe similar to the kayak. Even if he was the founder of this sport, he always preferred to stress the amateur aspect of canoeing rather than the racing one. In 1866 he founded the first canoe club, which became, in 1873, the Royal Canoe Club. On 22 April 1867 the first canoe race was held on the River Thames over a distance of 1 mile. In 1900 the kayak was adopted by the majority of European countries. The first treatise on paddling dates back to this year and was written by the Norwegian Nansen. The pioneer period ended in 1936 when, at the Olympic games in Berlin, canoeing became an Olympic speciality. At present, this sport is regulated by the ICF (International Canoe Federation) and by various national federations. Canoeing has been developed as a sport with two main specializations: *Olympic* (in calm water) and *whitewater* (in rough water). There are other specialities, such as polo canoeing, sail canoeing and marathon canoeing.

Olympic canoeing includes parallel races in calm water. The classic races are over distances of 500, 1000 and 10000 m. The following types of craft are used: kayaks (K1, K2, K4 according to the number of crew members) and Canadian canoes (C1, C2, C4) (Fig. 50.1).

Whitewater canoeing includes races that descend a river with rapids, or slalom in a river with falls, on which has been installed a racing field with obligatory 'gates' (doors) to be passed by either stem or stern. The crafts used are the kayak (K1) or Canadian canoe, which has a different design to the Olympic canoe; whitewater canoes are less rapid but more steady.

The materials from which paddles and canoes are made, and their shape, have evolved over time. The paddles have changed from wood to synthetic material such as kevlar and carbon, and from a flat blade to the most recent wing-shaped type.

Biomechanics

Kayak technique

The following description is valid both for Olympic canoeing in calm water with different crews and for whitewater canoeing in rough water. To make the technique easier, four fundamental phases can be distinguished:

1 *Position of attack* or beginning of the paddling cycle. The trunk is in a position of maximum rotation; the attacking shoulder is stretched forward and the corresponding arm is extended and horizontal. The active shoulder moves backward behind the head; the arm and the forearm are flexed at about 90°. The pelvis rotates forwards on the attack side and the corresponding leg flexes at around 130°.

2 *Passage in the water.* The first phase is dominated by the pushing of the leg corresponding to the traction and opposing rotation of the trunk, so that the traction arm, remaining extended, receives and transmits to the paddle the power resulting from the above-mentioned thrust. In the second phase the rotation of the

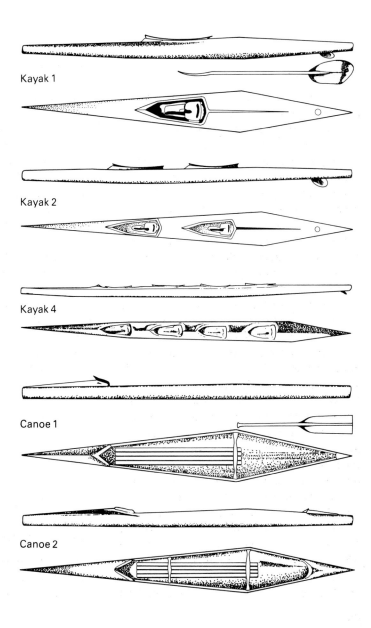

Fig. 50.1 Various types of kayak and Canadian canoe.

trunk and the thrust of the leg continue, while the rotation of the traction arm begins until the forearm reaches a minimum angle of 90°. The active arm completes the extension at the same time.

3 *Extraction*. After passage through the water, made with a rapid outward rotation of the traction arm, the extraction phase begins. This is also called return phase.

4 *Aerophase*. In this phase, a paddle cycle ends and the next one begins. As in extraction, this is made by the traction arm, which completes the outward rotation. This rotation and upward movement permits the paddle to achieve the semirotation necessary to change sides.

Canadian technique

Here we can also distinguish four phases in the paddling cycle:

1 *Position of attack*. Both arms are extended; the trunk is in a position of maximum rotation and flexion; and the forward leg maintains the angle of the basic position. The angle formed between the paddle and the water surface in the phase of attack is about 65°.

2 *Phase of traction*. From the position of attack, while maintaining extension of the arms, an opposing rotation and extension of the trunk is effected until returning to the basic position. The active arm makes a downward pressure on the paddle, trying to keep this pressure perpendicular. The uppermost arm, by moving the wrist, makes the paddle rotate outwards until the extraction phase.

3 *Phase of extraction*. In this phase, the extracting fist is at the level of the hip and the semiflexed arm moves rapidly outwards.

4 *Aerophase*. In this phase, the athlete passes from the basic position to the position of attack, keeping the arms extended and achieving a torsion of the body, with the trunk flexed.

Figure 50.2 shows the forces applied during the paddling cycle both in the kayak canoe and in the Canadian canoe, as registered by means of a dynamometric paddle (Perri *et al.*, 1990).

Anthropometry

Height: The ideal paddler is generally 2–8 cm taller than average, as has been demonstrated by Hirata (1977) in Olympic winners. Hirata has also shown that there is a height difference of about 3.5 cm between the best kayakers and the best canoeists, the former being the taller.

Body mass: According to Sidney and Shephard (1973), junior competitors are relatively light. On the other hand, senior competitors carry a substantial excess mass (on average 5.8 kg in men and 9.5 kg in women) which influences performance. The correlation between lean body mass and overall ability is 0.72.

Hirata (1977) showed that the gold medal winners in the Montreal Olympics were 3–10 kg heavier than the average contestant.

Muscle fibres: Canoeists present an unusual body composition, with 63% slow-twitch fibres in the deltoid, compared with 44% in a student population (Gollnick *et al.*, 1972; Tesch & Karlsson, 1985). The 'ideal' composition would be 50%, 65% and 70% of slow-twitch fibres for distances of 500, 1000 and 10 000 m respectively (Shephard, 1987).

Force

Canoeists' isometric forces reach high values in the handgrip, in elbow flexion and in knee extension. The coefficient of correlation with overall performance is, however, low: 0.58 for knee extension, 0.29 for handgrip and 0.11 for elbow flexion (Sidney & Shephard, 1973).

Some researchers have not found high values in the muscular regions of the trunk, especially in extension. In this region the peak force is only 29% higher than in untrained students (Cermak *et al.*, 1975).

We studied the force–velocity curve using an isokinetic ergometer for the upper limbs, at an angular velocity similar to the stroke frequency of a competition. We observed that

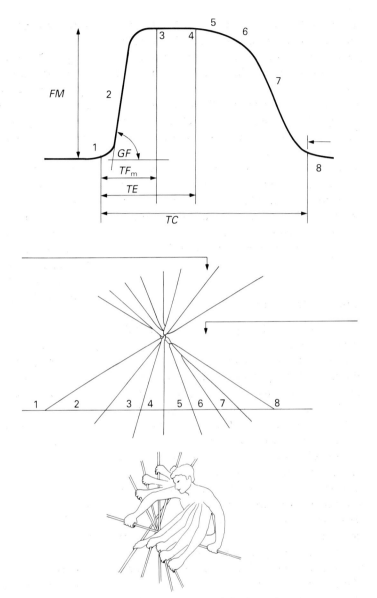

Fig. 50.2 (a) Strength graphics during kayak paddling, as registered with a dynamometric paddle. *FM*, maximal strength; *GF*, strength angle; *TC*, paddling time; *TE*, effective time; *TF*ₘ, time to reach maximal strength.

canoeists reach their maximum power at about 70 r.p.m. (Table 50.1).

Studies carried out by Armand (1983) and Vandewalle *et al.* (1983) have demonstrated that the force–velocity relationship plotted with data from tests on an arm ergometer give higher figures for canoeists than for athletes practising other sport disciplines (Table 50.2).

Anaerobic metabolism

In this section we will examine the maximum accumulation of blood lactate after upper limb ergometer exercise.

The literature gives conflicting data, perhaps depending on the type of test and ergometer used and on the motivation of the subjects.

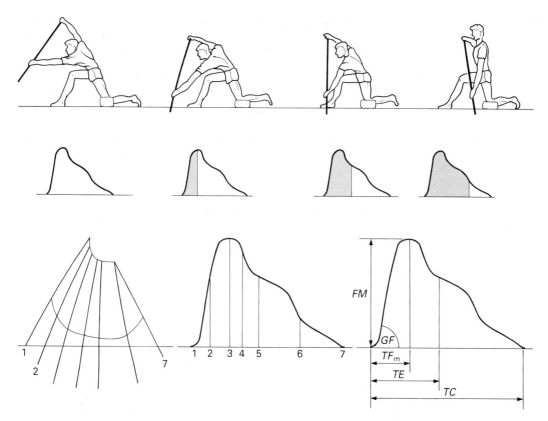

Fig. 50.2 (b) Strength graphics during Canadian canoe paddling, as registered with a dynamometric paddle. For abbreviations see caption to (a).

Cermak *et al.* (1975) observed blood lactate readings as high as 18.4 mmol·l^{-1} in men and 16.8 mmol·l^{-1} in women. Tesch and Lindberg (1984) had measurements of 5 mmol·l^{-1} (males) and 6 mmol·l^{-1} (females). Dal Monte (1983) observed 14 mmol·l^{-1} in a test that simulated a competition. In a laboratory test simulating the duration and energy output of races over a distance of 500 and 1000 m in Olympic kayak canoes and kayak ergometers ('Modest' kayak ergometer), Colli *et al.* (1990) obtained blood lactate measurements of 12.7 mmol·l^{-1} and 11.7 mmol·l^{-1}, respectively.

Table 50.3 presents data on tests conducted in the laboratory simulating the same distances. Notice that the blood lactate, excluding the basal reading, reaches a high level after the first

minute and then maintains a constant value for the rest of the test. One interpretation could be that the athlete does not produce lactate in the muscles. However, the metabolic intensity is far beyond the anaerobic threshold and close to the $\dot{V}_{O_2\,max}$. This indicates that the measurement of blood lactate concentration alone could give misleading information about anaerobic glycolytic activity. In 500 and 1000-m competitions of highly specialized athletes, we obtained values of 16.0 (s.d. ±0.70) mmol·l^{-1} and 13.5 (s.d. ±0.47) mmol·l^{-1} respectively (Colli *et al.*, 1990).

By comparing test data on two groups of top-level canoeists, the first group ($n = 14$) evaluated on the cycle ergometer and subsequently on the paddle ergometer, and the second

Table 50.1 Average isokinetic data: the canoeists reached their maximum power at about 70 strokes·min^{-1}.

	Maximum velocity (r.p.m.)	Maximum force (N)	Maximum power (W)	No. of subjects
Junior kayak (male)	70	514	705	4
Senior kayak (male)	70	674	928	7
Senior kayak (female)	70	393	471	5

Table 50.2 Force—velocity relationship for various types of athlete, using an arm ergometer.

Reference	Sport	Maximum velocity (r.p.m.)	Maximum force (N)	Maximum power (W)
Vandewalle et al. (1983)	Canoe/kayak			
	men	243	165	948
	women	218	103	549
	Handball (men)	230	134	768
	Boxing (men)	240	124	768
	Tennis (men)	237	112	662
	Sedentary (men)	222	104	578
Armand (1983)	Senior kayak (male)	226	122	1045
	Junior kayak (male)	216	171	698
	Senior canoe (male)	233	147	916
	Junior canoe (male)	213	180	642
	Senior canoe/kayak (female)	211	187	583
	Junior canoe/kayak (female)	193	222	413

Table 50.3 'Fractionated' laboratory test simulating the distances of 500- and 1000-m races in Olympic kayak canoes.

Time of work (4 min)	Mechanical work (kJ)	Mechanical power (W)	Oxygen comsumption during test (l·min^{-1})	Blood lactate mmol·l^{-1*}	Blood lactate mmol·l$^{-1\dagger}$
Total test (0—4 min)	94.10	392	15.03		
I min (0—1 min)	26.26	437	1.82	6.70	6.70
II min (1—2 min)	21.80	363	4.36	8.00	1.3
III min (2—3 min)	—	366	4.40	8.12	0.12
IV min (3—4 min)	—	401	4.45	8.44	0.32

* Lactate concentration: difference between maximal blood lactate value and resting value.
† Difference between peak blood lactate concentration and peak value the minute before.

group ($n = 10$) on the treadmill and paddle ergometer, Heller *et al.* (1984) measured values of 8.6 mmol·l^{-1} and 8.8 mmol·l^{-1} (not significantly different) for the first group and 13.2 and 12.5 mmol·l^{-1} ($p < 0.01$) for the second group. These figures suggest that in canoeists there are notable muscular and metabolic adjustments; in fact, when using the specific ergometer, and thereby activating a relatively small muscular mass, the lacatate value is similar to that obtained on the treadmill or cycle ergometer.

We have also carried out studies on whitewater canoeists, both during slalom performance and during specific tests, in order to study maximum lactate production (D'Angelo *et al.*, 1987). The 'figure of eight' distance (Fig. 50.3) had to be completed as many times as possible in 1 min, and the distance covered was calculated according to the landmarks between the two gates. When that slalom had ended, we found mean figures of 7.0 (s.d. ± 0.51) mmol·l^{-1}, while during specific tests in water we found a maximum of 13.2 (s.d. ± 1.11) mmol·l^{-1}. Field studies on Canadian canoeists have indicated values similar to those for kayakers. The only difference found was between the two racing distances, i.e. 500 and 1000 m, with values of 14.9 (s.d. ± 0.78) mmol·l^{-1} and 13.0 (s.d. ± 0.95) mmol·l^{-1} of lactate, respectively (not significantly different) (Colli *et al.*, 1990; personal data).

Anaerobic threshold

Cerretelli *et al.* (1979) and Tesch and Lindberg (1984) have noted a high anaerobic threshold in paddlers. Possible factors include the kinetics of $\dot{V}o_2$ at the onset of exercise, a high capillary density in the shoulder muscles, and a high oxidative power (Gollnick *et al.*, 1972) or a low lactate dehydrogenase activity.

Bunc *et al.* (1981) examined anaerobic thresholds using various ergometric tests. They found that paddlers tested on the treadmill had a threshold at 79% of $\dot{V}o_{2\,max}$, while the value on the kayak ergometer was around 86% of $\dot{V}o_{2\,max}$ (Tesch *et al.*, 1976). Colli *et al.* (1990) recorded the threshold on the kayak ergometer by an incremental test. They applied the 4 mmol·l^{-1} method (Mader, 1976) to the best Italian canoeists, differentiating them according to the various specialities (Table 50.4).

Threshold heart rate also reaches high figures. During an incremental test on the treadmill, with a constant slope of 5% and speed increments of 1 km·h^{-1}·min^{-1}, Bunc *et al.* (1981) found a threshold heart frequency of 177 beats·min^{-1} in relation to a maximum heart frequency of 192 beats·min^{-1} in top Hungarian

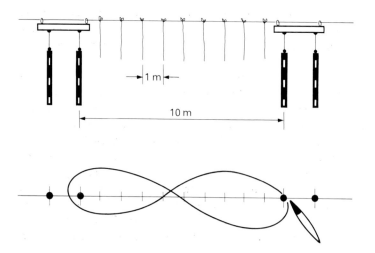

Fig. 50.3 Specific test for wild water canoeing: plan of the course.

Table 50.4 Anaerobic threshold of the best five Italian paddlers, applying Mader's test on the kayak ergometer.

	Power (W)	%$\dot{V}o_{2\,max}$	Heart rate (beats·min^{-1})	No. of subjects
500-m kayak (male)	268	79	178	1
1000-m kayak (male)	356	86	179	1
500-m kayak (female)	225	88	181	1
500-m canoe (male)	260	77.5	180	1
1000-m canoe (male)	299	87.3	177	1

male canoeists. Corresponding values were 182 and 195 beats·min^{-1}, respectively, in women.

Aerobic metabolism

Various tests and ergometers have been used to study aerobic metabolism. Many data have been recorded using the treadmill. Sidney and Shephard (1973) obtained values of 3.8 l·min^{-1} in junior males, 4.5 l·min^{-1} in senior males, and 2.8 l·min^{-1} in women whitewater paddlers. Vaccaro et al. (1984) recorded a mean of 4.7 l·min^{-1} in whitewater canoeists of the US national team. Heller et al. (1983) reported values of 5.2 l·min^{-1} in male senior canoeists and kayakers, and 3.3—3.4 l·min^{-1} in females; Horvath and Finney (1969) reported a mean of 3.8 l·min^{-1}. Many authors (Cermak et al., 1975; Vrijens et al., 1975; Tesch et al., 1976; Dransart, 1977; Rusko et al., 1978) using different leg ergometers, have obtained mean values ranging from 5.3 to 5.6 l·min^{-1}. Data referring to winners are better: Tesch et al. (1984) reported figures of 4.9 l·min^{-1} in Swedish junior males, 5.0 l·min^{-1} in senior males, and 5.4 l·min^{-1} in a world champion. Dransart (1977) presented exceptional data, 5.6 l·min^{-1} (85 ml·kg^{-1}·min^{-1}) in a French competitor. While the best athletes attain the same values with both the treadmill and the kayak ergometer, this is not the case with medium-level athletes or specializing athletes (Colli et al., 1990).

In canoeing, ergometers that can simulate paddling must be used. If they are not available, ergometers for upper limbs can be used. The canoeist provides a classic example of a fundamental feature of living beings: adaptability. The athlete continuously modifies her or his morphofunctional characteristics in relation to the specific requirements of the sport. The canoeist develops the upper part of the body, so opposing the evolutionary law which privileges the upright position of humans and thus the morphofunctional difference between upper and lower limbs. In this case values of $\dot{V}o_2$ are very interesting. Dal Monte et al. (Dal Monte & Leonardi, 1975) carried out a study comparing the kayak ergometer and the cycle ergometer on high-level canoeists, and found a difference (in ml·kg^{-1}·min^{-1}) of only 7.3% in favour of the cycle ergometer test. Heller et al. (1983) obtained a value of 4.45 l·min^{-1} with the cycle ergometer vs. 4.16 l·min^{-1} with the kayak ergometer. Such differences are slightly larger if comparison is made with the results of treadmill tests: in the above-mentioned study, Heller et al. obtained a value 4.87 l·min^{-1} with the treadmill compared with 4.01 l·min^{-1} with the kayak ergometer.

When Dal Monte's kayak ergometer was used on members of the Italian national kayak team, a mean value of 4.69 (s.d. $\pm$ 0.43) l·min^{-1} was obtained, with an anaerobic threshold at 82% (s.d. $\pm$ 6.3%) of $\dot{V}o_{2\,max}$ (Paselli et al., 1986). Many authors agree that sedentary people reach only about 70% of the maximum oxygen intake attained during running when they exercise on an ergometer for upper limbs, while canoeists obtain much higher values (Table 50.5).

The specificity of both the ergometer and

Table 50.5 Percentage of leg $\dot{V}o_{2\,max}$ developed by paddlers. From Shephard (1987).

Reference	% leg $\dot{V}o_{2\,max}$
Vrijens *et al.* (1975)	
Paddlers	89
Controls	81
Cermak *et al.* (1975)	
Male paddlers	95
Female paddlers	100
Dransart (1977)	77
Tesch & Lindberg (1984)	
Paddlers	87
Vaccaro *et al.* (1984)	89

the tests is important. They must reproduce, as far as possible, the behaviour during a race. In in a laboratory simulation of Olympic canoe races over a distance of 1000 m, and over a distance of 300 m and non-specific tests, Colli *et al.* (1990) found that the amount of energy released in aerobic ($\dot{V}o_2$) and anaerobic (lactate) metabolism was the same, both in high-level canoeists who participated in the Seoul Olympic games and in a group of canoeists belonging to the national team who were also canoeists of a high standard. The mechanical power differed between the groups, indicating a coordinative, technical and muscular specific adaptation that can be detected only by means of specific tests that reproduce the race situation (Tables 50.6–50.8).

Cardiovascular system

Echocardiography has produced some interesting data on heart volumes and ventricular mass. Values are similar to those of athletes who practise middle-distance running events (Table 50.9). Similar results are obtained when data are related to body surface area (Fig. 50.4) (Pelliccia & Spataro, 1988).

Sidney and Shephard (1973) have noted that the resting heart rate of canoeists is relatively high: they reported 71 beats·min^{-1} in juniors, and 60 and 67 beats·min^{-1} in men and women, respectively.

The systolic blood pressure is relatively high, around 135 mmHg. Armand (1983) attributes this to a high stroke volume and to a blockage of the peripheral circulation by the thoracic ribcage during paddling. The lung volumes are not particularly remarkable and are within the average anthropometric range. However, Sidney and Shephard (1973) found a relatively high correlation between lung volumes and performance (0.64 for the absolute vital capacity and 0.69 for the percentage according to age and height standards).

Table 50.6 Comparison between top-level and good-level athletes using non-specific tests. The performance of top-level athletes in running, traction and pushing with weights did not differ from that of good-level athletes.

	Top level	Good level	p	Student's t test
Swimming 100 m (s)	77 ± 8	90 ± 15	0.05	2.22
Swimming 300 m (s)	284 ± 38	327 ± 56	0.05	1.82
Running 1200 m (s)	247 ± 27	231 ± 8	n.s.	1.51
Tractions on bench (rep·50 kg^{-1}·60 s^{-1})	40.4 ± 5	40.4 ± 6.8	n.s.	0.02
Push on bench (rep·50 kg^{-1}·60 s^{-1})	34.6 ± 9.8	33.6 ± 4.8	n.s.	0.24
Tractions on bar (rep·60 s^{-1})	43.8 ± 6.8	47.1 ± 12	n.s.	0.69

Values are mean ± standard deviation; n.s., not significant; rep, repetitions.

Table 50.7 Comparison between top-level and good-level athletes in two kayak ergometer tests simulating distances of 1000 and 300 m.

	Top level	Good level	p
1000 m			
$W \cdot kg^{-1}$	3.66 ± 19	3.37 ± 0.34	0.05
$J \cdot paddle^{-1} \cdot kg^{-1}$	2.129 ± 3.6	2.016 ± 0.12	0.05
r.p.m.	102.7 ± 3.6	100 ± 1.0	n.s.
300 m			
$W \cdot kg^{-1}$	5.01 ± 0.24	4.62 ± 0.57	0.05
$J \cdot paddle^{-1} \cdot kg^{-1}$	2.360 ± 0.15	2.310 ± 0.10	n.s.
r.p.m.	127.0 ± 7	119 ± 10	0.05

Values are mean ± standard deviation; n.s., not significant; r.p.m., revolutions per min.

Table 50.8 Comparison between metabolic parameters in top-level and good-level athletes during kayak ergometer tests simulating the distance of 1000 m (duration 4 min). The only statistically significant difference is in efficiency.

	Top level	Good level	p
Oxygen consumption ($ml \cdot kg^{-1}$)			
0–1 min	21 ± 3	21 ± 4	n.s.
1–2 min	52 ± 4	51 ± 4	n.s.
2–3 min	54 ± 3	53 ± 4	n.s.
3–4 min	53 ± 3	53.5 ± 5	n.s.
Efficiency (%)	14.6 ± 0.74	13.4 ± 0.51	0.005

Values are mean ± standard deviation; n.s. not significant.

Training

Training must be specially devised for both junior and senior athletes. Account must be taken of whether the athletes have already specialized in a particular race distance and whether they are already 'top-level' athletes.

For a distance of 1000 m, in both kayak and Canadian canoes, the factors that limit performance seem to be lack of a good maximum aerobic power, the ability to oxidize the lactate produced, the capacity to tolerate a low pH and to maintain a high level of mechanical power as close as possible to the maximum. For a distance of 500 m, anaerobic capacity, good tissue and blood buffering capacity, oxygen kinetics and high mechanical power levels are fundamental, and are more important than $\dot{V}o_{2\,max}$.

Based on experience acquired from specific adaptation in top-level athletes, training must continuously and progressively simulate the race situation. This cannot be obtained if muscular dynamics differ from those performed in races, such as training with swimming, jogging or weights. On the contrary, aerobic and anaerobic exercises must be performed either in the vessel, or out of the water, with precisely simulated movements (kayak ergometers or similar devices) able to involve in the

Table 50.9 Left ventricular end-diastolic volume and left ventricular mass (mean value ± standard deviation) in aerobic sports. From Pelliccia & Spataro (1988).

	Left ventricular end-diastolic volume (ml)	Left ventricular mass (g)
Male		
Cross-country skiing	167 ± 14	314 ± 46
Walking	121 ± 6	255 ± 20
Marathon	162 ± 16	332 ± 42
Long-distance running	151 ± 22	258 ± 12
Middle-distance running	163 ± 8	336 ± 28
Canoeing	162 ± 14	388 ± 52
Rowing	168 ± 23	365 ± 55
Cycling	164 ± 30	355 ± 80
Control	118 ± 22	197 ± 36
Female		
Cross-country skiing	111 ± 16	213 ± 31
Marathon	122 ± 30	228 ± 19
Long-distance running	104 ± 10	183 ± 18
Middle-distance running	115 ± 10	227 ± 22
Cycling	121 ± 12	251 ± 19

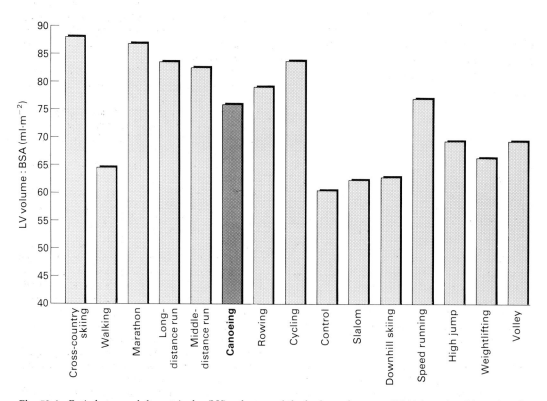

Fig. 50.4 Ratio between left ventricular (LV) volume and the body surface area (BSA) in male athletes (aerobic and anaerobic sports).

Table 50.10 Variations in mechanical parameters during the training season.

	60-s test (W·kg^{-1})	120-s test (W·kg^{-1})
Starting test	3.67	2.92
Second test (after a period of strength training and mixed aerobic/anaerobic training)	4.24 (+ 15.5%)	3.63 (+24.3%)
Third test (after a period of lactic acid training)	4.60 (+8.4%)	3.59 (−1.1%)
Fourth test (after a period of 'race rhythm' training)	4.61 (+0.2%)	3.93 (+9.4%)

same order the muscles and muscle fibres used for propulsion and those used to remove the lactate.

In conclusion, thanks to laboratory and field experiments (Colli *et al.*, 1990), we can affirm that methods aimed only at increasing the aerobic power and the anaerobic threshold are not correct from a methodological point of view. In support of this view, Table 50.10 stresses the difference in power observed in different phases of the training of top-level athletes during 'intensive' tests of 60 s and during specific tests that simulate the race.

References

Armand, J.-C. (1983) *Surveillance medicale de l'entrainement d'une equipe de canoe kayak de haut niveau de performance*. MD thesis, Université de Paris Ouest.

Bunc, V., Leso, J., Heller, J., Novak, J., Strejckova, B. & Novotny, V. (1981) Anaerobic threshold by specific and non specific load. *Lekar a TV* **3**, 35−37.

Cermak, J., Kuta, I. & Parizkova, J. (1975) Some predispositions for top performance in speed canoeing and their changes during the whole year training programme. *J. Sport Med. Phys. Fitness* **15**, 243−251.

Cerretelli, P., Pendergast, D., Paganelli, W.C. & Rennie, D.W. (1979) Effects of specific muscle training on $\dot{V}o_2$ on-response and early blood lactate. *J. Appl. Physiol.* **47**, 761−769.

Colli, R., Faccini, P., Schermi, C., Introini, E. & Dal Monte, A. (1990) Dalla valutazione funzionale all'allenamento del Canoista. *SDS, Rivista di Cultura Sportiva* **18**, 26−37.

D'Angelo, R., Coan, G., Mazzanti, L., Perli, C.P. &

Trompetto, M. (1987) Costruzione ed analisi dei test da campo. *Canoa Ricerca* **2**(6), 9−14.

Dal Monte, A. (1983) *La Valutazione Funzionale dell 'Atleta*. E.D. Sansoni, Florence.

Dal Monte, A. & Leonardi, L.M. (1975) Sulla specificita' della valutazione funzionale negli atleti: esperienze sui canoisti. *Medicina dello Sport* **28**(8), 213−219.

Dal Monte, A. & Leonardi, L.M. (1976) Functional evaluation of kayak paddlers from biomechanical and physiological viewpoints. In: Komi, P. (ed.) *Biomechanics V.B.*, pp. 258−267. University Park Press, Baltimore.

Dransart, G. (1977) *Contribution à la connaissance du canoe kayak*. Thesis, National Institute of Sport and Physical Education, Paris.

Federazione Italiana Canoa Kajak (1989) *Canoa, Manuale per l'Istruttore*. La Fiaccola, Rome.

Gollnick, P.D., Armstrong, R.B., Saubert IV, C.W., Piehl, K. & Saltin, B. (1972) Enzyme activity and fiber composition in skeletal muscle of trained and untrained men. *J. Appl. Physiol.* **33**, 312−319.

Heller, J., Bunc, V. & Kuta, M. (1983) *Functional Predisposition for Top Canoe and Kajak Performance*, p. 15 (abstract). International Congress on Sport and Health, Maastricht.

Heller, J., Bunc, V., Novak, J. & Kuta, I. (1984) A comparison of bicycle, paddling and treadmill spiroergometry in top paddlers. In: Lollgen, H. & Mellerowicz, H. (eds) *Progress in Ergometry: Quality Control and Test Criteria*, pp. 236−241. Springer, Berlin.

Hirata, K. (1977) *Selection of Olympic Champions*, Vols 1 and 2. Karger Publishers, Basel.

Horvath, S.M. & Finney, B.R. (1969) Paddling experiments and the question of Polynesian voyaging. *Am. Anthropol.* **71**, 271−276.

Mader, A. (1976) Zur Beurteilung der sportartspezifischen Ausdauerleistungsfähigkeit im Labor. *Sportartzt Sportmed.* **27**, 80−112.

Paselli, L., Dal Monte, A., Faccini, P. & Faina, M. (1986) Fosfati e prestazioni fisiche. *Canoa Ricerca* **1**(1), 3–11.

Pelliccia, A. & Spataro, A. (1988) Studio sulla morfologia e della funzione ventricolare sinistra negli atleti praticanti diverse discipline sportive. *Rassegna Internazionale di Medicina dello Sport* **3**(13), 1–8.

Perri, O., Dal Santo, A., Hazsik, E. & Toth, A. (1990) La tecnica di pagaiata in kajak e canadese. *Canoa Ricerca* **5**(16), 5–15.

Rusko, H., Havu, M. & Karvinen, E. (1978) Aerobic performance capacity in athletes. *Eur. J. Appl. Physiol.* **38**, 151–159.

Shephard, R.J. (1987) Science and medicine of canoeing and kayaking. *Sports Med.* **4**, 19–33.

Sidney, K.H. & Shephard, R.J. (1973) Physiological characteristics and performance of the white-water paddler. *Eur. J. Appl. Physiol.* **32**, 55–70.

Tesch, P. & Karlsson, J. (1985) Muscle fiber type and size in trained and untrained muscles of elite athletes. *J. Appl. Physiol.* **59**, 1716–1720.

Tesch, P. & Lindberg, S. (1984) Blood lactate accumulation during arm exercise in world class kayak paddlers and strength-trained athletes. *Eur. J. Appl. Physiol.* **52**, 441–445.

Tesch, P., Piehl, K., Wilson, G. & Karlsson, J. (1976) Physiological investigations of Swedish élite canoe competitors. *Med. Sports* **8**, 214–218.

Vaccaro, P., Clarke, D.H., Morris, A.F. & Gray, P.R. (1984) Physiological characteristics of the world champion whitewater slalom team. In: Bachl, N., Prokop, L. & Suckert, R. (eds) *Current Topics in Sport Medicine*, pp. 637–647. Urban & Schwarzenberg, Vienna.

Vandewalle, H., Peres, G. & Monod, H. (1983) Relation force–vitesse lors d'exercises cyclique realisés avec les membres supérieurs. *Motricité Humaine* **2**, 22–25.

Vrijens, J., Hoestra, P., Bouckaert, J. & Van Vytvanck, P. (1975) Effects of training on maximal work capacity and haemodynamics response during arm and leg exercise in a group of paddlers. *Eur. J. Appl. Physiol.* **36**, 113–119.

Chapter 51

Rowing

NIELS H. SECHER

Introduction

Rowing combines intense dynamic exercise with a need for development of a large force during each stroke. Accordingly, the circulation has to adapt not only to a large cardiac output but also to the increase in blood pressure following the Valsalva-like manoeuvre performed at the 'catch'. These demands are reflected in the hearts of rowers, which show large internal diameters and wall thickness. At the same time, the way in which rowers apply simultaneous pressure of the right and left leg against the stretcher may be unique to human motion and points to the neurophysiological problems involved in coordination (Secher, 1983). In contrast to many other sports, rowing is associated with few injuries. The main medical problems are concerned with extreme fatigue, although chronic low back pain may be a problem for some rowers, besides more trivial blisters. For reviews of the biomechanics and physiology of rowing see Schneider (1980), Secher (1983; 1990), Hagerman (1984), Körner and Schwanitz (1985), Hartmann (1987) and Steinacker (1987).

Rowing competitions

Competitions are divided into two distinct, yet related, disciplines: sweep rowing and sculling. In sweep boats, each rower uses a single oar approximately 4 m long, while in sculling they use two smaller (approximately 3 m) sculls on each side of the boat. Both types of boat are rowed, with the back towards the direction of the course, by pulling the oar at a cadence of between 34 and 38 strokes·min^{-1}. In contrast to traditional rowing boats, as well as to the first racing shells, the stroke is made more efficient by the use of a sliding seat, thereby adding leg extension to the work performed with the upper body and arms. In sweep rowing the boats may include two, four or eight rowers. In addition, pairs and fours are rowed both with and without a coxswain, while a coxswain is always present in the eights (Table 51.1). Sculls are rowed without a coxswain and encompass single, double and quadruple boats. The minimum body mass of the coxswain is 50 kg for the male and 40 kg for the female events.

Regattas

Race rowing started on the River Thames in England, with the 'Doggett's Coat and Badge' race, for professional watermen (1715) and for 'gentlemen', with the Oxford and Cambridge Boat Race (1829) and the Henley Royal Regatta (1839). Championships have been arranged by the Fédération Internationale des Sociétés d'Aviron (FISA) since 1893. In 1900 rowing appeared on the Olympic programme. FISA championships for women were added in 1954, and unofficial lightweight (maximum weight 72.5 kg; mean weight 70 kg) championships were introduced in 1974 and made 'official' in 1985. Lightweight championships for women

Table 51.1 Minimum boat weight allowed in FISA championships and the FISA competitions arranged for men and women including lightweights.

	Boat type*							
	4+	2×	2−	1×	2+	4−	4×	8+
Boat weight (kg)	51	26	27	14	32	50	52	93
Men	●	●	●	●	●	●	●	●
Male lightweights		●		●		●	●	●
Women		●	●	●		●	●	●
Female lightweights		●		●		●		

* Digits indicate number of rowers; +/− denotes the presence of a coxswain; × indicates scull boats. ● are the current events.

(maximum weight 59 kg; mean weight 57 kg) were added in 1985 after an unofficial regatta in 1984, and the distance rowed by women was increased from 1000 m to the 2000 m rowed by men. Of note, weighing may take place much earlier than the regatta, and the normal weight of the lightweight rower in the race is usually above the one 'allowed'.

Improvement of results

Since the first FISA regatta took place, the mean result has improved by about 0.7 s (range 0.6–0.9 s) per year (Fig. 51.1). It is possible to detect a similar 0.6 s (range 0.2–2.1 s) per year improvement in the results for the women over

1000 m. The improvement in rowing performance represents a composite effect of an increase of the size of the population in general and changes in training and selection of rowers; a contribution has also been made by the technical modifications in the construction of boats as well as the effort by the 1958–89 president of FISA, Thomas Keller, to standardize racing courses. Currently FISA has also standardized the weight of the boats to those presented in Table 51.1.

Duration of competitions

The median results in FISA regattas from 1974 to 1989 indicate a race duration of 6.5 min

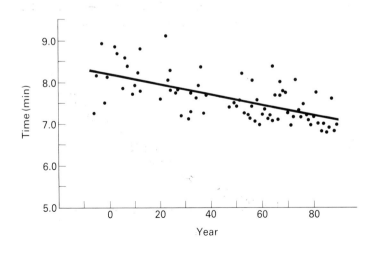

Fig. 51.1 Results obtained by FISA regatta winning single scull over 2000 m from 1893 to 1989. The regression line is shown, with 1900 as the starting point.

(range 5.8–7.2 min), and 6.6 min (range 5.9–7.3 min) for lightweights. In 2000-m races for women the times are 7.1 min (range 6.4–7.9 min) or 10% longer than for the men in similar events. The difference between the two types of women's race is larger (12%) suggesting that the 'cut' separating lightweight women and men is different. However, for both men and women the highest weight allowed in lightweight events is 74–75% of the average weight of the rowers in the open classes, 94 and 79 kg respectively. Values indicate a difference between results obtained in the similar open and lightweight events of 2.5% for men and 5% for women, supporting the need for a division of races into weight categories but also indicating that the quality of the lightweight women's races does not yet meet that of their male counterparts.

Biomechanics

The biomechanics of rowing is complex with a need for integrated movement of the boat, oars and body. The peak force in the stroke exceeds 1000 N in both male and female sweep rowing and is little more than 500 N in the scull boats (Körner & Schwanitz, 1985). Power is generated primarily to overcome the drag force of the water, wind resistance being of minor importance. Water resistance of the boat increases with speed to the second power when a smooth velocity is applied (Fig. 51.2). However, the velocity of the boat changes by approximately

30% during the stroke cycle (Körner & Schwanitz, 1985). Contrary to what might be expected, the highest boat velocity is reached when the oar is out of the water and the heavy bodies of the rowers are moving in the opposite direction to that of the shell (Körner & Schwanitz, 1985). Similarly, the movement of the bodies in the direction of the boat during the stroke decreases propagation of the shell. Only when the total system is taken into consideration, including both rowers and shell, is the highest velocity reached at the end of the stroke.

Muscle strength

Rowers are large and strong individuals, but their ability as rowers is not related in any simple way to their muscle strength. Only when measured in a simulated rowing position does muscle strength (2000 N) separate the best rowers from groups of lesser qualified rowers with a 'rowing strength' of approximately 1800 and 1600 N, respectively (Secher, 1983). Nevertheless rowing does require an ability to develop a large peak force during the stroke, and it may be argued that this requirement can be fulfilled only if rowing strength is close to that of the best rowers.

The best rowers tend to have many slow-twitch muscle fibres, with an average of about 70% (Körner & Schwanitz, 1985). Moreover, the size of the muscle fibres of rowers is large: for the leg muscles, an average of 3970 μm^2 vs.

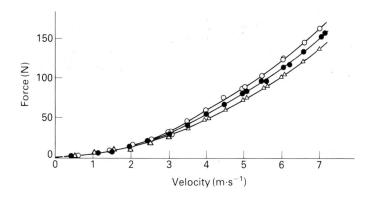

Fig. 51.2 Drag force applied to a single scull at different velocities. Three loads on the shell are presented. ○, 120 kg; ● 100 kg; △, 80 kg. From Balukow (1964).

3330 μm² in controls. The muscle fibres of rowers also have many capillaries around fibres: 7.3 vs. 3.1 in controls. These values point to the importance of local muscle adaptation in rowing. This consideration is especially relevant when training on the water is impossible and indoor training must be undertaken. The use of rowing ergometers and tank rowing is recommended.

Aerobic metabolism

An increase in ideal boat resistance with boat velocity to the second power suggests that the metabolism of rowers should increase with boat velocity to the third power (Secher, 1983). Yet, oxygen intake increases only with the speed of rowing to a power of about 2.4 (Fig. 51.3). At the present speed of competitive rowing, the metabolic cost of rowing may be calculated to be 6.7 l·min⁻¹ for men, 5.9 l·min⁻¹ for lightweight men, 5.3 l·min⁻¹ for women and 4.9 l·min⁻¹ for lightweight women. These high metabolic rates are reflected in the metabolic capacity of rowers as expressed by their maximal oxygen intake, being 6.1 l·min⁻¹ for men, 5.1 l·min⁻¹ for lightweight men, and 4.3 l·min⁻¹ for women (Secher, 1990). Moreover, a direct relationship has been demonstrated between results obtained in a FISA championship and the crew's average maximal oxygen intake

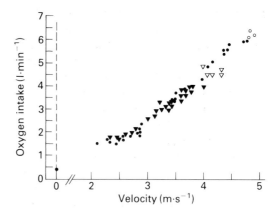

Fig. 51.3 Oxygen intake during rowing a single scull for two oarsmen. Values indicated with open symbols were not included in the regression. $\dot{V}O_2 = 0.1944 \, v^{2.21} + 0.28$.

(Fig. 51.4). In fact an almost perfect relationship ($r = 0.99$) can be demonstrated when the metabolic capacity of the crew is balanced with boat resistance and compared with results obtained in FISA regattas.

The results when rowing are correlated to the maximal oxygen intake of rowers expressed in l·min⁻¹ and not as ml·kg⁻¹·min⁻¹ (Secher, 1983). On the other hand, if values of maximal oxygen intake are to be compared between subjects, the dimensions of the athlete should be taken into consideration and a unit based on body

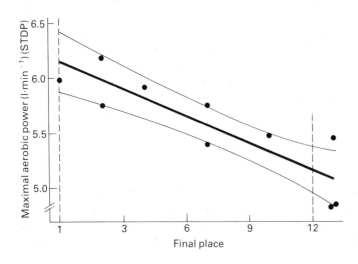

Fig. 51.4 Regression line between average maximal oxygen uptake of a crew and its placing in a FISA championship regatta (1971). The 95% confidence limits of the regression line are also shown. From Secher (1983).

surface area (or kg$^{-2/3}$) may be applied. When expressed in terms neutral to body dimensions, rowers' maximal oxygen intake is only approximately 300 ml·kg$^{-2/3}$·min^{-1} for men and 250 ml·kg$^{-2/3}$·min^{-1} for women, while the best runners, cyclists and skiers may approach 370 ml·kg$^{-2/3}$·min^{-1} and 270 ml·kg$^{-2/3}$·min^{-1}, respectively. Applying these figures to rowers, a maximal oxygen intake of 7.5 l·min^{-1} for men (6.2 l·min^{-1} for lightweight men) and 5.0 l·min^{-1} for women should be obtainable with associated improvements of performance. The data also indicate that while women rowers are within 10% of the best international female skiers and runners with respect to maximal oxygen intake, there is a 20% discrepancy between the best male rowers and the international élite athlete.

Anaerobic metabolism

Traditionally, anaerobic metabolism is indicated by a high peak blood lactate concentration, which increases with the muscle mass involved in exercise as well as the motivation of the rowers. Values of 11 mmol·l^{-1} have been reported after treadmill running, 15 mmol·l^{-1} after a national regatta, and 17 mmol·l^{-1} following a FISA championship. Accordingly the buffering system of the blood (bicarbonate) decreases from 26 to 13 mmol·l^{-1} after all-out rowing, and bicarbonate may in fact be eliminated from the blood. This means that the pH of the blood decreases from its normal value of 7.4 to 7.1 after all-out rowing. The pH was 6.8 in a rower in whom no bicarbonate was measured after all-out rowing.

These values give little indication of the amount of anaerobic metabolism. For that purpose the 'oxygen deficit' can be calculated. Oxygen deficit is the part of metabolism that is not covered by oxygen intake during exercise. In rowers, the oxygen deficit has been reported to be 88−97 ml·kg^{-1} or substantially larger than reported in runners. Rowers also have the highest plasma catecholamine values measured during exercise. However, the anaerobic con-

tribution to metabolism has not been determined for the duration of races, and even for 6-min all-out ergometer rowing, estimates vary between 21% and 30% (Secher, 1990).

Interest has also focused on the 'anaerobic threshold' or the work rate that elicits a blood lactate concentration of 4 mmol·l^{-1}. This work rate increases with training, and it seems to depend on the muscle fibre composition of the rower; those with many slow-twitch fibres are able to exercise at a high intensity with a blood lactate value of no more than 4 mmol·l^{-1} (Körner & Schwanitz, 1985).

Circulation

In 1920 cardiac output was measured during rowing in ordinary rowing boats by Liljestrand and Lindhard (1920), showing values of only 13−17 l·min^{-1}. However, cardiac output has not been determined during rowing with a sliding seat. A special problem during rowing is the involvement of many muscle groups. Thus different groups of muscle may compete for their share of the cardiac output when they have all been activated at maximal intensity (Secher, 1983). Variation in blood pressure is related to the cardiac cycle, resulting in a pulse pressure of approximately 45 mmHg (6 kPa) at rest. During rowing, blood pressure also varies with the rowing cycle, giving rise to a 'pulse pressure' of more than 100 mmHg (13.3 kPa). This means that the systolic pressure may approach 200 mmHg (26.7 kPa) during maximal rowing. Heart rate has been determined repetitively during rowing and is currently used to guide training intensity of rowers, often with the aim of applying an intensity close to that which elicits a blood lactate value of 4 mmol·l^{-1}.

Ventilation

As during other types of exercise, ventilation increases linearly with oxygen intake until approximately 80% of the rower's maximal oxygen intake is reached. At higher work rates the increase in ventilation becomes steeper with a higher recorded value of 243 l·min^{-1} (Secher, 1983). The vital capacity of rowers is also large, 6.8 litres (male mean), and a highest value of 9.1 litres has been measured.

The high ventilation rate during intense rowing indicates a marked increase in alveolar oxygen tension. Yet the large cardiac output elicited during maximal exercise makes saturation of haemoglobin critical, especially when exercise involves large muscle groups. Thus, during maximal arm exercise there is no decrease in haemoglobin saturation, but during 'all-out' rowing, a 7% reduction takes place. It may be speculated that the decrease in haemoglobin saturation during rowing is due to the decrease in pH of the blood, but arterial oxygen tension also decreases from a resting value of 105 mmHg (14 kPa) to 83 mmHg (11 kPa). This finding points to a decrease in diffusion of oxygen across the alveolar membrane. Indeed, a decrease in pulmonary dif-

fusion capacity takes place 2 h after exercise when cardiac output is comparable to that at rest (Fig. 51.5). The decrease in pulmonary diffusion capacity continues for at least 6 h but the normal value is re-established after 1 day.

Training

With the strong correlation between performance and the metabolic capacity of rowers, training should be directed towards increasing anaerobic and especially aerobic power and capacity. The maximal oxygen intake of rowers increases in proportion to the work performed, from 400 to 700 h·year^{-1} (approximately 1.1–2.2 h·day^{-1}), but with more prolonged training it becomes increasingly difficult to develop a further increase (Körner & Schwanitz, 1985). Large work rates may increase the work intensity which corresponds to a blood lactate concentration of 4 mmol·l^{-1}. It is also suggested that this variable offers the best physiological estimate of the performance of rowers, but data are not yet available to evaluate this notion.

Altitude training

With the difficulty of increasing maximal oxygen intake in well-trained athletes, altitude training has remained popular among some rowers and is carried out immediately before the FISA championship of the year. Early studies, involving mainly untrained subjects, showed a dramatic increase in maximal oxygen intake following altitude training. But such an effect has been more difficult to demonstrate in well-trained individuals, and in athletes it has been difficult to maintain even the prealtitude maximal oxygen intake (Secher, 1990). Yet, the amazing performance by East African nations in middle- and long-distance track events at sea level has made a lasting impression.

Performance on a rowing ergometer has not been demonstrated to increase following altitude training. Furthermore, in a controlled study (B. Levine, personal communication) the same increase was noted in maximal oxygen

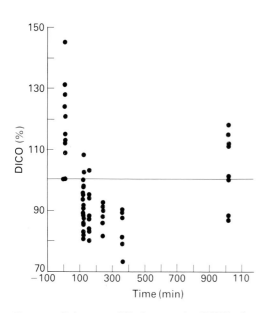

Fig. 51.5 Pulmonary diffusion capacity (DICO) after 'all-out' rowing on an ergometer. Immediately after rowing DICO increases markedly due to an elevated cardiac output. When cardiac output is similar to the prerowing value, DICO decreases for up to at least 6 h. The horizontal line indicates the pre-rowing value.

intake when training at altitude and at sea level. However, endurance at sea level increased more (68%) than at altitude (46%) in the group that trained at sea level. Conversely in the altitude training group, endurance was more enhanced at altitude (73%) than at sea level (43%). These results strongly indicate that competitions at sea level should be preceded by training that is also performed at sea level.

References

Balukow, C.N. (1964) Hydrodynamische Charakteristik der Sport-Ruderboote (German translation by E. Schatté). *Katera i Yachti* **3**, 187–191.

Hagerman, F.C. (1984) Applied physiology of rowing. *Sport Med.* **1**, 303–326.

Hartmann, U. (1987) *Querschnittuntersuchungen an Leistungsruderern im Flachland und Längsschnittuntersuchungen an Eliteruderern in der Höhe mittels eines zweistufigen Tests auf einem Gjessing-Ruder-ergometer*. Hartung-Gorre Verlag, Konstanz.

Körner, T. & Schwanitz, P. (1985) *Rudern*. Sportsverlag Berlin, Berlin.

Liljestrand, G. & Lindhard, J. (1920) Zur Physiologie des Ruderns. *Skand. Arch. Physiol.* **39**, 215–235.

Schneider, E. (1980) *Leistungsanalyse bei Rudermannschaften*. Verlag, Bad Homburg.

Secher, N.H. (1983) The physiology of rowing. *J. Sports Sci.* **1**, 23–53.

Secher, N.H. (1990) Rowing. In: Reilly, T., Secher, N.H., Snell, P. & Williams, C. (eds) *Physiology of Sports*. pp. 259–285. E. & F.N. Spon, London.

Steinacker, J.M. (1987) *Rudern*. Springer-Verlag, Berlin.

Chapter 52

Cross-Country Ski Racing

ULF BERGH AND ARTUR FORSBERG

Introduction

Cross-country skiing has been practised for at least 4000 years, most of the time for basic transportation. Nowadays, activities such as recreational touring and racing are the more common reasons for such skiing. As a result, skiing equipment has become more specialized and the level of performance has increased. This chapter focuses on cross-country ski racing, particularly performance at a very advanced level. The data presented are mostly taken from the literature but some of the authors' as yet unpublished results are included.

Skiing competitions

Cross-country skiing competitions for adults are performed over distances ranging from 5 to 90 km. In the world championships, the Olympic games and the world cup, the distances for individual races range from 5 to 30 km for females and from 10 to 50 km for males. Relay races consist of 4×5 km and 4×10 km events for females and males, respectively. In the individual events, the competitors usually start at 30-s intervals. However, in the world cup, a 30-km race divided into two 15-km races performed on two consecutive days has been tried and this format will be included in the 1991 world cup programme. The event starts with an ordinary 15-km race. The following day there is a 'pursuit race'; the start is arranged based on the competitors' time intervals obtained on the

first day, and the first to finish is the winner. In relay races, all teams start at the same time. The duration these races is, at present, approximately 15–100 min for females and 25–150 min for males.

As in most sports, the results in cross-country skiing have improved over the decades (Fig. 52.1). This is due to better equipment, better preparation of courses, and greater physical capacity of the skiers. There are considerable variations in this overall trend within relatively narrow timespans (a few years), probably resulting from differences in factors such as snow conditions and altitude. The results have improved more in cross-country skiing than in some other endurance events (Fig. 52.2). This is probably due to the fact that there has been room for considerable improvement in at least four areas of cross-country skiing: courses, equipment, skiing technique and physical capacity of skiers, whereas in other sports major contributions to a better performance have been possible in only one or two of these areas.

According to the rules, a racing course should contain uphill, downhill and flat terrain in equal proportions. Usually, more than half of the racing time is spent skiing uphill, and 10–15% skiing downhill (Frost et al., 1984). Consequently, one would expect the major part of the time differences between skiers to occur in the uphill parts of the course. This has been confirmed by timing the participants in various races (Frost et al., 1984). However, if one com-

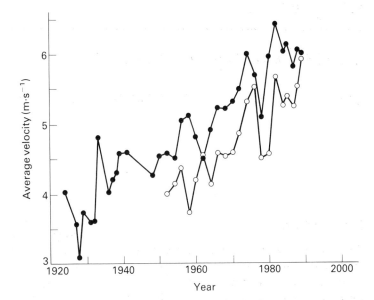

Fig. 52.1 Average speed in world championships and Olympic games in the men's shortest individual event (18 km up to 1948 and thereafter 15 km) (●) and the women's 10-km event (○).

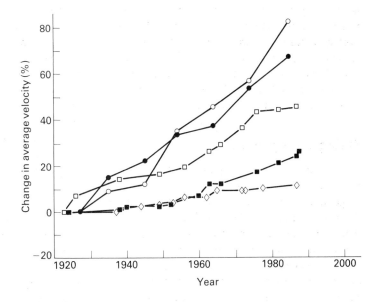

Fig. 52.2 Relative improvement of the results in some endurance sports, calculated according to the expression $100\cdot(v_i - v_0)\cdot v_0^{-1}$, where v_i is the speed for a given year and v_0 is the speed at the earliest of the illustrated competitions. For cross-country skiing, the calculations are based on the winning results in Olympic games and world championships. These values are presented as averages for each decade. For the other events, the world records are used to indicate performance. ○, Cross-country skiing (50 km); ●, cross-country skiing (15 km); □, swimming (1500 m); ■, speed skating (10 km); ◇, running (10 km).

pensates for differences in duration between uphill and downhill skiing the data become conflicting. Thus, there are data indicating that the fraction of the total time difference (compared with the winner) for a specific part of the course is directly proportional to the fraction of total racing time spent in this section of the course (Frost *et al.*, 1984). In contrast, a study based on four events in the 1989 world championships (A. Forsberg, unpublished data) indicates that the fraction of the time differences occurring in the uphill segments is much greater than its fraction of the total racing time.

Occasionally, 'mass starts' are used in

individual events. These races are usually quite long (60–90 km) and the courses are flatter. A number of these races are part of the so-called 'world loppet', which is a long-distance equivalent of the world cup.

In events such as swimming and running, the average velocity is lower over longer distances. This is mainly due to the fact that the available power declines with increasing duration of exercise (Åstrand & Rodahl, 1986). Hence, such a pattern would also be expected in cross-country skiing. The winning results in Olympic games and world championships from 1978 to 1985, indicate that the average velocity decreases as the distance increases for males, but not for females. During this time, the same technique was used over all distances. However, the anticipated distance–velocity relationship in cross-country skiing is obscured by the fact that courses may differ considerably with regard to snow conditions and total climb. Moreover, the total climb per unit of distance tends to be greatest in the shortest races, which decreases the average velocity.

The difference in skiing performance between males and females can be estimated by comparing the average racing speed (U. Bergh, unpublished data). The regression equations for average racing velocity as a function of chronological time indicate that males are skiing approximately 14% faster than females. Distance–velocity relationships based on (i) winning results in Olympic games and world championships, (ii) the fastest Olympic games or world championship race ever recorded for each distance, and (iii) the results from 10 races in the world cup, produced sex differences of 13%, 14% and 15%, respectively. These figures tend to be somewhat higher than those reported for other endurance events (Åstrand & Rodahl, 1986).

Generally, the performance in events such as cross-country skiing is determined by the difference between the forces acting in the forward direction and forces acting in the opposite direction. The former are limited by the rate of energy yield (motor power) of the skier (and in

downhill segments the force of gravity) and the capability to utilize this energy in the forward direction (technical skill).

The skier has to expend energy to: (i) overcome the friction between the ski and the snow; (ii) overcome the air resistance; (iii) elevate the centre of gravity during each stride and in uphill skiing; and (iv) accelerate the body's centre of mass (translational kinetic energy) and the mass of various body segments (rotational kinetic energy). The ability to release energy can be increased by training but it is strongly influenced by genetic factors. The friction between ski and snow can be influenced by the condition of the snow surface, waxing of the ski and by pressure-distribution characteristics (Ekström, 1980). Air resistance can be diminished by the design and material of the skier's outer garment and also by the skier's body position. The skiing technique aims at directing the largest possible fraction of the available metabolic power (and in skiing down hills the force of gravity) in a forward direction, parallel to the track while minimizing the resisting forces.

Energy yield

The duration of ski races is such that the energy source is predominantly (85–99%) aerobic metabolism (Åstrand & Rodahl, 1986). Oxygen intake is quite often close to its maximum in uphill segments of the race, judging from observed heart rate values (Bergh, 1982). Skiing can induce a higher oxygen intake than uphill running (Strömme et al., 1977). For these reasons, a very high maximal oxygen intake is likely to be a prerequisite for success in international cross-country ski racing (see Fig. 7.2). The anaerobic energy yielding system may be taxed substantially during racing conditions, judging from the blood lactate levels obtained at the finish of races (Åstrand et al., 1963; U. Bergh, unpublished data). However, the anaerobic capacity is generally of minor importance for cross-country skiing performance, especially in longer events, and can be decisive only if the differences in other functions are small.

The main substrates for muscular activity are fat and carbohydrates. The latter are stored as glycogen in the skeletal muscles and in the liver. If the racing time exceeds 1 h, there is a risk of emptying these stores, in which case the tempo will drop dramatically. This is not infrequent in races of 50 km or longer, where minutes may be lost within a few kilometres. Glycogen cannot be moved from one muscle to another and therefore some muscles may become depleted of glycogen, while others are far from empty. Carbohydrates can be supplied to the skier during a race. These carbohydrates primarily serve the very important purpose of maintaining an adequate blood glucose concentration, but may also decrease the rate of glycogen degradation, although to a limited extent (see Chapter 30). Hence, the vast majority of the glycogen needed during a race must be stored in the body of the skier before the start of the race.

Racing styles

At present, skiing competitions are classified into two styles: classic skiing (Figs 52.3a & 52.3b) and freestyle (Fig. 52.3c). In classic skiing three main techniques are used: diagonal (Fig. 52.3a), double pole, and kick double pole (Fig. 52.3b). In the freestyle events, skating is by far the most frequently used technique; classic skiing is hardly used at all. Skating can be performed in many different ways, but two main techniques can be identified: the double skate (V-skate) and the one leg skate (marathon-skate) of which the former is the dominating choice in freestyle events. Skating is approximately 10% faster than classic skiing (Stray-Gundersen & Ryschon, 1987). The question is: why? There are a number of possible explanations: (i) the attainable aerobic power is higher in skating than in classic skiing; (ii) for a given metabolic rate skating develops a greater power in the forward direction; and

(iii) the forces resisting the forward progression are lower in skating.

Comparison of the diagonal technique and the V-skate during maximal uphill skiing in nine male skiers of international calibre did not reveal any significant difference in oxygen intake between techniques (Table 52.1). In contrast, with six female skiers of national calibre, the diagonal technique produced significantly higher values than the V-skate (Table 52.1). Hence, these observations do not indicate that the superiority of skating is due to a higher aerobic power. On the other hand, there are indications that higher oxygen intake values can be attained in skating compared with the kick double pole technique (Nilsson & Löfstedt, 1984). However, the latter technique is used mainly on flat terrain, where the oxygen intake is not usually taxed to its maximum (Bergh, 1982). It is therefore not possible to state whether the attainable oxygen intake over an entire race will be higher in skating compared with classic skiing.

For a given velocity, skating has been reported to be metabolically approximately 10% less costly than classic skiing (Zupan et al., 1988). Skating has also been found to produce a higher velocity at a given blood lactate concentration than classic skiing (Nilsson & Löfstedt,

Table 52.1 Oxygen intake and heart rate during maximal uphill skiing. Approximately 3 min of all-out effort preceded by at least 30 min of warm-up skiing. The male skiers were all of international calibre; most of the females were not, although all of them belonged to the Swedish national team. From Forsberg et al. (1988) and unpublished data.

	Diagonal	Skate
Males ($n = 9$)		
Oxygen intake ($l \cdot min^{-1}$)	5.65 ± 0.61	5.59 ± 0.60
Heart rate (beats·min^{-1})	177 ± 8	177 ± 8
Females ($n = 6$)		
Oxygen intake ($l \cdot min^{-1}$)	3.41 ± 0.18	3.27 ± 0.21
Heart rate (beats·min^{-1})	178 ± 5	179 ± 4

Values are mean ± standard deviation.

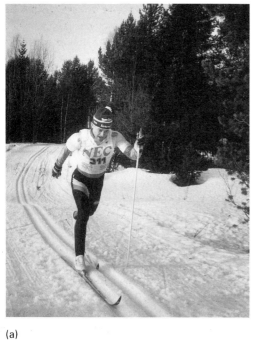

(a)

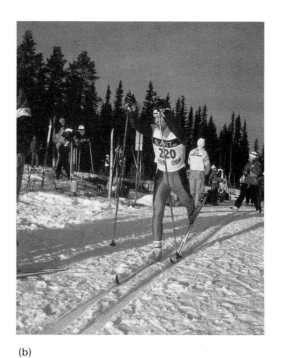

(b)

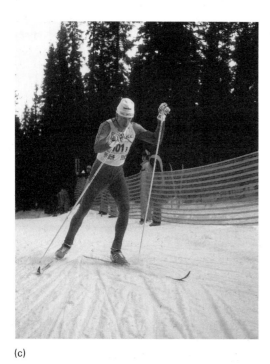

(c)

Fig. 52.3   (a) Diagonal technique. (b) Kick/double
pole technique. (c) V-skate (double skate) technique.

1984), which further supports the theory that skating is less costly than other cross-country skiing techniques. Hence, one probable explanation why skating is faster than classic skiing is that the metabolic rate for a given skiing velocity is lower in skating than in classic skiing; for a given aerobic power, skating produces a higher speed. The question is again: why? There are several possibilities: (i) resisting forces (air resistance and friction between the ski and the snow) are less; (ii) less work is performed against gravity; (iii) increases in kinetic energy are smaller; and (iv) there is a better transformation of energy between body segments. Factors (ii), (iii) and (iv) would increase the fraction of the available power directed forwards. There are no data on the air resistance for different racing styles. However, the body position is a crucial factor, and when conditions allow the skier to skate without using the poles, the V-skate may allow a more crouched posture, as in speed skating. In addition, skating can be performed without kick waxes and that reduces the frictional force. The glide becomes better, which is an advantage in almost all parts of a racing track. This may also contribute to a lowering of air resistance by reducing slowing on flats after downhill segments, thus allowing the skier to stay longer in a crouched position. Another possible difference between classic and skating techniques is that the work against gravity within a step-cycle may be lower in skating, since the vertical displacement of the centre of gravity, as well as the frequency of cycles, appears to be less than in classic skiing.

On the other hand, if the course is very soft the V-skate may be more costly than both the kick/double pole technique and the marathon-skate (Nilsson & Löfstedt, 1984). This may be due to the fact that the skis are tilted during skating so that the edges cut rather deeply into the snow during the planting and the thrust.

Among classic techniques, the kick/double pole technique has been found to demand either less oxygen than the diagonal technique (Westergren & Nylander, 1977; U. Bergh,

unpublished data) or more (MacDougall et al., 1979). The latter result is not compatible with the fact that the kick/double pole technique is the predominant one on flats, at least among élite skiers.

Skiing techniques differ with regard to the velocity attained over a distance of 90 m (Nilsson & Löfstedt, 1984). The V-skate is significantly faster (9%) than the kick/double pole technique, which in turn tends to be slower than the marathon-skate (3%).

Characteristics of élite cross-country skiers

Top skiers can vary considerably in body mass (Table 52.2). World-class male skiers during the 1970s and early 1980s differed by approximately 30 kg (Bergh, 1987). Thus, the influence of body size appears to be no greater than the differences in quality (the variation in capacity for a given body size), in contrast to the situation in many other sports, even endurance events, e.g. rowing (Secher, 1983). Cross-country skiers tend to be heavier than long-distance runners (Bergh et al., 1978), but lighter than rowers (Secher, 1983).

Maximal oxygen intake is extremely high, both in absolute volume and relative to body mass (Åstrand, 1955; Saltin & Åstrand, 1967; Hanson, 1973; Bergh et al., 1978) (Table 52.3). World-class skiers have significantly higher maximal oxygen intake than less successful skiers (Bergh, 1987). Among world-class skiers, the greatest variation appeared when expressing the values in $l \cdot min^{-1}$, while the unit $ml \cdot min^{-1} \cdot kg^{-2/3}$ produced the smallest variation (Bergh, 1987). Without an oxygen intake of at least 350 $ml \cdot min^{-1} \cdot kg^{-2/3}$ for males and 290 $ml \cdot min^{-1} \cdot kg^{-2/3}$ for females, the probability of winning gold medals in individual events in the Olympic games or world championships seems to be quite low (Bergh, 1987). This is supported by data on Swedish male medallists in individual events (Table 52.3). The medallists in the junior world championships had lower values for maximal oxygen intake (Table 52.3)

Table 52.2 Age, height, body mass and body mass index of cross-country skiers of international calibre during the season 1989−90.

	Age (years)	Height (cm)	Body mass (kg)	Body mass index (kg·m^{-2})
Males				
Mean	29	180	72	22.3
Standard deviation	4	6	6	1.4
Range	23−40	169−188	58−83	20.3−24.8
Females				
Mean	27	170	59	20.4
Standard deviation	4	5	4	1.0
Range	21−38	162−179	52−65	18.0−21.8

Table 52.3 Body mass and maximal oxygen intake in Swedish male medallists in Olympic games or world championships and in junior world championships.

	Body mass (kg)	Maximal oxygen intake		
		l·min^{-1}	ml·min^{-1}·kg^{-1}	ml·min^{-1}·kg$^{-2/3}$
1960s* ($n = 4$)	68 ± 3	5.56 ± 0.27	82.0 ± 2.27	335 ± 9
1970s* ($n = 4$)	72 ± 7	6.14 ± 0.46	84.9 ± 6.44	353 ± 20
1980s[†] ($n = 4$)	73 ± 5	6.33 ± 0.51	87.2 ± 1.61	363 ± 14
Juniors				
1979−89* ($n = 5$)	70 ± 3	5.53 ± 0.22	78.7 ± 2.56	324 ± 8

Values are mean ± standard deviation.
* Maximal oxygen intake measured during uphill running on a treadmill.
[†] Maximal oxygen intake measured during uphill skiing which produces approximately 3% higher values than uphill running (Strömme et al., 1977).

and none of them had won a medal in a world championship or the Olympic games while of junior age.

The oxygen cost of skiing at a given speed has been found to be lower in élite than in non-élite cross-country skiers (Harkins, 1978), indicating that élite skiers are technically superior. In contrast, another study comparing skiers of national calibre with recreational skiers did not confirm this finding (MacDougall et al., 1979). The latter study indicated a considerable difference within the group of élite skiers, in line with data on subjects whose skiing capability ranged from being next to national level down to recreational level (Wehlin et al., 1970). In contrast, a much lower variation was found among skiers of international calibre (Åstrand et al., 1963). Variation seems to be less at the international level, which is logical since individuals with unfavourable qualities will not reach this high level of performance.

Muscle fibres in leg muscles appear to be predominantly slow-twitch fibres, although the variation is considerable (Rusko, 1976; Bergh et al., 1978). A predominance of slow-twitch fibres is logical for several reasons: (i) slow-twitch fibres display a more complete glycogen depletion than fast-twitch fibres in both arm and leg muscles (Tesch et al., 1978) during cross-country skiing, indicating that the demands of this sport involve slow-twitch more than fast-twitch fibres; (ii) metabolism during cross-country skiing is predominantly aerobic and slow-twitch fibres have a high oxidative capacity; (iii) the number of capillaries per fibre is higher in slow-twitch fibres which enhances the oxygen transport; and (iv) slow-twitch fibres consume less glycogen for a given energy output (see Chapter 5).

Predicting performance from physiological variables

Table 52.4 displays the correlation coefficients between a number of variables and different performance criteria. As expected, no single variable fully explains the observed differences in skiing performance. Hence, it is hardly possible to predict the outcome of a ski race from physiological data. However, some characteristics show a considerable covariation with skiing performance. Maximal oxygen intake is one of these, and the skiing velocity at a given fraction of maximal oxygen intake is another, while oxygen intake at a given speed displays less covariation with skiing performance. This differs little from what has been found in running, where maximal oxygen intake explained 61% of the variation in marathon-running performance and the fraction of maximal oxygen intake utilized during treadmill running at a given speed explained 88% of the variation, while oxygen intake at a given running velocity accounted for 55% of the variation (Sjödin & Svedenhag, 1985). Corresponding figures for the performance in 5000-m running were 35%, 88% and 53%, respectively (Sjödin & Schéle, 1982). This discrepancy between running and skiing is probably explained by the fact that the subjects used only one skiing style during the measurements of oxygen intake, while additional styles were used during other parts of the race. Hence, in the skiing experiments the measured oxygen intake reflected only one aspect of the skiers' technical skill, whereas in running a single measurement is likely to be more representative of the oxygen cost, because the intraindividual

variation of style during a race is much less than in skiing. Therefore, in order to establish valid figures for the individual differences in the oxygen cost of skiing under racing conditions, one would need to make measurements for all of the actual combinations of skiing techniques and terrain, preferably at racing speed. Moreover, one must know for what fraction of the racing time the skier uses each of the different techniques. Hence, available data on the correlation between performance and the oxygen cost of skiing are hardly representative of the influence of technical skill on skiing performance.

Among variables other than physiological characteristics, the amount of cross-country skiing training seems to be a valuable predictor of performance, since it explains the vast majority (90%) of the variation in performance between individuals (Holm et al., 1976). A much lower figure (31%) was found for ski racing experience (Niinimaa et al., 1978).

Training

Cross-country skiing is characterized by repeated muscle contractions of a number of muscles over extended periods of time. Sometimes the active muscle mass is large enough to tax the cardiopulmonary system maximally, while in other instances the active muscle groups are too small. For small muscle groups, the attainable oxygen intake can vary substantially without any change in the maximal oxygen intake (Holmér, 1974; Clausen, 1976), and the performance in exercise with small muscle groups may vary considerably for a given maximal oxygen intake (Holmér, 1974; Clausen, 1976). Hence, there is a need both for a high maximal oxygen intake and a high aerobic power of the muscles engaged in the various skiing styles. These qualities can be considerably improved by training. Furthermore, it is important not to empty the glycogen stores in muscles active during the race. Endurance training, where intensities below maximal aerobic power are

Table 52.4 Correlation between cross-country skiing performance and different variables.

Performance criterion	No. of subjects	$\dot{V}O_{2\,max}$ (ml·kg⁻¹·min⁻¹)	$\dot{V}O_2$ at a given speed	$\dot{V}O_2 \cdot \dot{V}O_{2\,max}^{-1}$ at a given speed	Muscle fibre composition (% ST fibre)	Muscle strength (N·m·kg⁻¹)	Racing experience (years)	Training*	Reference
Rank†	4	1.00							Åstrand (1955)
Rank†	5	0.40	0.23	0.30					Åstrand et al. (1963)
Rank†	6	0.89							Bergh (1982)
Speed	3	0.98							Bergh (1982)
Speed (medium)	11	0.72	0.16	0.75					Wehlin et al. (1970)
Speed (high)	11			0.86					Wehlin et al. (1970)
Speed	11	0.89			0.26			0.93	Holm et al. (1976)
Speed	11					0.35			
Rank†,‡	6	0.03							Forsberg (unpublished)
Rank†	11	0.70							Forsberg (unpublished)
Racing success	10	0.40					0.56		Forsberg (unpublished) Niinimaa et al. (1978)

* Kilometres of skiing during the year of the race.
† Position to finish, Spearman's rank correlation coefficient is used.
‡ Women.

maintained for hours, causes adaptations in the muscles that increase fat metabolism, sparing glycogen (see Chapters 5 and 12).

The ability to convert the available energy into a forward motion of the body, i.e. the individual's skiing skill, is likely to be important, although the correlation between racing performance and the oxygen cost of skiing is not very impressive (Table 52.4). Another potentially important quality is the ability to choose the most effective racing style with regard to prevailing conditions. This is especially difficult in events with individual starting times, since there is then limited feedback as to what style is the most effective one.

Consequently, the training should include exercises that: (i) induce a high load on the cardiovascular system to increase maximal oxygen intake; (ii) involve all muscles that are used during competitive skiing in order to increase the attainable oxygen intake in skiing styles that only involve relatively small muscle groups, and to increase the capacity to spare glycogen; and (iii) improve the technical skill in order to increase skiing velocity at a given metabolic rate.

The attainable oxygen intake is of similar magnitude in running and in roller skiing (Bergh, 1982). Ski-walking (walking up a fairly steep hill using poles to imitate uphill skiing) and cross-country skiing have been shown to produce slightly higher values compared with running in subjects trained for cross-country skiing (Hermansen, 1973; Strömme et al., 1977). One advantage of roller skiing compared with running is that the upper body is also engaged in training in a manner similar to that of actual skiing (Petterson et al., 1977). It is important that muscles participating in poling are very durable since this movement contributes substantially to most racing styles (Ekström, 1980). Moreover, a high aerobic power of the muscles of the upper body facilitates the attainment of maximal oxygen intake during combined arm and leg exercise (Bergh et al., 1976).

One disadvantage of roller skiing might be that the skis can roll quite fast without much effort from the skier. Thus, the load on the oxygen transporting system may not be sufficient since the skiers do not seem to compensate fully for a decreased rolling resistance by increasing their speed, either on flat or uphill terrain (Forsberg & Karlsson, 1987). Therefore, skiers whose off-snow training consists predominantly of roller skiing should not always use fast roller-skis.

Skiing technique should be learned by skiing, because exercises such as roller skiing and ski-walking do not require identical patterns of motion (Petterson et al., 1977). Training of skiing technique ought to have priority with youngsters since it seems harder for adults to achieve the necessary coordination.

The top skiers of today train so much and so hard that only a well-trained body can endure this. Since the body needs time to adapt to high levels of physical stress, it takes several years of increased training volume and intensity before reaching the necessary level (Table 52.5). This partly explains why junior skiers rarely compete successfully in Olympic games and world championships, and why the average age of international-calibre skiers is almost 30 years (see Table 52.2). Moreover, the body adapts not only to increases in training but also to decreases. Therefore, the increments in training should be rather gentle and long breaks in training should be avoided, unless the individual's medical status dictates otherwise.

The content of training varies both between and within groups. There are, however, three main activities: cross-country running, roller skiing, and cross-country skiing. In the off-snow season, roller skiing accounts for 40–70% of the time devoted to endurance training. The intensity of this training also varies partly because skiers most often train on hilly terrain, where it is hard to keep a constant work rate. Skiers tend to exercise at a higher metabolic rate uphill than on flat terrain both during running and roller skiing (Forsberg & Karlsson, 1987). There are also seasonal variations. After the competitive season, high intensities ought

Table 52.5 Approximate amount of training for cross-country skiers in different age groups. Exercises such as warm-up and stretching are not included in the figures, which are representative of the present (1990) situation in Sweden.

	Age (years)	Amount of training (h·year^{-1})	
		Males	Females
Seniors	<20	650–750	500–700
Juniors	16–20	400–550	300–550
Youth	12–16	250–350	250–350

to be avoided, especially at the beginning of the off-snow season (when there is a risk of overuse injuries; see Chapter 32). High-intensity training is performed just before the competitive season, while the greatest amounts of training are carried out a few weeks after the beginning of the on-snow season. The intensity is usually such that blood lactate concentration is increased, but it rarely approaches the levels attained immediately after skiing competitions (Bergh, 1982).

Heat balance

Cross-country skiing is frequently performed in comparatively cold weather, and a substantial body heat loss as well as cold injuries might be expected. The temperature of a body tissue is the result of the balance between the sum of the heat production plus heat gain on one hand and the heat loss on the other. For the body as a whole, the metabolic heat production during ski racing is usually greater than the heat loss due to convection, conduction and radiation, and therefore the skier must sweat to maintain the heat balance of the body. In spite of this, certain parts of the body, e.g. nose, ears and feet, can become quite cold, and sometimes even suffer cold injuries. This may seem paradoxical, but it is explained by the fact that the local heat loss can be higher than the sum of the local heat production and heat gained via the warm blood. The rate of local heat loss is

high because the velocity of the wind is added to the velocity of the skiers. Furthermore, the convective and evaporative heat losses are considerably elevated on body parts facing the wind. To reduce these problems competitions should not be held at temperatures below −20°C. However, there are risks of cold injuries even at temperatures above these limits, especially in strong winds and/or if the course contains long downhill segments. Another problem is that the skier inhales thousands of litres of cold, dry air, which may cause irritation of the respiratory tract (see also Chapter 16).

The skier sweats during racing. The volume of sweat may, at least in longer races, amount to 4% of body mass (Holm *et al.*, 1976) and may exceed that which can be tolerated without a reduction in performance capability. Consequently, there is a need for fluid replenishment during cross-country ski racing over longer distances.

References

Åstrand, P.-O. (1955) New records in human power. *Nature* **176**, 922–923.
Åstrand, P.-O., Hallbäck, I., Hedman, R. & Saltin B. (1963) Blood lactates after prolonged severe exercise. *J. Appl. Physiol.* **18**, 619–622.
Åstrand, P.-O. & Rodahl, K. (1986) *Textbook of Work Physiology*, 3rd edn. McGraw-Hill, New York.
Bergh, U. (1982) *Physiology of Cross-country Ski Racing*. Human Kinetics, Champaign, Illinois.
Bergh, U. (1987) The influence of body mass in cross-country skiing. *Med. Sci. Sports Exerc.* **19**, 324–331.
Bergh, U., Kanstrup, I.-L. & Ekblom, B. (1976) Maximal oxygen uptake during exercise with various combinations of arm and leg exercise. *J. Appl. Physiol.* **41**, 191–196.
Bergh, U., Thorstensson, A., Sjödin, B., Hultén, B., Piehl, K. & Karlsson, J. (1978) Maximal oxygen uptake and muscle fiber types in trained and untrained humans. *Med. Sci. Sports* **10**, 151–154.
Clausen, J.P. (1976) Circulatory adjustments to dynamic exercise and effect of physical training in normal subjects and in patients with coronary disease. *Prog. Cardiovasc. Dis.* **18**, 459–495.
Ekström, H. (1980) *Biomechanical research applied to skiing: a developmental study and an investigation of cross-country skiing, alpine skiing and knee ligaments.* Linkoping Studies in Science and Technology,

dissertation no. 53. University of Linkoping, Sweden.

Forsberg, A. & Karlsson, E. (1987) Rullar det för lätt? (Are roller-skis too fast for aerobic training?) *Svensk Skidsport* 7, 48–50.

Forsberg, A., Palmgren, L.-E. & Karlsson, E. (1988) Konditionsträna båda stilarna. (Use both classic and skating techniques in aerobic training.) *Svensk Skidsport* 10, 44–46.

Frost, P., Gabrielsson, L. & Jalderyd, G. (1984) *Kapacitetsanalys av svenska damjuniorer.* (Analysis of racing capacity in Swedish junior female cross-country skiers.) Phys. Ed. student thesis. Report 1984:16, Gymnastik-och idrottshögskolan, Stockholm, Sweden.

Hanson, J. (1973) Maximal exercise performance in members of the US nordic ski team. *J. Appl. Physiol.* 35, 592–595.

Harkins, K.J. (1978) Metabolic cost comparison of cross-country skiing between élite and non élite. *Can. J. Sport Sci.* 3, 186 (abstract).

Hermansen, L. (1973) Oxygen transport during exercise in human subjects. *Acta Physiol. Scand.* Suppl. 399.

Holm, I., Sjödin, B., Nilsson, J., Tesch, P. & Forsberg, A. (1976) Muskelfunktionens förändring under Vasaloppet. (Changes in muscle functions during long distance skiing, Vasaloppet.) *Svensk Skidsport* 8, 27–30.

Holmér, I. (1974) Physiology of swimming man. *Acta Physiol. Scand.* Suppl. 407.

MacDougall, J.D., Hughson, R., Sutton, J.R. & Moroz, J.R. (1979) The energy cost of cross-country skiing among élite competitors. *Med. Sci. Sports* 11, 270–273.

Nilsson, C. & Löfstedt, M. (1984) *Effektivitetsanalys av några av skidorienteringens olika åksätt.* (Analyses of different cross-country skiing-techniques in ski-orienteering.) Phys. Ed. student thesis. Report 1984:19, Gymnastik-och idrottshögskolan, Stockholm, Sweden.

Niinimaa, V., Dyon, M. & Shepard, R.J. (1978). Performance and efficiency of intercollegiate cross-country skiers. *Med. Sci. Sports* 10, 91–93.

Petterson, L.-G., Skogsberg, L. & Zackrisson, U. (1977) *Muskel-aktivitet under olika träningsformer för längdåkning på skidor.* (EMG activity during cross-country skiing.) Phys. Ed. thesis, College of Physical Education, Stockholm.

Rusko, H., (1976) *Physical Performance Characteristics in Finish Athletes.* Studies in Sports, Physical Education and Health no. 8, University of Jyväskylä, Jyväskylä.

Saltin, B. & Åstrand, P.-O. (1967) Maximal oxygen uptake in athletes. *J. Appl. Physiol.* 23, 353–358.

Secher, N.H. (1983) The physiology of rowing. *J. Sports Sci.* 1, 23–53.

Sjödin, B. & Schéle, R. (1982) Oxygen cost of treadmill running in long distance runners. In: Komi, P. (ed.) *Exercise and Sport Biology,* pp. 61–67. Human Kinetics, Champaign, Illinois.

Sjödin, B. & Svedenhag, J. (1985) Applied physiology of marathon running. *Sports Med.* 2, 83–99.

Stray-Gundersen, J. & Ryschon T. (1987) Economy of skating versus classic roller skiing. *Med. Sci. Sports Exerc.* 19, 46 (abstract).

Strömme, S.B., Ingjer, F. & Meen, H.D. (1977) Assessment of maximal aerobic power in specifically trained athletes. *J. Appl. Physiol.* 42, 833–837.

Tesch, P., Forsberg, A. & Karlsson, J. (1978) Selective muscle glycogen depletion during cross-country skiing. *J. U.S. Ski Coaches Assoc.* 2, 12–17.

Wehlin, S., Agnevik, G., Sjödin, B. & Saltin, B. (1970) Fysiologiska undersökningar under Engelbrektsloppet. (Physiological studies during the Engelbrekt ski race.) *Svensk Idrott* 15–16, 1–6.

Westergren, T.-G. & Nylander, P. (1977) *Spannhårdhetens inverkan på start-och glidfriktion samt på energikravet vid olika åksätt.* (Influence of camber stiffness on starting and gliding friction and on energy cost for different skiing techniques.) Phys. Ed. student thesis. Gymnastik-och Idrottshögskolan, Stockholm, Sweden.

Zupan, M.F., Shepard, T.A. & Eisenman P.A. (1988) Physiological responses to nordic tracking and skating in élite cross-country skiers. *Med. Sci. Sports Exerc.* 20, 81 (abstract).

Chapter 53

Cycling

GEORG NEUMANN

Cycling events

Cycling comprises several disciplines (Table 53.1), with road and track cycling as the main ones. There are also trick cycling, veloball, bicycle cross, stayer races (cycling behind a motorcycle), BMX races and bicycle touring. As a combined sport, the triathlon is important. In the triathlon, cycling follows the swimming, and running comes at the end.

Both men and women engage in cycling. Different types of bicycle are used for the various events. The bicycle used for road cycling weighs about 9 kg; it has two brakes which function separately from each other and a gear-change (usually 10 gears). The bicycle frame is made from a special light metal or carbon fibre. Spoke wheels are increasingly being replaced by disc wheels. In track cycling, a lighter bicycle (about 6 kg) without brakes or gear-change is used. The pedalling power is transmitted via a rigid gear. Braking is carried out by using the incline of the track. Cycling tracks are between 170 and 400 m long. They are covered with cement or wood.

Exercise physiology of cycling

Cycling is a typical endurance-based sport. Competitions are carried out over a wide range of times. However, in track cycling, the typical duration of a competition is between 62 and 300 s (1000–4000 m), whereas the times in road cycling vary between 2 and 4 h. Extreme efforts

occur in triathlon ('iron man'). Here male and female competitors complete 3.8-km swimming, 180-km individual cycling, and finally a marathon run. Cycling induces different stress levels in the motor and cardiovascular systems as well as in metabolism.

Performance structure

Continuously improving top-class sports performances, which in cycling lead to an annual increase in speed of about 1%, result from changes in the training programmes. Strength endurance, in particular, must be improved because as speed increases, air resistance increases as its square. Technical improvements of the bicycle (mass, tyres) reduce the rolling resistance and a low sitting position reduces the air resistance (Fig. 53.1).

Athletic training is an essential part of the performance (Fig. 53.2; Tables 53.2 & 53.3). Changing the content of the training programme, or the structure of training and exercise, can have a permanent effect on the performance. The competitive result reflects the level of adaptation reached by the functional systems through athletic training as well as the athlete's inherent talent and improvements in equipment. The structure of athletic training is highly changeable; it allows many variants. The value of a particular training programme is clearly revealed by the athletic performance in high-level international sports competitions.

Table 53.1 Cycling events.

Event	Short-term endurance (1–2 min)	Medium-term endurance (2–10 min)	Long-term endurance			
			I (10–35 min)	II (35–90 min)	III 90–360 min)	IV (>360 min)
Track cycling	1000 m	Sprint (11–25 s and 2-min preload) 4000-m pursuit cycling (individual) 4000-m pursuit cycling (team) 3000-m pursuit cycling (women, individual)				
Road cycling				30–50-km individual competitions	100-km team competitions 80–180-km individual competitions	> 200-km competitions
Triathlon				30–50 km	180-km ironman (men and women)	
Tourism				20–50 km	50–120 km	
BMX	270–320-m course					
Mountain bikes (MTB)			5–20 km	30–50 km	50–70 km	

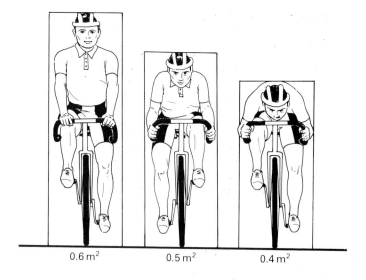

0.6 m²   0.5 m²   0.4 m²

Fig. 53.1 Air resistance surface in different cycling positions.

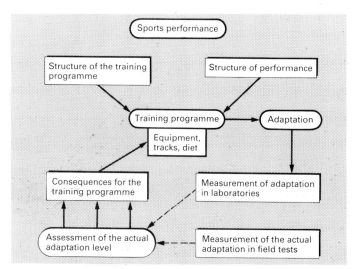

Fig. 53.2 Effect of the training programme (structure of training and exercise) on adaptation of the organism. Adaptation should be evaluated by means of laboratory and field tests and the training programme corrected according to the data measured.

Table 53.2 Comparison of different race resistances during uphill cycling and on a flat course. Body mass 70 kg, bicycle mass 10 kg, rolling resistance coefficient 0.004, friction forces in the power–transmission coefficient 0.006, air resistance 0.0207. Adapted from Müller (1988).

Parameter	50-km flat course	5-km uphill
Time (min)	64	12
Performance (km·h^{-1})	47	25
Air resistance (N)	34.43 (82%)	9.52 (12%)
Rolling resistance (N)	3.14 (7%)	3.14 (4%)
Frictional forces in power transmission (N)	4.71 (11%)	4.71 (6%)
Slope resistance (N)	—	60.43 (78%)

Table 53.3 Air resistance in cycling. Adapted from Taubmann (1983).

	Air resistance (%)*		
	Group of 4	Group of 3	Group of 2
First cyclist	94	97	97
Second cyclist	48	50	67
Third cyclist	37	45	—
Fourth cyclist	34	—	—

* Air resistance is 100% for an individual rider. Air resistance in a large group of riders (field) is only 30–35%. Example: first position 41 km·h⁻¹, *c.* 380 W (290 W are necessary to overcome air resistance); second position 230 W; third position 197 W; fourth position 189 W.

An increase in riding speed is possible only if the mean pedalling power, which is dependent on the pedal rate, is increased (Fig. 53.3). Coast *et al.* (1986) found that optimum pedal rates vary with power outputs; higher power outputs demand higher optimum pedal rates. By choosing the wrong combination of pedal speed and load, a rider may be at a disadvantage of 5–10% compared with others using an optimum pedal rate (120 or 80 r.p.m, both of which are often used in cycling).

Not all the qualities of an athlete can be changed by means of physical training. Among the hereditary qualities that characterize an athlete are body composition, the proportion of muscle fibres, and psychic qualities such as the ability to mobilize oneself and to will endurance. In cycling, the distribution of muscle fibres is an important precondition for an athlete who wishes to become a road or track cyclist (Tables 53.4 & 53.5). Characteristics of the body composition (body mass and height) may differ more widely than in running, because the bicycle provides the transport for excess body mass. Body fat in male cyclists is about 8–12%; in female cyclists it is 11–15%. To achieve top-level athletic performance in cycling, 8 ± 2 years of training are required. The age for top-class results in cycling is about 24 ± 2 years (s.d.). With an appropriate social motivation, top results are possible for about 10 years.

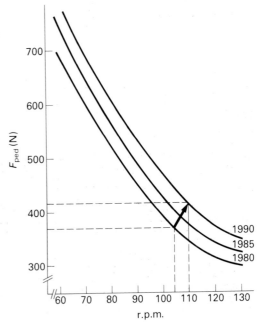

Fig. 53.3 Dependence of mean pedal power on pedalling frequency in athletes of the same performance level. In the future, it will be necessary to develop both abilities if an athlete is to remain competitive. From Kettmann (1983).

Demands on functional systems in short-term and medium-term endurance exercise

THE MOTOR SYSTEM

Short-term endurance exercise lasts between 1 and 2 min, and medium-term endurance

Table 53.4 Mean body mass, height, $\dot{V}_{O_2 max}$ and athletic performance of road and track cyclists of national élite in former East Germany (1980–1988).

Sport	No. of cyclists	Body mass (kg)	Height (m)	$\dot{V}_{O_2 max}$ (ml·min^{-1}·kg^{-1})	Ergometer performance-incremental work rate (W)	500-m sprint (s)
Men						
Track cyclists						
Sprinters	5	82	1.82	64.0	300	34.2
1000-m track	5	76	1.76	66.0	320	34.7
4000-m track	10	75	1.82	76.0	350	37.8
Road cyclists	20	72	1.79	78.0	400	40.0
Women						
Road and track cyclists	10	62	1.71	63.0	320	—

Table 53.5 Proportion and cross-sectional area of fibres in vastus lateralis muscle of national (East German) élite cyclists.

Sport	No. of cyclists	$\dot{V}_{O_2 max}$ (ml·min^{-1}·kg^{-1})	Fibre type (%)			Cross-sectional area (μm^2)	
			I (STF)	II (FTF)	IIa (FTG)	STF	FTF
Track cyclists							
Sprinters	5	64.0	65	35	30	9000	13 500
1000-m track	5	66.0	72	28	25	8500	12 000
4000-m track	10	76.0	78	22	22	8000	10 000
Road cyclists	20	78.0	80	20	20	7000	8 000
Female cyclists*	7	50.0	51	49	—	5500	5 220
US Olympic road team 1976		72.6	64	36	—	—	—
World sprint cycling champion 1976		55.0	47	53	—	—	—

* From Burke *et al.* (1977).
STF, slow-twitch fibres; FTF, fast-twitch fibres; FTG, fast-twitch glycolytic fibres.

exercise lasts between 2 and 10 min. For sprinting (3 min at low effort and 20 s at maximum effort) and for competition performances in 1000 and 4000-m track cycling, high activation of the central nervous system is required. In these track-cycling exercises the motor programme is provided by a predominant recruitment of fast-twitch muscle fibres. Among track cyclists, sprinters have the highest proportion of fast-twitch fibres, about 35–65%. Inten-

sive training programmes change the metabolic qualities of the fast-twitch fibres. Strength training leads to hypertrophy of muscle fibres, especially the fast-twitch fibres (Table 53.5).

ENERGETIC BASIS OF PERFORMANCE

For short-term endurance performance in track cycling, mainly local energy stores are used. In particular, adenosine triphosphate (ATP), phosphocreatine and glycogen are required to accelerate the bicycle from standstill (Fig. 53.4). The production of glucose in the liver and its delivery via the blood vessels takes 1 min and may produce an effect only in 4000-m competitions. Because start and finish follow each other within a few seconds, the energy can be supplied only via the alactic energy potential. In competitions of 1–5-min duration, 50% (reducing to 20%) of the energy is supplied under anaerobic conditions. These values are similar to those obtained by Åstrand and Rodahl (1986) and Medbø and Tabata (1989). In efforts that last for longer (up to 10 min) aerobic processes dominate (Table 53.6).

The high anaerobic proportion can be measured indirectly as the lactate concentration but cannot be exactly quantified. In competitions of between 1000 and 4000 m, blood lactate concentrations of 18–22 mmol·l^{-1} can be measured. In track-cycling performance, the energy exchange per unit of time is also high. Due to their intensive training, track cyclists have a higher anaerobic power than road cyclists, as may be concluded from the higher activity of anaerobic enzymes (Table 53.7). In 1000-m time-trials, anaerobic metabolism provides about 160 kJ·min^{-1} (38 kcal·min^{-1}), and in 4000-m team competitions it is about 140 kJ·min^{-1} (33.5 kcal·min^{-1}).

The high degree of central nervous system activation required in heavy track-cycling efforts also results in an increased release of catecholamines. The elevated levels of adrenaline and noradrenaline induce glycolysis, lipolysis and proteolysis. The resulting increase in free fatty acids and amino acids is of no use to metabolism in the short-term endurance workouts.

CARDIOVASCULAR BASIS OF PERFORMANCE

In short-term and medium-term endurance performances, the cardiovascular system is maximally activated. The maximal oxygen intake ($\dot{V}_{O_2 max}$) can be fully utilized only after a latency of 40–60 s. In order to raise the metabolism to a higher level, athletes perform a prestart warm-up.

In a few minutes of exercise, the cardiovascular system cannot establish a complete

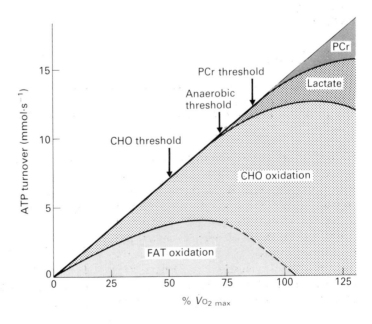

Fig. 53.4 Metabolic thresholds (carbohydrate (CHO), aerobic–anaerobic, and phosphocreatine (PCr)) related to adenosine triphosphate (ATP) turnover (Sahlin, 1986).

Table 53.6 Utilization of the functional systems of athletes during intensive endurance exercise of differing durations. Own data, from mixed endurance sports in former East Germany; anaerobic power data are estimates (see Åstrand, 1976).

Functional system	Measured value	STE (1–2 min)	MTE (>2–10 min)	LTE I (>10–35 min)	LTE II (35–90 min)	LTE III (90–360 min)	LTE IV (>360 min)
Circulation	Heart rate (beats·min^{-1})	185–200	190–210	180–190	175–190	150–180	120–170
Oxygen intake	% $\dot{V}o_{2\,max}$	95–100	95–100	90–95	80–95	60–85	50–60
Energy exchange	% Aerobic	50	80	85	95	98	99
	% Anaerobic	50	20	15	5	2	(1)
Energy consumption	kJ·min^{-1}	160	120	110	105	80	75
	kJ (total)	160–320	320–1200	1200–3700	3900–8400	8400–25 300	>27 000
Breakdown of glycogen	% Glycogen in muscle	10	30	40	60	80	95
Metabolism	Free fatty acids (mmol·l^{-1})	0.5	0.5	0.8	1.0	2.0	2.5
	Lactate (mmol·l^{-1})	18	20	14	8	4	2
	3-Hydroxybutyrate (µmol·l^{-1})	50	50	80	150	500	700
	Urea (Δ mmol·l^{-1})	0	1	1–2	2–3	3–6	4–8
	Alanine (µmol·l^{-1})	500	500	400	350	250	200
	Tyrosine (Δ µmol·l^{-1})	20	20	30	35	40	10
	Cortisol (µmol·l^{-1})	400*	400*	350*	(300)	(400)	(500)

* Stress.

STE, short-term endurance; MTE, medium-term endurance; LTE I–IV, subdivisions of long-term endurance.

Table 53.7 Enzyme activity of vastus lateralis muscle in national élite cyclists in former East Germany.

Enzyme activity (μmol·s^{-1}·kg^{-1} wet muscle)	Road cyclists ($n = 19$)	Track cyclists ($n = 12$)	p
Glycogen synthetase	127 ± 23	68 ± 35	0.002
Phosphoglycerate kinase	2900 ± 800	4270 ± 1000	0.001
Pyruvate kinase	1720 ± 360	2880 ± 800	0.001
Lactate dehydrogenase	3820 ± 120	6500 ± 190	0.001
Citrate synthetase	720 ± 189	490 ± 169	0.005

Values are mean ± standard deviation.

metabolic steady state. Proof of this is seen in the continuous increase in venous blood lactate concentration, which reaches its maximum value only after the competition, in the 5th to 10th minute of recovery. This delay occurs because there is an imbalance between the accumulation and removal of lactate in short-term and medium-term endurance exercise.

Utilization of functional systems in long-term endurance exercise

THE MOTOR SYSTEM

Long-term endurance exercise lasts from 10 min to several hours (see Table 53.6). Due to the highly different motor, energy and psychic demands, endurance exercises are grouped in several time spans. Neumann (1984) has described the following groups: long-term endurance II (35–90 min), long-term endurance III (90–360 min) and long-term endurance IV (> 360 min). In long-term endurance performance, the potential power of the muscles is particularly dependent on fatigue-resistant slow-twitch fibres. It is not by accident that successful road cyclists have a high proportion of slow-twitch fibres (70–95%). To sustain bicycle exercise for several hours, a motor stereotype is required. This stereotype is developed by prolonged training and is characterized by the dominant recruitment of slow-twitch fibres. A stable motor stereotype considerably restricts motor readjustments. The motor varia-

bility only increases if fast-twitch fibres are again included in the motor programme by short-term exercise bouts. If cycling is combined with strength training exercises (for instance cycling uphill), the slow-twitch fibres will become hypertrophic. The cross-sectional area of slow-twitch fibres enlarges to about 7000–8000 μm^2. Endurance training improves the blood supply of the muscles because capillarization is increased.

ENERGETIC BASIS OF PERFORMANCE

The glycogen stores in the muscles and liver are only sufficient for intensive efforts lasting up to 90 min (Table 53.6). In long-term group III endurance exercise additional food and fluid intake is necessary during exercise. In long-term endurance exercise, free fatty acids are the main substrate (Fig. 53.5).

In road cyclists, the triacylglycerol content in the muscle is elevated. The triacylglycerol content serves as a stable fat reserve. Long-term endurance trained athletes store more fat in the slow-twitch fibres, in droplets located near the mitochondria (Hoppeler, 1986). After only 3 days of extensive cycling exercise (4.5 h·day^{-1}) the triacylglycerol content of the muscles declines significantly (Brouns et al., 1989). Probably 50% of the free fatty acids oxidized during exercise is derived from local energy stores (Paul & Holmes, 1975). During prolonged exercise, free fatty acids from adipose tissue may account for up to 60% of the total energy

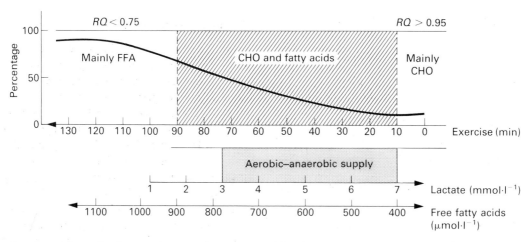

Fig. 53.5 Relationship between lactate concentration and free fatty acids (FFA) when cycling under aerobic conditions. Below a lactate concentration of 3 mmol·l^{-1} mainly FFA are metabolized, and above 7 mmol·l^{-1} lactate mainly carbohydrates (CHO) are metabolized. *RQ*, respiratory quotient.

needs (Hultman & Sjöholm, 1983). Fat metabolism spares muscle glycogen.

In cycling exercises lasting for several hours, the availability of carbohydrates is always limited. At first the muscle breaks down glucoplastic amino acids for gluconeogenesis (Wahren *et al.*, 1971). The rising concentration of serum urea reveals elevated protein catabolism. The longer the duration of exercise, the greater the increase in serum urea (see Table 53.6). The concentration of ketones also rises because the decreased availability of carbohydrate augments fat metabolism (Neumann, 1983).

THE CARDIOVASCULAR SYSTEM

In cycling exercise of several hours' duration the heart rate lies between 140 and 170 beats·min^{-1}. The increase in core temperature caused by the active muscles is of great importance with regard to the increase in heart rate. Due to an increasing dehydration the transport of heat to the body surface is impeded. With increasing muscle fatigue, the heart rate rises further. In long-term endurance exercises only about 70% of $\dot{V}o_{2\,max}$ is utilized.

This means, in road cycling, that an athlete with a body mass of 72 kg and a $\dot{V}o_{2\,max}$ of 78 ml·min^{-1}·kg^{-1} at a speed of 37 km·h^{-1} will utilize approximately 54 ml oxygen·min^{-1}·kg^{-1}.

Assessment of functional capacity

Laboratory tests

In cycling the most important device for laboratory testing is the cycle ergometer. The power is measured in Nm·s^{-1} = 9.81 W. In our laboratory the exercise starts between 100 and 150 W, and is increased by steps of 30−50 W. Individual steps may last for 2−4 min. One test in wide use is described in Fig. 53.6, and it may be performed as an incremental test and/or as steady state test. A combination of both improves the evaluation (Fig. 53.7). Important data recorded during the test include heart rate, oxygen intake, pulmonary ventilation, and blood lactate concentration. Significant parameters for evaluation of power are $\dot{V}o_{2\,max}$, the work rate at a lactate concentration of 3 mmol·l^{-1}, and the percentage of $\dot{V}o_{2\,max}$ at a lactate concentration of 3 mmol·l^{-1}.

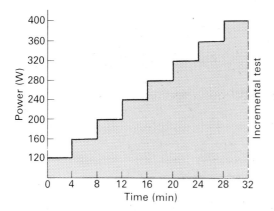

Fig. 53.6 An incremental test track for road cyclists.

Maximal oxygen intake

The endurance-related fitness level exerts a decisive influence on $\dot{V}_{O_2\,max}$. Élite cyclists achieve a $\dot{V}_{O_2\,max}$ of $75-80$ ml·min^{-1}·kg^{-1}. Several years of performance-oriented training is necessary to achieve such high values (Fig. 53.8). However, the hereditary predispositions for excellence in endurance-based sports have considerable influence. Depending on the content of the training programme, $\dot{V}_{O_2\,max}$ may vary from 8 to 12 ml·min^{-1}·kg^{-1} within the training year. Only in an ideal case can cyclists achieve their individual $\dot{V}_{O_2\,max}$ at the time of a world championship. If the proportion of intensive exercise training increases (work rate

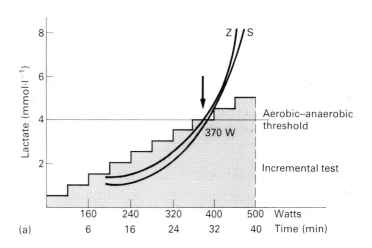

Fig. 53.7 Comparison of (a) incremental test results in two cyclists (Z and S) with (b) the performances achieved in a 30-min workout in the aerobic–anaerobic transition, at a lactate concentration of 4 mmol·l^{-1} in the first test. The 30-min test provides better information on the stability of endurance than incremental testing alone.

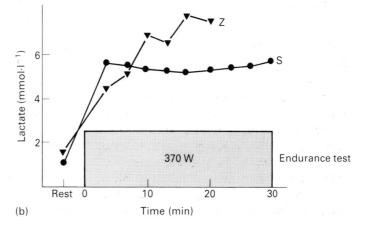

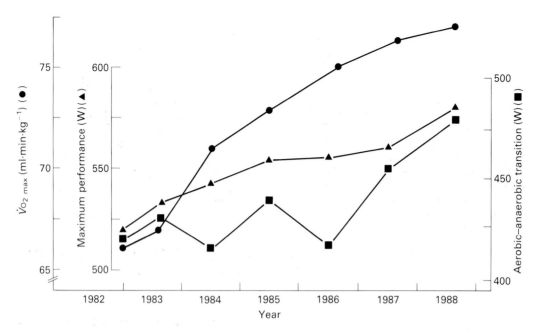

Fig. 53.8 Longitudinal study of six top level road cyclists (mean values). $\dot{V}_{O_2 max}$ (●), the maximum ergometer performance in the incremental test (▲) and the performance at the aerobic–anaerobic transition (■). The distance covered in training sessions increased from 30 000 to 35 000 km·year^{-1} during the period under observation (A. Berbalk & S. Kettmann, unpublished data, 1989).

in the aerobic–anaerobic transition), $\dot{V}_{O_2 max}$ will drop again.

One reliable parameter is to calculate the performance (P) at a lactate concentration of 3 or 4 mmol·l^{-1}. The P_3 or P_4 result allows a better differentiation of the aerobic power than $\dot{V}_{O_2 max}$ (Neumann & Schüler, 1989). With an increase in aerobic capacity, the lactate performance curve shifts to the right (Fig. 53.9). Additional information may be obtained if the stepwise increase in power is supplemented by a 30-min steady state test (see Fig. 53.7).

Ability may be evaluated by measuring the increase in lactate concentration. While track cyclists reach a lactate value of 10–14 mmol·l^{-1} in laboratory tests, road cyclists reach only 6–10 mmol·l^{-1} lactate. In road cyclists, training reduces the level of anaerobic enzymes (Table 53.7).

Training exercises are performed at about 70–80% of $\dot{V}_{O_2 max}$.

Field tests

An incremental test may also be performed under field conditions. Distances may vary between 3 and 5 km. The velocities set may increase from 70%, 80%, 85%, 90% up to 100% of the maximum riding speed. Between these steps a break of 2 min is required to measure lactate concentration. Lactate is measured 1 min after the effort. As in all step tests, four steps are considered a minimum and five steps are a desirable optimum.

Follow-up during the training process

To evaluate the intensity and volume of exercise, fitness level and the degree of recovery, such parameters as heart rate, lactate, serum urea and creatine kinase concentrations are suggested.

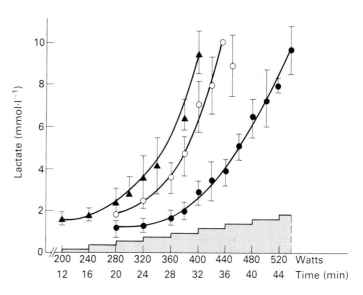

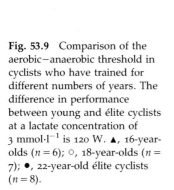

Fig. 53.9 Comparison of the aerobic–anaerobic threshold in cyclists who have trained for different numbers of years. The difference in performance between young and élite cyclists at a lactate concentration of 3 mmol·l^{-1} is 120 W. ▲, 16-year-olds ($n = 6$); ○, 18-year-olds ($n = 7$); ●, 22-year-old élite cyclists ($n = 8$).

Training intensity

Adaptation to cycling is facilitated by performing training in aerobic, aerobic–anaerobic and anaerobic metabolic states. The data necessary to control the intensity of exercise are listed in Table 53.8. The heart rate, in particular, is an appropriate parameter for individual differentiation of the effort intensity in an aerobic metabolic state (lactate 3 mmol·l^{-1}). The predominant part of training is performed at the level of basic endurance (Table 53.8). From 70% to 80% of training (30 000–35 000 km·year^{-1}) is performed at this aerobic level.

A new method of evaluating the intensity of cycling, especially the effect of heavy training, is to measure the activity of creatine kinase. Heavy-interval training or strength training elevates the level of creatine kinase up to 1–6 μmol·s^{-1}·l^{-1}. If a level of > 10 μmol·s^{-1}·l^{-1} is reached, the rate of exercise must be reduced or the recovery period prolonged.

Protein catabolism

Measurement of serum urea can give an indication of considerably elevated protein metab-

olism and breakdown. Depending on the fitness level and the duration of the exercise the concentration of serum urea is increased at rest. Training may induce resting serum urea levels of 5–7 mmol·l^{-1}. If the level of serum urea during rest rises to 9 mmol·l^{-1}, the work rate must be reduced (Lorenz & Gerber, 1979) or the high protein catabolism will impede the process of adaptation. The serum urea concentration immediately after long-term endurance exercise must be assessed differently. A rise of up to 12 mmol·l^{-1} is possible. A recovery period of approximately 15 h causes a decline of serum urea concentration of 2–3 mmol·l^{-1}.

The influence of recovery

Replenishment of the energy stores, especially the glycogen deposits, is of central significance in cycling. In prolonged daily training on the road (> 180 km) or in tour races, the glycogen stores cannot be replenished within 24 h if the athlete remains on a 'normal' diet. For cyclists the distribution of energy carriers in the food is important. The percentage of carbohydrate in their food should be 55–60%, the share of fat being 20–25% and of protein 15–18%. A significant glycogen sparing, as well as super-

Table 53.8 Follow-up of élite cyclists during the training process.

	Basic endurance	Basic endurance and intensity	Intensity	Short-term endurance intervals
Distance	100–200 km	60–100 km	30–50 km	200–1000 m
Velocity (km·h^{-1})	28–33	32–37	37–40	42–50
Frequency (pedalling rate·min^{-1})	100	105	90–110	110–120
Energy exchange	Aerobic	Aerobic–anaerobic	Aerobic–anaerobic	Alactacid–lactacid
Measurement of actual adaptation in field tests				
Lactate (mmol·l^{-1})	2–3	3–4	4–7	>7
Heart rate (beats·min^{-1})	120–150	140–160	160–180	180–200

compensation within 24 h of recovery, was observed after consumption of a high-maltodextrin and low-fructose beverage (Brouns et al., 1989). If catabolism predominates, body mass will decrease. Saris et al. (1989) found an average energy intake of 25–26 MJ·day^{-1} (5900–6200 kcal·day^{-1}) during the Tour de France. The highest energy intake was 32.7 MJ·day^{-1} (7780 kcal·day^{-1}). The energy intake *during* the race was 40–50% of daily intake. In case of high environmental temperatures, the athlete's fluid requirements may rise up to 10 l·day^{-1} with 6 litres being ingested during the race. Accordingly, road cycling

Table 53.9 Daily intake of energy, protein, carbohydrate, fat and micronutrients from food and energy-containing food supplements, and the percentage intake during the Tour de France. From Saris et al. (1989).

Cyclists ($n = 5$)	Mean daily intake ± s.d.	Intake during race (%)
Energy (MJ)	24.3 ± 5.3	49
Protein (g)	217 ± 47	35
Carbohydrate, simple (g)	463 ± 159	61
Carbohydrate, complex (g)	386 ± 100	55
Fat (g)	147 ± 39	39
Calcium (mg)	3044 ± 1000	60
Iron, haem (mg)	5.3 ± 1.6	1
Iron, non-haem (mg)	24.9 ± 9.4	55
Vitamin B$_1$ (mg)	2.4 ± 0.7	44
Vitamin B$_2$ (mg)	5.0 ± 1.6	61
Vitamin B$_6$ (mg)	2.4 ± 0.7	46
Vitamin C (mg)	158 ± 146	29
Water (litres)	6.7 ± 2.0	61

* Mean body mass before and after race was 69.2 kg and 68.9 kg, respectively.

has high energy and fluid requirements compared with other sports. In normal training, if the energy consumption does not surpass 20 MJ·day^{-1} (about 4800 kcal·day^{-1}), recovery may be ensured by consumption of high carbohydrate food. Any higher energy consumption requires an additional intake of glucose concentrates, glucose fluids, vitamins and minerals (Table 53.9). One third of the carbohydrate requirements may be covered by carbohydrate-rich liquids. Blend-sugar (glucose, fructose, maltodextrin) can be recommended for its gastric tolerance. These polysaccharides prevent stomach disorders or diarrhoea during exercise. The amount of carbohydrate needed in cycling is 50 g glucose·h^{-1} exercise. If only 20 g of glucose are taken, a marked gluconeogenesis and ketogenesis may develop and hypoglycaemic reactions may occur.

A substantial glucose intake immediately before cycling is not advisable. Glucose feeding (75 g) 30–45 min before endurance exercise increases the rate of carbohydrate oxidation, impedes the mobilization of free fatty acids and reduces exercise time to exhaustion (Forster et al., 1979). A considerable glucose intake may also impede the utilization of free fatty acids (Essig et al., 1980; Sasaki et al., 1987).

References

Åstrand, P.-O. (1976) Aerobic and anaerobic work capacity. In: Jokl, E., Anand, R.L. & Stoboy, H. (eds) Advances in Exercise Physiology. Medicine and Sport No. 9, pp. 60–66. Karger, Basel.

Åstrand, P.-O. & Rodahl, K. (1986) Textbook of Work Physiology. McGraw-Hill Book Company, New York.

Brouns, F., Saris, W.H.M., Beckes, E. et al. (1989) Metabolic changes induced by sustained exhaustive cycling and diet manipulation. Int. J. Sports Med. 10, 549–562.

Burke, E.R., Cerny, F., Costill, D. & Fink, W. (1977) Characteristics of skeletal muscle in competitive cyclists. Med. Sci. Sports 9, 109–122.

Coast, W., Cox, R.H. & Welch, H.G. (1986) Optimal pedalling rate in prolonged bouts of cycle ergometry. Med. Sci. Sports Exerc. 18, 225–230.

Essig, D., Costill, D.L. & van Handel, P.J. (1980) Effects of caffeine ingestion on utilization of muscle glycogen and lipid during leg ergometer cycling. Int. J. Sports Med. 1, 86–90.

Forster, C., Costill, D.L. & Fink, W.J. (1979) Effects of pre-exercise feedings on endurance performance. Med. Sci. Sports Exerc. 11, 1–5.

Hoppeler, H. (1986) Exercise-induced ultrastructural changes in skeletal muscle. Int. J. Sports Med. 7, 187–204.

Hultman, E. & Sjöholm, H. (1983) Substrate availability. In: Knuttgen H., Vogel, J.A. & Poortmans, J. (eds) Biochemistry of Exercise, pp. 63–75. Human Kinetics, Champaign, Illinois.

Kettmann, S. (1983) Zur Entwicklung von Hauptleistungsfaktoren im Straßenradrennsport als Voraussetzung für die Steigerung der Wettkampfleistung. Dissertation, Research Institute for Physical Culture and Sport, Leipzig.

Lorenz, R. & Gerber, G. (1979) Harnstoff bei körperlichen Belastungen: Veränderung der Synthese, der Blutkonzentration und der Ausscheidung. Medizin und Sport 19, 240–248.

Medbø, J.I. & Tabata, I. (1989) Relative importance of aerobic and anaerobic energy release during short-lasting exhausting bicycle exercise. J. Appl. Physiol. 67, 1881–1886.

Müller, P. (1988) Steigerung der Bergfahrleistung im Straßenradrenn Sport durch zielgerichtete Trainingsbelastungen im Kraftausdauer- und Wettkampfspezifischen Training. Dissertation, Research Institute for Physical Culture and Sport, Leipzig.

Neumann, G. (1983) Metabole Regulation bei Langzeitausdauerbelastungen. Medizin und Sport 23, 169–175.

Neumann, G. (1984) Stoffwechselprobleme beim Ausdauerlauf. Medizin und Sport 24, 49–56.

Neumann, G. & Schüler, K.-P. (1989) Sportmedizinische Funktionsdiagnostik. J.A. Barth, Leipzig.

Paul, P. & Holmes, W.L. (1975) Free fatty acid and glucose metabolism during increased energy expenditure and after training. Med. Sci. Sports Exerc. 7, 176–184.

Sahlin, K. (1986) Metabolic changes limiting muscle performance. In: Saltin, B. (ed.) Biochemistry of Exercise VI, pp. 323–343. Human Kinetics, Champaign, Illinois.

Saris, W.H.M., van Erp-Baart, M.A., Brouns, F., Westerterp, K.R. & ten Hoor, F. (1989) Study on food uptake and energy expenditure during extreme sustained exercise: the Tour de France. Int. J. Sports Med. 10, S25–S31.

Sasaki, H., Maeda, J., Usui, S. & Ishiko, T. (1987) Effect of sucrose and caffeine ingestion on performance of prolonged strenous running. Int. J. Sports

Med. **8**, 261–265.

Taubmann, W. (1983) *Tabellen und Formelbuch Radrennsport*, Part II. German College for Physical Culture, Leipzig.

Wahren, J., Ahlborg, G., Fehling, P. & Jorfeed, L. (1971) Glucose metabolism during exercise in man. In: Pernow, B. & Saltin, B. (eds) *Muscle Metabolism during Exercise*, pp. 179–203. Plenum Press, New York.

Chapter 54

Triathlon Training and Competition

JACK T. DANIELS

Introduction

Multievent competition is not a new type of sporting event; the ancient Olympic games included a pentathlon, which involved a long jump, javelin throw, discus throw, running and wrestling (Schaap, 1963). When the modern Olympics became a reality, at the turn of the 20th century, new multievent sports became part of the Olympic games, and today we still have a decathlon for men, heptathlon for women and modern pentathlon for men and women as summer events, and a biathlon in the winter games.

In 1978, the first Hawaii Ironman triathlon competition was staged; there were 15 starters and 12 finishers in that event, which included an ocean swim, a long bicycle road race and a full 42.2-km marathon run (O'Toole & Douglas, 1989). Today, the Hawaii Ironman World Championship Triathlon '...is synonymous with ultraendurance exercise and typifies the increasing popularity of these events' (O'Toole & Douglas, 1989). The 1988 race had 1275 starters (of over 20 000 applicants) and 1189 finishers (O'Toole & Douglas, 1989).

Although triathlons can and do exist which involve competition in almost any three events imaginable, the swim−cycle−run triathlon is the one most usually contested. The popularity of the Hawaii Ironman, and many other shorter (and sometimes longer) triathlons, has led to considerable discussion and concern regarding training, safety and even the order of events.

Triathletes are known for their ability not only to perform well in three different disciplines, but also to endure continuous physical exercise for many hours.

Typically, the cycling portion of a triathlon competition takes more time to complete than either of the other segments of the race. Swimming, on the other hand, makes up the shortest portion, by far. In the case of the Ironman triathlon, the swim is 3.86 km (2.4 miles); the cycle event covers 180 km (112 miles); and the run is a standard marathon of 42.2 km (26.2 miles).

Top triathletes have been found to have attributes similar to other athletes who specialize in the individual sports of swimming, cycling and running, with $\dot{V}o_{2\,max}$ values equal to or greater than those of swimmers, when expressed in $ml \cdot kg^{-1}$ body $mass \cdot min^{-1}$, and somewhat less than is typical for élite cyclists and élite runners (O'Toole et al., 1987). Élite female triathletes compare more favourably with élite runners and cyclists than do their male counterparts (Roalstad, 1989) and both male and female triathletes have physiques most similar to cyclists (O'Toole et al., 1987).

In their characterization of triathletes, Holly et al. (1986) found that the top finishers have a higher $\dot{V}o_{2\,max}$ and spend more time training in all events, than do slower performers, certainly not unlike what holds true for competitors in many endurance events. Kohrt et al. (1987) reported moderate correlations between $\dot{V}o_{2\,max}$ and run (-0.68) and cycle (-0.78) times;

597

the swim time and swim $\dot{V}o_{2\,max}$ correlation was somewhat less powerful (-0.50). As is the case among runners, swimmers and cyclists, there seems to be a somewhat typical triathlete physique and physiological make-up, with some outstanding performers who do not fit the mould and some 'ideal specimens' who do not race particularly well.

Training

Training for three different endurance events offers advantages and disadvantages over single-event training. To develop the skills and peripheral physiological adaptations needed for optimal performance in each of the events, some time must be set aside for refining each skill — there must be a fair degree of specificity of training. This demands considerable time, which, of course, can be beneficial to the development of a strong central component of endurance fitness.

O'Toole (1989) reported that mean weekly training amounts for triathletes preparing for the Ironman competition included 11.6 km of swimming, 365 km of cycling and 72.4 km of running each week. These distances consumed 3.5 h of swimming, 12.3 h of cycling and 5.75 h of running each week. This training regimen requires the triathlete to average a little over 3 h of training per day, with many spending much more time than that. Most of the triathletes studied by O'Toole (1989) performed each of the three events 4 or 5 days per week and included some interval training in each event every week.

It is obvious that serious training for a triathlon competition demands considerable time and energy, and attention must be given to avoiding injury and to obtaining adequate rest and proper nutrition. Applegate (1989), in her discussion of the nutritional concerns of ultraendurance triathletes, says that the athletes must consider carefully the nutritional needs of training and of competition, both as it relates to prerace meals and feedings during a race (see Chapters 12 and 30).

There are triathlons of greatly varying distances and durations; some are truly ultraendurance in nature, while others last for 1 h or less. However, because of the need to spend time training for each of three different events, even those athletes who prefer shorter competitions find themselves spending considerable time in training. Still, the athletes should make every attempt to practise sound training principles for the optimization of performance in each discipline and to prepare for the total triathlon event as well. In other words, there must be a thoughtful combination of quality training to improve efficiency and economy of exercise, with a constant reminder that the total event is an endurance one which demands a submaximal effort throughout. The total performance must always be foremost in the mind of the triathlete to avoid overtraining in any one of the individual events.

Kohrt et al. (1989) studied a group of triathletes over a period of 8 months of training and found that $\dot{V}o_{2\,max}$ improved only in the cycling event (apparently as a result of these particular subjects having more room for improvement in the peripheral development of cycling musculature). However, improvements in lactate threshold were significant in both cycling and running, suggesting that improvements in economy or mechanical efficiency were still possible beyond the point that $\dot{V}o_{2\,max}$ improved and that more emphasis should be placed on the types of training that elicit improvements in these parameters and on those that allow for prolonged performance at increasingly higher fractions of $\dot{V}o_{2\,max}$.

Safety and event order

Injury and medical concerns

Hiller (1989) has stated that dehydration is the most common reason for a triathlete to need medical attention in an Ironman competition; hyponatraemia is the most common electrolyte disturbance in races lasting for more than 8 h (Hiller et al. 1986; Hiller, 1989). It is recommended that for races lasting for more than 4 h, athletes should practise some form of sodium replacement (Hiller *et al.*, 1987; Hiller, 1989). Intravenous fluid therapy for races longer than 4 h should be 5% (280 mmol·l^{-1}) dextrose in normal saline; the same concentrations or 5% dextrose in 0.5 normal saline solution is recommended for races of less than 4 h duration (Hiller, 1989). Triathletes who are slower in performing their races expose themselves to greater chances of dehydration and hyponatraemia than do the faster competitors, because of the time spent exercising. It is advisable to have fluid stations more readily available than is typical at marathon running events. Every 2 km would seem to be a desirable frequency for fluid stations during the running event.

Laird (1989) reported that swimming accounts for 1–3% of the medical visits among ultraendurance triathletes; 10% of injuries are from cycling, with the remainder of medical visits associated with the run or after the finish of the event. It is not clear whether the proliferation of problems associated with the run is a function of the run itself or the fact that the run comes after considerable stress has already taken place in the first two events. Laird (1989) also confirmed that dehydration and exhaustion account for the majority of primary medical diagnoses.

O'Toole *et al.* (1986) showed that many triathletes break down red blood cells during races and that haemolysis may contribute to a chronic iron deficient state. O'Toole *et al.* (1988) found that 18 of the 46 male Ironman triathletes they studied had haemoglobin concentrations of less than 140 g·l^{-1}; one of 11 males competing in 2–3-h triathlons was in this 'anaemia' range. Of the 38 females studied only two were clinically anaemic (haemoglobin < 120 g·l^{-1}). 'Overall, 95% of the 95 triathletes studied showed evidence of red blood cell breakdown during the course of a triathlon, as judged by decreases in serum haptoglobin, ... with a range of 4% to 83% decrease' (O'Toole *et al.*, 1988). There were no differences between males and females in the amount of decrease in haptoglobin, nor in the renal excretion of iron, which was present in 28.3% of the athletes studied (O'Toole *et al.*, 1988).

Event order

It is important to explore the impact of different orders of performing the three triathlon events, as they apply to safety and race performance. Although the swim–cycle–run order is the most popular, other orders have been used.

Swimming is normally placed first for safety reasons, even though swimming after cycling or running may give the body a cooling break and a chance to rest leg muscles. The jobs of officials monitoring the swimmers would be lengthened considerably if the swim were to come after several hours of cycling or running, and medical problems, which might occur during the swim as the result of an earlier fatiguing run or cycle, would be more difficult to address in the water. In very long triathlons, placing the swim later in the schedule could mean that competitors would be in the water after daylight was over, a situation that would be particularly difficult to monitor. There certainly can be problems with having the swim first. For example, in mass starts of large groups of competitors there can be considerable contact, with resultant loss of performance. If better swimmers start first, this can help the congestion problem, but this adds another dimension to keeping track of who is where in the race and may limit spectator interest. In long races, where fatigue and dehydration can become a real factor later in the race, swimming after other events would present poor options for the athlete in trouble — there is no possibility of slowing to a walk or getting off the bicycle as is possible in the other two events.

As attractive as a first event of running might be, from a standpoint of thinning out the field and completing the most demanding event early in the competition, the safety of the competitors may be greater if the swimming is placed first, at least in longer triathlons with limited fields of entry.

A more legitimate controversy is whether to run or cycle last. Proponents of the cycle-last theory feel that running is a more demanding event and should be performed while the competitors are still fairly fresh and well hydrated. The earlier swim would not detract from the glycogen supply of the running muscles and the following cycling event would allow for rehydration and more carbohydrate consumption than is possible during the run. Cooling during the cycle might also be better at a time when thermoregulation is of considerable concern.

Those who feel that running should be last believe it is safer to run during this time of greater fatigue because medical problems are more easily addressed than they might be if the athlete is moving along at a fast pace on a bicycle. It is also possible that the opportunity to replenish fuel and fluid during a (middle) stage of cycling would allow the participant to enter the final (running) stage in better condition.

There is no doubt that the safety of the participants must be of primary concern, and there is not adequate data regarding the benefits and hazards of any particular order of events. It is certainly possible that what is best for a long triathlon event is not best for shorter races. Further research must be conducted to determine what order of events will provide for the safest, fairest and fastest triathlon races over a variety of distances.

Concluding remarks

Triathlon competitions continue to gain in popularity around the world. Many of the attributes of the competitors, their nutritional and training needs, and injury and medical concerns are similar to those exhibited and confronted by other (single-sport) athletes. On the other hand, triathletes have attributes and concerns that are unique to them, and they have emerged as a group of athletes who do not have to be compared to other athletes. A triathlon is a single sporting event, just as a long jump or high jump is a single event, and even though it is useful to analyse the parts of any whole, the whole is what is important.

References

Appelgate, E. (1989) Nutritional concerns of the ultra-endurance triathlete. *Med. Sci. Sports Exerc.* **21**(5) (Suppl.), 205–209.

Hiller, W.D.B. (1989) Dehydration and hyponatremia during triathlons. *Med. Sci. Sports Exerc.* **21**(5) (Suppl.), 219–221.

Hiller, W.D.B., O'Toole, M.L., Laird, R.H. *et al.* (1986) Electrolyte and glucose changes in endurance and ultraendurance exercise: results and medical implications. *Med. Sci. Sports Exerc.* **18**(2) (Suppl.), 62–63.

Hiller, W.D.B., O'Toole, M.L., Laird, R.H. & Smith, R. (1987) Hyponatremia in triathletes: a prospective study of 270 athletes in events of 2 hours to 34 hours duration. *Med. Sci. Sports Exerc.* **19**(2) (Suppl.), 71.

Holly, R.G., Barnard, R.J., Rosenthal, M., Applegate, E. & Pritikin, N. (1986) Triathlete characterization and response to prolonged strenuous competition. *Med. Sci. Sports Exerc.* **18**(1), 123–127.

Kohrt, W.M., Morgan, D.W., Bates, R. & Skinner, J. (1987) Physiological responses of triathletes to maximal swimming, cycling and running. *Med. Sci. Sports Exerc.* **19**(1), 51–55.

Kohrt, W.M., O'Connor, J.S. & Skinner, J.S. (1989) Longitudinal assessment of responses by triathletes to swimming, cycling and running. *Med. Sci. Sports Exerc.* **21**(5), 569–575.

Laird, R.H. (1989) Medical care at ultraendurance triathlons. *Med. Sci. Sports Exerc.* **21**(5) (Suppl.), 222–225.

O'Toole, M.L. (1989) Training for ultraendurance triathlons. *Med. Sci. Sports Exerc.* **21**(5) (Suppl.), 209–213.

O'Toole, M.L. & Douglas, P.S. (1989) Introduction: the ultraendurance triathlete: physiologic and medical considerations. *Med. Sci. Sports Exerc.* **21**(5) (Suppl.), 198–199.

O'Toole, M.L., Hiller, W.D.B., Crosby, L.O. & Douglas, P.S. (1987) The ultraendurance triathlete: a physiological profile. *Med. Sci. Sports Exerc.* **19**(1), 45–50.

O'Toole, M.L., Hiller, W.D.B., Roalstad, M., DeTorre, J.B., Laird, R.H. & Massimino, F. (1986) Hemolysis during triathlon races. *Med. Sci. Sports Exerc.* **18**(2) Suppl. 87.

O'Toole, M.L., Hiller, W.D.B., Roaldstad, M.S. & Douglas, P.S. (1988) Hemolysis during triathlon races: its relation to race distance. *Med. Sci. Sports Exerc.* **20**(3), 272–275.

Roalstad, M. (1989) Physiologic testing of the ultra-endurance triathlete. *Med. Sci. Sports Exerc.* **21**(5) (Suppl.), 200–204.

Schaap, R. (1963) *An Illustrated History of The Olympics*, pp. 29–30. Alfred A. Knopf, New York.

Chapter 55

Mountaineering

ROBERT B. SCHOENE AND THOMAS F. HORNBEIN

Introduction

Mountaineering encompasses a broad range of physical activities, from the intense muscular conditioning and gymnastic agility of the rock climber to the durability and endurance of the high-altitude mountaineer. Common to all forms of mountaineering, from fast and difficult short ascents of artificial or real rock walls to remote ascents in unexplored regions, is the element of verticality, i.e. high-angle terrain where error or unforeseen events can result in death. Therefore, common to all forms of mountain climbing are such elements as difficulty, a variable quantum of risk and the need for skill, knowledge and judgment.

Aside from the elements of risk and uncertainty, the physical demands upon the human body are analogous to those of other sports, such as gymnastics, skiing and endurance running. The unique element of mountain venture derives from the decrease of barometric pressure and the partial pressure of inspired oxygen. For example, at the summit of Mount Everest, the barometric pressure is but one third of that at sea level. The resulting hypoxia impedes performance and places special demands on the human body with regard to strength, endurance and nutrition. Certain illnesses caused by hypoxia may at times be fatal.

In this chapter we will limit our discussion to the effects of high altitude upon human performance. We shall review the physiological

adaptations to hypoxia, discuss the limits to maximum exercise at extreme altitude, define endurance in this environment, and consider attributes that are conducive to better performance at high altitude. Additionally, we shall briefly discuss nutritional requirements and make suggestions for training.

The environment

While the high-altitude environment includes other environmental stresses such as cold and exposure to intense ultraviolet radiation which may have an impact on elements of performance such as muscle fatigue, dehydration, malnutrition and mental fatigue, the decreasing barometric pressure with increasing altitude is the unique problem for the high-altitude mountaineer (Table 55.1). Because of a variety of physiological adaptations, oxygen delivery to the tissues is remarkably well maintained in spite of the decreased partial pressure of oxygen (Po_2) in the inspired air (Fig. 55.1). Adaptation minimizes the magnitude of steps in the oxygen cascade, helping to maintain an adequate delivery of oxygen to the mitochondria. Without any adaptation, a sudden exposure to severe hypoxia can result in a loss of consciousness and even in death.

Adaptation

The body adjusts to hypoxia with changes in ventilation, gas exchange from the alveoli to

Table 55.1 Mean ± s.d. values for resting ventilation and arterial blood gases in seven subjects, measured during a simulated 40-day ascent of Mount Everest, in a chamber (Operation Everest II). Modified from Goldberg & Schoene (1990).

Altitude		Barometric pressure (Torr)	Partial pressure of inspired oxygen (Torr)	Pulmonary ventilation ($l·min^{-1}$)	pH	Partial pressure of carbon dioxide (Torr)	Partial pressure of oxygen (Torr)	Oxygen saturation (%)
Feet	Metres							
0	0	760	150	11.0 ± 1.0	7.43 ± 0.04	33.9 ± 3.5	99.3 ± 9.3	97.6 ± 0.1
15 000	4570	429	80	14.6 ± 2.7	7.46 ± 0.02	25.0 ± 2.2	52.4 ± 4.0	84.8 ± 4.0
20 000	6100	347	63	20.9 ± 6.3	7.50 ± 0.04	20.0 ± 2.8	41.1 ± 3.3	75.2 ± 6.0
26 500	8080	282	49	36.6 ± 7.9	7.53 ± 0.03	12.5 ± 1.1	36.6 ± 2.2	67.8 ± 5.0
29 029	8840	240	43	42.3 ± 7.7	7.56 ± 0.03	11.2 ± 2.1	30.3 ± 2.1	58.0 ± 4.5

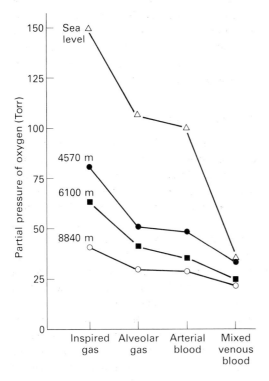

Fig. 55.1 The cascade of oxygen partial pressures at four different altitudes.

Ventilation

With the initial exposure to high altitude, breathing increases (Weil, 1986). The hyperventilation (relative to sea level) is initiated by the peripheral chemoreceptors, notably the carotid body (Lahiri et al., 1981), although there is much variability between individuals in the magnitude of this response. Much of the increased ventilation occurs within the first few days after ascent, but a steady level of ventilation at a particular altitude may not develop for several weeks. Many years of residence at high altitude can result in a decrease of ventilation (Fig. 55.2) (Weil, 1986). Hyperventilation results in a decrease of alveolar P_{CO_2} and an increase of alveolar P_{O_2} which is reflected by an increased arterial P_{O_2} and oxygen content of arterial blood (West et al., 1983b). Ventilatory acclimatization is associated with renal bicarbonate excretion in compensation for the respiratory alkalosis, but compensation is never complete, for there is a persistent respiratory alkalaemia.

Pulmonary function

Upon initial ascent, lung compliance, vital capacity and air flow decrease and gas trapping increases (Coates et al., 1979; Jaeger et al., 1979; Gautier et al., 1982). These changes are attributed to an increase in interstitial lung water,

the blood, haemoglobin affinity for oxygen, red blood cell mass and transfer of oxygen from the capillaries to the mitochondria (Schoene & Hornbein, 1988). The most important recipients of oxygen are the exercising muscle and the central nervous system.

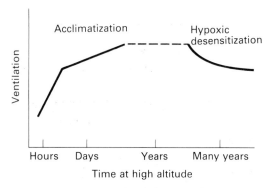

Fig. 55.2 Course of ventilatory response to acclimatization to high altitude at different durations of exposure, from hours to a lifetime. From Weil (1986), with permission.

which normally resolves within the first day or two at altitude. Life-long residence at high altitude results in an increase of lung volume and diffusion capacity, documented in high-altitude natives of the Andes and Himalaya (Remmers & Mithoefer, 1969; Frisancho et al., 1973; Vincent et al., 1978).

Gas exchange

Alveolar hypoxia results in an increase in pulmonary arterial pressure, which at rest improves perfusion of non-dependent regions of the lung and therefore decreases physiological dead space ventilation. Prolonged stay at high altitude can result in severe pulmonary hypertension, leading to chronic mountain sickness (Monge's disease), characterized by pulmonary hypertension, polycythaemia, mental slowing and cor pulmonale (Monge, 1928; Winslow & Monge, 1987).

Diffusion

Transfer of oxygen from the air to the blood is decreased because of the lower driving pressure of oxygen in alveolar gas (Fig. 55.3) (West & Wagner, 1980). This limitation to oxygen transfer from the air to the blood is accentuated during exercise, when a higher cardiac output

results in a shorter transit time for the red blood cell across the pulmonary capillary and a briefer opportunity for end-capillary Po_2 to approach that in the alveoli (Fig. 55.3). The arterial oxygen desaturation that occurs with exercise at high altitude can be quite profound (Fig. 55.4) (West et al., 1983a).

Blood

Two adaptations of oxygen transport occur at high altitude: (i) an increase in red blood cell production) and (ii) changes in the affinity of haemoglobin for oxygen (Fig. 55.5) (Winslow et al., 1984). The first adaptation is mediated by the hormone, erythropoietin, which increases rapidly upon ascent to high altitude (Abbrecht & Littell, 1972). An initial increase in haematocrit is probably secondary to haemoconcentration. Increases in red blood cell volume and total blood volume require several weeks to complete (Sanchez et al., 1970). There is marked variability in this response in both sojourners and high-altitude natives. An increase in haemoglobin concentration increases oxygen-carrying capacity but if the increase is too great (haemoglobin >190 $g \cdot l^{-1}$), blood viscosity also increases and a decrease in blood flow and oxygen delivery may result. Both sojourners and native highlanders who seem best adapted to high altitude maintain haemoglobin concentrations in the range of 160–180 $g \cdot l^{-1}$ (normal sea level value 130–150 $g \cdot l^{-1}$) (Beall & Reischman, 1984). Chronic mountain sickness is one example of the adverse consequence of a surfeit of red blood cell production (Winslow & Monge, 1987).

The affinity of haemoglobin for oxygen influences both loading of oxygen at the lung and unloading at the tissues. At moderate altitudes a rightward shift of the oxyhaemoglobin dissociation curve enhances unloading of oxygen to the tissue (Aste-Salazar & Hurtado, 1944; Moore & Brewer, 1981). While the arterial Po_2 is high enough to minimize the effect of the shift on arterial oxygen saturation, at very high altitudes (where alveolar Po_2 is much less), a

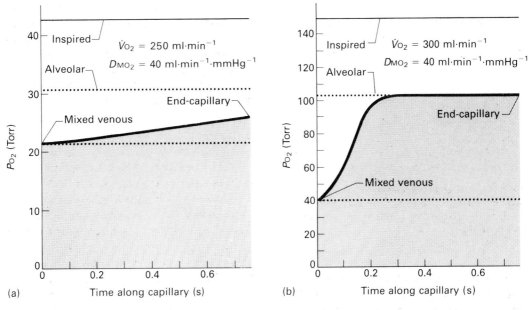

Fig. 55.3 Comparison of the calculated time-course of P_{O_2} in the pulmonary capillary of a climber at rest on the summit of Mount Everest (P_B 250 Torr, $P_{I_{O_2}}$ 43 Torr) (a) to sea-level values (P_B 760 Torr, $P_{I_{O_2}}$ 150 Torr) (b). From West (1980), with permission. $D_{M_{O_2}}$, membrane diffusion capacity for oxygen; P_B, barometric pressure; $P_{I_{O_2}}$, inspired partial pressure of oxygen.

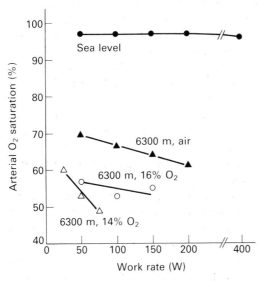

Fig. 55.4 Arterial oxygen saturation (%) does not decrease with exercise at sea level but drops progressively more rapidly with higher levels of exercise at greater altitudes. From West *et al.* (1983a), with permission.

left-shifted curve might better optimize intake of oxygen at the lung (Fig. 55.5) (Winslow *et al.*, 1984). Some animals who live or birds that fly at very high altitude have left-shifted oxy-haemoglobin dissociation curves (Swan, 1970; Faraci *et al.*, 1984), and the marked respiratory alkalosis noted in humans at extreme altitude also results in a leftward shift of the curve (Winslow *et al.*, 1984).

Tissue adaptation

Adaptation at the cellular level is less well understood. Some studies suggest that several weeks exposure to high altitude results in increases in capillary and mitochondrial density as well as decrease in cell size, all of which would decrease the radial diffusion distance for oxygen from the capillaries to the mitochondria (Ou & Tenney, 1970; Tenney & Ou, 1970; Banchero, 1975). There is controversy about what occurs to oxidative enzymes upon ascent

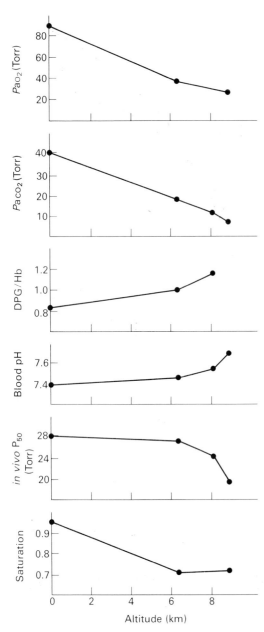

Fig. 55.5 Effectors of oxygen–haemoglobin (Hb) affinity. The net result at extreme altitude is a protected arterial oxygen saturation. DPG, diphosphoglycerate. From Winslow *et al.* (1984), with permission.

to high altitudes (Hochachka *et al.*, 1982; Green *et al.*, 1989), but the sum total of all these mentioned changes is presumably beneficial to oxidative metabolism.

Limitation to exercise

Although little is known about endurance performance at high altitude, a great deal is known about maximum work capacity. Maximum oxygen intake ($\dot{V}o_{2\,max}$) decreases with increasing altitude (West *et al.*, 1983a; Reeves *et al.*, 1987; Cymerman *et al.*, 1989). Studies both in the field and in a high altitude chamber have shown that at the summit of Mount Everest (barometric pressure of approximately 250 Torr) $\dot{V}o_{2\,max}$ is about 20% of the sea level value (Fig. 55.6) (West *et al.*, 1983a; Cymerman *et al.*, 1989). Interestingly, even though individuals may start with different values of $\dot{V}o_{2\,max}$ at sea level, those who have been studied have similar values when exercising at a barometric pressure equivalent to that at the summit of Mount Everest.

The cause of the decrease in exercise performance is probably multifactorial, including impaired diffusion of oxygen from air to blood in the lung and consequently a lesser availability of oxygen to the exercising muscles and brain (Gale *et al.*, 1985; Torre-Bueno *et al.*, 1985; Wagner *et al.*, 1986; 1987). At very high altitude, diffusion of oxygen to the tissues may also be compromised by the low Po_2.

The ventilatory response to exercise at high altitude is a marked increase in ventilation. This helps maintain arterial oxygen saturation (Fig. 55.7) (Schoene, 1984), but is not sufficient to reverse the diffusion limitation and the subsequent desaturation of arterial blood. In the high-altitude sojourner, a greater ventilatory response results in less arterial oxygen desaturation (Schoene *et al.*, 1984), while in high-altitude natives who have a more blunted ventilatory response, desaturation is minimized in part by an increased surface area for oxygen transfer (diffusion capacity) (Dempsey *et al.*, 1971).

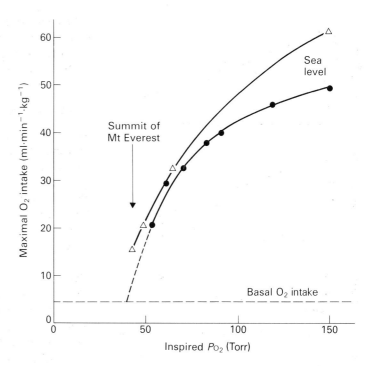

Fig. 55.6 Maximal oxygen intake ($\dot{V}O_{2\,max}$) against inspired PO_2. There is a predictable decrease in $\dot{V}O_{2\,max}$ at high altitudes. From West *et al.* (1983a). △, 1981 expedition; ●, from Pugh *et al.* (1964).

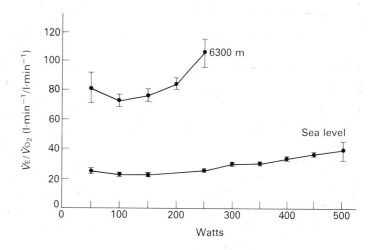

Fig. 55.7 The ventilatory response expressed as the ventilatory equivalent ($\dot{V}E/\dot{V}O_2$) in subjects at sea level (PB 755 Torr) and at 6300 m (PB 350 Torr), demonstrating that the ventilatory response for a given metabolic rate is almost four times the sea level value. From Schoene (1984).

For a given work rate, cardiac output is, for the most part, similar at high altitude to that at sea level (Reeves *et al.*, 1987). After exposure of several weeks or longer at moderate to extreme altitude, maximal heart rate is decreased (West *et al.*, 1983a). Inhalation of oxygen results in an increase in maximum heart rate and in work capacity, although values remain well below those at sea level. The mechanism for this lower maximum heart rate is not understood.

Limits to short bouts of intense exercise may reflect a failure of oxygen delivery to the brain rather than muscle. Hypoxia may impair central nervous system function. Numerous accounts exist of climbers at these heights who upon further exertion hallucinate, have narrowed or blurred vision, or come close to losing consciousness. Several studies have shown neurobehavioural dysfunction after return from extreme altitude (Cavaletti *et al.*, 1987; Hornbein *et al.*, 1989; Regard *et al.*, 1989). This is particularly notable in individuals with a more vigorous ventilatory response to hypoxia, an attribute that correlates with a better physical performance while at high altitude (Hornbein *et al.*, 1989). The authors speculate that the greater ventilatory response results in more profound hypocapnia and cerebral vasoconstriction, and consequently a larger decrease in oxygen delivery to the brain.

Endurance performance at high altitude

For high-altitude mountaineering, endurance is defined not in hours, but in days, weeks or months. Therefore, data taken from brief, maximal exercise may not predict performance at high altitude. Much information on the effect of high altitude on athletic performance was obtained in the 1960s at the time of the Mexico City Olympics (altitude 2300 m). For events lasting for more than 2 min, some period of acclimatization is necessary for optimal performance. Most studies looked at $\dot{V}o_{2\,max}$ or performance time over measured distances (Dill *et al.*, 1966; Buskirk *et al.*, 1967; Grover *et al.*, 1967), but improvement in submaximal exercise performance rather than intense exercise to exhaustion is more pertinent to high-altitude climbing (Maher *et al.*, 1974). Here little objective information exists. As any high-altitude mountaineer can relate, at altitudes up to 5000 m, performance improves with time. One study suggested that endurance time at 75% of $\dot{V}o_{2\,max}$ was greater at day 12 than at day 2 of exposure at 4300 m (Maher *et al.*, 1974). This improvement was associated with decreased blood lactate concentrations, suggesting that improved exercise capacity resulted from better tissue oxygenation. No similar longitudinal studies have been performed above 6000 m.

Based on anecdotes, an altitude of 5500 m, where the barometric pressure is half that at sea level, appears to represent the limit of permanent human habitation. Above that altitude, performance deteriorates after the initial period of acclimatization. It has become fashionable during expeditions to extreme altitude to acclimatize at moderate altitude with occasional short forays to extreme altitude before making a final rapid ascent. This approach may optimize the adaptive processes while minimizing the deleterious effects of extreme altitude.

Training

Although aerobic fitness is generally associated with greater speed of travel and thus safety in the mountains, it is not clear whether maximal aerobic power correlates with performance at extreme altitude. Aerobic training at low altitude or intermediate altitude is still the most beneficial way to enhance performance at high altitude. Gains may be achieved by optimization of ventilation, haematological response, cardiovascular fitness and peripheral tissue adaptation, the benefits of which are common both to low and high-altitude performance. Of these adaptations, those of the blood and tissues may be particularly important. At low altitude a modest increase in haemoglobin concentration is associated with improved endurance performance (Buick *et al.*, 1980). One might presume that the high-altitude sojourner would gain similar benefits. All of these adaptations occur spontaneously at high altitude over days to weeks. In order to optimize performance, the mountaineer should ascend at a comfortable pace that will allow adaptation to take place while minimizing the possibility of incurring altitude illness.

The élite climber

Unlike most sports in which élite performers have many common characteristics, the élite mountaineer cannot be so simply described. Several researchers have studied some physiological markers of mountaineers who have climbed on one or more occasions to 8000 m or higher (Schoene, 1982; Masuyama et al., 1986; Oelz et al., 1986). Factors, such as hypoxic ventilatory responses, aerobic power, strength, muscle fibre type and biomechanics, were investigated to see whether any of these characteristics predicted climbing performance at extreme altitude (Oelz et al., 1986). Most, but not all, of the climbers had high $\dot{V}o_{2\,max}$ values ($>$60 ml·kg^{-1}·min^{-1}). On the other hand, one of the world's best climbers had a $\dot{V}o_{2\,max}$ that was only moderately greater than the normal expected value (48 ml·kg^{-1}·min^{-1}). Previously, a very high $\dot{V}o_{2\,max}$ was thought to be a requisite for the Himalayan climber. Perhaps the efficient climber may be able to climb for prolonged periods of time at a high percentage of their $\dot{V}o_{2\,max}$, similar to long-distance runners. The absolute value of $\dot{V}o_{2\,max}$ at sea level may not be a relevant predictor of performance at extreme altitude, because the factors limiting $\dot{V}o_{2\,max}$ at sea level (primarily cardiovascular) are not those that limit performance at extreme altitude — diffusion limitation either at the lung and/or the peripheral tissues becomes the critical factor.

A number of studies have found that many successful climbers to extreme altitude have moderate to high ventilatory responses (HVR) to hypoxia (Schoene, 1982; Masuyama et al., 1986; Oelz et al., 1986) and exercise (Oelz et al., 1986). A greater alveolar ventilation ensures a higher alveolar Po_2 and subsequently minimizes the arterial oxygen desaturation during exercise (Schoene et al., 1984). This characteristic is probably only important for those who go to extreme altitudes, where a slight increase in ventilation can make a substantial difference in oxygen saturation. On the other hand, some individuals with blunted HVR and ventilation upon ascent appear to be more prone to mild and severe altitude illness (Hackett et al., 1982; 1988). A higher breathing response may, therefore, be a helpful but not essential attribute of the high-altitude climber.

These studies have not found any characteristic common to all élite climbers. What may be more important are some of the less tangible traits without which no mountain can be climbed. A strong psychological drive, tenacity, patience, team work, knowledge, skill, judgment and joy in the activity are all prerequisites that are difficult to define by objective data.

Nutrition

Although many of the physiological responses to high altitude are well described, another key element to success or failure with prolonged stay at high altitude is nutrition. The well-described shift in food preference from fats and carbohydrates primarily to carbohydrates as one ascends may reflect the body's needs. A unique factor found in high-altitude climbers is malabsorption in both the small and large intestines (Boyer & Blume, 1984). This has been documented at altitudes above 6000 m. Carbohydrates are probably better absorbed than other fuels; thus to optimize performance carbohydrates should be ingested to the point of tolerance to ensure adequate blood glucose, muscle glycogen and free fatty acid and triglyceride stores. Although weight loss is generally the rule in individuals climbing at high altitude for weeks or more, there is individual variability in this response which may reflect the difference in preferences and tolerance for food (Boyer & Blume, 1984).

Both field and high-altitude chamber studies have documented a decrease in muscle mass, while fat stores (although decreased from sea level) are still present (Boyer & Blume, 1984; Green et al., 1989). These findings reflect muscle catabolism, which suggests utilization of gluconeogenesis to maintain blood glucose and muscle glycogen. Interestingly, studies even at extreme altitude show adequate muscle glycogen stores (Green et al., 1989).

Summary

Physiological adaptations to high altitude optimize aerobic power in an environment characterized by a diminished oxygen supply.

Although these adaptations improve aerobic capacity during a stay at moderate altitude, sea-level capacities are never restored. Even less information is known about endurance performance for the high-altitude mountaineer during prolonged exposure to altitude. Much anecdotal evidence suggests that at moderate altitude, continual activity and adequate nutrition are the key elements in sustaining endurance and performance. At extreme altitude much more individual variability may exist based on psychological rather than physiological characteristics.

References

Abbrecht, P.H. & Littell, J.K. (1972) Plasma erythropoietin in men and mice during acclimatization to different altitudes. *J. Appl. Physiol.* **32**, 34–58.

Aste-Salazar, H. & Hurtado, A. (1944) The affinity of hemoglobin for oxygen at sea level and high altitude. *Am. J. Physiol.* **142**, 733–743.

Banchero, N. (1975) Capillary density of skeletal muscle in dogs exposed to similated altitude. *Proc. Soc. Exp. Biol. Med.* **148**, 435–439.

Beall, C.M. & Reischman, A.B. (1984) Hemoglobin levels in the Himalayan high altitude population. *Am. J. Phys. Anthropol.* **63**, 301–306.

Boyer, S.J. & Blume, F.D. (1984) Weight loss and changes in body composition at high altitude. *J. Appl. Physiol.* **57**, 1580–1585.

Buick, F.J., Gledhill, N., Froese, A.B., Sprite, L. & Meyers, E.C. (1980) Effect of induced erythrocythemia on aerobic work capacities. *J. Appl. Physiol.* **48**, 636–642.

Buskirk, E.R., Collias, J., Akers, R.F., Prokop, E.K. & Reategui, E.P. (1967) Maximal performance at altitude and on return from altitude in conditioned runners. *J. Appl. Physiol.* **23**, 259–266.

Cavaletti, G., Moroni, R., Garavaglia, P. & Tredici, G. (1987) Brain damage after high altitude climbs without oxygen. *Lancet* **i**, 101.

Coates, G., Gray, G., Mansell, A. *et al.* (1979) Changes in lung volume, lung density, and distribution of ventilation during hypobaric decompression. *J. Appl. Physiol.* **46**, 752–755.

Cymerman, A., Reeves, J.T., Sutton, J.R. *et al.* (1989) Operation Everest II: maximal oxygen uptake at extreme altitude. *J. Appl. Physiol.* **66**, 2446–2453.

Dempsey, J.A., Reddun, W.G., Birnbaum, M.L. *et al.* (1971) Effects of acute through life-long hypoxic exposure in exercise pulmonary gas exchange.
Respir. Physiol. **13**, 62–89.

Dill, D.B., Myrhe, L.G., Phillips, E.E., Jr & Brown, D.K. (1966) Work capacity in acute exposure to altitude. *J. Appl. Physiol.* **21**, 1168–1176.

Faraci, F.M., Kilgore, D.L., Jr & Feddle, M.R. (1984) Oxygen delivery to the heart and brain during hypoxia: Peking duck versus bar-headed goose. *Am. J. Physiol.* **247**, R69–R75.

Frisancho, A.R., Velasquez, T. & Sanches, J. (1973) Influence of developmental adaptation on lung function at high altitude. *Hum. Biol.* **45**, 583–594.

Gale, G.E., Torre-Bueno, J.R., Moon, R.E., Saltzman, H.A. & Wagner, P.D. (1985) Ventilation-perfusion inequality in normal humans during exercise at sea level in simulated altitude. *J. Appl. Physiol.* **58**, 978–988.

Gautier, H., Peslin, R., Grassino, A. *et al.* (1982) Mechanical properties of the lungs during acclimatization to altitude. *J. Appl. Physiol.* **52**, 1407–1415.

Goldberg S. & Schoene, R.B. (1990) Mountain sickness and other disorders at high altitude. In Aghabadian, R.V. (ed.) *Emergency Medicine*. Little Brown & Company, Boston (in press).

Green, H.J., Sutton, J.R., Young, P., Cymerman, A. & Houston, C.S. (1989) Operation Everest II: muscle energetics during maximal exhaustive exercise. *J. Appl. Physiol.* **66**, 142–150.

Grover, R.F., Reeves, J.T., Grover, E.B. & Leathers, J.E. (1967) Muscular exercise in young men native to 3100 meters altitude. *J. Appl. Physiol.* **22**, 555–564.

Hackett, P.H., Rennie, D., Hofmeister, S.E., Grover, R.F., Grover, E.B. & Reeves, J.T. (1982) Fluid retention and relative hyperventilation in acute mountain sickness. *Respiration* **43**, 321–329.

Hackett, P.H., Roach, R.C., Schoene, R.B., Harrison, G.L. & Mills, W.R. Jr. (1988) Abnormal control of ventilation in high altitude pulmonary edema. *J. Appl. Physiol.* **64**, 1268–1272.

Hochachka, K.W., Stanley, C., Merkt, J. & Sumar-Kalinowski, J. (1982) Metabolic meaning of elevated levels of oxidative enzymes of high altitude adapted animals: an interpretive hypothesis. *Respir. Physiol.* **52**, 303–313.

Hornbein, T.F., Townes, B.D., Schoene, R.B., Sutton, J.R. & Houston, C.S. (1989) The cost to the central nervous system of climbing to extremely high altitude. *N. Engl. J. Med.* **321**, 1714–1719.

Jaeger, J.J., Sylvester, J.T., Cymerman, A., Berberich, J.J., Denniston, J.C. & Maher, J.T. (1979) Evidence for increased intrathoracic fluid volume in man at high altitude. *J. Appl. Physiol.* **47**, 670–676.

Lahiri, S, Edelman, N.H., Cherniack, N.S. & Fishman, A.P. (1981) Role of carotid chemoreflex in respiratory acclimatization to hypoxia in goat and sheep. *Respir. Physiol.* **46**, 367–382.

Maher, J.T., Jones, L.G. & Hartley, L.H. (1974) Effects of high altitude exposure on submaximal endurance capacity of men. *J. Appl. Physiol.* **37**, 895–898.

Masuyama, S., Kimura, H., Sugita, T. *et al.* (1986) Control of ventilation in extreme altitude climbers. *J. Appl. Physiol.* **61**, 500–506.

Monge, M.C. (1928) La enfermadad de los Andes. Sindromes eritremicos. *Ann. Fac. Med.* (Univ. San Marcos, Lima) **11**, 1–16.

Moore, L.G. & Brewer, G.J. (1981) Beneficial effect of rightward hemoglobin-oxygen dissociation curve shift for short-term high altitude adaptations. *J. Lab. Clin. Med.* **98**, 145–154.

Oelz, O., Howard, H., di Prampero, E. *et al.* (1986) Physiological profile of world-class high altitude climbers. *J. Appl. Physiol.* **60**, 1734–1742.

Ou, L.C. & Tenney, S.M. (1970) Properties of mitochondria from hearts of cattle acclimatized to high altitude. *Respir. Physiol.* **8**, 151–159.

Reeves, J.T., Groves, B.M., Sutton, J.R. *et al.* (1987) Operation Everest II: preservation of cardiac function at extreme altitude. *J. Appl. Physiol.* **63**, 531–539.

Regard, M., Oelz, O., Brugger, P. & Landis, T. (1989) Persistent cognitive impairment in climbers after repeated exposure to extreme altitude. *Neurology* **39**, 210–213.

Remmers, J.E. & Mithoefer, J.C. (1969) The carbon monoxide diffusing capacity in permanent residents at high altitude. *Respir. Physiol.* **6**, 233–244.

Sanchez, C., Merino, C. & Figallo, M. (1970) Simultaneous measurement of plasma volume in cell mass in polycythemia of high altitude. *J. Appl. Physiol.* **28**, 775–778.

Schoene, R.B. (1982) The control of ventilation in climbers to extreme altitude. *J. Appl. Physiol.* **53**, 886–890.

Schoene, R.B. (1984) Hypoxic ventilatory response in excercise ventilation at sea level and high altitude. In: West, J.B. & Lahiri, S. (eds) *Man at High Altitude.* American Physiologic Society Clinical Physiology Series. Waverly Press, Baltimore.

Schoene, R.B. & Hornbein, T.F. (1988) Respiratory adaptation to high altitude. In: Murray, J.F. & Nadel, J.A. (eds) *Textbook of Respiratory Medicine,* pp. 196–220. W.B. Saunders, Baltimore.

Schoene, R.B., Lahiri, S., Hackett, P.H. *et al.* (1984) Relationship of hypoxic ventilatory response to exercise performance on Mt. Everest. *J. Appl. Physiol.* **56**, 1478–1483.

Swan, L.W. (1970) Goose of the Himalaya. *Nat. Hist.* **79**, 68–75.

Tenney, S.M. & Ou, L.C. (1970) Physiological evidence for increased tissue capillarity in rats acclimatized to high altitude. *Respir. Physiol.* **8**, 137–150.

Torre-Bueno, J.R., Wagner, P.D., Saltzman, H.A., Gale, G.E. & Moon, R.E. (1985) Diffusion limitation in normal subjects during exercise at sea level in simulated altitude. *J. Appl. Physiol.* **58**, 989–995.

Vincent, J., Hellot, M.F., Vargas, E., Gautier, H., Pasquis, P. & Lefrancois, R. (1978) Pulmonary gas exchange, diffusing capacity in natives and newcomers at high altitude. *Respir. Physiol.* **34**, 219–231.

Wagner, P.D., Gale, G.E., Moon, R.E., Torre-Bueno, J.R., Stolp, B.W. & Saltzman, H.A. (1986) Pulmonary gas exchange in humans exercising at sea level in simulated altitude. *J. Appl. Physiol.* **61**, 280–287.

Wagner, P.D., Sutton, J.R., Reeves, J.T., Cymerman, A., Groves, B.M. & Malconiun, N.K. (1987) Operation Everest II: pulmonary gas exchange during a simulated ascent of Mt. Everest. *J. Appl. Physiol.* **63**, 2348–2359.

Weil, J.V. (1986) Ventilatory control at high altitude. In: Fishman, A.P., Cherniack, N.S., Widdicome, J.G. & Gieger, S.R. (eds) *Handbook of Physiology. The Respiratory System, Section 3, Vol. II, Control of Breathing, Part 1.* pp. 730–727. American Physiologic Society, Bethesda, Maryland.

West, J.B. & Wagner, P.D. (1980) Predicted gas exchange on the summit of Mt. Everest. *Respir. Physiol.* **42**, 1–16.

West, J.B., Boyer, S.J., Graber, D.J. *et al.* (1983a) Maximal exercise at extreme altitudes on Mt. Everest. *J. Appl. Physiol.* **55**, 688–702.

West, J.B., Hackett, P.H., Maret, K.H., Milledge, J.S., Peters, R.M. Jr., Pizzo, C.J. & Winslow, R.M. (1983b) Pulmonary gas exchange on the summit of Mt. Everest. *J. Appl. Physiol.* **55**, 678–687.

Winslow, R.M. & Monge, C.C. (1987) *Hypoxia, Polycythemia, and Chronic Mountain Sickness.* Johns Hopkins University Press, Baltimore.

Winslow, R.M., Samaja, M. & West, J.B. (1984) Red cell function at extreme altitude on Mt. Everest. *J. Appl. Physiol.* **56**, 109–116.

Chapter 56

The Physiology of Human-Powered Flight

ETHAN R. NADEL AND STEVEN R. BUSSOLARI

Introduction

Humans always have been fascinated with the concept of flight, yet throughout history the actuality of flight has been relegated to winged animals or assigned to the realm of myth. Only in very recent times have the understanding of the requirements of flight and the development of strong and light structures enabled flight to be accomplished under human power alone.

The first record of human-powered flight was from the ancient Greek civilizations. As first reported by Homer around the 8th–7th century BC, a Mycenean craftsman and inventor named Daedalus fashioned wings from feathers and wax and flew under his own power from a hillside cleft in King Minos' Labyrinth, in which he was imprisoned, across the Aegean Sea to his freedom. According to later versions of the myth, Daedalus flew with his son, Icarus, who, ignoring his father's advice, flew too close to the sun and fell to his death when the heat of the sun melted his wings.

Drela and Langford (1985) have charted the progress of human-powered flight since the time of Daedalus. They noted that only within the past 30 years or so has human-powered flight progressed beyond the realm of extended glides from a catapult takeoff. This was undoubtedly because the early human-powered aircraft required more power to maintain steady flight than the pilot could produce. Progress in the realm of human-powered flight was stimulated by the challenge of competition for

monetary prizes established by the British industrialist Henry Kremer in 1959. The first Kremer prize, awarded for flying a human-powered aircraft around a 1-mile (1609 m), figure-of-eight course under human power alone, was not claimed until 1977 by Bryan Allen, flying the Paul MacCready-designed *Gossamer Condor*. The second Kremer prize of £100 000 went to the same team when Bryan Allen pedalled the *Gossamer Albatross* across a 37-km strait of the English Channel in 1979. This was indeed an endurance event; the flight time was nearly 3 h. In 1988, *Daedalus*, designed by a team of engineers from the Massachusetts Institute of Technology, flew under human power from the north coast of Crete to the island of Santorini, a distance of 119 km, in just under 4 h.

Aeroplane aerodynamics

To understand the reasons why human-powered flight has become possible only in recent times, it is important to appreciate the basics of aeroplane aerodynamics (for an expanded discussion see Shevell, 1983). Four forces — lift, weight, thrust and drag — are the determinants for flight. As an aircraft moves through the air, the shape of its wing imparts differential velocities to the air passing over its upper and lower surfaces, creating a higher pressure beneath the wing and a lower pressure above the wing. This results in a net upward force called lift. In level flight, lift is balanced by the downward force of gravity, the aircraft weight. A horizontal thrust force is furnished by the propeller which is driven by the aircraft engine. In level, unaccelerated flight, thrust balances the total horizontal resistive force, drag, which is produced by a combination of the movement of air past the exposed surfaces of the aircraft (form and parasite drag) and the disturbance of the air caused by the wing as it produces lift (induced drag).

The power required for flight is the product of thrust and velocity, or, in level flight, drag and velocity. Since form and parasite drag increase roughly as the square of the velocity, the power (force × velocity) required to overcome these components of drag will increase as the cube of velocity. Thus, doubling the airspeed of a given aircraft would require roughly an eightfold increase in the power applied by the engine (the human engine in the case of a human-powered aircraft). A more exact relationship between power required and aircraft design parameters may be obtained by consideration of the equations that describe the production of lift and induced drag:

$$\text{Power} = [2/\rho S]^{1/2} \; W^{3/2} \; C_D/C_L^{3/2}$$

where ρ is the air density, S is the wing area, W is the total weight of the aircraft including payload (in a human-powered aircraft, the pilot is a significant fraction of W), and C_D and C_L are coefficients of drag and lift that depend on the aircraft shape. The above equation confirms that it is important for the aircraft designer to minimize weight and drag while maintaining a high lift and a large wing area to keep the required power low.

Design strategies

Over the years, human-powered aircraft designers have attempted to solve the problem of reducing the power requirement to that which a human could be expected to maintain by adopting several strategies. One strategy was to design a very light structure with a large wing area by using external wire bracing. The high parasite drag of the wire bracing was compensated for by keeping the design airspeed (velocity) low to minimize its contribution to the power required. The success of the *Gossamer* human-powered aircraft was the result of this design strategy. The disadvantage of this type of aircraft is its low speed, which requires its pilot to remain aloft for a long period of time to cover a given distance. The development of strong, lightweight graphite—epoxy and other composite materials permitted designers to eliminate the external wire bracing while maintaining a large wing area with little weight penalty. The *Daedalus* aircraft (Fig. 56.1), with its 34.1-m semicantilever wingspan, is an example of this design strategy.

Power requirements for flight

The outcome of aerodynamic and materials innovations led to the design of a low-power, moderate-speed aircraft that was able to be flown for extended periods. Preliminary calculations and measurements, derived largely from tow tests of the aircraft, showed that the mechanical power requirement to fly the *Daedalus* was about $3.0-3.5$ W·kg^{-1} pilot weight at the design speed of 24 km·h^{-1}. Assuming the pilot's ability to convert 24% of the potential energy of stored fuels to mechanical work in the muscle machinery (Åstrand & Rodahl, 1986), the pilot must maintain a fuel conversion rate of nearly 15 W·kg^{-1}, requiring an oxygen intake of about 45 ml oxygen·min^{-1}·kg^{-1}, to generate mechanical power at 3.5 W·kg^{-1}. This metabolic cost is approximately the same as that required to pedal a bicycle over level ground at a speed of 37 km·h^{-1} (Whitt & Wilson, 1982). Based upon knowledge of performance characteristics, the metabolic cost of flying the *Gossamer Albatross* at its design speed of 18 km·h^{-1} has been estimated to be 20% higher, a remarkable output to maintain throughout the English Channel crossing. (Note: A human-powered aircraft is flown like any aircraft; the pilot adds power to gain altitude and decreases power to descend. Because the human-powered aircraft

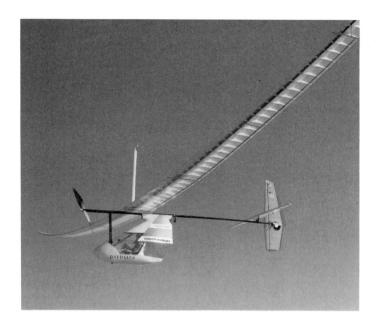

Fig. 56.1 The *Daedalus* undergoing flight-testing at Edwards Air Force Base in California. In April 1988, K. Kanallopoulos flew the *Daedalus* between the Greek islands of Crete and Santorini, a distance of 119 km, in just under 4 h. The distance and duration are the current world records for human-powered flight. Photo courtesy of the Daedalus Project, Massachusetts Institute of Technology.

Table 56.1 Characteristics of the 25 final pilot candidates.

Parameter	Mean ± s.d. value
Maximal oxygen intake (semirecumbent position) (ml oxygen·min^{-1}·kg^{-1})	69.2 ± 5.2
Maximal mechanical power output (W·kg^{-1})	5.25 ± 0.53
70% maximal power output (W·kg^{-1})	3.54 ± 0.36
Mechanical efficiency (%)	24.1 ± 3.7

flies within 6 m of the surface, the loss of altitude due to a reduction in power for more than a few seconds will cause the aircraft to land, or worse.)

As human-powered aircraft designers have refined their designs and used lighter and stronger materials, the power requirements for flight have come into the realm of the possible for more than just the élite endurance athlete. It is notable that the *Daedalus* pilot team of five athletes was selected from more than 300 initial applicants (Nadel & Bussolari, 1988). The maximal mechanical power production of the 25 athletes who were invited for objective test-ing was 5.25 W·kg^{-1} (Table 56.1). The 70% maximum power, which most fit people should be able to sustain aerobically for extended periods, was therefore 3.54 W·kg^{-1}, higher than the most conservative estimate of power required to maintain steady flight in the *Daedalus*. The ability to generate power at this rate is the critical factor for extended flight. Factors that can limit prolonged flight include hyperthermia, dehydration and/or hypoglycaemia, the same factors that can limit other endurance exercise bouts (for a discussion of the strategies to limit the development of these factors during the *Daedalus* flight, see Nadel & Bussolari, 1988).

References

Åstrand, P.-O. & Rodahl, K. (1986) *Textbook of Work Physiology*. McGraw-Hill, New York.

Drela, M. & Langford, J.S. (1985) Human-powered flight. *Sci. Am.* **253**, 144–151.

Nadel, E.R. & Bussolari, S.R. (1988) The Daedalus project: physiological problems and solutions. *Am. Sci.* **76**, 351–360.

Shevell, R.S. (1983) *Fundamentals of Flight*. Prentice Hall, New Jersey.

Whitt, F.R. & Wilson, D.G. (1982) *Bicycling Science*. MIT Press, Cambridge, Massachusetts.

Chapter 57

Endurance in Other Sports

PER-OLOF ÅSTRAND

Individual sport events with demands for endurance during training and competition have been discussed in preceding chapters. *Orienteering* was mentioned only in passing, but it is certainly an endurance sport because it involves long distances of cross-country running (the 'ideal' time is about 1 h 30 min for men and about 1 h for women). Armed with a compass and a map, the competitor must find her or his way to checkpoints in the terrain. Many countries have annual meetings with up to 5 days of competitions. In Sweden more than 20 000 people participate, with classes from beginners up to élite, and age groups from children up to master athletes. The endurance training follows the same principles discussed in Chapter 52. Orienteering is also a popular sport when performed on skis.

Many other events are time consuming with regard to both training sessions and competition time. However, physical activity during competition is often not continuous but intermittent, i.e. short bursts of vigorous exercise are followed by rest or low-intensity activity. The physiology of this type of exercise was briefly discussed in Chapter 2. A few examples of such events are given below.

Several studies on *soccer* have been carried out (see Ekblom, 1986). On average the players cover about 10 km during the 90-min game, and it has been estimated that top-class performers of British first-division teams walk and run 13.5 km in total (see Ekblom, 1986). Soccer involves high-intensity, intermittent exercise

although the total number of tackles in a game is only some 15–20, with 10–15 headings. Even so, the heart rate is often high and close to the player's maximum. Ekblom estimated that the average oxygen intake during the game could be about 80% of the maximum. The maximal aerobic power of players in good national teams seems to be around 65–67 ml·kg^{-1}·min^{-1} with individual values exceeding 70 ml·kg^{-1}·min^{-1}. Peak blood lactate concentrations above 12 mmol·l^{-1} have frequently been measured. It is evident that soccer players must devote time to endurance training. In the recent world championships many games were extended by 2 × 15-min periods.

Other games with high-intensity, non-continuous, intermittent exercise are *European handball, basketball, volleyball, netball, field hockey, ice hockey* and *water-polo.*

A high maximal aerobic power can lower the demand on anaerobic energy yield. The importance of oxygen stored in the myoglobin was discussed in Chapter 2 (see Fig. 2.1). However, training does not seem to increase the myoglobin concentration in human skeletal muscle. One aspect of the importance of separate endurance training for players is the fact that training sessions often last for 2–2.5 h.

We have a similar situation in racket sports. A *tennis* match can last for up to 4 h or more, sometimes in a hot environment. In *table tennis* the three sets may take from 20 to 30 min. In the Swedish national team, including world champions, the maximal oxygen intake averaged 65 ml·kg^{-1}. The mean oxygen intake during games was about 70% of the maximum. At big tournaments a player often must play several matches per day.

Fencing is another event with many matches per day, which complicates food and water intake. A competition often lasts for 2 days and the fencers are usually active for 10–12 h on each day of competition. The six members of the Swedish national épée team have been studied. Altogether, the fencers won 13 gold, one silver and four bronze medals in world championships and Olympic games. The mean maximal oxygen intake was 5.2 l·min^{-1} and 67.3 ml·kg^{-1}·min^{-1} (Nyström *et al.*, 1990). Endurance training is considered an important part of their training. It is interesting to note that the muscle mass was significantly larger in the 'forward leg' than in the contralateral leg, although the fibre composition was similar.

This list could be much longer. The conclusion is that the training of aerobic power is of importance for all athletes, not least because habitual physical activity is essential for optimal function. In addition, there is the health aspect. Many studies have shown convincingly that training of the oxygen transport system can significantly reduce the morbidity and mortality from cardiovascular disease (for references see Powell *et al.*, 1987; Åstrand, 1988).

References

Åstrand, P.-O. (1988) From exercise physiology to preventive medicine. *Ann. Clin. Res.* **20**, 10–17.

Ekblom, B. (1986) Applied physiology of soccer. *Sports Med.* **3**, 50–60.

Nyström, J., Lindwall, O., Ceci, R., Harmenberg, J., Svedenhag, J. & Ekblom, B. (1990) Physiological and morphological characteristics of world class fencers. *Int. J. Sports Med.* **11**, 136–139.

Powell, K.E., Thompson, P.D., Caspersen, C.J. & Kendrick, J.S. (1987) Physical activity and the incidence of coronary heart disease. *Ann. Rev. Public Health* **8**, 253–287.

Index